Understanding Homoeopathy

A simple and new approach to the fundamentals and basis of the method

By
Dr. Trevor Smith
M.A.,M.B.B.Chir.,D.P.M.,M.F.Hom.

Insight Editions,
Worthing, Sussex, England

ISBN 0 946670 00 5

Typesetting and origination by
Alan Sutton Publishing Limited.
Printed in Great Britain by Dotesios
(Printers) Ltd., Bradford-on-Avon.

A New Introduction to Homoeopathy

1. What is homoeopathy — some initial definitions and explanations. (p. 1)
2. Origins. (p. 7)
3. The homoeopathic conception of illness and disease. (p. 11)
4. The basic causation of illness. (p. 16)
5. The indications for homoeopathy. (p. 28)
6. The action and functions of homoeopathy. (p. 33)
7. Dilution and disease. (p. 40)
8. The advantages of the homoeopathic approach. (p. 44)
9. Some limitations. (p. 49)
10. More indications for homoeopathy. (p. 52)
11. Preparation of the remedies. (p. 58)
12. Making a start. (p. 62)
13. Homoeopathy and the home. (p. 68)
14. First aid. (p. 73)
15. The twenty basic remedies and their usage. (p. 87)
16. Some useful addresses and places of contact. (p. 97)

CHAPTER ONE

Some initial definitions and explanations

Homoeopathy is a form of prescribable treatment for various illness conditions using extracts of naturally occuring materials chosen and prepared for the individual in a way that is unique in medicine. The basic materials come from various sources, the majority are of plant origin but others are also derived from animal and mineral material. In addition there are some important remedies called nosodes, acting like vaccines, but without their risks and side-effects and these are prepared from diseased tissue and cell material. For example *Pertussin* used in the treatment and prevention of whooping-cough is made from the mucous of throat swabs of whooping-cough sources.

The word homoeopathy takes its origin from classical Greek and its roots — homeos and pathos, mean 'equal suffering'. This gives the clue to the action and approach of the method which is to treat 'suffering' or illness using remedies that can in their natural, unprepared state produce 'equal' or similar physical and psychological symptoms to those of the patient.

Deadly Nightshade, for example, from which the remedy *Belladonna* is prepared, when taken in its crude, wild form from the hedge-row, produces an intensely toxic reaction. There is collapse, burning pains, a flushed red face, dilated pupils and a bounding pulse. The temperature is often raised and nausea or vomiting is frequent. The least jolt or movement usually aggravates all the symptoms. This poison-reaction closely resembles the clinical picture of a severe scarlet-fever reaction with a scalding skin rash, raised temperature and burning pains usually worse for jarring, noise or disturbance of any kind. Such symptoms clearly resemble those of *Belladonna* before it is extracted from Deadly Nightshade and it is this similarity which is used as the principle in choosing the remedy which best treats and cures the particular scarlet-fever reaction.

In general, homoeopathy tends to use substances which in their original and raw state have the ability to irritate the body in various areas of organ-functioning. It is this power to stimulate the organism, creating a reaction in certain specific areas, which is retained by the medicines in their homoeopathic form and is an intrinsic part of their potential to treat and cure the patient.

Research studies called 'Provings', toxicity recordings and clinical experience are all used to form an overall symptom-profile of each remedy and give an accurate prediction of the clinical state most likely to be effectively treated by a remedy at the time.

However Homoeopathy is not primarily concerned with an automatic-cure for a condition such as scarlet-fever, but seeks to treat and support the type of individual response to their condition, varying enormously from one person to another. This concern for the individual and each unique pattern of response is characteristic of the whole homoeopathic approach. *Belladonna* may be perfectly appropriate for one member of the family with a severe and acute toxic scarlatinal reaction, but in another, the reaction may be quite different. The rash may be mild — the predominant problem a chest condition with a dry persistant irritating cough preventing sleeping, so that *Bryonia* — the extract of the wild hop is more indicated. In another child, the throat is the major problem without either a toxic state and much rash or involvement of the chest to any great extent. Where the throat is purple so that the least swallowing becomes painful and agonising, then neither of the two remedies are appropriate and *Phytolacca* — the extract of the poke-root plant is indicated — however much *Belladonna* is considered as a specific for scarlet-fever. In the last clinical analysis, it is always the individual symptom-pattern and the patient that decides the remedy, not a diagnostic label or a clinical entity or any assumptions on a 'scientific' or theoretical basis, leading to a theoretical, non-personal prescription and practise of medicine.

Homoeopathy is more than just an effective treatment for the individual. It is an overall way of looking at the patient. Every aspect of the person is taken into account when assessing and considering the most appropriate remedy for a problem and most likely to be of help. However physical the complaints — perhaps a problem of eczema, hiatus hernia, 'blood pressure', varicose veins or haemorrhoids, the patient's psyche and psychological make-up is also considered in detail as part of understanding the totality of the illness and totality of make-up.

However psychological and seemingly emotional the problem — perhaps an anxiety-state, depression or agitation with insomnia, the patient's physical health is given equal weight as the more obvious psychological aspects. This includes the natural energy and physiological patterns and body rhythms, to give an overall picture with a maximum of information in all areas. In homoeopathy the aim is clarity of diagnosis and knowledge of the total person as an aid to understanding all the relevant factors causing and contributing to the illness. A remedy may then be chosen which includes to a maximum the patient's complex yet unique psychological and physical profile.

Homoeopathy is also a philosophy of cure in the sense that it doesn't see disease as just something that arrives and implants itself in an unsuspecting organ or cellular area of the body. The whole disease-process must be seen as part of an overall totality in the development and evolution of the individual, so that his vulnerability and susceptibility at that particular time has sense and meaning. Illness is usually far more than just a passive act of infiltration by a virus organism or simple invasion by a 'germ' — whatever form it takes. In most case, the illness or dis-ease is not an act of chance or a blow-of-fate which happened — one wet and blustery afternoon, but relates to an overall state of both body and mind. Often over a period of months or even years preceding the acute illness, there have been a whole chain of minor problems. These were not necessarily illnesses-in-themselves, but pointers that all was not right within as an abnormal susceptibility and weakness developed externally. The eventual illness is often the end-product of a long chain of depleting events — both psychological as well as physical.

As you can now see, homoeopathy puts a lot of emphasis on the mental attitudes of the individual and the underlying emotional health and satisfaction of the individual. Whatever the problem, it has always been considered of fundamental importance to help both the deeper psychological aspects as well as the more apparent physical and external symptoms and events. The mind can influence all things, and in homoeopathy it is often key to many of the problems — however apparently simple and physical they seem to be. The remedies act very deeply in this sphere and it is one of their major advantages, since when properly prescribed, homoeopathy helps both areas in depth.

Case report
A woman of 55 came for a consultation this week. I have known her for several years and had not seen her for some six months. There was no previous history of skin troubles and in the past I had treated her for joint and rheumatic problems. This time however there were none of the usual symptoms and instead she complained of an odd but severe facial allergic rash which caused intolerable irritation and itching discomfort, mainly over the left side of the face and to a lesser extent over her whole body generally. The problem was present most of the day but was definitely aggravated by heat and the warmth of the bed-clothes. There was not much to go on as far as diagnostic causes were concerned and she associated the rash herself with the use of a detergent and with a household-name 'natural' bath foam and soap which she had however used over the years. The condition had also come on again with severity when she had worn a pair of woolen socks, washed in her usual detergent, but in her mind, probably not sufficiently and thoroughly rinsed.

It was all a great mystery. I then said that in all allergic cases, although the disease in itself was not psychological, nevertheless there was always an underlying psychological component which often acted as a trigger to the more acute allergic reaction to occur. My patient thought for a moment and then after a meaningful pause said — well, over the period of the skin trouble, I very nearly lost my daughter-in-law and her baby from severe hypertension (blood-pressure) during her pregnancy. She was in hospital at the time and there was certainly a great deal of worry and stress occuring which she had not previously referred to.

Whether in fact, the stress she referred to was in any way a causative factor is difficult to prove, but it seems possible and likely. It is also interesting that she only gave me the new information about deeper psychological matters in response to my giving her my own experience about some of the underlying factors in allergy. The case illustrates the close links between physical reactions and deeper psychological happenings — not always admitted or available to the patient.

As a matter of interest, the remedy emerging from the material given is likely to be either *Sulphur* or *Pulsatilla*, the former having stronger skin affiliations than the latter. In order to be certain as to which remedy is the 'right' one, you would need more information to go on.

CHAPTER TWO

Origins

Samuel Hahnemann, the German physician (1755–1843) developed ancient homoeopathic principles into a full comprehensive science with a broad new range of medical applications. A brilliant scholar since his early years and linguist, in his early thirties after nearly a decade of medical experience in general and specialised practise, he became disenchanted with conventional medicine and what he regarded as its barbaric practises, devoting himself entirely to writing and translating. During this period of withdrawal, he became involved in translating the major work of the eminent Scottish physician Cullen, who in 1789 had just completed the second edition of his Materia Medica. In this volume Cullen describes the action of Peruvian *Cinchona* bark or Quinine on Malaria. Hahnemann had first-hand experience of the dreaded illness from clinical work in the Low Countries shortly after qualifying and was not convinced about Cullen's conclusions as to *Cinchona* and its mode of action. He decided to experiment with the bark on himself, taking a tincture of *Cinchona*. Within hours, the previously healthy Hahnemann had developed all the symptoms of a malaria-like condition which discontinued when he stopped taking the quinine.

From these small beginnings Hahnemann developed the insights which led him to conclude that remedy-substances can cause similar symptoms in the healthy as those which it can cure in the sick. This first 'proving' experiment of Hahnemann became the link which led to other remedies being developed and 'proven' by symptom-free volunteers and a charting of the symptoms produced gave an accurate guide to the therapeutic potential of the substances used and indications for their eventual use in the treatment of illness.

Although Hahnemann developed the Homoeopathic method and introduced a series of very important remedies, the Homoeopathic principle is almost as old as medicine itself. Certainly Hippocrates, the Greek physician (born 460 b.c.) father of medicine and originator of the Hippocratic oath, used the principles and his writings recommended that like be treated by like. Paracelsus the great renaissance scholar and philosopher of the 15th century (1490–1541) knew of the same principles and researched and recommended them. But his was a lone voice and he was a man before his time, and it was not until nearly 200 years later that Hahnemann re-discovered the principles although meeting with as much opposition for his revolutionary approach as had Paracelsus, and the method finally became accepted and established.

Similar principles can be seen in primitive tribes. Fear of the wrath of omnipotent Gods was appeased by creating fearsome replicas, especially masks and totums of awesome figures in order to avoid their feared retributions. Action to avoid the threat of drought or flooding in primitive communities is sometimes taken by the local power or medicine man who creates by ritualistic dance — catastrophes-in-miniature, to bring the urgently needed rain to crops or to subdue the driving rain threatening already swollen rivers. The old principle of 'a hair of the dog' has been known for generations and needs no explanation or elaboration.

Until relatively recently and certainly prior to the 'pharmaceutical revolution', homoeopathy was the normal approach to health and used by a majority of doctors. It is still quite common to meet today patients who can clearly recall taking *Arnica* for bruising and *Rhus Tox* for sprains as a child, the whole family treated homoeopathically whatever their age and generation.

Initially Hahnemann found that using the mother tinctures in treatment could in some cases give toxic effects to the patients although their indications were correct and the remedies were given homoeopathically. Hahnemann experimented by diluting the tinctures to the point where they could be given more safely without losing their therapeutic potential. To his amazement dilution did not diminish the power of the remedies but increased their scope and depth of action and the greater the dilution the more powerful and effective the remedy was found to be. Succussion, or vigorous shaking of each dilution formed is essential to 'stamp' upon the solution its therapeutic qualities and this was also one of Hahnemann's fundamental and unique discoveries.

Nevertheless Hahnemann was consulted by some patients where the remedies, even in their diluted and dynamised form were without effect. These were the problems of chronic illness and Hahnemann worked for many years on such problems, culminating in his volume 'Chronic Diseases' which set out his new theories of miasms. He grouped chronic illness into three main headings due to miasm, which he saw as containing certain characteristics of the original illness occuring within the family, perhaps several generations previously. The miasm is the 'ghost' of the original illness. Psora was the most widespread and important, linked to earlier scabies or 'the itch'. Sycosis was related to Gonorrhoeal illness in an earlier generation and Syphilis to a previous syphilitic infection affecting subsequent generations to some degree. This was the theory and not everyone accepts it, but it does provide a useful way of thinking about and looking at the ever-present problems of chronic illness. The major remedies associated with the miasmic illness are for Psora — *Sulphur,* for Sycosis *Thuja* and for Syphilis — *Mercurius.*

CHAPTER THREE

The Homoeopathic conception of disease and illness

For centuries philosophers have seen man as a microcosm or reflection of the universe. By his habits and patterns, periods of energy-spurts and activity — but also his need for quiet, hibernation and withdrawal, man has natural rhythms and seasons of growth which lead on to maturity and a harvesting of fruits — not only of work-labour but also of being and thinking.

In health, man is centred — in a position of balance, a dynamic combination of tonicity and relaxation — not just simply tension and passivity. There is a gentle un-awareness, without withdrawal or denial — the knowing that the heart is beating, the lungs functioning, the limbs moving without palpitation, breathlessness, spasm or stiffness. The body surface contains a sufficient quantity of moisture without drenching sweats or unpleasant dry-ness, which does not lead to either a flakey skin-complaint or constipation with hard and bullet-like stools. This state of balance is in constant movement and adjustment as the vital processes of body-absorption, energy-extraction, drainage and excretion of waste-matter goes on. There is a constant supply and distribution where necessary with-out interfering at the same time with essential psycholo-

11

gical processes of communication, thinking both intuitively and logically or the subtle process of sensing and 'knowing' as the day moves through its inevitable 'ups and downs' of successes and failures.

Illness occurs when there is an interference with such natural patterns so that man becomes alienated from his natural birthright of instincts and self-knowledge. All the pressures and demands of an essentially non-rhythmic modern society — the concrete jungle as it has been called more than once, undermine and drain resources and reserves so that a sense of naturalness and timing becomes non-existant.

Just as we eat oranges all the year round — whether they are in season or not, so too we are expected to function in the same way, day after day, year after year, with no allowances made for the needs and cycles of expansion and diminution which are fundamental to mankind. The needs of consumer-demand must be adhered to, rather like our conforming behaviour on the holiday fortnight allotted, with no place or understanding made for the varying make-up and patterns of the individual.

Illness is imbalance within the psyche as much as within the functionings of the physical body. All too often there is nervous tension taking the place of healthy tonicity and tone, leading to discomfort and pain as tensions accumulate. These remain un-dispersed, because the organism has no natural, ready-made effluent drainage-pathways at its immediate disposal to cope with such artificial build-ups which were never intended to take place. This is why, when tension-states occur they so easily become chronic and a severe problem. They are very much a by-product of pressurised modern man and unrelated to the physiological build-up of natural tone and energy which when in excess, can be easily disposed of by the body's energy pathways and drives.

Every symptom is of prime importance to the homoeopath, reflecting the health and strength of the vital or life-energies. Usually when there is a sudden acute illness there has also been a period of malaise or vague ill-health preceding the obvious disease as the vital energy is slowly depleted before clear-cut symptoms occur. Homoeopathy considers that illness begins in the most central parts of the person, namely the mind or psyche, with depression, irritability and lack of energy to name some of the commonest expressions. The most central of all elements is undoubtedly the spiritual core and when this is also affected, as well as psychological depletion there is frequently a deep crisis of faith with loss of belief and trust in any overall pattern or meaning to life which gives an added depth to the common sense of isolation, or loneliness which occurs.

Symptoms are the essential key to prescribing and basis of the homoeopathic prescription, determined by matching the patient's overall 'problem-picture' to that of the remedies. Often the individual's life-style has become distorted beyond recognition so that there is an unnatural compromise between true aims, ideals and principles and even codes of beliefs to the service of 'financial necessities'. All too often, true to Parkinson's Law — the more we have the more we want, creates an unending spiral leading to chronic illness and ill-health. Such unnatural life-styles create conflicts with unbearable frustrations for many. The psychologically and environmentally abnormal lives, remote from true self, real motivation and need, create psychological havoc and spiritual devastation and emptiness, expending precious and irreplaceable reserves of life and energy.

Under such circumstances, demands and pressures, any natural balance is quickly lost and problems of malaise, fatigue, constipation and insomnia occur — even in the very young. For many, the underlying dissatisfactions are a cry for help, as life becomes so complicated that no longer does the dog wag the tail, but the tail the dog and by any measure of vitality and health, this is a recipe for disaster.

A sore throat or recurrent ear infection may not necessarily reflect any profound psychological state, but at times the lowering of resistance cannot be explained in any other terms than a diminution of natural vital resistance by pressures of a change of school or anxiety about an impending examination or how well a sibling is achieving in another class or school.

Case Reports

A woman of 32 came this week with a severe recurrence of genital herpes. She was quite clear that the condition had been aggravated by recent examination fears and the breakdown of the relationship with her boyfriend. Also this week a man of 78 with recurrent prostatic difficulties was certain that a recent aggravation was because of business pressures and the need for redundancies in staff who had served him faithfully for many years.

The symptom is the normal healthy response to pressure and stress of some kind and is a reaction to it as the body attempts to correct the balance, the scales tipped against it by underlying pressures. These vital and individual expressions are however important reactions to be conserved and fostered by the homoeopathic approach rather than something to be eradicated or suppressed because they are a reaction of life itself. It takes a certain strength to create a symptom however negative it may

appear, that reflects and to a degree contains the underlying conflict — having an essentially preservative
function basically healing, however obscure this may
appear initially.

For the majority, symptoms are the very intimate and
personal expressions of the individual so that the child
with a tendency to be quick and impatient, may be equally
acute and rapid in the pattern of their illnesses, quickly
severely ill with pain and high temperature but just as
quickly becoming well and responding quickly. Another
member of the same family, much more sluggish to
develop and generally slow in all things, with a tendency
to hold back and slow to reveal themselves, generally
has a pattern of illness which is more drawn-out and
taking longer to treat and to cure. The overall tendency
to sluggish reactions and passivity of growth and thinking
holds true for the way that body-symptoms develop and is
an aspect of overall personality and pattern of responding
or opposing life, as much highlighted during a physical
illness as at any other time.

CHAPTER FOUR

The Basic Causation of illness and disease

Whatever the precipitating causes, all illness is inevitably the product and combination of external pressures and internal psychological changes. Normal balanced physiological functioning is dependent upon healthy workings of both external and internal interchange. In illness there is a lack of liaison physiologically between these two fundamentals and inbalance or dis-ease is the result. When an individual is psychologically depleted by underlying anxiety or depressive problems of stress of any kind, then this is likely to have a draining effect and to be debilitating to energy supplies and body functioning. Particularly the digestive functioning is interfered with, which means that the break-down of our energy-providers or foods is affected with consequent lessening of available power-resources. At the same time, the excretory channels of the bowel may become much less efficient, with all the risks of toxic-reabsorbtion, constipation and general discomfort.

In a similar way, when there is primarily an external or physical problem as for example — varicose veins, recurrent sinusitis, or chronic catarrh, such varied and different problems may affect the underlying psyche, confidence, poise and attitudes generally, the emotional responses and drive sapped by a predominantly physical disturbance.

In every case, whenever the underlying psychological state is interfered with in any way, with feelings and emotions that cannot be adequately or easily contained this depletes energy and natural resistance and paves the way for a possible physical reaction and illness.

The following factors are often instrumental either directly or indirectly in the development of disease and are usually explored during the homoeopathic initial and subsequent interviews and consultations in the search to understand both the precipitating causes and overall meaning of an acute or chronic illness.

Inherited factors

These are the areas of inherited constitutional flaws, which we all have to some extent. Adler called them the areas of 'organ weakness' which run through families, giving a tendency to skin problems, chest weakness, infection in certain parts of the body and sometimes migraine attacks. The problem is an inherited one, but different from the more obvious chromosomal and predictable transmitted diseases as haemophilia, because the links are more subtle and tenuous. Homoeopathy called these more subtle flaws-of-disease the Miasms.

Case Reports

An example occurred recently with a colleague. She had developed a worrying problem of an irritating summer dry cough which was very troublesome and tended to recur year after year for no apparent cause. There was a strong history of tuberculosis however in the family which involved several members over more than one generation, although the patient herself had never been directly involved in any way with the disease and exhaustive tests had always been completely negative. When the nosode of the tuberculosis illness — *Tuberculinum* was given however, the patient made a rapid recovery from all her symptoms where all conventional medicine had consistently failed to evoke any positive response whatsoever. We must assume that here there was the typical tuberculosis miasm at work which was controlled by its nosode or homoeopathic vaccine. My colleague needed the *Tuberculinum* yearly to control the symptoms which recurred less acutely for three years and she has not required the nosode since.

Another example of inherited factors at work and causing disease was the case of the identical twins who came this week. One brother needed help for a chronic problem, the other had a back problem. Both were aged 65. What was most striking was that both had developed a right-sided hernia or rupture the previous year, needing surgery, within a few weeks of the other at a time when they were living many miles apart and unaware that the other had developed a similar weakness at exactly the same time.

Exhaustion
Weakness from excessive wear and tear is daily seen by every doctor as a precipitating factor in the development of disease. Such exhaustion often follows a period of prolonged and excessive demand and effort as may occur after the nursing of a sick relative or friend over many weeks or months. It is quite usual to find that there are underlying feelings of psychological resentment present and sometimes guilt involved which adds to the fatigue. A relative is often difficult and demanding and often there

are many mixed feelings about the advisability of nursing-home admission, particularly with the elderly. Usually a lot of tension is present which adds to the physical load and can finally deplete all the reserves with a sense of exhaustion and at the same time insomnia despite the fatigue. A depressive breakdown can occur unless it is prevented in time by good sense and at least some relief from the physical burden.

Allergic factors
The commonest are seen in hay-fever, eczema or asthma, although at times non-specific conditions may also occur with a general swelling of the face and fingers or the whole body after certain foods and in some, exposure to a dust-loaded environment. The allergic factors are typically those of pollen, house-dust, cat and animal hair, certain foods, especially the gluten of wheat, dairy products, particularly cow's milk with allergy developing in the infant in some cases or even with breast-feeding when the allergen is transmitted across the natural barrier of the mother to the child and becomes present in the breast milk. The attacks are always rather paradoxal and unpredictable, with no known and definite pattern, often varying also with social situation as much as the pollen count. There is nearly always a lot of anticipation and fear of the attacks occuring and in many cases, undoubtedly a powerful psychological element is at work as well as a more straight-forward allergic one. In many cases however strict the desensitizing diet or the injections, these are ineffective because they do not take into account the full depth of the problem.

Psychological factors
Shock, rejection, anger, misunderstanding, rivalry, com-

petition and jealousy can all provoke severe feelings which at times are uncontrollable. These feelings need to be expressed and given life in order that they may be reasonably satisfied and dealt with at the time and to avoid the canker of underlying resentment further developing with its inherent destructiveness. Avoidance of the occurrence of conversion-symptoms is also important for the individual as when these occur they take with them a great deal of energy and drive belonging to the problem when it is re-sited in what is usually an inappropriate physical area. When this happens in the chest it may cause asthma or chronic bronchitis, within the bowels it may be a cause of colitis, and when the skin is used to contain the emotion, then a psoriasis or eczema problem may occur. Excessive emotional tension in the duodenum or alimentary tract may result in duodenal ulceration. Such physical developments referred to above, do nothing to relieve or resolve the underlying psychological basic hurt and only further complicate life because there is the added worry of an often dangerous physical problem eating-up vitality and the healthy functioning of the organ involved and when severe even threatening life itself.

Epidemic factors
At times, often where preventative hygiene has become non-existant, certain diseases of viral or bacterial causation develop. They are often animal-carried and create multiple attacks within a large area so that an epidemic occurs. Often the cause is not clearly known and it seems that yet another new strain of virus has appeared, resistant to all known antibiotics which can devastate the health of thousands, particularly the elderly, although it may occur at any age. Examples are influenza, typhoid, cholera, plague.

Mechanical factors
Any form of blockage or interference to normal physiological functioning from any cause — either displacement or non-alignment of the spine, scarring and blockage leading to narrowing of normal channels and interference with elimination, absorption and drainage causes pain and discomfort. Physical damage from any form of trauma as a traffic accident, chronic ulcer or the breakdown of a wound after surgery, comes into this category because of the formation of eventual scar-tissue which at a later date may contract and cause distortion of neighbouring tissues.

Parasitic factors
These are important in certain tropical countries where the invasion of bowel and tissues by tape, round and thread worms is endemic. The latter are also especially common in this country and it is now quite common to see adults as well as children troubled by problems of anal irritation in the night or evening hours due to this cause and perpetuated by self-infection. Round worms, hydatid cysts and bilharzia are seen in many middle Eastern and tropical countries and have become much more common with the age of rapid jet-travel to all parts of the world and they are a constant factor to be considered whenever chronic disease is not responding to the usual measures.

Poisoning factors
These are on the increase with lead levels now at a peak in many of our cities and carbon monoxide levels at times beyond the safety limit. Babies and the young child are especially vulnerable to such environmental hazards. Poisoning may be environmental, accidental, industrial or deliberate and each needs special consideration. Asbestos

poisoning is an example of industrial hazard and the risks of certain occupations.

In recent years, drugs of the stimulant variety as cocaine, morphine-derivatives as heroin, marihuana, and certain hallucinogenic drugs as L.S.D. have become common toxic factors in varying age-groups and occupations in a search for a contrived exit to seemingly insoluble languor and boredom, but which only creates alternative and in many ways more severe problems.

Iatrogenic factors (doctor-induced illness)
There is little doubt that the complications of modern allopathic medicines is one of the major factors in patient-complaints and illness in our time. Drug-induced illness and dependency is now a major problem in every surgery throughout the country and the number of patients who are addicted to sedatives, tranquillizers, purgatives, anti-depressants and pain-killers probably runs into millions and even tens of millions if the European population is considered and the pattern of prescriptions looked at closely. These are people who have no psychological illness of addiction or dependency in the main, but having started a course of treatment and become more or less free from symptoms, they are quite unable to give up their medicines from fear of a relapse and often because they feel that they need to 'take' something to remain well. Withdrawal of such drugs is often impossible in a busy surgery because of the time required for each individual's anxieties. The tendency is to go on for a further month or perhaps another three months, with the patient at a low-par level of well-being and energy, but without dramatic side-effects being present. When this occurs the tendency is not to stop the treatment and to observe the patient for a time, but to switch to a similar related-drug

in the hope that no reaction will be forthcoming — other than the usual dependency one — now increasingly accepted as normal and no longer a response-of-disease and an abnormality.

Particularly the anti-depressants, the blood-pressure depressants or hypotensive drugs and the contraceptive 'pill', also the hormone therapies, especially the oes-trogens and the steroid group of suppressants are the major culprits.

Their action outside the therapeutically desired one is often broad-ranging, involving the heart and ciculation, the immuned defensive system, the vital organs of the liver and kidneys, which may be all effected by a variety of side-effects and dysfunction. Such remedies although important and of value, may nevertheless when over-prescribed, cause the very same symptoms which they are trying to cure and serve to reinforce the original illness. This has been quite clearly shown to occur with certain tranquillizers, prescribed by the billion, causing symp-toms of tension and anxiety in their own right and even the vital anti-spasmodics used for asthma have been shown to provoke bronchial spasm when there is an allergic reaction to the synthetic colorants used in the pill-coating.

Socially-induced factors

These are the other illnesses of addiction, so common-place and subtle in many cases as to be accepted as normal, but where the symptoms and the consequences are often enormously important for the overall health and vitality of the person. I am thinking here of such social-addictions and government-revenue earners as cigarettes and alcohol as causes of disease. The former, with the proven action of tobacco on the lungs, heart and circulation and also growth of the young foetus, provoking a much smaller placenta, umbilical cord and birth weight and chest problems of the neonate. There are also grave implications for cancer in adults and circulatory disease for every young woman on the 'pill'. Despite the warning notices, in general the public has not been fully warned of their dangers and a minimum has been done to put over clearly that these are potential killers. In spite of this the advertising goes on and more and more young people still use cigarettes or their attractive packaging as either a social-prop or a symbol of their new-found maturity.

Alcohol is also one of the major disease-inducers of our time, a poison to the delicate cells of the liver, heart and brain when taken in excess and regularly. I am not referring here to the often advantageous tonic action of social drinking or wine in moderation with meals.

I still see lonely, isolated people, both men and women, from a variety of social levels, often of mature years and who drink regularly to obliterate or forget. Depressed and lonely, often feeling hopeless, they don't eat adequately at such times and with each successive bottle taken, they feel more and more trapped and depressed and down, yet are unable to find or go for help or advice so that they slowly destroy themselves both physically and psychologically.

The other social causes are the diseases caused by an excess of coffee and tea or sugar, all of which are addictive and undesirable and in excess they cause a combination of either hypoglycaemia or energy-vitality collapse, restlessness and nervous tension. Often the caffeine-containing drinks may affect quite fundamental areas of a person's physiology, including the menstrual cycle. The role of such dubious but widespread practise of using additives as colorants, preservatives, stabilisers, oxidisers and artificial flavour and sweetner agents in basic foods is still uncertain. Many have been withdrawn because of their association with possible cancer-formations and fortunately they are under constant scrutiny. Doubtless we are not yet at the end of the list of those due for withdrawal and their whole purpose to artificially prolong storage and shelf-life and to give an apparent freshness is highly questionable, only justifiable on financial grounds but not those of the individual and any quality of food or life. Even the so-called 'harvest-foods' all too often contains such additives if the labels are carefully scrutinized. Their role in disease formation is one to be constantly on the watch for in the press and be prepared to discard any suspect foodstuffs should a warning be given.

Dietary factors
Most people now eat a poorly balanced meal, far too rich in starches, sugars and often protein for the sedate adult's needs. It is often lacking in essential fibre-content, natural vitamins, minerals and adequate raw-foods as fresh fruit. This is especially true of the elderly but also the teenager. The former live alone, neglecting themselves, because it is difficult to cook and buy for one person and a bun and jam is easiest to make, especially a frozen or pre-cooked one. The latter want hamburgers, chips, coke and a milk-shake with chocolate because their taste-buds are formed by the media and no longer by nutritional requirements and instinctive vitality-needs.

Stress factors
Distinct from psychological factors as outlined earlier, this section could equally be called diseases of modern living or modern times. Here illness is caused by subtle

indefinable factors as constant pressures, wear-and-tear, rush, lack of rhythm, noise and tension-pace generally. The general concept underlying stress is the now frequent assumption that 'time is money' or that 'a minute gained is a minute saved'. But unfortunately if you ask the individual what they have done with all the minutes saved — too often the reply is vaguely negative. Discord, lack of balance, purposeless competative drives all take their toll both psychologically and physiologically with tension across the shoulders, low-back pain, pain in the elbows and shoulders common at all ages. Fibrositis, rheumatism, indigestion, constipation, high blood-pressure, strokes, peptic ulcer and gall-bladder disease are but a few of the common diseases of our time and civilisation. They are all very common and their exact cause is often from a variety of pressures and stresses combined with poor dietary intake and psychological factors all combining to undermine vitality and to allow the easy entry and development of disease and premature degenerative changes.

Environmental factors
These are now common in all parts of the world. For many, crowded, inadequately heated offices and workshops, poorly illuminated with no natural daylight is the norm. Open-plan offices create an environment of being surrounded by too many people in large noisy and smokey impersonal spaces with little privacy which creates depression and undermines health. Over-heating is a factor in certain modern office or home blocks with a dry atmosphere and often the stress and tension of an hour or more of tiring commuting to the office in pressurised over-crowded conditions, sometimes standing packed like sardines before the day starts. It is not surprising that

many young people are already tired before their day begins. The result is that heart-attacks are occuring in both men and women at an increasingly young age and that nervous breakdowns, all the addictions discussed, obesity, or its counterpart anorexia is now frequently seen.

At the end of the day there is an unhealthy, jaded sense of fatigue and collapse. Some are too tired to eat properly even and another snack meal is often the pattern. More and more people are leading mindless, passive, purpose-less lives glued to the television or isolated under head-phones. They are often full of good intentions but just too exhausted and tired to carry them through into reality. Such pressures are soon translated into physical changes, recognizable disease and symptoms in one form or another. Prevention by early diagnosis and homoeopathy should be the first priority and the patient treated at the early jaded, low and exhausted, irritable or depressed stage of illness — well before physical and often irreversi-ble cellular changes occur. Many have however often run the gauntlet of conventional treatments before homoeopathy is given a trial — not infrequently in desperation and as a last resort, rather than as a first line of safe and effective treatment.

CHAPTER FIVE

The indications for Homoeopathy

For convenience these have been grouped into acute and chronic problems, but there are really no fixed or firm dividing lines where people are concerned and each problem must be dealt with on merit according to the degree of dis-ease and individual make-up.

Acute Problems

Psychological problems

Because of its unique action in the mental sphere homoeopathy has a deep-acting therapeutic role to play in all the emotional and psychological problems that now occur so frequently. The latest estimates are that there are about 15 million cases of depression present in this country (U.K.) and there are probably at least as many cases of anxiety-tension being treated. About one case in three seen at any surgery has a weighted psychological element to it when the symptoms are not clearly emotional from the start. The commonest problems seen are a sense of confusion and sadness or overwhelming tension or depression with either a clear 'down' in the mental area with lack of drive, libido and energy or the depression is expressed physically by a chronic low-back problem or chronic indigestion. Covert or hidden depression often presents as any recurrent, 'dragging-down' problem of any form which cannot be either clearly diagnosed or treated by any satisfactory means. All of these problems are eminently suitable for the homoeopathic approach and the majority respond speedily and with total or near-total recovery.

Allergic Problems

Homoeopathy has an important and effective part to play in all the allergic conditions, particularly hay-fever, migraine, allergic rhinitis and eczema. Because it can re-align any excessive and inappropriate physiological reaction at a protein level as well as incorporating a balancing or psychological function, a single remedy, when well-chosen to fit the patient, may help quickly resolve an often long-standing allergic disability.

First-aid

Homoeopathy has proved invaluable over the years in the treatment of all the common first-aid emergencies that commonly occur in the home. These naturally vary with the people and personalities involved, particularly in acute problems. In general homoeopathy is remarkably effective in a wide variety of situations which may vary from an insect sting, cut or graze to the treatment of infections, wounds, splinters, burns and scalds. In all cases it is the degrees of damage or trauma that is key and judgement is required to match the correct remedy-profile to that of the patient's symptoms with a minimum of delay. Severe cases require hospitalisation or treatment in a specialised unit, as with an extensive burn or severe road accident, with homoeopathy playing a less direct and more supportive, secondary, but nevertheless important role, to stimulate healing and a swift return to recovery.

Casualty or Surgical Conditions
Where the problem is one which requires specialised care and treatment beyond the home and common first-aid approach then homoeopathy acts to support and strengthen, minimising infection or reactions generally, other than the essential vital one, which it supports as throughout homoeopathy. In the surgical emergency, homoeopathy speeds the cure by limiting shock from an adverse reaction to either the initial accident or the surgical intervention with possible loss of blood or fluids. It makes for a more responsive patient, confident and relaxed, with recovery-time kept to a minimum according to the individual needs of the patient.

Exhaustion States
In itself, homoeopathy cannot provide and replace depleted reserves. It can however stimulate repose and essential relaxation so that a return to healthy functioning occurs with a replenishment of bodily reserves from food, the environment and where possible, a healthy atmosphere, providing that it is available. Both psychological as well as physical depletions are occuring with increasing frequency and both need to be regularly replenished for life to continue at a high-level and to cope with demands. In such states, homoeopathy has a lot to offer and can make more energy available to storage organs such as the spleen and liver for the essential build-up of reserves which is often the key to a return to vitality and more effective functioning in general.

Infections

These respond well to homoeopathy particularly those of the bladder as with cystitis, the chest as bronchitis, laryngitis, sore throat or asthma. Other common infective problems where there is a rapid response are skin problems, especially chronic recurrent conditions, infective wounds, hang-nail problems and sinusitis. In all cases, provided that the infection falls within the 'normal' or usual limits and is not one of overwhelming or epidemic proportions, or involving an elderly person with diminished vitality, then the response is nearly always favourable. Pneumonia of the elderly, especially of the acute and viral type is a difficult problem for any form of treatment and in general it is best treated by antibiotics with homoeopathy playing a supportive, back-up role. Similarly with the major epidemics, or more unusual highly infectious conditions as cholera, typhoid, meningitis and smallpox – these are best treated in hospital with antibiotics and homoeopathy reserved as a background support and particularly important in the convalescent phase of treatment.

Chronic Problems

These are often recurrent problems that have failed to respond satisfactorily to any conventional approach and have become resistant to often long-standing repeat-prescriptions of either steroids or antibiotics over the years. Such problems include the chronic allergies as asthma, hay-fever or the difficult 'civilisation' diseases like hiatus hernia, peptic-ulcer, raised blood pressure, colitis, angina. Homoeopathy is helpful in all of these unless urgent surgery is required or the conditions have been left and neglected without any treatment so that the patient is in danger — as with an imminent and severe haemorrhage or an uncontrollable infection — perhaps peritonitis.

Case History

A patient was seen recently with a history of heart attacks and increasingly severe anginal pain, occuring every hour of the day and night. The patient could not move or speak without chest pain, and the least movement to undress or even to describe the pain caused intolerably severe pain. The patient was far too ill for a homoeopathic consultation and should have been in an acute cardiac unit several weeks previously, possibly on continuous anticoagulant therapy.

It is unrealistic to expect homoeopathy to act as a miracle-cure — in a perilous condition which has been left to reach a dangerous level — where the patient lacks the vitality and the strength for a healing reaction to occur. In general it is better in almost every condition to bring the patient for treatment as early as possible rather than to wait until the very last possible moment or until they are in crisis.

CHAPTER SIX

The Action and Function of Homoeopathy

Homoeopathy has a unique action both physically and psychologically. Its main sphere of action is directly on the vital energy flow and reserves within the physical body as well as the mental sphere, acting deeply on both counts. This action is best summarised by the following unique and special properties of the homoeopathic prescription.

The Balancing function

Homoeopathy has an important role to play in correcting or balancing of physiological functioning. Excesses of secretion and flow, whatever their cause, lead to problems often with pain, spasm or colic and flatulence. All of this can be relieved or prevented by the homoeopathic approach which stimulates the body towards equilibrium, harmony and balance rather than passivity and stasis, where an unsatisfactory state of intestinal or glandular inactivity prevails with indigestion or constipation the inevitable outcome. The excessive build-up of either acidity and gas or tension, anger and resentment can be released as balancing occurs both psychologically as well as physiologically with increased relaxation and flow occuring at both levels. The lessening of emotional tension and anxiety leading to an overall more balanced perspective is inseperable from the closely related glandular and intestinal functioning.

The Strengthening function

Homoeopathy has a definite strengthening role. This can be clearly seen where there is a chronic back problem with weakness and pain. Often after a single prescription the patient may say 'look how much more I can do and how much more agile and strongly I can move, get out of a chair, bend or sway — I couldn't do that a week ago — my back was far too weak'. Psychologically it also strengthens confidence. *Arnica* is one of the best remedies to increase strength with *Arsenicum* a close second.

The Supportive function

Homoeopathy supports vital energies without dissipation or depletion. Nor does it leave the patient exhausted or feeling worse than before starting the treatment or worse than the original problem that brought them to the doctor initially. Especially it is supportive of the individual patient's needs and quite naturally acts where most needed and in the major areas of weakness and lack. It will not however act where there is no requirement of either support or stimulus to functioning.

Preservative functioning

Essentially this is the preservation and storage — both physiologically as well as psychologically, of vital energy reserves, so that these can be further added-to and built-up. Homoeopathy never depletes essential reserves, thereby creating exhaustion. It does have the power to mobilise, concentrate and re-distribute whatever vitality the individual has at their disposal and to direct such strengths to the areas most needed. At the same time it creates an overall sense of well-being and relaxation.

Un-locking function
All too often problems get locked-away in areas of the body like motor-way slipways which cannot be dealt with and a chronic situation is created. In fact, the problem is just beneath the surface, but inaccessible to natural healing responses which are unable to function. The problem is contained, but cannot be released. This is seen particularly whenever there has been a prolonged treatment by one of the steroid drugs. The disease is kept immobilised, partially paralysed, just under the body's defensive layer — as can be clearly seen in many cases of chronic eczema or psoriasis. The condition neither evolves and cures or clears-up, nor is it apparently getting worse as long as the tablets and creams are continued. However if these are missed for more than a few days, the whole problem breaks-through the surface with a vengeance and irritating severity, only to be pushed back and down again with a different steroid or higher dose of the original drug. This tendency for disease to 'have out', to come out and to express themselves is perfectly natural using the vital reaction. After stopping suppressant therapy, such emergent reactions may be much more severe and are sometimes a source of considerable anxiety to the patient. With homoeopathy these chronic patterns and processes can often be unlocked and made available to the natural healing powers of the body — which the remedy stimulates. But when there has been a long history of suppression, from whatever cause, then the initial healing reaction is likely in all cases to be a strong one until a state of healthy harmony and balance is

re-established by the patient.

Curative function

By unlocking and bringing to surface — either in the mental sphere or the physical organs, homoeopathy frees disease from its chains and makes it accessible to the processes of cure which are within every healthy individual. It will not free the disease or an underlying condition so that it becomes rampant and overwhelming, however. Homoeopathy respects the needs of the individual and will not release a negative process unless it is in the interests of the person and can be adequately dealt with by the defenses at the time. In general the homoeopathic stimulus acts on the defensive and immune-response resistance areas, mobilising them to efficient activity and thus frees the hitherto bound-up disease process which has been impairing the health of the individual and perpetuating a chronic state of ill-health.

The Centreing function

There is another major function of the remedies that is not always appreciated — that of centreing the patient so that a more overall and less distorted viewpoint can be taken helping relaxation and keeping priority-of-need more in focus. In this way, the patient is less prone to be overwhelmed by relatively trivial and insignificant happenings and can worry, be concerned, with real issues rather than neurotic areas which are negative ultimately, often repetitive and usually relatively insignificant. I have seen this happen many times with the high potency remedies and this is unique to the homoeopathic response.

Case Reports

A woman came with a double problem — she had a strangulated haemorrhoid or 'pile', the size and appearance of a ripe victoria plum, painful in the extreme and making sitting impossible, walking difficult. But she was also severely depressed — quite unrelated to her painful venous condition. Within a few hours of receiving *Pulsatilla* in the IOM dosage, the pile had shrunk to a small size and was far more comfortable and bearable. At the same time confidence had returned following a long talk with her boy-friend about a matter that had been troubling her and a cause of conflict for several weeks. This problem had been both worrying and depressing her for too long and had eventually undermined her basic confidence. She was able to suddenly feel herself for the first time in months, resolve the psychological situation and regain confidence so that she almost immediately felt better, more of a total person and more in balance. The condition was completely resolved in both areas with a single treatment and no further help was required or other remedies.

Another patient came with a severe anxiety-tension state, unable to sleep or to relax. At the same time there was the most severe urinary condition of intense irritation with cystitis so intense that there was painful frequency of urination every 15 minutes of the day and night. A single dose of *Sycotico 30* was given — one of the bowel nosodes. Within minutes, the patient experienced relief, for the first time in weeks, the psychological state becoming more relaxed at the same time as the bladder condition. My patient fell into a deep refreshing sleep within minutes of taking the remedy and both bladder and tension state completely cleared from that time with no repeat of the remedy being required.

The Dynamic function of cure

The law of cure is well-known and is clearly seen throughout homoeopathic treatments. It is often most noticeable in skin and arthritic conditions or where there is a rheumatic problem. Most recent symptoms respond initially to treatment and those problems that have been present for long periods respond only later to the potencies — the remedy going 'back in time' so to speak and roots-out step by step the deepest and initial causes of a problem. Homoeopathy often brings to the surface during cure old and long-forgotten symptoms that just as rapidly disappear as quickly as they arise — either quite spontaneously or with the helping hand of a remedy. The recurrence of such symptoms does not mean that the patient is getting worse or having a recurrence of an old problem, but it does mean that the remedy is acting dynamically and deeply so that remnants of earlier conditions — not dealt with adequately at the time, or suppressed then, can now be finally and thoroughly eradicated from the body's vital energy resources and brings back a welcome boost to vitality which was previously being sapped and drained-away. Once out in the 'open', such symptoms are quite naturally eradicated by natural healing resources. Symptoms are also normally relieved from the top of the body downwards — from scalp to trunk and finally the feet in keeping with the direction of energy flows. Recovery also occurs from more centrally affected organs as the heart, kidney, liver or lungs to more peripheral and relatively insignificant areas as a joint-capsule or muscle. A heart condition as angina may clear up, but the patient says that they are no better or even feel worse because they have developed a return of an old problem of indigestion or a frozen shoulder, but the heart is healthier, the patient free from cardiac pain on walking.

But the process of homoeopathy is such that it will unerringly flush-out at the same time any disease process in its pathway at the particular depth and resonence of the remedy and potency used and according to the dynamic logic of the pathways which are being cleared.

Some further general points about the action of the remedies

Note that the specific action of the homoeopathic remedies is to 'throw out' all that is repressed or suppressed, beneath the surface or unavailable to the patient at either a physical or psychological level. The remedy brings out these physical symptoms to the surface, making them 'available' to the body for resolution and cure. The remedy does not and will not differentiate between the elements that it liberates, either good or bad, positive and desirable or what may be undesirable or painful. At times a remedy may also throw-out feelings of bitter grievance, anger and resentment as well as bringing out equally deep and repressed alienated feelings of attachment, libidinal drive, or long-denied sentiments of grief and loss as also lost creative drives. This is all part of the uniqueness of the homoeopathic response and is why it is particularly important to follow-up closely and carefully after the initial prescriptions, especially a high-potency one because the patient may need guidance with the psychological reactions — either positive or negative which may emerge. Caution is only necessary, as in all cases of medical treatment or healing where there is a previous history of severe or chronic disease, particularly a poorly resolved and immured old T.B. condition, previous psychiatric history and breakdown, also cancer.

CHAPTER SEVEN

Dilution and Disease

Homoeopathy operates according to profound physiological principles throughout nature and both animal and human life. These principles are clearly expressed by the Schultz law of stimulus and growth which states that where there are healthy living and growing cells, these are stimulated by a small stimulus, inhibited by a medium stimulus and that a strong stimulus destroys all growth completely. Much of this work was carried out by the experimental physiologists Arndt and Schultz, working with yeast cells and the effect of arsenic on their growth proliferation. Arsenic as *Arsenicum* in its homoeopathic form, is a very powerful remedy and used extensively in acute conditions.

There is no doubt about the importance of this principle. The trace elements are essential to healthy functioning and the body, which can synthesise most things is unable to produce its trace-substances as copper and cadmium. These are needed in minute amounts for the healthy formation of blood and other cell-tissues. Without them, the body may become prone to certain obscure and chronic diseases. It is also well-known that both copper and cadmium are extremely toxic in large doses to the body, but in their minute stimulating dietary 'homoeopathic' amounts, they are absolutely essential to health.

Homoeopathic remedies are always given in small dosages because these can be most easily responded to and taken-up by the body. They are used by the body as 'pointers' to areas of tension or lack, directing vitality to areas of most need and opening-up dis-eased areas to the body's intrinsic and natural healing powers. Where there is a mineral or vitamin deficiency, the substance in its diluted or potency form can be most easily taken-up and absorbed without excessive loss of the substance in the stools or causing intolerable irritation to the lining mucosa of the stomach or bowel.

Homoeopathy acts by the principle of minimal dilution repeated as infrequently as possible. The aim in homoeopathy is one only — to stimulate a vital healing response in the area affected so that a break-through of energy-activity may occur, and then to stop the remedy.

Originally the remedies were given in their mother-tincture, or undiluted form by Hahnemann and his followers, which although provoking a powerful vital reaction, had undesirable side-effects from the strength of the tinctures used. He then began experimenting with weaker solutions and increasing serial dilutions, to find a suitable dilution that would be effective without side-effects. To the amazement of Hahnemann, he found that the remedies were enhanced in their action by serial dilution. The more he diluted — rather than weaking the homoeopathic action, it was increased. This chance finding, seemingly paradoxal at the time, led to a whole new dimension of thinking and homoeopathic development for both patient and doctor.

By bringing life and healing circulation and warmth to areas previously inert and non-active, the remedies can transform areas of dis-ease into more healthy tissue again. A non-functioning area, with loss of tone or spasm with pain and blockage, may return to become healthy tissue within a short period of time. Once the healing reaction has occurred, the homoeopath has done his job by restoring vitality where previously there was more tension than the body could either eliminate or contain without symptoms and interference with normal functioning. This vital reaction can in most cases be relied upon to continue and carry-on to complete the work. Homoeopathy acts rather like a key — opening a door and pointing the way in areas where previously there was no way-apparent, no lock or even key-hole visible in what seemed an impossible situation. This is why patients are so often completely astounded by their speed of response to the remedies, particularly when the higher dilutions of 30c or more are given.

The lower dilutions of the 6c or 3x potencies usually act at a purely physical and tissue level with any more general and constitutional or psychological benefits being secondary to the peripheral ones.

When the higher dilutions of 30c and more are used, there is more stimulus of general activity, with responses at both the mental as also the physical levels. Where the problem is apparently at a shoulder level only, due to penetration of cold or damp into the joint, then *Sanguinaria, Rhus tox, Dulcamara,* according to the symptoms, in their lower, 'local' potencies is perfectly adequate. However when the problem is one of a frozen shoulder with clearly psychological under-tones — since the loss of a close relative or from an unhappy marriage, with anger, rage and resentment barely controlled or even repressed, then the prescription has to be thought about carefully. In cases where such underlying feelings are present, at the expense of health, then in all cases the higher 30 or even 200c potencies give better results and enable any underlying depression to be resolved more speedily.

The minimal dose or 'atomic' level of dilution is becoming more and more important in other related fields other than in pure medicine. In agriculture and in the prevention of toxic damage to plants and animals it has become increasingly recognized as an important area of research and disease-prevention. A recent paper (1979) in the Annals of Human Biology describes the importance of garlic in plant health as an effective fungicide and pesticide at dilutions of one part in a hundred — which is the beginning of our centisimal scale in homoeopathy. In Smarden (Kent), an outbreak of poisoning occurred in the early 60's where many cattle had to be slaughtered and burned. There was a small leak from a nearby manufacturing company into a stream which was an animal water-supply. Fluoracetamide was being manufactured and a dilution of this substance of one part in 10 million or 10^{-7} was lethal. The level of dilution is such as to be equivalent to the higher dilutions used in homoeopathy and confirms directly that such dilutions not only act as a stimulus but in certain cases — as with fluoracetamide, they can be effectively lethal too.

Such dangers are fortunately not the case where standards of purity and safety are those of international requirement. Stringent safe-guards are in operation to ensure total non-toxicity. This is why there are no known side-effects of the method and from the remedies used so that their safety is assured at all ages and in all dosages.

CHAPTER EIGHT

The advantages of the homoeopathic approach

1. It is a natural method using simple principles and remedies, unlike most modern drugs, which are basically pure and non-synthetic — not artificial in origin. Many of our most advanced and modern treatments have unpredictable results, stimulating a temporary and often shifting 'synthetic' cure which is out of phase with the needs and total expressions of the patient. Homoeopathy is in resonance with the total person, the total man and the treatments as the cure, forms part of an overall meaningful and harmonious unity.

2. Homoeopathy stimulates the natural resources of the body to bring about a cure in its own time, in its own rhythms, without imposing a pattern of responses which the individual is unable to cope with, or set within a time limit. Each patient proceeds according to their vital energy resources and reserves and although some may establish a rapid and energetic vital response, others respond more slowly and gently in keeping with their overall patterns — the speed of their psychological and physiological reactions in toto. No pattern is brought to bear, no standards or pressures are laid down and the body is simply stimulated along certain predictable path-

ways of response and then allowed to proceed at its own pace. This is why the question 'How long will it take doctor'? is so very difficult to answer unless there is already experience of the patient and knowledge of his responses — perhaps to a particular remedy, often a constitutional one, over the years. Whenever the patient is in a convalescent state, the remedies still work, but more time is needed and a slower response is the norm.

3.   It is effective at all ages — from the child of a few weeks old to the most elderly member of the family. The whooping cough prophylactic nosode is effective in the youngest infant, but equally the prostatic remedy *Sabal Serr*, is effective in the octogenerian or when an elderly lady has a spot of bladder weakness with a tendency to 'leak' slightly on rushing or with excitement. Whatever the age, the well-indicated remedy will always strengthen and act to some degree, however much the calendar has turned since infancy. All age groups are seen in a busy practise and often several generations of the same family, each with their characteristic problem common to their age-group. I commonly see families like this in consultation, the grand-parents, mums and dads and the children — all responding well and often equally quickly, the single remedy just as effective in the elderly as with the baby.

4.   The remedies stimulate a general state of well-being and of confidence generally without leaving the patient more depleted and in a worse state than before, worse than the original condition being treated — as can frequently happen with some vaccination reactions in the young child.

5.   The remedies are pleasant to take, usually made-up in lactose or sugar of milk and quite acceptable to the youngest infant or the most difficult child. Once swal-

lowed they do not lead to a foul taste or breath, a coated tongue or have any after-taste or after-effects other than the intended ones of the remedy.

6. There are no side-effects of the remedy — no diarrhoea, nausea, weakness, circulatory effects, haemorrhagic tendencies, drowsiness which could be either overwhelming or dangerous. Sometimes the remedy stimulates an aggravation of the underlying problem temporarily — as part of the vital reaction which the homoeopathic is aiming for and this may give sometimes some discomfort temporarily before an improvement occurs. However such responses-to-treatment are quite different from a side-reaction to a drug treatment where there is intolerance or allergy to some aspect of the remedy. This does not occur in homoeopathy and such aggravations as occur are usually understood and felt by the patient to be positive and a part of cure.

7. There is no danger from the homoeopathic remedies because of the degree of dilution aimed at giving the patient a minimal stimulus and prepared to the most stringent pharmaceutical codes of purity. Because the aim is always a minimal dose, this is also a safe one with a minimum of external or outside interference upon body functioning, creating and emphasising a maximum of 'self' and natural cure and confidence, fully supported by the homoeopathic remedies.

8. The remedy does not have to be taken for tedious, endless periods with a maintainance dosage to sap the best-developed confidence and promote psychological dependency and undermine health over the years. As soon as there is a recovery from symptoms and a return to normal functioning whatever the problem, the remedy is stopped and the body's natural functioning is encouraged to resume as it was before treatment was required.

9. The remedies can be used preventatively or prophylacticly in certain problems. For example in german measles during pregnancy, scarlet fever, whooping cough or measles — when the individual is in an especially low or vulnerable state or when the disease is particularly virulent and epidemic at a time when there is a potential danger to health as with the elderly or in pregnancy.

10. Homoeopathy acts deeply and will eradicate whenever possible the roots of a disease, even when chronic and present since birth or with a family-tendency to the condition. Especially it has this ability to 'sweep' cleanly and deeply within the tissues the remnants of earlier, and often inadequately treated or suppressed problems. At the time they seemed cured but nevertheless have recurred in one form or other over the years as a constant irritant lowering vitality and health. This 'cleaning-out' role of homoeopathy brings to the surface elements of such former illnesses. A condition, long since forgotten, yet also 'hanging around' over the years, comes out like a skeleton from the cupboard as a familiar symptom, to be finally eradicated and cured — either by new-found vitality or the appropriate remedy.

11. In chronic disease and where there is an inherited tendency and weakness, homoeopathy offers a radical cure to many conditions even where the symptoms do not form a recognizable clinical disease.

12. Homoeopathy gets to the causes of a problem by acting on its roots, stimulating a healthy vitality and response at the deepest level of underlying illness, preventing recurrence. It does not just act on the symptoms to relieve them in a palliative, seemingly reassuring way, but leaving the underlying causes unaffected and intact.

13. Homoeopathy does not deplete the patient or leave him more exhausted by the cure than before the

illness. It supports the immune-defence system of vitality within the patient, bringing and restoring confidence in the patient's own ability to heal and play a positive role in healing because it balances and harmonises at the very deepest levels of being.

CHAPTER NINE

Some limitations too

In reality these are relatively few and mainly centred around those problems which are obstructive or surgical in origin, or where the intrinsic individual vitality, for whatever reason, is abnormally weak and feeble.

1. The method is not recommended for any condition primarily surgical as an acute appendicitis, or where there is a severe abdominal infection with the risk of peritonitis occurring. Also where an acute and severe haemorrhage has occurred or an imminent danger or in any condition whatsoever which requires surgery, then in the majority of cases homoeopathy should be in a supportive role only. Homoeopathy acts as a gentle stimulus to the body's healing powers, but when an acute condition has arisen for whatever reason and is overwhelming, entering deeply into the organs or eroding tissues, then usually the homoeopathic approach has been left too late and immediate surgical or antibiotic treatment should be used to help the patient over the immediate crisis and possible danger to life. In such cases homoeopathic remedies play a secondary role and background to other immediate treatments and the underlying reason as to why the tissues have become so weak and

feeble can be left to a later post-convalescent time and dealt with if possible by the homoeopathic approach at that time.

2.   When there is an acute crisis illness, as with an overwhelming infection, where the body is not responding in a strong, healthy way with a temperature and inflammatory reaction within reasonable limits. Where the patient is markedly toxic or weak and elderly, lacking in reserves and vital energy, then a homoeopathic approach should not be used for the acute stages and conventional treatments given.

3.   In general, whenever the usual vital, defensive reactions of the body to contain, limit and localise an inflammatory response is not present or when vitality is low as may occur in a convalescent or post-operative condition, then homoeopathy is not usually the ideal treatment at this stage. A period of time is needed to build-up energy reserves which may take several weeks. During this period of build-up, the patient is dangerously vulnerable and homoeopathy is sometimes best left until the crisis is well and truly over.

4.   Homoeopathy is not a panacea or a cure-for-all. Anyone who pretends it is does not understand the method fundamentally and does the treatment a disservice. It is always important that the indications are clear-cut, logical and take into account the patient's ability to respond to the remedies and the length of time that this is likely to take. In general, the tablets should not be handled because the medicine is on the surface and this lessens their efficacy or may neutralise them completely. They are best not taken during a period of steroid treatment or immediately after it. Also the excessive intake of tea or coffee reduces their action during a course of treatment. In general, any form of suppressant treat-

ment taken at the time of a homoeopathic consultation, also precludes a homoeopathic approach because it has a neutralising and opposite effect upon any remedies that may be prescribed or taken.

CHAPTER TEN

More indications for homoeopathy

Homoeopathy is most efficient in those conditions where — either physically or psychologically, over a period of weeks and months, there has been a build-up of stress and tension. In general, to be effective, the underlying problem should not be one which is either mechanical or surgical in origin or due to an acute and overwhelming infection.

Invasive tumours and cancers are conditions where natural immunity and resistance to chaos-provoking cellular elements has been lost. They are usually the result of chronic long-standing conditions or attitudes, often neglected or denied over months and years. When they occur, a multiple approach is required, including diet and surgery with homoeopathy playing a supportive role during the acute stages. Such conditions, whenever possible, are always best treated by prevention before the acute condition has manifested. The condition is not hopeless however and what the body can produce — the body can also cure, given the correct drive, stimulus, diet and way of life. Most important of all is a correct attitude to self and others and help may be needed to look more sensibly at this area.

Cancer treatment, when it is necessary, must use every modern technique available, including x-ray treatment, irradiation, modern drugs, surgery, conventional remedies, diet, visualisation techniques and possibly psychotherapy. In all cases the supportive homoeopathic approach makes the patient more at ease, more relaxed and comfortable with a lessening of tension and suffering and usually a better outlook which is so very fundamental in every case.

First-aid conditions respond well provided they are not severe and extensive with major lacerations. A severe burn or scald or extensive wound or haemorrhage that requires suturing must have hospital treatment, but all other cases respond well to simple homoeopathic approach. If an ambulance is necessary, homoeopathy supports the patient before it arrives, reducing shock and helping to prevent complications. In many cases homoeopathy will reduce infection and haemorrhage. But in every first-aid case it is important to be realistic and to use judgement as to the extent of the injury and whether or not it is an injury suitable for homoeopathy. Where there is doubt and uncertainty get another opinion from the nearest casualty department without loss of time, or where there is no immediate response to the remedies.

Homoeopathy is used effectively for menstrual disorders, problems of heart and circulation including blood-pressure, digestive difficulties and urinary problems. Muscular cramps, rheumatism and arthritis respond well and are frequently relieved or cured. Other important areas of action are infections of the skin, nose, throat and chest. Many of the common skin conditions as acne and psoriasis often clear completely with homoeopathy.

Emotional conditions of tension and dis-ease is one of the foremost indications for homoeopathy, especially where diminished vitality and a build-up of fatigue, exhaustion and apathy has occurred. These emotional stress conditions diminish resistance and the body's natural immune-defences as much as any prolonged physical condition or chronic illness where vitality is minimal and the body cannot defend itself at all adequately against the external hazards that threaten at all times to undermine healthy reserves and organ functioning. During a convalescent period, or after a 'bad' attack of influenza, pneumonia, or perhaps a viral hepatitis or glandular fever, reserves are low and particular care must be taken to avoid either a recurrence or a new penetrating illness.

At such times, homoeopathy, when correctly applied, can work wonders to pull the person round from a particularly vulnerable position or where recovery seems prolonged or even impossible to attain after a severe infection which has 'emptied all the batteries'.

Circulatory problems or gastric catarrhal conditions respond well and peptic ulceration is frequently helped provided that the condition is not one that has been neglected to the point of perforation or where scar tissue over the years has created a chronic obstruction which only surgery can remedy. Such complications although rare, must be ruled out at the time of consultation and examination and where there is doubt, a barium meal or other radiological investigation may be essential to give background information for an overall homoeopathic approach and to be certain that a surgical approach is not more indicated and more in the best interests of the patient. Duodenitis, duodenal ulceration, hiatus hernia, gall-bladder dysfunction can all respond very positively but where gall-bladder symptoms are due to a large stone causing obstruction, colic and impaired healthy flow of bile along its duct, then surgery is recommended with homoeopathy in a secondary back-up role.

All the so-called stress diseases of civilisation also respond well to homoeopathy. They are unfortunately as much seen in our domestic pets as in humans, which is perhaps one of the reasons why vetinary homoeopathy has become so popular and sought-after because the results are often just as convincing as with their owners. This very clear-cut response from animals of all kinds most definitely scuttles the usual criticism of the method, based on ignorance or mis-information, which suggests that homoeopathy is only a matter of suggestion and placebo-response without any proven or definite specific healing response by the individual.

The 'diseases of civilisation' include all the common circulatory problems especially varicose veins, angina, heart disease in general, degenerative conditions and hardening of the arteries or premature arterioschlerosis, rather than from old age. Blood-pressure or hypertension, the chronic peptic and indigestion syndromes already mentioned, especially obesity and many problems of chronic nasal and throat congestion and catarrh also come into this category.

Eczema, psoriasis, chronic skin infective conditions and fungal states, give in general a marked positive response, sometimes following an initial aggravation of symptoms, especially where topical or local steroid creams have been used over the years. Herpes — either as shingles (herpes zoster), or its genital form, is becoming increasingly a matter for concern but especially the latter with many young people, because of its frequency and that many carriers are symptom-free. Both forms are largely incurable by conventional methods but respond well to homoeopathy. The other common form of herpes is much more benign although common and unpleasant — I refer to oral herpes or the common cold sore of the lips and mouth, which according to its exact position and site indicates its specific homoeopathic treatment.

Many of the common Private and 'personal' intimate difficulties of the couple in the sexual sphere of their relationship respond well to the homoeopath approach when combined with sufficient time and an overall look at the problem jointly. This is also true for nervous problems in general because of the depth of action of the remedy in the psychological sphere of the individual. I regard this as one of the unique advantages of homoeopathy and all too often insufficiently appreciated by both practitioner and patient alike.

Homoeopathy can be important in the prevention of epidemics. An epidemic of poliomylitis was controlled by a New Zealand practitioner by *Gelsemium* with outstanding results. Other less dramatic epidemic conditions can be also effectively treated or prevented by using either the appropriate remedy or the nosode obtained from pathological material to form a homoeopathic no-risk vaccine. This is often used for such problems as whooping-cough, measles, mumps, influenza, german-measles and glandular-fever.

All the allergic problems respond well, especially asthma, eczema, urticaria and hay-fever. The latter is often best treated in the early season by specific remedies, appropriate for the individual type of problem before the pollen-count builds up to a level which produces severe symptoms. An autumn type of hay-fever also occurs, associated with tree moulds and for this a homoeopath may use mixed autumn pollens (*M.A.P.*).

Arthritis of every type is helped — either osteo-arthritis and degenerative disease of the elderly or the more acute inflammatory immune-disease reactions of the younger person, known as rheumatoid arthritis. Similarly gouty inflammations and painful conditions usually react positively to homoeopathy. In some of the arthritic cases reported, even where severe changes have been seen on the x-rays, later films have shown regeneration of new bone development around the joint area, as the remedy works to stimulate vitality and new circulation in the region affected. Where there is organ degeneration, especially of the liver after chronic alcohol abuse or viral hepatitis, a return to more normal functioning can be sometimes clearly seen and demonstrated by improved liver-function tests where the correct and specific remedy has been used. Similarly some of the continental animal experiments using rats and mice, have shown that poisoned liver cells, nearly destroyed by carbon tetrachloride can clearly and demonstrably regenerate by being given the appropriate homoeopathic remedy. Although I do not necessarily approve of such methods and homoeopathy has been built-up over the years by research on healthy human volunteers in the 'proving' experiments and their response to treatment during clinical work — nevertheless, it is also of considerable interest to have such tangible proof of how poisoned toxic cells can recover when given their appropriate potency and remedy.

CHAPTER ELEVEN

Preparation of the remedies

Using well-tried methods, developed over many years, the homoeopathic pharmacist uses his expertise to put the basic homoeopathic substances into solution so that serial dilutions or potencies can be developed to medicate the homoeopathic granules or tablets. The remedies are in general of plant, animal or mineral origin. Many are perfectly soluble and can be made up immediately from the fresh plant tinctures with an alcohol mixture to form the mother-tincture containing the pharmacologically active alkaloids. From these all other dilutions are prepared.

Some remedies are however quite insoluble in their crude form. These include minerals as *phosphorus* and silica (*Silicea*) and such base metals as copper (*Cuprum*), iron (*Ferrum*), zinc (*Zincum*), lead (*Plumbum*). Hahnemann discovered an entirely new process called trituration which for the first time in medical history was able to put into solution previously insoluble substances. The method he used was a process of grinding-up the innert insoluble substance with lactose granules and repeating the process several times until the mixture became soluble so that it became possible to create the same serial dilutions as with the soluble remedies. The use of the salts of these substances in their gross and less active form was in this way, finally improved upon.

In this country (U.K.) tinctures are usually diluted according to the decimal or centisimal scale, the latter being most common. Using the centisimal dilutions and the Hahnemannian method of one drop of the remedy-tincture added to 99 drops of dilutant fluid, usually alcohol-based, the mixture is ready for succussing. It is vigorously shaken, traditionally about 30 times on a firm base as a book to succuss or dynamise the substance. This forms the first centisimal potency. One drop of this in 99 drops of dilutant, once succussed, forms the second centisimal potency and so on. When the remedy has been diluted in this way six times, it becomes the sixth or 6c potency. With the decisimal potencies, one drop of the remedy-tincture is diluted in 9 drops of the dilutant fluid to form the potency, succussed at every stage. After three stages of the dilution, the common potency of 3x is formed.

Standards of purity are always stringent and laid down by European pharmaceutical standards to ensure the highest standards of control and purity in the preparation of the remedies for the satisfaction of both doctor and patient alike. At all stages carefully sterilised neutral glass tubes are used for the serial fluids, which are prepared by hand up to 200c. For the higher potencies and dilutions up to the M (thousand), IOM (ten thousand) and CM (one hundred thousand) potencies a mechanical potentiser is used.

The tinctures in potency are added to sugar of milk (lactose) crystals, tablets or globules to 'hold' the remedy for use by the patient. Using high-potency 95% alcohol solutions for medication ensures that the whole of the lactose tablets, when agitated, come into contact with the chosen potency in their usual 7 gram phial prepared by the pharmacist.

It is important to realise that the remedy lies predominantly on the surface or outside of the pill or tablet used. For this reason they should not be handled when taken and one only shaken into their container lid and crushed or swallowed on the tongue. In particular no remedy should be handled for another person when prescribed. They should always be taken well away from food, tea or coffee and stored in a clean glass jar, preferably a new one, not near any strongly perfumed items as soaps, perfumes, menthol or camphor. The container should not have been used previously for other medicines — either allopathic or homoeopathic, as there is a risk of neutralising the remedies and making them ineffective.

There is another method of preparing the potencies which finds favour on the continent although less so here in the U.K. This is also an early method which does not use serial tubes but relies upon a single container whereby the 99 to one ratio is strictly kept to, but where the one drop is considered to adhere to the inside of the container after succussing. In this Korsakov method the dilutant fluid is thrown out of the same jar each time after succussion and a further 99 drops added each time to complete the serial ratios. The same bottle is used for each potency until the required one is achieved.

Note that all the 'finished' remedies look, taste, and small alike and cannot be differentiated in any way by the naked eye. The mother tinctures can be differentiated by crystallography or chromatography methods at this stage in our knowledge and research is continuing to be able to differentiate the potencies by these and related methods.

In the U.K. many practitioners follow the guide-lines

laid down by the great American homoeopath Kent who soundly recommended taking only one single remedy at a time and continuing with that remedy for as long as it is benefiting the patient and there is a healing response and an improvement. He recommended a change of remedy only when improvement stopped or when there was no reaction of a dynamic kind to the potency given or simply when nothing happened. When symptoms abate and are completely cleared, then the remedy should be omitted completely and the patient take nothing at all, letting the body's natural defences and vitality 'take the wheel'.

CHAPTER TWELVE

Making a start

The first step is always the longest and most difficult and so it may seem in homoeopathy too — but the method is not so complicated and the principles once grasped are simple and logical. In order to familiarise yourself with the method nevertheless takes a period of time to get confidence in a new approach and new remedies. To gain this experience it is advisable to begin with the following four simplest remedies from the list of twenty listed and recommended in chapter twenty. Begin with remedies in the 6th centisimal or 6c potency and start as outlined below. Always buy your remedies from an established and preferably recommended pharmacy, but in all cases get to know your pharmacist — the sources of your remedies must be of the highest quality at all times.

Arnica is the most commonly prescribed remedy of all and probably the most useful and basic for the beginner. Use it in any situation of painful bruising and swelling after a trauma — for example from a fall or tumble, a heavy knock or any similar cause. It is also valuable for psychological hurts and shocks as well as the physical ones. Sometimes there is the quite spontaneous development of 'bruised' — often left-sided pain in a rib or costal muscle, occuring after strain in that region — as from carrying an unaccustomed weight of a heavy suitcase or changing from an electric typewriter back to a manual one. What is important in the choice of *Arnica* as the indicated remedy is the quality of the bruised and swollen feeling in the area affected. Muscular strain responds well as after lifting a heavy weight and being suddenly caught off-balance. The unaccustomed use of a ladder — in late summer for fruit-picking, or when winter-pruning or decorating in the home may cause pain and a bruised aching situation — just the type of pain for *Arnica* and giving rapid relief. Any situation that puts strain on unusual areas of tendon and muscle leading to pain or an actual bruise developing is where the remedy is most indicated. For a very painful condition it may be given hourly but with the majority of conditions, thrice daily is adequate.

Aconitum is the great remedy for fear reactions of any kind especially acute ones. It is valuable for sudden chills from exposure to an East wind or from cold and draughts. Neuralgic pains often occur as a result of such exposures, and provided they are caught within the first 48 hours by the remedy, such painful conditions are quickly resolved. There may be an acute headache, or a sore throat from a cold with pains in the scalp, neck and facial area. *Aconitum* is of value for reactions of acute shock, especially those of fear, fright or panic at the time — the person caught psychologically off-balance and unprepared leading to agitation and restlessness. In such conditions of either physical or psychological exposure, then *Aconitum* is invaluable. Always use the remedy as early as possible, especially during the first 48 hours after exposure —

whatever its source and you will find that given the correct indications, that *Aconitum* gives quick and almost immediate results.

Calendula is unique in stimulating healthy healing and the formation of granulation tissue to protect and cover a wound or cut. A severe wound needs suturing, one acutely infected or where there is foreign matter within the lesion requires treatment in the nearest casualty department but *Calendula* can still be safely given in the 6th potency internally and also applied locally as a tincture when generally cleaning-up the area. Use it for all cuts, abrasions and wounds — its power to stimulate healing is often astonishing.

Rhus Tox is indicated for conditions of muscular or tendon strain where there is spasmodic aching or painful conditions as lumbago, from exposure to cold and damp, or sudden strain with cold air on an area of 'pulled' muscle especially where sweating has made the area vulnerable to cooling and chill. Sprains, strain, any form of muscular swelling with tenderness, — frequently from trauma indicates *Rhus tox*. It often follows *Arnica* and is also useful for itchy, red, eczematous conditions with a limited local or small areas of eruption. In all cases when the remedy is indicated the condition is usually better for warmth and often local heat and generally made worse by cold cool air and damp. Generally movement rather than immobility gives relief and comfort so that the patient tends to move a lot or fidget, wanting to be up and moving about, rather than resting in bed or sitting in a chair. This motion gives relief from tension and any spasm present.

Start to think homoeopathicly in your overall general approach to any problem which you intend to treat yourself. Don't just think so much of treating a 'cold' or a 'headache', but think of the person and a more overall type of problem and complaint rather than quickly giving a name to it. This 'naming' is more of a barrier to homoeopathy than an aid. Jot down the symptoms — the things complained of by the individual. Try to see clearly the type of head-cold for example complained of. If there are three children in the family, all down with a cold, almost certainly each one will have a slightly distinct but varying symptom-pattern. Note how the cold came on and anything that caused or aggravated it. Note also anything that is especially desired or disliked — for example a craving for hot drinks or ice-cold ones. Some patients have an intense, almost obsessional dislike of the least draught or cool air because it aggravates their condition, yet others crave fresh air and want all the doors and windows open.

Note also the colour, pattern and characteristics of any discharge occuring. A nasal discharge may be continuous, thin and watery or it may be yellow or greenish, thick and full of mucous. Some secretions are excoriating or burning to neighbouring tissues causing pain and discomfort. With others the discharge is more dry and stringy. In general note the factors which tend to make the condition worse as the time of day when symptoms are most severe as well as most eased — for example morning or better at the end of the day.

All of this gives an overall viewpoint and helps ensure that a correct remedy is chosen for the particular individual's needs at the time. The more accurate the prescription, the more efficient the remedy. An approximate, close-fitting remedy may give a degree of symptom relief but is unlikely to affect a cure. Some relief often occurs but often the results are disappointing to both patients and prescriber — in many cases blaming the method rather than inaccurate prescribing. In general — approximately is not good enough for homoeopathy and a lasting cure. So make sure of this overall way of looking and thinking, then you can be sure of far better results on each occasion. Try to make this overall-looking, thinking and approach to homoeopathic prescribing a discipline so that you can gradually learn with experience more and more of the response to the remedies, their characteristics and build on this experience. Especially gain skill by practise, using the twenty basic remedies initially so that your results and ability-to-prescribe is assured with increasing certainty and confidence.

When learning to prescribe and to familiarise yourself with the common remedies always be aware of laterality — or the side of the body affected. Whether a tonsillar infection is predominantly left or right-sided, or a lumbago, painful knee, or gouty condition is important and note too if the condition commenced on one side and then moved over to later involve the other side of the body. The laterality of the major remedies must be known and those remedies which are primarily right-sided as those where the action is on the left part of the body.

Right-sided remedies include *Lycopodium, Bryonia, Belladonna, Nux. Vom.*

Left-sided remedies include *Lachesis, Kali Carb, Graphites, Sepia, Sulphur.*

The key psycholigical aspects of each basic remedy must be clearly known as it is indispensable to good and accurate prescribing. These are the 'mentals' and they include —

The irritability of *Nux Vom*
The fear of *Aconitum*

The indifference of *Sepia*
The pride of *Platina*
The jealousy of *Lachesis*
The resentment of *Staphisagria*
The passivity and tearfulness of *Pulsatilla*

Try also to get quite clear the distinguishing mobility factors of each major remedy you are using and working on, such as

The restless and agitation of *Rhus tox, Arsenicum, Zincum Met.*

The immobility of *Bryonia.*

The other factors to be quite clear about and which often 'make' or clinch the diagnosis are

Thirst — absent in *Pulsatilla, Apis*

Thirst — frequent in *Calcarea* and *Phosphorus* (for ice-cold drinks).

Whether the patient is sweating or not and if the perspiration is offensive.

Absence of sweating- *Lycopodium.*

Profuse sweating — *Calcarea, Thuja, Mercurius, Ipecacuanha, Silicea.*

The general metabolism and heat output of both patient and remedy should be familiar in order to make an accurate choice of prescription.

For example *Belladonna, Sulphur* — both burning hot.

Arsenicum, Silicea and *Calcarea* always very cold and chilly, craving heat.

But *Pulsatilla* is also always chilly and cold but aggravated by the least heat.

CHAPTER THIRTEEN

Homoeopathy and the home

Homoeopathy has never been a second-class citizen in the treatment stakes and many families have used homoeopathy effectively for varied conditions over several generations. It is a well-tried first-line treatment approach. Many use homoeopathy however when conventional treatments fail or are still unsatisfactory after frequent trials. In many ways this is a wrong use of homoeopathy because such methods have all too often depleted and jaded the patient beyond all limits, quite separately from any diminishing effects of their illness. Under such conditions, homoeopathy is slower to act because of a depleted or sluggish vitality from drug side-effects, which may take several weeks to recover from and to remove from the system.

Because of its effectiveness, in the majority of cases, there is no reason why homoeopathy should not be used as the front-line approach to illness. The method can be curative at all ages naturally depending upon the type of constitution and condition treated, its severity and duration. In the child, the remedies can be used preventatively for all the common childhood conditions where there is a special risk as with some outbreaks of measles, whooping-cough, chicken pox and mumps — using the nosode or homoeopathic vaccine-equivalent without the increasingly recognized risks of conventional vaccination. It is helpful in young babies for the common teething problems or where there is wind or digestive discomfort. In the nursing mother many of the common feeding problems which arise — as soreness of a breast or nipple can be quickly dealt with and eased. Such childhood complaints as eczema, asthma, — the common infective illnesses of the child, sore throat, hay-fever, allergic rhinitis with a continual blocked nose or ear problems, not responding to ever-changing antibiotic after antibiotic give way to homoeopathy.

Chronic conditions also of both child and adolescent like acne, rheumatoid arthritis, tonsillitis, are within the curative range of the well-chosen remedy. The common adult problems of peptic ulcer, hiatus hernia, blood-pressure or angina of effort usually respond remarkably well and long periods of pain and discomfort relieved. Menstrual problems with hot flushes, drenching sweats, period pains and pre-menstrual tension are daily treated by homoeopathy with good results.

The elderly have their own areas of particular problems which respond given good-will and patience. The commonest difficulties are the arthritic ones, seen at all ages and in all degrees. Prostatic problems, or those of bladder weakness and prolapse are also common. All the above areas of problem can show a positive and noticeable response to homoeopathic treatment and quite frequently improvement occurs without a long pause or delay.

When there is an overwhelming problem of meningitis, pneumonia, influenza-of-the-elderly, appendicitis, collapse, stroke, any form of severe haemorrhage or severe infection where antibiotics are valuable and well and truly indicated, then homoeopathy should be used to support the patient until the doctor comes or until the patient is moved to hospital. Both *Arnica* and the Bach rescue remedy drops are invaluable. Such methods effectively help to relieve any shock and moreover act as a valuable and often essential back-up supportive therapy to conventional treatments and surgery when it is required.

Stress illness of the adult or child in any form usually responds well and quickly to the potencies when carefully chosen and treated early. Homoeopathy can give a rapid resolution to many acute problems and a rapid return to a more relaxed and balanced self. If the problem is an overwhelming one or due to very severe shock, then more time for healing must obviously be expected and allowed for in every case.

I have already mentioned the nosodes in the prevention of childhood illness but they also have a role where an adult is especially vulnerable or at risk. I am thinking particularly of such exposures as an adult male in contact to a child with mumps where the adult has no natural immunity from a previous childhood infection so that mumps orchitis and possible sterility is a real risk and the specific nosode gives welcome protection. Similarly the early pregnant mother must be protected from all contacts and risks of infection with rubella or german measles — indeed with any viral epidemic illness during the key early weeks of pregnancy. The rubella nosode is useful prophylactically where a suspected contact may have unwittingly occurred or only discovered in retrospect. In an elderly person too who is convalescent and therefore especially vulnerable and where influenza is a possibility, or where there is a history of earlier chronic bronchitis or emphysema, then the influenza nosode may be given to both protect and lessen the impact of any infection that does occur. In this way the risks of complications occuring in an already vulnerable and weakened constitution are markedly reduced.

Chronic problems especially the psychological ones respond well to homoeopathy but it is also of value in certain more physical and mechanical conditions if surgery is either undesirable or impossible or where it may have failed for a variety of reasons. In such cases — for example of hiatus hernia, prolapse, rupture (hernia), these may respond well in terms of symptom-relief even where the external mechanical problem is not markedly changed. I have however had good results with prolapse of the elderly in many cases where over a period of months the uterine prolapse has no longer 'come down' so severely as before the homoeopathic treatment had been prescribed.

In all cases, should a prolapse or hernia either become twisted upon itself or strangulated and irreducible, so that the blood supply is cut-off causing a risk of gangrene occuring, then surgery is immediately indicated whatever the state of general health.

Any hernia that is no longer reversible or reducible, having previously been easily pushed back with ease, should be the subject of an immediate medical consultation without delay because of the risks and possibility of strangulation occuring. Homoeopathy should never be used as an alternative to surgery in such cases as appendicitis or where it is suspected and a surgical opinion must be always sought at any age. In general the best treatment of all disease and illness is prevention and early diagnosis. Especially where there is a problem of severe organic disease or cancer, the most modern proved techniques must be combined with traditional homoeopathic treatments — often as a secondary back-up treatment unless conventional treatment has failed or is no longer indicated, when homeopathy can be used as the total approach and used in a variety of potencies as best fits the symptoms as they occur and the patterns of organic dysfunction caused by the disease.

Never be tempted to regard homoeopathy however as a panacea and a cure-all. As with any form of treatment, however advantageous, it has both its indications and its limitations. There are periods when homoeopathy must be used in the background. However enthusiastic you may be, don't go 'overboard' over homoeopathy — for a problem that requires either surgery or a traditional approach. When in doubt ask your doctor, get a consultation and a proper professional opinion.

Homoeopathy implies a totality of overall approach and viewpoint which should not be dogmatic or a rigid one. Your flexibility of mind is most important. There is no need to try and create magic with homoeopathy — the method just does not need it and this is not how it is meant to be used. There are specific indications for homoeopathy and when these are not present then another method should be used or considered. In the final diagnosis it is always the patient who matters most of all and not the principles or method of cure however much you are in favour of them. A particular approach — even a homoeopathic one must be right for the patient if not it will fail and it is not wholistic.

CHAPTER FOURTEEN

First Aid

Cuts and wounds

Clean the area very carefully with *Calendula* lotion, removing any foreign material of any kind which is present. All bleeding must be stopped by local pressure in the area using clean gauze or cotton wool. If a tourniquet is used, it must be released frequently. When in any way severe give *arnica 6* for shock hourly or the Bach rescue remedy, 5 drops to be repeated hourly until shock is no longer present. Keep the patient warm and covered whenever the patient is in shock and give warm drinks usually. *Calendula* should be applied both locally to the wound area and given internally in the 6th potency hourly for the first few hours and then three times daily. Honey is often a useful dressing to apply as an alternative to calendular and the dressing need not be removed for several days before being replaced by a similar one. *Hypericum* is indicated in the 6th potency whenever there is damage to nerve tissue with bruising or shooting nerve pains going up the limbs from the hand or foot. When the wound involves tendons, *Ruta* or *Bellis Perennis* should be used as soon as the initial shock period has passed. If the area involved is muscle, give *Rhus tox 6* and when the main area affected is bone, or periosteum — the fine tissue sheath covering the bone, give *Symphytum* 6 three times daily.

Foreign bodies
Essentially these are irritants to local tissue and must always be removed to avoid a severe infective reaction. They may occur in any of the orifices of the body including the eyes and must be removed gently and with care to avoid damage to the delicate tissues in the area. A protective inflammatory reaction usually occurs almost immediately. Having removed the object from the nostril, ear, eye, or on occasions genital area, apply *Calendula* locally if there are any signs of an inflammatory-reaction, and give either *Calendula* 6 internally three times daily for three days or use *Arnica* if there is evidence of any marked swelling or bruising in the area.

Black Eye
Due to a blow or injury. Initial treatment should be *Arnica 30* for shock repeated hourly until there is an improvement. When there has been an acute or severe fear reaction give *Aconitum* 6 three times daily for three days. *Ledum* (Marsh tea) is an excellent remedy when the areas are red rather than black, the patient chilly and cold, often in a cold sweat. They are improved by a local cold compress to the area affected. *Hamamelis* 6 is of value when the haemorrhagic area is much darker and blacker than with the *Ledum* type of eye. Use *Ruta* (rue) in the 6th potency when there is much pain in the areas of bruising of bone causing pain or discomfort. If the eyeball itself is affected and painful use *Symphytum* 6 three times daily and if it persists a specialist unit should be consulted to exclude any damage to the eye which may require

surgical or other specialised treatment.

Falls and sprains

The major immediate remedy should be *Arnica 6* for the swelling and bruising to tissues in the area. *Hypericum* is useful for pain of bruised and stretched delicate nervous tissue which is so often associated, or when there are shooting pains. In general a firm supportive bandage is recommended, often a cold application to the part to reduce swelling. *Ruta* is indicated for tendon and particularly bone pain or tenderness. Use *Rhus tox* when there is muscular stiffness afterwards, better for heat. When there is severe pain in the area, worse for the least movement use *Bryonia* instead of *Rhus tox. Belladonna* is only indicated when the area is extremely reddened and sensitive to the very least movement or jarring sensation. *Bellis perennis* is a fine remedy where there is swelling and pain from strain, usually worsened and aggravated by damp and cold and with marked weakness and exhaustion and a need to lie down. Recurrent sprains, especially of the ankles might indicate *Calcarea* if there is a chilly disposition and weakness with obesity. For a tendency to accident-proneness generally, with sprains part of an overall pattern consider *Kali Carb* as a useful remedy.

Puncture wounds from bites and stings

As is always the case in homoeopathy the remedy depends upon the symptom-picture. When there has been a simple puncture-wound which is clean and uncomplicated as from a cat-bite or other small animal, then the best remedy is *Ledum 6* three times daily. When there is pain and swelling use *Calendula* locally and *Hypericum* when the pain is severe and shooting-in character. For a bee sting use *Apis 6* and for a painful wasp sting — either

Arnica or *Rhus tox* — the latter when there is considerable redness and irritation. If the area affected is very swollen and irritating with blister formation after a bite — as occurs with an allergic reaction to a sting, use *Urtica 6* hourly if severe, or three times daily if less so. Should the reaction to a bite or sting be more severe with redness, inflammation spreading up the arm or leg use *Belladonna 6* as for *Urtica*. If the condition is dark red, swollen and painful almost with a blue tinge, an intolerance of any pressure or covering to the area, give *Lachesis 6* hourly until there is relief. After a snake bite, try to remove the venom by sucking the area and spitting out afterwards. The patient should be removed to hospital at the earliest opportunity. Use *Arnica* for shock. When the patient is ill, cold and collapsing give *Carbo Veg.* instead of *Arnica* to revive.

Nose Bleeding (epistaxis)
These are common in some children and may occur quite spontaneously or associated with agitation and restlessness. In the adult it may be a sign of raised blood-pressure when recurrent and it is generally a signal to have a complete physical check-up. Use simple local pressure or packing of the nostril to control the bleeding. *Hamamelis* (witch hazel) is the most useful remedy for recurrent conditions in the child. When the cause is from a fall or tumble use *Arnica 6* hourly until there is relief. When the cause is much more emotional then give *Ignatia* if associated with tears or loss in any form. Use *Natrum Mur.* if the emotion is more general. When associated with fainting and heat give *Pulsatilla 6*.

Bruises
Usually the result of a simple traumatic happening with

blueness and swelling. In general *Arnica* covers the majority of cases and there is rapid relief. If not, consider *Bellis Perennis* (the common daisy) for cases associated with pain, swelling and a feeling of exhaustion. In some instances the bruising is quite spontaneous and independent of any injury. In such cases consider *Phosphorus* and if recurrent a check-up and blood profile is recommended to clarify the causes of any small, recurrent bleeding-tendency into the skin or nearby tissues.

Hiccough

The common condition of recurrent brief spasmodic contractions of the diaphragm, usually digestive in origin. Most cases respond well and quickly to *Nux Vom* 6 given every ten minutes until there is relief. When associated with an emotional upset *Natrum Mur.* is preferable in the 30th potency and repeated after half an hour if there is no relief. *Arsenicum* can be used when associated with a sudden chill and shivering. Use *Pulsatilla* when the condition is linked with a child or adult getting over-heated and exhausted, often after tears.

Fainting

This is another common 'household emergency', and it can be often quite worrying to onlookers when the faint is severe. The commonest cause is from a hot and airless situation when *Pulsatilla* usually gives a quick response. The best general remedy to use is the Bach rescue drops as an immediate emergency measure, 5 drops on the tongue. When due to weakness and exhaustion use *China* 6. If due to emotion at the sight of blood give *Nux. Vomica*. Where the patient is cold, marble-white, chilly and covered with sweat give *Carbo Veg* or *Veratrum Alb*. Fainting from fear needs *Aconitum* to correct it. When associated with prolonged standing and immobility give *Alumina 30*.

Diarrhoea

This is a common problem for both adult and child. It is most dangerous to the young baby because of the risks of dehydration and in this age group treatment is best given by a physician. There are many possible remedies available for this type of problem and they need to be carefully differentiated by the overall condition as well as the type of stool. A watery unformed stool may require *Sulphur*, *Podophyllum*, *Nux vom* or *Mercurious*. Where the stool is more varied, *Pulsatilla* may be indicated. If blood is present *Phosphorus* or *Hamamelis* may be required and a green stool is often an indication for *Chamomilla*. A pale watery stool suggests *Calcarea* and a more yellow stool *Chelidonium*. In all the diarrhoeal problems the general state often gives the clue to the appropriate remedy when prescribing. Any suggestion of dehydration or shock or collapse may require immediate hospitalisation.

Vomiting

One of the most common household emergencies. Try and ascertain the cause whatever the age of the person and be especially careful in an adult or where the problem is repetitive or relatively 'out of keeping' with the person. For the vomiting of pregnancy consider *Kreosotum*, *Tabacum* or *Nux vom*. Important general remedies for vomiting include *Aconitum*, *Lobelia*, *Nux vom*, *Arsenicum*, *Antimonium Tart*. Try and get a clear picture of the pattern of vomiting, any aggravating factors and its overall taste, colour and frequency. Note also any key times and relate these to the remedy. For example early morning suggests *Hepar sulph*; mid-morning sickness — *Psor-*

inum; Noon vomiting — *Mag. Carb.;* afternoon problems – *Sulphur;* evening sickness – *Carbo Veg.* Later night-time vomiting includes such remedies as *Calcarea* or *Ferrum Met.*

Toothache
The most valuable general remedies are *Coffea, Chamomilla, Staphisagria, China, Belladonna, Hepar sulph.* All of these should be known and be differentiated. It is not the purpose of this present volume to differentiate the remedies in detail but each one has its appropriate site of pain type and time of aggravation which is important for accurate prescribing.

Indigestion and flatulence
The major general remedies include *Argentum Nit, Lycopodium, Nux vom,* and these should be familiar to the prescriber. Indigestion on waking may indicate *Sulphur* or *Lachesis.* Morning problems often respond well to *Baptisia* whilst afternoon dyspepsia with flatulence, about 4.00pm. responds best to *Lycopodium.* The late evening indigestions often indicate *Pulsatilla* where the general features fit the remedy. When symptoms occur in the early hours, about 3 or 5.00am. then the remedy is more likely to be *Kali Carb.* For general flatulence and discomfort, *Cargo Veg.* is often highly dependable. In all cases, a careful overall look at the person must be made, especially for 'first time' indigestion or change of eating-patterns in the adult. Also any loss of appetite or weight-loss, inexplicable general malaise — like any odd and bizarre symptoms is an indication for a proper professional check-up. When symptoms persist, or fail to respond, or get worse with homoeopathy, this is also an indication for a full physical examination, especially when a seemingly

well-prescribed and a well-indicated remedy has been given. If the response to prescribing is at all poor or disappointing, there may be an underlying organic lesion, which makes a homoeopathic response impossible or short-lasting. All of these features indicate a professional check-up. An alternative to the professional examination is a check at one of the diagnostic centres which several of the private insurance companies have made generally available for a nominal fee and the results sent to the general practitioner. In this way a stress problem or one of simple dysfunction and a temporary matter can be differentiated from any more serious underlying organic disease which may require a different or additional treatment to the homoeopathic one.

Temperature
In all cases where there is a raised temperature above the normal of 98·4 F or 37 C, the cause should be ascertained. Usually the reason is an infection somewhere or other — perhaps of the ear, throat, teeth or due to a common cold. But there are exceptions and a stress illness can also equally produce a temperature. Remedies include *Hepar Sulph, Belladonna, Pyrogen, Mercurius, Aconitum, Phytolacca*. The site of infection, side of a throat infected or which ear is relevant to the remedy eventually chosen as also the degree of sweating, restlessness, pain and psychological attitudes. All are important in chosing the right remedy and when well-chosen, the results are often dramatic. But in all cases, the patient is best kept in bed and given fluids only until the temperature subsides. When a raised temperature heralds one of the more general childhood infective illnesses, then the specific nosode of that disease may be required as well as one of the above.

Hang-over

Strictly speaking a 'hair of the dog' is homoeopathic and perhaps the reason for its popularity with many alcoholics on waking and before they can begin their day. In general however it is not recommended because it simply reinforces the habit and a remedy that provokes similar, but not exactly identical symptoms is preferable. *Avena Sat.* (oats) is often highly recommended by many, but I prefer either *Nux Vom* or *Sulphur* for such symptoms combined with a naturally high vitamin dietary regime and vitamin B in potency, which if given additionally, tends to improve results.

Headache

Where the pain is over the forehead, of a dull heavy nature, then *Bryonia* or *Belladonna* is useful. Pain at the back of the head in the occipital region responds to *Nux Vom* or *Carbo veg* and especially *Silicea* where it has moved backwards from the forehead region and settled in the occiput.

Pain in the temples is often helped by *Natrum Mur.* If the headache increases in severity or the back of the neck is stiff and there is high fever, the diagnosis of meningitis must be excluded by a doctor as soon as possible and hospitalisation arranged if the diagnosis is at all likely. A small haemorrhage or leakage from a cerebral aneurysm can also cause similar symptoms with irritability particularly in young adults. Where symptoms fail to respond, and are getting worse, then get a medical opinion as soon as possible. In this latter case a lumbar puncture may be essential to reduce intracranial pressure and to relieve headache. Most cases however are of the simple migrainous kind and there is a good response to the homoeopathic prescription giving a calming of agitation and relief of pain. Only when there is no response should a family be on their guard and think of alternative types of problem where the correct treatment is not homoeopathy but hospitalisation with conventional treatments and techniques.

Colic
The type of pain, site, time of day or night and area affected are all relevant to the best remedy. For colicy pain which bends the patient double, consider *Mag. Phos, Colocynth, Belladonna, Pulsatilla, Graphites,* or *Chamomilla.* All of these have their distinct diagnostic features, laterality and distinguishing hallmarks which help to decide the best remedy. Where colic is associated with flatulence then consider either *Nux vom* especially where irritability is marked or *Carbo veg.*

Sea-sickness
The best remedies are often *Tabacum, Cocculus, Kali Carb,* or *Petroleum.* Each must be differentiated according to the particular symptoms, the degress of problem and the amount of sweating, collapse, mucous production and vertigo present.

Acute throat conditions
One of the most common household first-aid emergencies, especially of the young school-child when every few weeks a vulnerable child can miss school because of recurrent illness with high temperature and sore throat. Often the lymph nodes of the area are tender and swollen and there is loss of appetite and energy. Repeated antibiotics, course after course, seem to be of no real assistance and usually tend to undermine the child's natural immune resistance further. Many parents turn in despera-

tion to homoeopathy after yet another antibiotic has done nothing for the child. The response is very often encouraging with homoeopathy and the major remedies include *Belladonna, Phytolacca, Causticum, Sulphur, Hepar Sulph, Nitric acid* and *Mercurius.* Where the problem is definitely worse on one side, consider *Lachesis* for left-sided tonsillar infections when raw and tender and *Lycopodium* for a similar right-sided problem. For suppuration or definite pus formation give either *Silicea* or *Mercurius* — especially for abscess formation (or quinsy) in the tonsillar area. If the condition worsens at all, and there is the least indication of difficult or obstructed breathing, call an ambulance and get the child to hospital immediately without delay.

Acute ear problems
Belladonna is often the best remedy, or *Pulsatilla* for less severe and less 'hot' type of problem which has more variable and changeable symptoms. *Chamomilla* is indicated for very severe pain and both *Phosphorus* and *Hepar sulph* are also useful. Make sure that there is not a foreign body in the ear causing blockage and infection. If in doubt and it cannot be easily removed get expert professional help. In general right-sided acute ear problems respond well to *Belladonna* or *Fluoric Acid* and left-sided infections more to *Aconitum, Graphites* or *Dulcamara.*

Sleeplessness
When there is inability to get off to sleep from an over-active mind then *Lycopodium* is helpful. But where the insomnia occurs in the early morning hours, waking about 5.00am with restless, vague anxiety, then *Kali carb.*

is more indicated. Sudden waking with fear and agitation at about midnight or just after, especially with a feeling of chill indicates *Arsenicum*. Where wakefulness occurs a little later, about 2–3.00 a.m., this time with a sense of heat, the need to pass water, throw off the covers, push the feet out of the bed-covers, but no sooner out then freezing cold, a need for a cool drink or biscuit, then the remedy is *Pulsatilla*. Another useful general remedy, where there is tension and agitation and restlessness is *Coffea*. More general wakefulness from anxiety and vague apprehension may need *Natrum Mur* and if the underlying problem is one of fear and grave insecurity then consider *Aconitum* as the remedy of choice. *Ignatia* is indicated for insomnia of the recently widowed and where grief and mourning is the major factor.

Lumbago
Remedies include *Rhus Tox, Bryonia, Rhododendron, Nux Vom, Dulcamara*. Each has its specific and distincitve type of symptomatology which should be known. The cause is also important — whether from strain *(Rhus tox)*; exposure to damp *(Pulsatilla)*; due to a change of weather *(Dulcamara)*; exposure to a cold dry wind *(Bryonia)*; associated more with a uterine problem and pains referred into the back region *(Sepia)*. Some forms of lumbago are markedly relieved by heat and rubbing *(Rhus tox)* yet others are not helped at all or even worsened *(Bryonia)*. Other types of discomfort need firm local support and pressure to obtain relief from pain and here *Natrum Mur.* should be thought about.

The Common Cold
The best remedy at an early stage is often *Aconitum*, if the condition can be caught within the first 48 hours. Follow-

ing this I usually like to use either *Nux Vomica, Arsenicum* or *Gelsemium,* depending upon the symptom pattern of the individual, the degree of chillyness or weakness. When there is a 'flu' epidemic in the area, give the specific nosode *Influenzinum.* For severe nasal congestion consider *Kali Bic* or *Kali Carb.* and where the discharge is green, yellow or variable, give *Pulsatilla.* A continuous watery, drip-discharge may need *Allium cepa* for relief. If the temperature is raised consider *Hepar Sulph.* and in general keep the patient on fluids only until the fever subsides.

Boils
The common localised infection of the skin with pus formation, redness and usually severe lancing pain. *Belladonna* is best for the acute stage and it may be followed by *Sulphur* if the condition persists. Where there is an associated toxic condition or a raised temperature, think of *Mercurius* or possibly *Hepar sulph.* Should the condition worsen, enlarge and discharge frank pus or form a deep crater becoming a carbuncle, then *Anthracinum* is more the remedy of choice, followed by *Silicea* or *Arsenicum.*

Breathlessness
This is an important condition and it is important to get the diagnosis right. If in any doubt do not hesitate to get medical advice. Where recurrent asthma is the reason, major remedies include *Medorrhinum, Phosphorus, Natrum Mur, Arsenicum* or *Ipecacuanha.* Chronic bronchitis may require *Sulphur* or *Kali Carb.* The time of onset of the attack is important. For morning breathlessness — *Sulphur* or *Sepia;* for onset in the early afternoon — *China.;* evening breathing difficulties — consider *Pulsatil-*

la or *Lycopodium*. After midnight *Arsenicum* may be required. In the early morning hours consider *Ammonium Mur* or *Kali Carb*. Where due to anger remember *Nux vom;* damp — *Dulcamara;* from an emotional outburst — *Natrum Mur;* exposure to chill — *Apis;* from a heat reaction — *Pulsatilla*.

CHAPTER FIFTEEN

The twenty basic remedies and their usage

The recommended basic remedies for the family homoeopathic chest are — *Aconitum, Arnica, Arsenicum Alb., Belladonna, Bryonia, Carbo Veg, Chamomilla, Gelsemium, Hepar Sulph, Hypericum, Kali Bic, Ledum, Lycopodium, Mag. Phos., Natrum Mur, Nux Vom, Sepia, Sulphur, Thuja.*

Aconitum
The most acute of all remedies and most efficient when given within the first 48 hours of the onset of symptoms. There is a mixture of fear, anxiety, uncertainty and agitation, with often pain, diarrhoea or headache. The commonest causative factors of the typical painful and often inflammatory condition is chill from cold or damp air. Often a seemingly strong and healthy-looking person, well-built and active is struck-down by acute bronchitis, or an alimentary infection. They are convinced that death is imminent and all symptoms are aggravated by heat, the bed coverings and at midnight. Where an illness is clearly the result of fear give *Aconitum* in the 30th potency even if many years have elapsed since the original fright.

Arnica

The greatest of all the remedies and the most easy to use so that it is ideally suited for the beginner to homoeopathy. Pain and swelling with bruising is the key to arnica and shock of either an emotional or traumatic cause with damage to tissues. It is indicated both pre- and post-operatively during the convalescent period. Also for dental interventions and after loss of blood with shock and weakness. The *Arnica* personality is typically sensitive but also physically so that they are intolerant of any discomfort and complain that 'the bed is too hard' — however soft it may in fact be.

Arsenicum Alb.

After *Aconitum*, this is one of the most acute remedies in the repertory — meaning that it is indicated for sudden acute conditions of recent onset. The make-up tends to be that of the thin restless type, rather fussy and fastidious to detail. Major symptoms giving the clue to the remedy are overwhelming weakness, collapse and chill. They crave heat and warmth of any kind — either from a fire or hot drinks. In this the remedy resembles *Rhus tox* which also has much of the restlessness, but *Arsenicum* is also deeply restless and unsatisfied in mind and often depressed and anxious.

Heat comes into another area of the remedy in that burning pains are characteristic coupled with great chilly-ness to the extent of wearing several layers of vests or long-johns on the warmest summer day. The body heat is always at a low level, in keeping with such common problems as prostration and exhaustion. Diarrhoea with rigors and shivers is frequent.

Belladonna (Deadly nightshade)
Another invaluable remedy for acute conditions. The typical picture is one of redness, inflammation and local heat. The area affected may be the skin as in scarlet fever or an infection as erysipelas or when a hang-nail infection is spreading up the arm in bright-red inflammatory streaks, pain and heat along the line of the infection. Sensitivity is another important feature with intolerance of the least noise or draught. Movement and jarring cause the most intense aggravation of pain. The sore throat is often worse for swallowing, ear-ache is aggravated by the least movement and the skin worse for pressure or touch. An examination may be resisted by floods of tears and also all symptoms are increased by lying down. An affected area is often immobilised by lying on it to control movement and pain. Typically the pupils are dilated when there is fever.

Carbo Veg (vegetable charcoal)
Of enormous value in general sluggish conditions of the body. There is a lack of vital protective energy reaction making the person slow and vulnerable to whatever infection is currently in the area — so that they are forever 'down' with a winter cold, 'flu, coughs or bronchitis. Typically they are tired and irritable with no energy. Their great problem is often burning indigestion pains with flatulence or a poor circulation, cold and chill and venous difficulties so that the ankles swell easily or varicose veins are marked. It is a most useful emergency remedy however for weakness, collapse and faintness — especially for the convalescent patient or when there is fatigue after a long period of strain like nursing a sick friend or relative for weeks or months without a break.

Chamomilla

An invaluable remedy for the oversensitive — both physically and mentally. There is a combination of low-pain threshold, irritability, and generally a grumbling, complaining attitude is present from the young child with teething problems to the adult with unbearable back or menopausal pain. In most cases pain is worse from any form of heat and a cool local compress brings relief. It is a classic treatment for teething or dental discomfort and typically a child cries as soon as put down and will only sleep or rest when constantly carried. It is important to understand *Chamomilla* as an adult remedy as well as one for teething and it is valuable for a variety of conditions of adult discomfort, unbearable or poorly tolerated painful conditions in general.

Gelsemium (Yellow Jasmine)

One of the best remedies for 'flu conditions, particularly where there is weakness, sluggish exhaustion with trembling and shaking of limbs — often due to rigors as the temperature rises. Indicated also for the anxiety condition of an examination, stage-fright or public-speaking. Weakness of certain muscle-groups as writers-cramp is relieved and after illness and surgery it stimulates a rapid return to activity. Most symptoms are aggravated by heat in any form.

Hepar Sulph (Calcium Sulphide)

I recommend this remedy for many of the common infective conditions where there is extreme sensitivity to touch or pressure and when the general disposition is one of anger and irritability. It is useful in throat conditions with a splinter-like sensation at the back of the throat and where the least exposure to cold dry air aggravates.

Cough due to cold, or bronchitis showing this same picture of worsening from cold air and over-touchiness indicates the remedy. Many skin infective conditions are helped especially where there is itching, ulceration, or a cheesy-like discharge. Constipation is common and adds to the general picture of impatience, intolerance and irritabilty.

Hypericum (St. John's Wort)

One of the most important of all the first aid remedies. It is indicated especially in the treatment of all wounds — both externally as a tincture or cream and internally in the 6th potency. The characteristic picture for prescribing is extreme tenderness and soreness with pain where bleeding has occurred or in puncture or more open wounds, especially those involving peripheral nerve damage or crushing, leading to shooting pains — radiating up the limbs. Such injuries may follow a crush wound to a finger tip or a blow to the shin where there is a minimum of protective covering. All symptoms are relieved by warmth and aggravated by cold which intensifies the pain, causing spasm and loss of function in the area. Pain is generally intensified by movement or examination of the part affected.

Kali Bic. (Potassium Bichromate)

This remedy has an important role to play in problems of congestion to mucous membrane anywhere in the body. It is particularly helpful in chronic or acute nasal and throat problems with blockage giving a stringy, mucous or jelly-like discharge. Troublesome problems of leucorrhoea (whites) are also relieved. Typically the discharges have a yellowish discolouration and the general condition is relieved by warmth and fresh air.

Ledum (Marsh tea)
I recommend this remedy for penetrating wounds and injuries where there is not much pain or sensitivity associated — otherwise *Hypericum* is more indicated. The wound is usually clean as from a bite or where a pin or nail has pierced the skin, the area freezing cold — like ice and with a characteristic purplish or bluish tinge to the surrounding skin. Paradoxically although the surrounding area is so cold, the patient is intolerant of any form of heat and craves a cool atmosphere for comfort. The results of old puncture-wounds, still causing discomfort and pain are often relieved by *Ledum,* many years after the original trauma.

Lycopodium (club moss)
Otherwise innert, until made up into its homoeopathic potency, *Lycopodium* is of greatest value in the intellectual type of make-up with little tendency to physical exercise or muscular development. The mind is strong and active, full of ideas and plans but the body is like an anchor and their weakest link to achievement. A remedy for all right-sided problems with typical early afternoon or evening aggravation of all symptoms. There are many chest, throat, kidney and digestive problems most of them beginning on the right side and only later causing trouble on the left. The skin is nearly always dry and sweating is rare. Nervousness and lack of confidence is common and it rivals *Gelsemium* for panic problems, especially where there is an audience or something new and unfamiliar on the horizon — although there are not usually any great problems on the day itself and they nearly always give a good account of themselves, because they are such achievers.

Mag. Phos. (Phosphate of magnesium)
Invaluable for all conditions where pain is associated with
spasm and colic. The underlying condition may be intestinal or gall-bladder colic which typically doubles-up the
patient, is improved by local heat but aggravated by cold
or draughts. Firm pressure also gives relief and this
combined with a hot water bottle may be the only way to
obtain relief until *Mag. phos.* is given.

Natrum Mur. (sodium chloride)
One of the deepest acting of all homoeopathic remedies,
especially in the mental sphere where for many conditions
it is unrivalled. It is a remedy for the isolated and solitary,
always worse for company where contact with others
causes an aggravation of any problem — whether the
watery diarrhoea, migraine headaches, or their depression. Easily tearful, walking in a wind, coughing or laugh-
ter nearly always brings a flow of tears. Excessive salt is
responsible for the common problem of water-retention,
clearly seen in the bloated face, fluid under the eyes and
often swelling of the ankles due to circulatory weakness.
Many of the painful complaints are the direct result of this
tendency to retain and a disturbed internal salt balance.
Most conditions are better for firm local pressure — as the
low back pain or ache. In general the sea has either a tonic
effect and brings an improvement or alternatively leads to
further aggravation.

Nux Vom. (poison nut)
Another of the greatest remedies in the homoeopathic
repertory. It is indicated for the over-worked and over-
fed executive, worn-out by work and the pressures of
travel, worries and generally 'burning the candle' at both
ends. Because of the typical *Nux* temperament, they can

do nothing in reasonable moderation, acting impatiently and zealously — too involved emotionally to reach reasonable and rational conclusions and never able to see when they are over-tired. Because of their temperament, they are unable to delegate responsibilities being typically perfectionistic and demanding of themselves as well as all others around them. They make difficult, 'impossible', unpopular bosses because they can give nobody any initiative without constantly checking and interfering. Their problems are nearly always the result of underlying tension and spasm, so that often they have problems of chronic back pain, indigestion or constipation with spasm, worse for noise, pressure and any demand. They are their own worst enemy in all areas.

Phosphorus
The range of action of this remedy is extraordinary. It is especially useful for intermittent complaints where there are brief flashes of pain, cough or discomfort. There is nearly always great restlessness and nervousness, the person typically pale, thin, sensitive, nervous and fearful needing constant reassurance. The remedy acts on all bright red haemorrhagic conditions of any type from piles to a sudden nose-bleed or for deeper disturbances like ulcerative colitis when the overall picture and temperament fits. Usually there is a craving for ice-cold drinks and thirst is intense. *Phosphorus* acts deeply on nearly all the tissues but is pre-eminent in chest problems from asthma to whooping cough and bronchitis. Whenever there are severe problems with the breakdown of tissue or even bone — as with a degenerative condition of a bed-ridden elderly person, *Phosphorus* is often the answer. It acts vigorously on the liver and is a remedy to learn and to be familiar with in all its depths. The results are often

outstanding in conditions that will respond to no other treatment.

Sepia (Ink of the cuttle fish)
A remedy for fatigue and depression especially where there is irritation and the need to be away from others — however close. The patient is typically angry, aggressive, worn-out and dragged-down by chronic pains and sufferings — as the aching low-back, constipation or period problems with flooding and exhausting low dragging pelvic pain. All symptoms are better for rest, warmth and frequently for dancing. There is nothing they enjoy more than a brisk walk or exercise — once they can be persuaded to participate, although without *Sepia*, such improvement is inevitably short-lasting and leads eventually to yet further tiredness and irritability.

Sulphur
One of the best remedies for chronic problems which have resisted all other treatment — even homoeopathic ones. Chronic infection is common, especially of the skin with eruptions and discharges, often of pus and invariably offensive and offensive-looking. The patient is exhausted, untidy, intolerant of both heat or cold and made worse by bathing and water. They are usually in a muddle, full of bright ideas which never materialise or are just unrealistic. Heat is a major problem and the patient nearly always feels too hot and sweats profusely. Indigestion is also common, usually with burning-type pains. Many chronic infections are helped by *Sulphur* especially if the skin is also involved. Quickly exhausted, they are nevertheless constantly hungry and warm food is often the only thing that gives comfort and relief — particularly fatty food, in spite of the offensive indigestion and diarrhoea that

inevitably follows.

Thuja (Tree of Life)

The remedy to use for the ill-effects of vaccination even if these occurred many years previously. It is also the recommended treatment for chronic warts of any part of the body — but especially of the anal or genital areas. The skin gives off a profuse, offensive sweat so that the feet tend to feel 'damp' inside both socks and shoes. Another problem area that *Thuja* helps is any chronic bladder problem — like cystitis, urethral discharges, irritation and frequency which recurs. The added presence of cauliflower-like chronic warts almost certainly confirms the prescription.

CHAPTER SIXTEEN

Some useful addresses and places of contact

Ainsworth's Homoeopathic Pharmacy,
38, New Cavendish Street, London W1M 7LH.
01 935 5330

The British Homoeopathic Association
27a, Devonshire Street, London W1N 6BY.
01 935 2163

Bristol Homoeopathic Hospital
Cotham, Bristol 6.
Bristol 312231

Freeman's Homoeopathic Pharmacy
7, Eaglesham Road, Clarkston, Glasgow.
041 644 1165.

Galen's Homoeopathic Pharmacy
1, South Terrrace, South Street, Dorchester, Dorset.
Dorchester 63996.

Gould's Homoeopathic Pharmacy
14, Crowndale Road, London NW1 1TT.
01 388 4752.

Hahnemann Society
217, Coldharbour Lane, London SW9 BRU.
01 737 3979.

The Homoeopathic Development Foundation
19A, Cavendish Square, London W1M 9AD
01 629 3204

Liverpool Homoeopathic Clinic
Mossley Hill Hospital.
051 724 2335.

Manchester Homoeopathic Clinic
Brunnswick Street, Ardwick, Manchester.
061 273 2446.

Nelson's Homoeopathic Pharmacy
73, Duke Street, Grosvenor Square, London W1M 6BY.

Tunbridge Wells Homoeopathic Hospital
Church Road, Tunbridge Wells.
0982 42977.

Weleda (U.K.) Ltd.
Heanor Road, Ilkeston, Derbyshire DE7 8DR.
0602 303151.

IMPORTANT

HERE IS YOUR REGISTRATION CODE TO ACCESS MCGRAW-HILL PREMIUM CONTENT AND MCGRAW-HILL ONLINE RESOURCES

For key premium online resources you need THIS CODE to gain access. Once the code is entered, you will be able to use the web resources for the length of your course.

Access is provided only if you have purchased a new book.

If the registration code is missing from this book, the registration screen on our website, and within your WebCT or Blackboard course will tell you how to obtain your new code. Your registration code can be used only once to establish access. It is not transferable.

To gain access to these online resources

1. **USE** your web browser to go to: **www.mhhe.com/faheybrief6e**

2. **CLICK** on "First Time User"

3. **ENTER** the Registration Code printed on the tear-off bookmark on the right

4. After you have entered your registration code, click on "Register"

5. **FOLLOW** the instructions to setup your personal UserID and Password

6. **WRITE** your UserID and Password down for future reference. Keep it in a safe place.

If your course is using WebCT or Blackboard, you'll be able to use this code to access the McGraw-Hill content within your instructor's online course.

To gain access to the McGraw-Hill content in your instructor's WebCT or Blackboard course simply log into the course with the user ID and Password provided by your instructor. Enter the registration code exactly as it appears to the right when prompted by the system. You will only need to use this code the first time you click on McGraw-Hill content.

These instructions are specifically for student access. Instructors are not required to register via the above instructions.

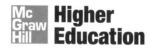

Thank you, and welcome to your McGraw-Hill Online Resources.

0-07-297381-1 t/a
Fahey
Fit & Well Brief, 6/E

WMXL-L3YU-UWD7-623G-X7ZY

REGISTRATION CODE
REGISTRATION CODE

The McGraw-Hill Companies

Mc Graw Hill Higher Education

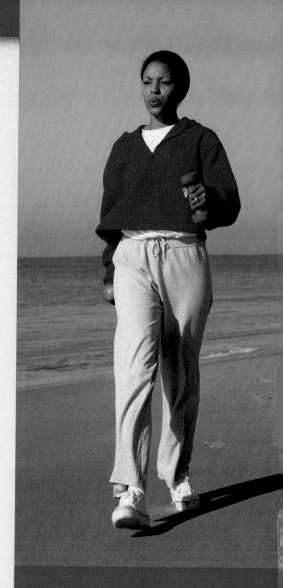

Fit & Well

SIXTH EDITION

Core Concepts and Labs in Physical Fitness and Wellness

Brief Edition

Thomas D. Fahey
California State University, Chico

Paul M. Insel
Stanford University

Walton T. Roth
Stanford University

McGraw Hill

Boston   Burr Ridge, IL   Dubuque, IA   Madison, WI   New York
San Francisco   St. Louis   Bangkok   Bogotá   Caracas   Kuala Lumpur
Lisbon   London   Madrid   Mexico City   Milan   Montreal   New Delhi
Santiago   Seoul   Singapore   Sydney   Taipei   Toronto

FIT & WELL: CORE CONCEPTS AND LABS IN PHYSICAL FITNESS AND WELLNESS, BRIEF EDITION
Published by McGraw-Hill, an imprint of The McGraw-Hill Companies, Inc., 1221 Avenue of the Americas, New York, NY 10020. Copyright 2005, 2003 by McGraw-Hill. Copyright 2001, 1999, 1997, and 1994 by Mayfield Publishing Company. All rights reserved. No part of this publication may be reproduced or distributed in any form or by any means, or stored in a database or retrieval system, without the prior written consent of The McGraw-Hill Companies, Inc., including, but not limited to, in any network or other electronic storage or transmission, or broadcast for distance learning.

Some ancillaries, including electronic and print components, may not be available to customers outside the United States.

This book is printed on acid-free paper.

4 5 6 7 8 9 0 QPD / QPD 0 9 8 7 6 5

ISBN 0-07-284434-5

Vice president and Editor-in-chief: *Emily Barrosse*
Publisher: *William R. Glass*
Sponsoring editor: *Nicholas R. Barrett*
Director of development: *Kathleen Engelberg*
Developmental editor: *Kirstan Price*
Developmental editor for technology: *Aric Bright*
Marketing manager: *Pamela Cooper*
Field publisher: *Jason Dewey*
Editorial assistant: *Julia Ersery*
Permissions coordinator: *Marty Granahan*
Media producer: *Lance Gerhart*
Media supplement producer: *Meghan Durko*
Production editor: *Brett Coker*
Production supervisor: *Randy Hurst*
Design manager: *Violeta Díaz*
Cover designer: *Yvo Riezivos*
Art manager: *Robin Mouat*
Illustration: *John and Judy Waller*
Manager, photo research: *Brian J. Pecko*
Print supplement producer: *Louis Swaim*
Compositor: *The GTS Companies*
Cover photo: © *Joel W. Rogers/Corbis*
Typeface: *10.5/12 Berkeley Book*
Paper: *45# Lighthouse Matte*
Printer and binder: *Quebecor-Dubuque*

Library of Congress Cataloging-in-Publication Data

Fahey, Thomas D. (Thomas Davin), 1947-
    Fit & well: core concepts and labs in physical fitness and wellness / Thomas D. Fahey,
    Paul M. Insel, Walton T. Roth.—6th ed., Brief.
        p. cm.
    Includes bibliographical references and index.
    ISBN 0-07-284434-5
        1. Physical fitness. 2. Health. I. Title: Fit and well. II. Insel, Paul M. III. Roth, Walton T. IV. Title.

GV481.F26 2004c
613.7'043—dc22

2004050475

The Internet addresses listed in the text were accurate at the time of publication. The inclusion of a Web site does not indicate an endorsement by the authors or McGraw-Hill Higher Education, and McGraw-Hill does not guarantee the accuracy of the information presented at these sites.

www.mhhe.com

Preface

For today's fitness-conscious student, *Fit and Well: Brief Edition* combines the best of two worlds. In the area of physical fitness, *Fit and Well* offers expert knowledge based on the latest findings in exercise physiology, sports medicine, and nutrition, along with tools for self-assessment and guidelines for becoming fit. This special Brief Edition contains the first 8 of the 15 chapters in the full version of *Fit and Well*. To create this book, we have drawn on our combined expertise and experience in exercise physiology, athletic training, personal health, scientific research, and teaching.

OUR AIMS

Our aims in writing this book can be stated simply:

- To show students that becoming fit and well greatly improves the quality of their lives
- To show students how they can become fit and well
- To motivate students to make healthy choices and to provide them with tools for change

The first of these aims means helping students see how their lives can be enhanced by a fit and well lifestyle. This book offers convincing evidence of a simple truth: To look and feel our best, to protect ourselves from degenerative diseases, and to enjoy the highest quality of life, we need to place fitness and wellness among our top priorities. *Fit and Well* makes clear both the imprudence of our modern, sedentary lifestyle and the benefits of a wellness lifestyle.

Our second aim is to give students the tools and information they need to become fit and well. This book provides students with everything they need to create their own personal fitness programs, including instructions for fitness tests, explanations of the components of fitness and guidelines for developing them, descriptions and illustrations of exercises, sample programs, and more. In addition, *Fit and Well* provides accurate, up-to-date, scientifically based information about key topics and issues in nutrition.

In providing this material, we have pooled our efforts. Thomas Fahey has contributed his knowledge as an exercise physiologist, teacher, and author of numerous exercise

science textbooks. Paul M. Insel and Walton T. Roth have contributed their knowledge of current topics in health as the authors of the leading personal health textbook, *Core Concepts in Health*.

Because we know this expert knowledge can be overwhelming, we have balanced the coverage of complex topics with student-friendly features designed to make the book accessible. Written in a straightforward, easy-to-read style and presented in a colorful, open format, *Fit and Well* invites the student to read, learn, and remember. Boxes, labs, tables, figures, artwork, photographs, and other features add interest to the text and highlight areas of special importance.

Our third aim is to involve students in taking responsibility for their health. *Fit and Well* makes use of interactive features to get students thinking about their own levels of physical fitness and wellness. We offer students assessment tools and laboratory activities to evaluate themselves in terms of each component of physical fitness and in the key area of nutrition.

We also show students how they can make difficult lifestyle changes by using the principles of behavior change. Chapter 1 contains a step-by-step description of this simple but powerful tool for change. The chapter not only explains the five-step process but also offers a wealth of tips for ensuring success. Behavior management aids, including personal contracts, behavior checklists, and self-tests, appear throughout the book. *Fit and Well*'s combined emphasis on self-assessment, self-development in each area of wellness, and behavior change ensures that students not only are inspired to become fit and well but also have the tools to do so.

CONTENT AND ORGANIZATION OF THE SIXTH EDITION

The basic content of *Fit and Well* remains unchanged in the sixth edition. Chapter 1 provides an introduction to fitness and wellness and explains the principles of behavior change. Chapters 2–7 focus on the various areas of fitness. Chapter 2 provides an overview, discussing the components of fitness, the principles of physical training, and the factors involved in designing a well-rounded, personalized exercise program. Chapter 3 provides basic information on how the cardiorespiratory system functions, how the body produces energy for exercise, and how individuals can create successful cardiorespiratory fitness programs. Chapters 4, 5, and 6 look at muscular strength and endurance, flexibility and low-back health, and body composition, respectively. Chapter 7 "puts it all together," describing the nature of a complete program that develops all the components of fitness. This chapter also includes complete sample exercise programs. Finally, Chapter 8 treats the key wellness area of nutrition.

For the sixth edition, each chapter was carefully reviewed, revised, and updated. The latest information from scientific and wellness-related research is incorporated in the text, and newly emerging topics are discussed. The following list gives a sample of some of the new and updated material included in the sixth edition of *Fit and Well:*

- New research on links between lifestyle and quality of life
- Physical activity recommendations from the Institute of Medicine, World Health Organization, and other organizations
- Dietary Reference Intakes for vitamins, minerals, energy macronutrients, water, and electrolytes
- New and alternative food pyramids and new food labeling requirements for trans fats
- Performance aids and dietary supplement safety and labeling issues
- Preventing and managing low-back pain
- Nutrition for athletes
- Diabetes and pre-diabetes
- Exercise in hot and cold weather

Research in the areas of health and wellness is ongoing, with new discoveries, advances, trends, and theories reported nearly every week. For this reason, no wellness book can claim to have the final word on every topic. Yet, within these limits, *Fit and Well* does present the latest available information and scientific thinking on important wellness topics. Taken together, the chapters of the book provide students with a complete, up-to-date guide to maximizing their well-being, now and through their entire lives.

WW To help students obtain the most current wellness information, each chapter in the sixth edition is also closely tied to the Web site developed as a companion to the text. Boxes, illustrations, tables, labs, terms, and sections of text marked with the special World Wide Web icon have corresponding links and activities on the *Fit and Well* Online Learning Center (www.mhhe.com/fahey).

FEATURES OF THE SIXTH EDITION

This edition of *Fit and Well* builds on the features that attracted and held our readers' interest in previous editions.

These features are designed to help students increase their understanding of the key concepts of wellness and to make better use of the book.

Laboratory Activities

To help students apply the principles of fitness and wellness to their own lives, *Fit and Well* includes **laboratory activities** for classroom use. These hands-on activities give students the opportunity to assess their current level of fitness and wellness, to create plans for changing their lifestyle to reach wellness, and to monitor their progress. They can assess their daily physical activity, for example, or their level of cardiorespiratory endurance, or they can design a program to improve muscular strength and endurance. Many labs end with a section labeled "Using Your Results," which guides students in evaluating their scores, setting goals for change, and moving forward. Labs are found at the end of each chapter; they are perforated for easy use.

WW The laboratory activities are also found in an interactive format on the *Fit and Well* Online Learning Center. For a complete list of laboratory activities, see pp. xiv–xv in the table of contents.

Illustrated Exercise Sections

To ensure that students understand how to perform important exercises and stretches, *Fit and Well* includes three **illustrated exercise sections,** one in Chapter 4 and two in Chapter 5. The section in Chapter 4 covers exercises for developing muscular strength and endurance, as performed both with free weights and on weight machines. One section in Chapter 5 presents stretches for flexibility, and the other presents exercises to stretch and strengthen the lower back. Each exercise is illustrated with one or more full-color photographs showing proper technique.

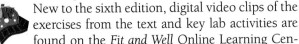 New to the sixth edition, digital video clips of the exercises from the text and key lab activities are found on the *Fit and Well* Online Learning Center. Look for the special video icon in the text to find out when to look online for corresponding video clips.

Sample Programs

To help students get started, Chapter 7 offers seven complete **sample programs** designed to develop overall fitness. The programs are built around four popular cardiorespiratory endurance activities: walking/jogging/running, bicycling, swimming, and in-line skating. They also include strength training and stretching exercises. Each one includes detailed information and guidelines on equipment and technique; target intensity, duration, and frequency; calorie cost of the activity; record keeping; and adjustments to make as fitness improves. The chapter also includes general guidelines for putting together a personal fitness program: setting goals; selecting activities; setting targets for intensity, duration, and frequency; maintaining a commitment; and recording and assessing progress.

Boxes

Boxes are used in *Fit and Well* to explore a wide range of current topics in greater detail than is possible in the text itself. Boxes fall into five different categories, each marked with a special icon and label.

 Take Charge boxes distill from the text the practical advice students need to apply information to their own lives. By referring to these boxes, students can easily find information about such topics as becoming more active, rehabilitating athletic injuries, exercising in hot weather, adding whole-grain foods to the diet, judging serving sizes, boosting motivation for behavior change, and many others.

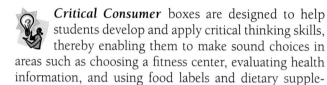 *Critical Consumer* boxes are designed to help students develop and apply critical thinking skills, thereby enabling them to make sound choices in areas such as choosing a fitness center, evaluating health information, and using food labels and dietary supplement labels to make informed dietary choices.

 Dimensions of Diversity boxes highlight fitness and nutrition concerns for particular population groups. Topics include fitness for people with disabilities, gender differences in muscular strength, and ethnic foods.

 Wellness Connection boxes explore the close connection between mind and body, looking at such topics as the effects of exercise on mood and mental functioning, and expressive writing.

 In Focus boxes highlight current topics and issues of particular interest to students. These boxes focus on such topics as the importance of lifestyle for young adults, exercise safety, exercise machines versus free weights, diabetes, and fitness and fatness.

Vital Statistics

Vital Statistics tables and figures highlight important facts and figures in an accessible format. From tables and figures marked with the Vital Statistics label, students learn about such matters as the leading causes of death for Americans and the factors that play a part in each one; the relationship between lifestyle and quality of life; public health achievements of the twentieth century; and the most popular fitness activities. For students who learn best when material is displayed graphically or numerically, Vital Statistics tables and figures offer a way to grasp information quickly and directly.

Common Questions Answered

Sections called **Common Questions Answered** appear at the ends of Chapters 2–8. In these student-friendly sections, the answers to frequently asked questions are presented in easy-to-understand terms. Included are such questions as, Do I need more protein in my diet when I train with weights? How can I safely increase exercise intensity? What is core strength training? Can a workout with an exercise ball be useful in preventing and managing low-back pain? and How can I tell if I'm allergic to a food?

Motivation for Change

New to the sixth edition, **Motivation for Change** sections provide strategies for beginning a behavior change program and maintaining healthy new habits over time. Motivation for Change strategies focus on such key aspects of behavior change as building self-efficacy, finding role models and social support, overcoming obstacles and lapses, changing environmental cues, giving rewards, and tracking program progress. These sections appear at appropriate points throughout each chapter.

Tips for Today

Chapter-ending **Tips for Today** sections provide a very brief distillation of the major message of each chapter, followed by suggestions for a few simple things that students can try right away. Tips for Today are designed to encourage students and to build their confidence by giving them easy steps they can take immediately to improve their wellness.

Quick-Reference Appendixes

Included at the end of the book are four appendixes containing vital information in an easy-to-use format. **Appendix A, Injury Prevention and Personal Safety,** is a reference guide to preventing common injuries, whether at home, at work, at play, or on the road. It also provides information on giving emergency care when someone else's life is in danger.

Appendix B, Nutritional Content of Common Foods, allows students to assess their daily diet in terms of 11 nutrient categories, including protein, fat, saturated fat, fiber, cholesterol, and sodium. **Appendix C, Nutritional Content of Popular Items from Fast-Food Restaurants,** provides a breakdown of the nutritional content of the most commonly ordered menu items at popular fast-food restaurants.

Appendix D, Monitoring Your Progress, is a log that enables students to record and summarize the results of the assessment tests they complete as part of the laboratory activities. With space for preprogram and postprogram assessment results, the log provides an easy way to track the progress of a behavior change program.

OTHER FEATURES AND LEARNING AIDS

At the beginning of each chapter, under the heading **Looking Ahead,** five or six statements preview the main points of the chapter for the student and serve as learning objectives. Each chapter also opens with **Test Your Knowledge**—a series of three multiple choice and true-false questions, with answers. These self-quizzes facilitate learning by emphasizing key points, highlighting common misconceptions, and sparking debate. Within each chapter, important terms appear in boldface type and are defined on the same or facing page of text in a **running glossary,** helping students handle new vocabulary.

Other features and learning aids are found at the end of each chapter. **For Further Exploration** sections offer suggestions for using the free student supplements that accompany the text—the Online Learning Center, the Daily Fitness and Nutrition Journal, and the HealthQuest CD-ROM—to build fitness and wellness. These sections also list recommended books, newsletters, organizations, hotlines, and Web sites. Finally, **chapter summaries** offer students a concise review and a way to make sure they have grasped the most important concepts in the chapter.

For more on the features of the book, refer to the illustrated **User's Guide to *Fit and Well,*** found on pp. xvii–xx.

TEACHING TOOLS

Available with the sixth edition of *Fit and Well* is a comprehensive package of supplementary materials designed to enhance teaching and learning.

Instructor's Resource CD-ROM (ISBN 0-07-284425-6)

The Instructor's Resource CD-ROM combines all the major electronic resources offered with the sixth edition of *Fit and Well.*

- The **Course Integrator Guide** includes learning objectives, extended chapter outlines, lists of additional resources, and many other teaching tools. It also describes all the print and electronic supplements available with the text and shows how to integrate them into lectures and assignments for each chapter. For the sixth edition, the guide was prepared by Julie Lombardi, Millersville University.
- One hundred **Additional Laboratory Activities** supplement the labs that are included in the text. These additional labs are also available to students on the Online Learning Center.
- The **test bank** includes nearly 1000 true-false, multiple choice, and essay questions. The questions are available as Word files and with the Brownstone **computerized testing software.** Brownstone provides a powerful, easy-to-use test maker to create a print version, a computer lab version, or an Internet version of each test. The Interactive Instructor CD-ROM includes the Diploma program for Windows users and Exam VI for Macintosh users; the Diploma program also includes a built-in gradebook.
- The **PowerPoint slides,** expanded for the sixth edition, provide a lecture tool that you can alter or expand to meet the needs of your course. The slides include key lecture points and images from the text and other sources.

Printed versions of key supplements—the Course Integrator Guide, Additional Labs, and test bank—are also available (ISBN 0-07-302495-3). The printed supplements are loose-leaf and three-hole-punched, ready to be placed in a binder.

Video Resources

A variety of video resources is available for use with the sixth edition of *Fit and Well.* The Online Learning Center described below includes brief digital video clips of key exercises and labs featured in the text. Other video resources include the following:

- The **McGraw-Hill Custom Video for Health** (ISBN 0-7674-2567-7) includes brief video segments with additional information on wellness topics such as nutrition, exercise, and heart disease.
- **Students on Health Custom Video** (ISBN 0-7674-0022-4) features students from college campuses across the country discussing how their daily lives are affected by their choices in such wellness areas as exercise, nutrition, and stress.
- The **Healthy Living Video Clips CD-ROM** (ISBN 0-07-238808-0) contains a collection of brief, digitized video clips that can be used to introduce a lecture or to spark classroom discussion. The segments are 2–4 minutes long.

Videos from Films for Humanities and from the award-winning series *Healthy Living: Road to Wellness* are also available.

Digital Solutions

The *Fit and Well* **Online Learning Center (www.mhhe. com/fahey)** provides many resources for both instructors and students. Instructor tools include downloadable versions of the Course Integrator Guide and the PowerPoint slides, links to professional resources, and a guide to using the Internet. For students, there are learning objectives, self-quizzes and glossary flashcards for review, interactive Internet activities, and extensive links. The Online Learning Center also includes many tools for wellness behavior change, including interactive versions of the Behavior Change Workbook as well as lab activities from the text and additional labs from the Course Integrator Guide. Through the Online Learning Center, students can also access **PowerWeb** (www.dushkin.com/online) resources, including articles on key wellness topics, study tips, and a daily news feed.

The **Online Lab Manual and Workbook,** developed in collaboration with Quia™, offers an electronic version of labs, assessments, and quizzes compiled from the text and its main supplements. This new online supplement provides students with interactive labs and assessments, self-scoring quizzes, and instant feedback. Benefits for instructors include a grade book that automatically scores, tracks, and records students' results; it also offers instructors the opportunity to review individual and class performance and customize activities for their course. To find out more about the Quia™ Online Lab Manual and Workbook, including how you can package it with *Fit and Well*, contact your local sales representative.

Classroom Performance System (CPS) brings interactivity into the classroom or lecture hall. CPS is a wireless response system that gives instructors and students immediate feedback from the entire class. Each student uses a wireless response pad similar to a television remote to instantly respond to polling or quiz questions. Contact your local sales representative for more information about using CPS with *Fit and Well*.

The **Health and Human Performance Web Site** (**www.mhhe.com/hhp**) provides monthly articles about current issues, downloadable supplements for instructors, a "how-to" technology guide, self-assessments, study tips, exam-preparation materials, and a wealth of other tools and resources for instructors and students. It also includes information about professional organizations, scholarship opportunities, conventions, and careers.

PageOut (**www.pageout.net**) is a free, easy-to-use program that enables instructors to quickly develop Web sites for their courses. PageOut can be used to create a course home page, an instructor home page, an interactive syllabus that can be linked to elements in the Online Learning Center, Web links, online discussion areas, an online grade book, and much more. The Online Learning Center can also be customized to work with products like WebCT and Blackboard.

For more information about McGraw-Hill's digital resources, including how to obtain passwords for PageOut and PowerWeb, contact your local representative and visit McGraw-Hill on the World Wide Web (www.mhhe.com/solutions).

Student Resources Available with *Fit and Well*

In addition to the materials on the Online Learning Center, there are many resources available with *Fit and Well* designed to help students learn and apply key concepts.

- The **Daily Fitness and Nutrition Journal** (ISBN 0-07-284432-9) is a handy booklet that guides students in planning and tracking their fitness programs. It also helps students assess their current diet and make appropriate changes. It is packaged free with each copy of the text.
- **HealthQuest 4.2** (ISBN 0-07-295116-8) is an interactive CD-ROM that helps students explore their wellness behavior. It includes tutorials, assessments, and behavior change guidance in such key areas as stress, fitness, nutrition, communicable diseases, cardiovascular disease, cancer, tobacco, alcohol, and other drugs. It is packaged free with each copy of the text.

- **NutritionCalc Plus** (ISBN 0-07-292084-X) is a dietary analysis program with an easy-to-use interface that allows users to track their nutrient and food group intakes, energy expenditures, and weight control goals. It generates a variety of reports and graphs for analysis, including comparisons with the Food Guide Pyramid and the Dietary Reference Intakes. The ESHA database includes thousands of ethnic foods, supplements, fast foods, and convenience foods; users can also add their own foods to the database. NutritionCalc Plus is available on CD-ROM (Windows only) or in an Internet version.
- The **Quick View Guide to the Internet for Students of Health, Physical Education, and Exercise Science, Version 2.0** (ISBN 0-7674-2062-4) provides step-by-step instructions on how to access the Internet; how to find, evaluate, and use online information about fitness and wellness; and many other topics.

Additional supplements and many packaging options are available; check with your local sales representative.

A NOTE OF THANKS

Fit and Well has benefited from the thoughtful commentary, expert knowledge, and helpful suggestions of many people. We are deeply grateful for their participation in the project.

Academic reviewers of the sixth edition:
Ann Arns, Wartburg College
Brian W. Bergemann, Campbell University
Evonne Bird, Truman State University
Lisa Borho, Clark College
Donna Campbell, Abraham Baldwin College
Trey Cone, University of Central Oklahoma
Gregory M. Dominick, Lander University
Michele L. Duffey, Pennsylvania State University
Mary Ann Erickson, Fort Lewis College
Tony Evans, Pacific Lutheran University
Kevin Hill, Wayne State College
Amy Howton, Kennesaw State University
Paulette W. Johnson, Virginia State University
Jennifer Jones, Vincennes University
Richard Krejci, Columbia College
Gary Liguori, North Dakota State University
Julie A. Lombardi, Millersville University
Derek Mann, University of Florida
Holly Molella, Dutchess Community College
Suzel Molina, Palo Alto College
Duston Morris, University of Arkansas
Leigh K. Murray, Kent State University
Steve Patrick, State University of New York, Cortland
Tim Patrick, Furman University
Douglas C. Porter, Olivet Nazarene University
John A. Richards, University of North Carolina, Greensboro

John Smith, Texas A&M University, Kingsville
Allan R. Thompson, Kalamazoo Valley Community College
Sonia Tinsley, Centenary College of Louisiana
Michael Webster, University of Southern Mississippi
Louise Whitney, Lansing Community College
Patricia A. Zezula, Huntington College

Special fitness consultants for the sixth edition:

Declan Connolly, University of Vermont
Marialice Kern, San Francisco State University
Scott O. Roberts, California State University, Chico

Special thanks are due to Rich Schroeder, DeAnza College, for hosting the photo and video shoots for several editions and to the many students at DeAnza College and California State University, Chico, who have participated in these shoots. We are also grateful to the *Fit and Well* book team, without whose efforts the book could not have been published. Special thanks to Nick Barrett, executive editor; Kirstan Price, developmental editor; Aric Bright, developmental editor for technology; Julia Ersery, editorial assistant; Pam Cooper, marketing manager; Jason Dewey, field publisher; Brett Coker, production editor; Melissa Williams, managing editor; Randy Hurst, production supervisor; Violeta Díaz, design manager; Robin Mouat, art manager; Brian J. Pecko, manager, photo research; and Marty Granahan, permissions editor.

Thomas D. Fahey
Paul M. Insel
Walton T. Roth

Brief Contents

CHAPTER 1   Introduction to Wellness, Fitness, and Lifestyle Management   1

CHAPTER 2   Basic Principles of Physical Fitness   27

CHAPTER 3   Cardiorespiratory Endurance   55

CHAPTER 4   Muscular Strength and Endurance   87

CHAPTER 5   Flexibility and Low-Back Health   133

CHAPTER 6   Body Composition   167

CHAPTER 7   Putting Together a Complete Fitness Program   189

CHAPTER 8   Nutrition   217

APPENDIX A   Injury Prevention and Personal Safety   A-1

APPENDIX B   Nutritional Content of Common Foods   B-1

APPENDIX C   Nutritional Content of Popular Items from Fast-Food Restaurants   C-1

APPENDIX D   Monitoring Your Progress   D-1

Index   I-1

Contents

Preface   iii

CHAPTER 1

Introduction to Wellness, Fitness, and Lifestyle Management   1

WELLNESS: THE NEW HEALTH GOAL   2
The Dimensions of Wellness   2
New Opportunities, New Responsibilities   3
Behaviors That Contribute to Wellness   4
The Role of Other Factors in Wellness   7
National Wellness Goals   8

REACHING WELLNESS THROUGH LIFESTYLE MANAGEMENT   9
Getting Serious About Your Health   9
Building Motivation to Change   10
Enhancing Your Readiness to Change   13
Developing Skills for Change: Creating a Personalized
    Plan   15
Putting Your Plan into Action   18
Staying with It   18
Being Fit and Well for Life   20
Tips for Today   20
Summary   20
For Further Exploration   21
Selected Bibliography   22
Lab 1.1   Your Wellness Profile   23
Lab 1.2   Lifestyle Evaluation   25

CHAPTER 2

Basic Principles of Physical Fitness   27

PHYSICAL ACTIVITY AND EXERCISE FOR HEALTH AND FITNESS   28
Physical Activity on a Continuum   28
How Much Physical Activity Is Enough?   31

HEALTH-RELATED COMPONENTS OF PHYSICAL FITNESS   32
Cardiorespiratory Endurance   32
Muscular Strength   33
Muscular Endurance   33
Flexibility   34
Body Composition   34
Skill-Related Components of Fitness   34

PRINCIPLES OF PHYSICAL TRAINING: ADAPTATION TO STRESS   34
Specificity—Adapting to Type of Training   34
Progressive Overload—Adapting to Amount of Training
    and the FITT Principle   35
Reversibility—Adapting to a Reduction in Training   37
Individual Differences—Limits on Adaptability   37

DESIGNING YOUR OWN EXERCISE PROGRAM   37
Medical Clearance   37
Assessment   37
Setting Goals   37
Choosing Activities for a Balanced Program   38
Guidelines for Training   40
Tips for Today   43
Summary   43
For Further Exploration   44
Selected Bibliography   46
Lab 2.1   Safety of Exercise Participation   47
Lab 2.2   Your Physical Activity Profile   49
Lab 2.3   Overcoming Barriers to Being Active   51

CHAPTER 3

Cardiorespiratory Endurance   55

BASIC PHYSIOLOGY OF CARDIORESPIRATORY ENDURANCE EXERCISE   56
The Cardiorespiratory System   56
Energy Production   58
Exercise and the Three Energy Systems   58

BENEFITS OF CARDIORESPIRATORY ENDURANCE EXERCISE 60
Improved Cardiorespiratory Functioning   60
Improved Cellular Metabolism   61
Reduced Risk of Chronic Disease   62
Better Control of Body Fat   63
Improved Immune Function   63
Improved Psychological and Emotional Well-Being   64

ASSESSING CARDIORESPIRATORY FITNESS   64
Assessment Tests   65
Monitoring Your Heart Rate   66
Interpreting Your Score   66

DEVELOPING A CARDIORESPIRATORY ENDURANCE PROGRAM   66
Setting Goals   67
Applying the FITT Equation   68
Warming Up and Cooling Down   70
Building Cardiorespiratory Fitness   71
Maintaining Cardiorespiratory Fitness   72

EXERCISE SAFETY AND INJURY PREVENTION   72
Hot Weather and Heat Stress   72
Cold Weather   74
Poor Air Quality   74
Exercise Injuries   74

Tips for Today   77
Summary   77
For Further Exploration   79
Selected Bibliography   80

Lab 3.1   Assessing Your Current Level of Cardiorespiratory Endurance   81
Lab 3.2   Developing an Exercise Program for Cardiorespiratory Endurance   85

CHAPTER 4

Muscular Strength and Endurance   87

BASIC MUSCLE PHYSIOLOGY AND THE EFFECTS OF STRENGTH TRAINING   88

BENEFITS OF MUSCULAR STRENGTH AND ENDURANCE   89
Improved Performance of Physical Activities   89
Injury Prevention   90
Improved Body Composition   90
Enhanced Self-Image and Quality of Life   90
Improved Muscle and Bone Health with Aging   90
Prevention and Management of Chronic Disease   90

ASSESSING MUSCULAR STRENGTH AND ENDURANCE   91

CREATING A SUCCESSFUL STRENGTH TRAINING PROGRAM   92
Static Versus Dynamic Strength Training Exercises   92
Weight Machines Versus Free Weights   94
Applying the FITT Principle: Selecting Exercises and Putting Together a Program   94
Intensity of Exercise: Amount of Resistance   94
The Warm-Up and Cool-Down   96
More Advanced Strength Training Programs   98
Weight Training Safety   98
A Caution About Supplements and Drugs   100

WEIGHT TRAINING EXERCISES   104

Tips for Today   119
Summary   119
For Further Exploration   120
Selected Bibliography   122

Lab 4.1   Assessing Your Current Level of Muscular Strength   123
Lab 4.2   Assessing Your Current Level of Muscular Endurance   127
Lab 4.3   Designing and Monitoring a Strength Training Program   131

CHAPTER 5

Flexibility and Low-Back Health   133

WHAT DETERMINES FLEXIBILITY?   134
Joint Structure   134
Muscle Elasticity and Length   134
Nervous System Activity   135

BENEFITS OF FLEXIBILITY AND STRETCHING EXERCISES   135
Joint Health   135
Prevention of Low-Back Pain and Injuries   135
Additional Potential Benefits   136
Flexibility and Lifetime Wellness   136

ASSESSING FLEXIBILITY   136

CREATING A SUCCESSFUL PROGRAM TO DEVELOP FLEXIBILITY   136
Applying the FITT Principle   136
Making Progress   139
Exercises to Improve Flexibility   139

PREVENTING AND MANAGING LOW-BACK PAIN   145
Function and Structure of the Spine   145
Causes of Back Pain   146
Preventing Low-Back Pain   146

Managing Acute Back Pain   148
Managing Chronic Back Pain   148
Exercises for the Prevention and Management of Low-Back
   Pain   149

Tips for Today   152
Summary   152
For Further Exploration   153
Selected Bibliography   154

Lab 5.1   Assessing Your Current Level of
Flexibility   155

Lab 5.2   Creating a Personalized Program for
Developing Flexibility   161

Lab 5.3   Assessing Muscular Endurance for
Low-Back Health   163

Lab 5.4   Posture Evaluation   165

CHAPTER 6

Body Composition   167

**WHAT IS BODY COMPOSITION, AND WHY IS IT
IMPORTANT?   168**
Overweight and Obesity Defined   168
Prevalence of Overweight and Obesity Among
   Americans   169
Excess Body Fat and Wellness   170
Problems Associated with Very Low Levels of Body Fat   172

**ASSESSING BODY MASS INDEX, BODY
COMPOSITION, AND BODY FAT DISTRIBUTION   173**
Calculating Body Mass Index   174
Estimating Percent Body Fat   175
Assessing Body Fat Distribution   177

SETTING BODY COMPOSITION GOALS   177

MAKING CHANGES IN BODY COMPOSITION   177

Tips for Today   178
Summary   178
For Further Exploration   178
Selected Bibliography   180

Lab 6.1   Assessing Body Mass Index and Body
Composition   181

Lab 6.2   Determining a Target Body Weight   187

CHAPTER 7

Putting Together a Complete Fitness
Program   189

DEVELOPING A PERSONAL FITNESS PLAN   190
1. Set Goals   190
2. Select Activities   190

3. Set a Target Frequency, Intensity, and Time (Duration)
   for Each Activity   194
4. Set Up a System of Mini-Goals and Rewards   196
5. Include Lifestyle Physical Activity in Your Program   196
6. Develop Tools for Monitoring Your Progress   196
7. Make a Commitment   196

PUTTING YOUR PLAN INTO ACTION   197

MAINTAINING YOUR PROGRAM: FIT FOR LIFE   198

**EXERCISE GUIDELINES FOR PEOPLE WITH SPECIAL
HEALTH CONCERNS   198**
Arthritis   199
Asthma   199
Diabetes   200
Heart Disease and Hypertension   200
Obesity   200
Osteoporosis   201

EXERCISE GUIDELINES FOR LIFE STAGES   201
Children and Adolescents   201
Pregnant Women   201
Older Adults   202

Tips for Today   202
Summary   202
For Further Exploration   202
Selected Bibliography   203

SAMPLE PROGRAMS FOR POPULAR ACTIVITIES   204
General Guidelines   204
Walking/Jogging/Running Sample Program   204
Bicycling Sample Program   207
Swimming Sample Program   209
In-Line Skating Sample Program   211

Lab 7.1   A Personal Fitness Program Plan and
Contract   213

Lab 7.2   Getting to Know Your Fitness Facility   215

CHAPTER 8

Nutrition   217

**NUTRITIONAL REQUIREMENTS: COMPONENTS OF
A HEALTHY DIET   218**
Proteins—The Basis of Body Structure   220
Fats—Essential in Small Amounts   221
Carbohydrates—An Ideal Source of Energy   225
Dietary Fiber—A Closer Look   227
Vitamins—Organic Micronutrients   228
Minerals—Inorganic Micronutrients   230
Water—A Vital Component   230
Other Substances in Food   231

NUTRITIONAL GUIDELINES: PLANNING YOUR DIET 233

Dietary Reference Intakes (DRIs) 233
The Food Guide Pyramid 234
Dietary Guidelines for Americans 237
The Vegetarian Alternative 241
Dietary Challenges for Special Population Groups 242

NUTRITIONAL PLANNING: MAKING INFORMED CHOICES ABOUT FOOD 244

Food Labels—A Closer Look 244
Dietary Supplement Labels—New Requirements 246
Food Additives—Benefits and Risks 246
Foodborne Illness—An Increasing Threat 246
Irradiated Foods—A Technique of Biotechnology 249
Organic Foods—Stricter Standards for a Booming Industry 249

A PERSONAL PLAN: APPLYING NUTRITIONAL PRINCIPLES 249

Assessing and Changing Your Diet 249
Staying Committed to a Healthy Diet 251

Tips for Today 251
Summary 251
For Further Exploration 253
Selected Bibliography 255

NUTRITION RESOURCES 256

Lab 8.1   Your Daily Diet Versus the Food Guide Pyramid 261
Lab 8.2   Dietary Analysis 265
Lab 8.3   Informed Food Choices 267

APPENDIX A   Injury Prevention and Personal Safety A-1
APPENDIX B   Nutritional Content of Common Foods B-1
APPENDIX C   Nutritional Content of Popular Items from Fast-Food Restaurants C-1
APPENDIX D   Monitoring Your Progress D-1

Index I-1

BOXES

TAKE CHARGE

Tips for Moving Forward in the Cycle of Behavior Change 14
Motivation Boosters 19
Becoming More Active 30

Exercising in Hot Weather 75
Rehabilitation Following a Minor Athletic Injury 77
Safe Weight Training 99
Safe Stretching 138
Stretches to Avoid 144
Good Posture and Low-Back Health 147
Getting Your Fitness Program Back on Track 198
Setting Intake Goals for Protein, Fat, and Carbohydrate 224
Choosing More Whole-Grain Foods 226
Eating for Healthy Bones 232
Judging Serving Sizes 236
Reducing the Fat in Your Diet 240
Eating Strategies for College Students 243

CRITICAL CONSUMER

Evaluating Sources of Health Information 11
Choosing a Fitness Center 45
Evaluating Home Exercise Equipment 70
Dietary Supplements: A Consumer Dilemma 103
Choosing Exercise Footwear 195
Using Food Labels 245
Using Dietary Supplement Labels 247

WELLNESS CONNECTION

Signs of Wellness 20
Exercise and Total Wellness 29
Exercise and the Mind 64
Expressive Writing and Chronic Conditions 148
Exercise, Body Image, and Self-Esteem 172
Sleep 199
Eating Habits and Total Wellness 219

DIMENSIONS OF DIVERSITY

Wellness Issues for Diverse Populations 9
Fitness and Disability 35
Benefits of Exercise for Older Adults 62
Gender Differences in Muscular Strength 91
The Female Athlete Triad 173
Ethnic Foods 250

IN FOCUS

Lifestyle Matters for Young Adults 12
Is Exercise Safe? 38
Exercise Machines Versus Free Weights 94
Can You Be Fit and Fat? 169
Diabetes 171

LABORATORY ACTIVITIES

Lab 1.1   Your Wellness Profile 23
Lab 1.2   Lifestyle Evaluation 25

Lab 2.1   Safety of Exercise Participation 47
Lab 2.2   Your Physical Activity Profile 49
Lab 2.3   Overcoming Barriers to Being Active 51
Lab 3.1   Assessing Your Current Level of
          Cardiorespiratory Endurance 81
Lab 3.2   Developing an Exercise Program for
          Cardiorespiratory Endurance 85
Lab 4.1   Assessing Your Current Level of
          Muscular Strength 123
Lab 4.2   Assessing Your Current Level of
          Muscular Endurance 127
Lab 4.3   Designing and Monitoring a Strength
          Training Program 131
Lab 5.1   Assessing Your Current Level of
          Flexibility 155
Lab 5.2   Creating a Personalized Program for
          Developing Flexibility 161

Lab 5.3   Assessing Muscular Endurance for Low-
          Back Health 163
Lab 5.4   Posture Evaluation 165
Lab 6.1   Assessing Body Mass Index and Body
          Composition 181
Lab 6.2   Determining a Target Body Weight 187
Lab 7.1   A Personal Fitness Program Plan and
          Contract 213
Lab 7.2   Getting to Know Your Fitness
          Facility 215
Lab 8.1   Your Daily Diet Versus the Food Guide
          Pyramid 261
Lab 8.2   Dietary Analysis 265
Lab 8.3   Informed Food Choices 267

Ww The Behavior Change Workbook and the laboratory activities are also found in an interactive format on the *Fit and Well* Online Learning Center (www.mhhe.com/fahey).

A User's Guide to *Fit and Well*

Are you looking for ways to improve your lifestyle and become fit and well? Do you need help finding reliable wellness resources online? Would you like to boost your grade? *Fit and Well* can help you do all this and much more!

LABORATORY ACTIVITIES

These hands-on self-assessments help you determine your current level of wellness and create plans for making positive changes in your lifestyle. The Using Your Results sections guide you in setting goals and moving forward based on the results of the assessments. Lab activities are included at the end of every chapter on easy-to-use perforated pages.

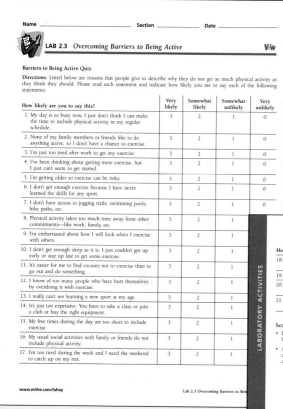

Vw *Fit and Well*
ONLINE LEARNING CENTER
(www.mhhe.com/fahey)

Look for the special World Wide Web icon throughout the text. Elements marked with the icon have corresponding activities and links on the *Fit and Well* Online Learning Center. The lab activities can be found online in an interactive format.

MOTIVATION FOR CHANGE

New to the sixth edition, Motivation for Change sections provide strategies for beginning a behavior change program and maintaining new healthy habits over time.

TIPS FOR TODAY

Tips for Today sections, found at the end of each chapter, provide a brief summary of the major message of the chapter, followed by suggestions for a few easy steps you can try right away to improve your level of wellness.

MOTIVATION FOR CHANGE! Are you one of the many people who choose fast food or packaged snack foods often because they are quick and convenient? You can't eliminate these choices from your environment, but you can increase your chances of making healthier choices by finding other options that are just as convenient. Review the menus of the restaurants you visit most often and identify choices that meet your dietary goals and that you enjoy. Next, locate other inexpensive restaurants or food sources that are near your campus or home. Finally, identify ready-to-eat foods like prewashed vegetables and fruit salad that could you stock at home and pack for an inexpensive bag lunch. Make a list of restaurants, stores, and specific food items that are convenient and that are a match for your dietary goals. When you are tempted by less healthy choices, refer to your list for both practical information and a motivation boost.

Staying Committed to a Healthy Diet

Beyond knowledge and information, you also need support in difficult situations. Keeping to your plan is easiest when you choose and prepare your own food at home. Advance planning is the key: mapping out meals and shopping appropriately, cooking in advance when possible, and preparing enough food for leftovers later in the week. A tight budget does not necessarily make it more difficult to eat healthy meals. It makes good health sense and good budget sense to use only small amounts of meat and to have a few meatless meals each week.

In restaurants, keeping to food plan goals becomes somewhat more difficult. Portion sizes in restaurants tend to be larger than serving sizes of the Food Guide Pyramid, but by remaining focused on your goals, you can eat only part of your meal and take the rest home for a meal later in the week. Don't hesitate to ask questions when you're eating in a restaurant. Most restaurant personnel are glad to explain how menu selections are prepared and to make small adjustments, such as serving salad dressings and sauces on the side so they can be avoided or used sparingly. To limit your fat intake, order meat or fish broiled or grilled rather than fried or sauteed, choose rice or a plain baked potato over french fries, and select a clear soup rather than a creamy one. Desserts that are irresistible can, at least, be shared.

Strategies like these can be helpful, but small changes cannot change a fundamentally high-fat, high-calorie meal into a moderate, healthful one. Often, the best advice is to bypass a large steak with potatoes au gratin for a flavorful but low-fat entree. Many of the selections offered in ethnic restaurants are healthy choices (refer to the box on ethnic foods for suggestions).

Fast-food restaurants offer the biggest challenge to a healthy diet. Surveys show that about 70% of 18- to 24-year-olds and 64% of 25- to 34-year-olds visit a fast-food restaurant at least once a week. Fast-food meals are often high in calories, total fat, saturated fat, trans fat, sodium,

and sugar; they may be low in fiber and in some vitamins and minerals (see Appendix C). If you do eat at a fast-food restaurant, make sure the rest of your meals that day are low-fat meals rich in fruits and vegetables.

Knowledge of food and nutrition is essential to the success of your program. The information provided in this chapter should give you the tools you need to design and implement a diet that promotes long-term health and well-being. If you need additional information or have questions about nutrition, be sure the source you consult is reliable.

Tips for Today

Eating is one of life's great pleasures. There are many ways to satisfy your nutrient needs so you can create a healthy diet that takes into account your personal preferences and favorite foods. If your current eating habits are not as healthy as they could be, you can choose equally delicious foods that offer both short-term and long-term health benefits. Opportunities to improve your diet present themselves every day, and small changes add up.

Right now you can

- Substitute a healthy snack—an apple, a banana, or plain popcorn—for a bag of chips or cookies.
- Drink a glass of water and put a bottle of water in your backpack for tomorrow.
- Plan to make healthy selections when you go to dinner, such as a baked potato instead of french fries or salmon instead of steak.
- Study the box on ethnic foods in this chapter and plan to order a healthy selection the next time you eat at your favorite ethnic restaurant. Do the same with the fast-food restaurants listed in Appendix C at the end of the book.

SUMMARY

- The six classes of nutrients are carbohydrates, proteins, fats, vitamins, minerals, and water.
- The nutrients essential to humans are released into the body through digestion. Nutrients in foods provide energy, measured in kilocalories (commonly called calories); build and maintain body tissues; and regulate body functions.
- Protein, an important component of body tissue, is composed of amino acids; nine are essential to a diet. Foods from animal sources provide complete proteins; plants provide incomplete proteins.
- Fats, a major source of energy, also insulate the body and cushion the organs; 3–4 teaspoons of vegetable oil per day supplies the essential fats. For most people, dietary fat intake should be 20–35% of total calories, and unsaturated fats should be favored over saturated and trans fats.

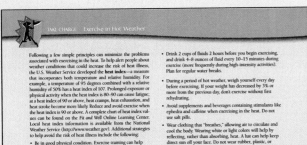

TAKE CHARGE *Exercise in Hot Weather*

Following a few simple principles can minimize the problems associated with exercising in the heat. To help alert people about weather conditions that could increase the risk of heat illness, the U.S. Weather Service developed the **heat index**—a measure that incorporates both temperature and relative humidity. For example, a temperature of 95 degrees combined with a relative humidity of 50% has a heat index of 107. Prolonged exposure or physical activity when the heat index is 80–90 can cause fatigue; at a heat index of 90 or above, heat cramps, heat exhaustion, and heat stroke become more likely. Reduce and avoid exercise when the heat index is 90 or above. A complete chart of heat index values can be found on the *Fit and Well* Online Learning Center. Local heat index information is available from the National Weather Service (http://www.weather.gov). Additional strategies to help avoid the risk of heat illness include the following:

- Be in good physical condition. Exercise training can help the body adapt to heat by increasing the sweat rate.
- Use caution when exercising in extreme heat or humidity (over 80°F and/or 60% humidity).
- Slow exercise or add rest breaks to maintain your prescribed target heart rate; as you become acclimatized, you can gradually increase intensity and duration.
- Exercise in the early morning or evening, when temperatures are lowest.

- Drink 2 cups of fluids 2 hours before you begin exercising, and drink 4–8 ounces of fluid every 10–15 minutes during exercise (more frequently during high-intensity activities). Plan for regular water breaks.
- During a period of hot weather, weigh yourself every day before exercising. If your weight has decreased by 3% or more from the previous day, don't exercise without first rehydrating.
- Avoid supplements and beverages containing stimulants like ephedra and caffeine when exercising in the heat. Do not use salt pills.
- Wear clothing that "breathes," allowing air to circulate and cool the body. Wearing white or light colors will help by reflecting, rather than absorbing, heat. A hat can help keep direct sun off your face. Do not wear rubber, plastic, or other nonporous clothing. "Sauna suits" cause loss of body water, not fat, and don't improve body composition.
- Rest frequently in the shade.
- Slow down or stop if you begin to feel uncomfortable. Watch for the signs of heat disorders listed below; if they occur, act appropriately.

Problem	Symptoms	Treatment
Heat cramps	Muscle cramps, usually in the muscles most used during exercise.	Stop exercising, drink fluids, and massage or stretch cramped muscles.
Heat exhaustion	Weakness, dizziness, headache, rapid pulse, profuse sweating, pale face, normal or slightly elevated temperature.	Cool the body. Stop exercising, get out of the heat, remove excess clothing, drink cold fluids, and apply cool and/or damp towels to the body.
Heat stroke	Hot, flushed skin (may be dry or sweaty), red face, chills, shivering, disorientation, erratic behavior, high body temperature, unconsciousness, convulsions.	*Get immediate medical attention,* and try to lower body temperature. Get out of the heat, remove excess clothing, drink cold fluids, and apply cool and/or damp towels to the body or immerse it in cold water.

When to Call a Physician Some injuries require medical attention. Consult a physician for head and eye injuries, possible ligament injuries, broken bones, and internal disorders such as chest pain, fainting, elevated body temperature, and intolerance to hot weather. Also seek medical attention for ostensibly minor injuries that do not get better within a reasonable amount of time. You may need to modify your exercise program for a few weeks to allow an injury to heal.

Managing Minor Exercise Injuries For minor cuts and scrapes, stop the bleeding and clean the wound. Treat injuries to soft tissue (muscles and joints) with the R-I-C-E principle: rest, ice, compression, and elevation. Immediately following the injury, rest the affected area and apply ice. Elevate the affected part of the body, and

heat stroke A severe and often fatal heat illness produced by exposure to very high temperatures, especially when combined with intense exercise; characterized by significantly elevated core body temperature.

hypothermia Low body temperature due to exposure to cold conditions.

frostbite Freezing of body tissues characterized by pallor, numbness, and a loss of cold sensation.

wind chill A measure of how cold it feels based on the rate of heat loss from exposed skin caused by cold and wind; the temperature that would have the same cooling effect on a person as a given combination of temperature and wind speed.

heat index A measure of how hot it feels; the temperature that would have the same heating effect on a person as a given combination of temperature and relative humidity.

Terms

TAKE CHARGE BOXES

Take Charge boxes, found throughout the text, provide practical advice that you can apply to your everyday life.

RUNNING GLOSSARY

Important terms appear in boldface type in the text and are defined in a running glossary on the same or facing page. A pronunciation guide to the glossary terms is found on the Online Learning Center.

CRITICAL CONSUMER BOXES

Critical Consumer boxes help you develop and apply critical thinking skills so you can make sound choices related to wellness. Additional resources for each Critical Consumer topic are found on the *Fit and Well* Online Learning Center.

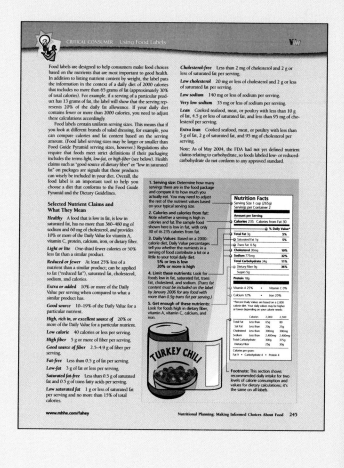

CRITICAL CONSUMER Using Food Labels

Food labels are designed to help consumers make food choices based on the nutrients that are most important to good health. In addition to listing nutrient content by weight, the label puts the information in the context of a daily diet of 2000 calories that includes no more than 65 grams of fat (approximately 30% of total calories). For example, if a serving of a particular product has 13 grams of fat, the label will show that the serving represents 20% of the daily fat allowance. If your daily diet contains fewer or more than 2000 calories, you need to adjust these calculations accordingly.

Food labels contain uniform serving sizes. This means that if you look at different brands of salad dressing, for example, you can compare calories and fat content based on the serving amount. (Food label serving sizes may be larger or smaller than Food Guide Pyramid serving sizes, however.) Regulations also require that foods meet strict definitions if their packaging includes the terms *light*, *low-fat*, or *high-fiber* (see below). Health claims such as "good source of dietary fiber" or "low in saturated fat" on packages are signals that those products can wisely be included in your diet. Overall, the food label is an important tool to help you choose a diet that conforms to the Food Guide Pyramid and the Dietary Guidelines.

Selected Nutrient Claims and What They Mean

Healthy   A food that is low in fat, is low in saturated fat, has no more than 360–480 mg of sodium and 60 mg of cholesterol, *and* provides 10% or more of the Daily Value for vitamin A, vitamin C, protein, calcium, iron, or dietary fiber.

Light or lite   One-third fewer calories or 50% less fat than a similar product.

Reduced or fewer   At least 25% less of a nutrient than a similar product; can be applied to fat ("reduced fat"), saturated fat, cholesterol, sodium, and calories.

Extra or added   10% or more of the Daily Value per serving when compared to what a similar product has.

Good source   10–19% of the Daily Value for a particular nutrient.

High, rich in, or excellent source of   20% or more of the Daily Value for a particular nutrient.

Low calorie   40 calories or less per serving.

High fiber   5 g or more of fiber per serving.

Good source of fiber   2.5–4.9 g of fiber per serving.

Fat-free   Less than 0.5 g of fat per serving.

Low-fat   3 g of fat or less per serving.

Saturated fat-free   Less than 0.5 g of saturated fat and 0.5 g of trans fatty acids per serving.

Low saturated fat   1 g or less of saturated fat per serving and no more than 15% of total calories.

Cholesterol-free   Less than 2 mg of cholesterol and 2 g or less of saturated fat per serving.

Low cholesterol   20 mg or less of cholesterol and 2 g or less of saturated fat per serving.

Low sodium   140 mg or less of sodium per serving.

Very low sodium   35 mg or less of sodium per serving.

Lean   Cooked seafood, meat, or poultry with less than 10 g of fat, 4.5 g or less of saturated fat, and less than 95 mg of cholesterol per serving.

Extra lean   Cooked seafood, meat, or poultry with less than 5 g of fat, 2 g of saturated fat, and 95 mg of cholesterol per serving.

Note: As of May 2004, the FDA had not yet defined nutrient claims relating to carbohydrate, so foods labeled low- or reduced-carbohydrate do not conform to any approved standard.

1. Serving size: Determine how many servings there are in the food package and compare it to how much you actually eat. You may need to adjust the rest of the nutrient values based on your typical serving size.

2. Calories and calories from fat: Note whether a serving is high in calories and fat. The sample food shown here is low in fat, with only 30 of its 235 calories from fat.

3. Daily Values: Based on a 2000-calorie diet, Daily Value percentages tell you whether the nutrients in a serving of food contribute a lot or a little to your total daily diet.
5% or less is low
20% or more is high

4. Limit these nutrients: Look for foods low in fat, saturated fat, trans fat, cholesterol, and sodium. (Trans fat content must be included on the label by January 2006 for any food with more than 0.5 g trans fat per serving.)

5. Get enough of these nutrients: Look for foods high in dietary fiber, vitamin A, vitamin C, calcium, and iron.

Nutrition Facts
Serving Size 1 cup (265g)
Servings per Container 2

Amount per Serving
Calories 235   Calories from Fat 30

	% Daily Value*
Total Fat 3g	5%
Saturated Fat 1g	5%
Trans Fat 0.5g	
Cholesterol 30mg	10%
Sodium 775mg	32%
Total Carbohydrate 34g	11%
Dietary Fiber 9g	36%
Sugars 5g	
Protein 18g	

Vitamin A 25%	•	Vitamin C 0%
Calcium 12%	•	Iron 20%

*Percent Daily Values are based on a 2,000 calorie diet. Your daily values may be higher or lower depending on your calorie needs:

	Calories	2,000	2,500
Total Fat	Less than	65g	80g
Sat Fat	Less than	20g	25g
Cholesterol	Less than	300mg	300mg
Sodium	Less than	2,400mg	2,400mg
Total Carbohydrate		300g	375g
Dietary Fiber		25g	30g

Calories per gram:
Fat 9 • Carbohydrate 4 • Protein 4

Footnote: This section shows recommended daily intake for two levels of calorie consumption and values for dietary calculations; it's the same on all labels.

www.mhhe.com/fahey

Nutritional Planning: Making Informed Choices About Food 245

Behavior Change Workbook

This workbook is designed to take you step by step through the process of behavior change. The first eight activities in the workbook will help you develop a successful plan—beginning with choosing a target behavior and moving through the program planning steps described in Chapter 1, including the completion and signing of a behavior change contract. The final seven activities will help you work through common obstacles to behavior change and maximize your program's chances of success.

Part 1   Developing a Plan for Behavior Change and Completing a Contract
1. Choosing a Target Behavior
2. Gathering Information About Your Target Behavior
3. Monitoring Your Current Patterns of Behavior
4. Setting Goals
5. Examining Your Attitudes About Your Target Behavior
6. Choosing Rewards
7. Breaking Behavior Chains
8. Completing a Contract for Behavior Change

Part 2   Overcoming Obstacles to Behavior Change
9. Building Motivation and Commitment
10. Managing Your Time Successfully
11. Developing Realistic Self-Talk
12. Involving the People Around You
13. Dealing with Feelings
14. Overcoming Peer Pressure: Communicating Assertively
15. Maintaining Your Program over Time

ACTIVITY 1   CHOOSING A TARGET BEHAVIOR

Use your knowledge of yourself and the results of Lab 1-2 (Lifestyle Evaluation) to identify five behaviors that you could change to improve your level of wellness. Examples of target behaviors include smoking cigarettes, not exercising regularly, eating candy bars every night, not getting enough sleep, getting drunk frequently on weekends, and not wearing a safety belt when driving or riding in a car. List your five behaviors below.

1. _____
2. _____
3. _____
4. _____
5. _____

For successful behavior change, it's best to focus on one behavior at a time. Review your list of behaviors and select one to start with. Choose a behavior that is important to you and that you are strongly motivated to change. If this will be your first attempt at behavior change, start with a simple change, such as wearing your bicycle helmet regularly, before tackling a more difficult change, such as quitting smoking. Circle the behavior on your list that you've chosen to start with; this will be your target behavior throughout this workbook.

www.mhhe.com/fahey

W-1

BEHAVIOR CHANGE WORKBOOK

The Behavior Change Workbook takes you step by step through the process of behavior change. It helps you target a specific behavior, set goals, create a plan, and overcome common obstacles to change. The Workbook is available in an interactive format on the Online Learning Center, and a printed copy is included in the full and alternate editions of the text.

USER'S GUIDE

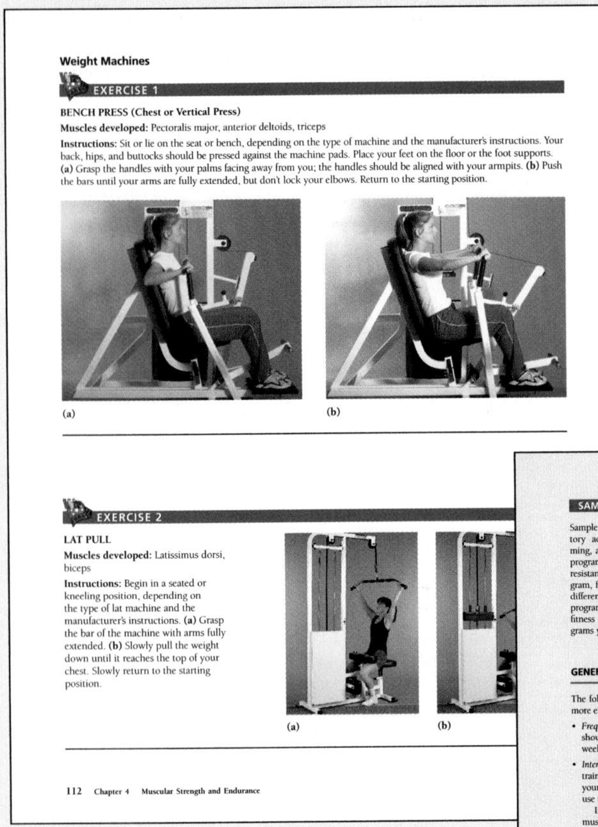
Weight Machines

EXERCISE 1

BENCH PRESS (Chest or Vertical Press)

Muscles developed: Pectoralis major, anterior deltoids, triceps

Instructions: Sit or lie on the seat or bench, depending on the type of machine and the manufacturer's instructions. Your back, hips, and buttocks should be pressed against the machine pads. Place your feet on the floor or the foot supports. **(a)** Grasp the handles with your palms facing away from you; the handles should be aligned with your armpits. **(b)** Push the bars until your arms are fully extended, but don't lock your elbows. Return to the starting position.

(a) (b)

EXERCISE 2

LAT PULL

Muscles developed: Latissimus dorsi, biceps

Instructions: Begin in a seated or kneeling position, depending on the type of lat machine and the manufacturer's instructions. **(a)** Grasp the bar of the machine with arms fully extended. **(b)** Slowly pull the weight down until it reaches the top of your chest. Slowly return to the starting position.

(a) (b)

112 Chapter 4 Muscular Strength and Endurance

SAMPLE EXERCISE PROGRAMS

Illustrated exercise programs in Chapters 4 and 5 show proper technique for exercises and stretches that develop muscular strength and endurance, flexibility, and low-back health; video clips of the exercises can be found on the Online Learning Center. The complete sample fitness programs in Chapter 7 are built around popular endurance activities such as walking, jogging, cycling, and swimming.

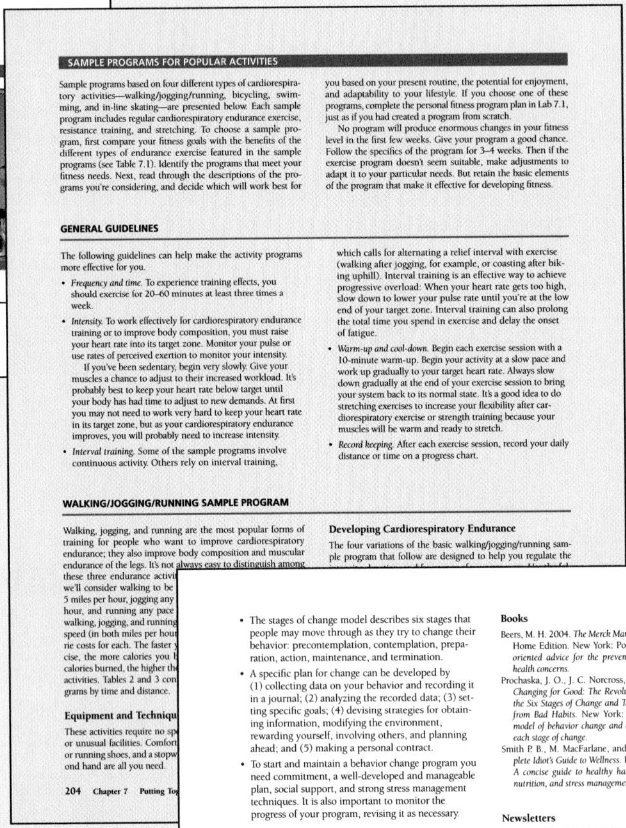
SAMPLE PROGRAMS FOR POPULAR ACTIVITIES

Sample programs based on four different types of cardiorespiratory activities—walking/jogging/running, bicycling, swimming, and in-line skating—are presented below. Each sample program includes regular cardiorespiratory endurance exercise, resistance training, and stretching. To choose a sample program, first compare your fitness goals with the benefits of the different types of endurance exercise featured in the sample programs (see Table 7.1). Identify the programs that meet your fitness needs. Next, read through the descriptions of the programs you're considering, and decide which will work best for you based on your present routine, the potential for enjoyment, and adaptability to your lifestyle. If you choose one of these programs, complete the personal fitness program plan in Lab 7.1, just as if you had created a program from scratch.

No program will produce enormous changes in your fitness level in the first few weeks. Give your program a good chance. Follow the specifics of the program for 3–4 weeks. Then if the exercise program doesn't seem suitable, make adjustments to adapt it to your particular needs. But retain the basic elements of the program that make it effective for developing fitness.

GENERAL GUIDELINES

The following guidelines can help make the activity programs more effective for you.

- *Frequency and time.* To experience training effects, you should exercise for 20–60 minutes at least three times a week.
- *Intensity.* To work effectively for cardiorespiratory endurance training or to improve body composition, you must raise your heart rate into its target zone. Monitor your pulse or use rates of perceived exertion to monitor your intensity.
  If you've been sedentary, begin very slowly. Give your muscles a chance to adjust to their increased workload. It's probably best to keep your heart rate below target until your body has had time to adjust to new demands. At first you may not need to work very hard to keep your heart rate in its target zone, but as your cardiorespiratory endurance improves, you will probably need to increase intensity.
- *Interval training.* Some of the sample programs involve continuous activity. Others rely on interval training, which calls for alternating a relief interval with exercise (walking after jogging, for example, or coasting after biking uphill). Interval training is an effective way to achieve progressive overload: When your heart rate gets too high, slow down to lower your pulse rate until you're at the low end of your target zone. Interval training can also prolong the total time you spend in exercise and delay the onset of fatigue.
- *Warm-up and cool-down.* Begin each exercise session with a 10-minute warm-up. Begin your activity at a slow pace and work up gradually to your target heart rate. Always slow down gradually at the end of your exercise session to bring your system back to its normal state. It's a good idea to do stretching exercises to increase your flexibility after cardiorespiratory exercise or strength training because your muscles will be warm and ready to stretch.
- *Record keeping.* After each exercise session, record your daily distance or time on a progress chart.

WALKING/JOGGING/RUNNING SAMPLE PROGRAM

Walking, jogging, and running are the most popular forms of training for people who want to improve cardiorespiratory endurance; they also improve body composition and muscular endurance of the legs. It's not always easy to distinguish among these three endurance activi... we'll consider walking to be ... 5 miles per hour, jogging any ... hour, and running any pace ... walking, jogging, and running ... speed (in both miles per hou... rie costs for each. The faster ... cise, the more calories you ... calories burned, the higher th... activities. Tables 2 and 3 con... grams by time and distance.

Equipment and Techniqu...

These activities require no sp... or unusual facilities. Comfort... or running shoes, and a stopw... ond hand are all you need.

204 Chapter 7 Putting To...

Developing Cardiorespiratory Endurance

The four variations of the basic walking/jogging/running sample program that follow are designed to help you regulate the ...

FOR FURTHER EXPLORATION

For Further Exploration sections at the end of each chapter describe books, newsletters, organizations, hotlines, and Web sites that you can turn to for additional advice and information. These sections also suggest ways to use the free tools available with *Fit and Well:*

- The Daily Fitness and Nutrition Journal gives you an easy way to plan and track a fitness program and a program for dietary improvement.
- The HealthQuest CD-ROM includes interactive tutorials, self-assessments, review questions, and many other resources.
- The *Fit and Well* Online Learning Center (www.mhhe.com/fahey) provides interactive study guide questions, learning objectives, chapter outlines, glossary flashcards, Internet activities, links, and other useful study aids.

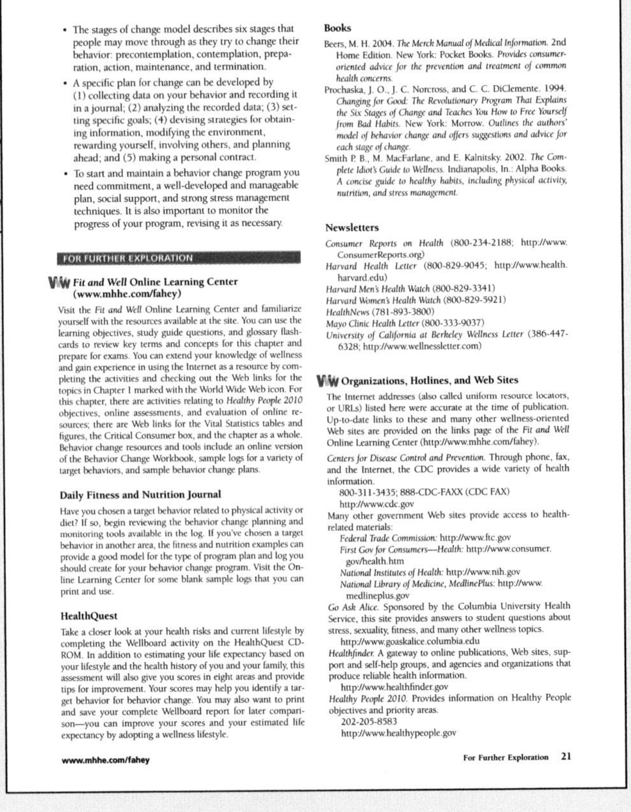
- The stages of change model describes six stages that people may move through as they try to change their behavior: precontemplation, contemplation, preparation, action, maintenance, and termination.
- A specific plan for change can be developed by (1) collecting data on your behavior and recording it in a journal; (2) analyzing the recorded data; (3) setting specific goals; (4) devising strategies for obtaining information, modifying the environment, rewarding yourself, involving others, and planning ahead; and (5) making a personal contract.
- To start and maintain a behavior change program you need commitment, a well-developed and manageable plan, social support, and strong stress management techniques. It is also important to monitor the progress of your program, revising it as necessary.

FOR FURTHER EXPLORATION

Fit and Well Online Learning Center (www.mhhe.com/fahey)

Visit the *Fit and Well* Online Learning Center and familiarize yourself with the resources available at the site. You can use the learning objectives, study guide questions, and glossary flashcards to review key terms and concepts for this chapter and prepare for exams. You can extend your knowledge of wellness and gain experience in using the Internet as a resource by completing the activities and checking out the Web links for the topics in Chapter 1 marked with the World Wide Web icon. For this chapter, there are activities relating to *Healthy People 2010* objectives, online assessments, and evaluation of online resources; there are Web links for the Vital Statistics tables and figures, the Critical Consumer box, and the chapter as a whole. Behavior change resources and tools include an online version of the Behavior Change Workbook, sample logs for a variety of target behaviors, and sample behavior change plans.

Daily Fitness and Nutrition Journal

Have you chosen a target behavior related to physical activity or diet? If so, begin reviewing the behavior change planning and monitoring tools available in the log. If you've chosen a target behavior in another area, the fitness and nutrition examples can provide a good model for the type of program plan and log you should create for your behavior change program. Visit the Online Learning Center for some blank sample logs that you can print and use.

HealthQuest

Take a closer look at your health risks and current lifestyle by completing the Wellboard activity on the HealthQuest CD-ROM. In addition to estimating your life expectancy based on your lifestyle and the health history of you and your family, this assessment will also give you scores in eight areas and provide tips for improvement. Your scores may help you identify a target behavior for behavior change. You may also want to print and save your complete Wellboard report for later comparison—you can improve your scores and your estimated life expectancy by adopting a wellness lifestyle.

Books

Beers, M. H. 2004. *The Merck Manual of Medical Information.* 2nd Home Edition. New York: Pocket Books. *Provides consumer-oriented advice for the prevention and treatment of common health concerns.*

Prochaska, J. O., J. C. Norcross, and C. C. DiClemente. 1994. *Changing for Good: The Revolutionary Program That Explains the Six Stages of Change and Teaches You How to Free Yourself from Bad Habits.* New York: Morrow. *Outlines the authors' model of behavior change and offers suggestions and advice for each stage of change.*

Smith P. B., M. MacFarlane, and E. Kalnitsky. 2002. *The Complete Idiot's Guide to Wellness.* Indianapolis, In.: Alpha Books. *A concise guide to healthy habits, including physical activity, nutrition, and stress management.*

Newsletters

Consumer Reports on Health (800-234-2188; http://www.ConsumerReports.org)
Harvard Health Letter (800-829-9045; http://www.health.harvard.edu)
Harvard Men's Health Watch (800-829-3341)
Harvard Women's Health Watch (800-829-5921)
HealthNews (781-893-3800)
Mayo Clinic Health Letter (800-333-9037)
University of California at Berkeley Wellness Letter (386-447-6328; http://www.wellnessletter.com)

Organizations, Hotlines, and Web Sites

The Internet addresses (also called uniform resource locators, or URLs) listed here were accurate at the time of publication. Up-to-date links to these and many other wellness-oriented Web sites are provided on the links page of the *Fit and Well* Online Learning Center (http://www.mhhe.com/fahey).

Centers for Disease Control and Prevention. Through phone, fax, and the Internet, the CDC provides a wide variety of health information.
800-311-3435; 888-CDC-FAXX (CDC FAX)
http://www.cdc.gov

Many other government Web sites provide access to health-related materials:
Federal Trade Commission: http://www.ftc.gov
First Gov for Consumers—Health: http://www.consumer.gov/health.htm
National Institutes of Health: http://www.nih.gov
National Library of Medicine, MedlinePlus: http://www.medlineplus.gov

Go Ask Alice. Sponsored by the Columbia University Health Service, this site provides answers to student questions about stress, sexuality, fitness, and many other wellness topics.
http://www.goaskalice.columbia.edu

Healthfinder. A gateway to online publications, Web sites, support and self-help groups, and agencies and organizations that produce reliable health information.
http://www.healthfinder.gov

Healthy People 2010. Provides information on Healthy People objectives and priority areas.
202-205-8583
http://www.healthypeople.gov

www.mhhe.com/fahey

For Further Exploration 21

1

Introduction to Wellness, Fitness, and Lifestyle Management

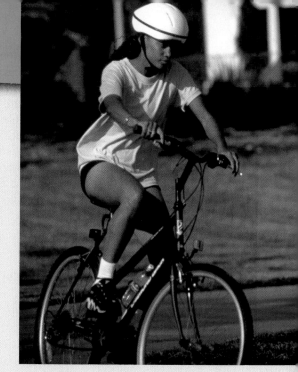

LOOKING AHEAD

After reading this chapter, you should be able to

- Describe the dimensions of wellness
- Identify the major health problems in the United States today, and discuss their causes
- Describe the behaviors that are part of a fit and well lifestyle
- Explain the steps in creating a behavior management plan to change a wellness-related behavior
- Discuss the available sources of wellness information and how to think critically about them

TEST YOUR KNOWLEDGE

1. Which of the following lifestyle factors is the leading preventable cause of death for Americans?
   a. excess alcohol consumption
   b. cigarette smoking
   c. poor dietary habits and lack of exercise

2. More than two-thirds of all college students make which of the following positive lifestyle choices?
   a. using safety belts
   b. not drinking and driving
   c. eating two or fewer high-fat foods per day
   d. not smoking cigarettes

3. Only 50% of health-related Web sites are nonpromotional and based on scientific information. True or false?

ANSWERS

1. B. Smoking causes about 435,000 deaths per year; poor diet and inactivity are responsible for about 400,000; and alcohol, about 85,000.

2. ALL FOUR. However, the majority of students do not exercise regularly, do not wear bicycle helmets, and eat few fruits and vegetables. There are many areas in which college students can change their behavior to improve their health.

3. FALSE. The number is closer to 35%. Most health-related Web sites sell products and/or are not based on scientific information.

W *Fit and Well* **Online Learning Center**   www.mhhe.com/fahey

Visit the *Fit and Well* Online Learning Center for study aids, online labs, additional information about wellness, links, Internet activities that explore the importance of a wellness lifestyle, and much more.

A first-year college student resolves to meet the challenge of making new friends. A long-sedentary senior starts riding her bike to school every day instead of taking the bus. A busy graduate student volunteers to plant trees in a blighted inner-city neighborhood. What do these people have in common? Each is striving for optimal health and well-being. Not satisfied to be merely free of major illness, these individuals want more. They want to live life actively, energetically, and fully, in a state of optimal personal, interpersonal, and environmental well-being. They have taken charge of their health and are on the path to wellness.

WELLNESS: THE NEW HEALTH GOAL

Wellness is an expanded idea of health. In the past, many people thought of health as being just the absence of physical disease. But wellness transcends this concept of health, as when individuals with serious illnesses or disabilities rise above their physical or mental limitations to live rich, meaningful, vital lives. Some aspects of health are determined by your genes, your age, and other factors that may be beyond your control. But true wellness is largely determined by the decisions you make about how to live your life. In this book, we will use the terms "health" and "wellness" interchangeably to mean the ability to live life fully—with vitality and meaning.

The Dimensions of Wellness

No matter what your age or health status, you can optimize your health in each of the following six interrelated dimensions. Wellness in any dimension is not a static goal but a dynamic process of change and growth (Figure 1.1).

Physical Wellness Optimal physical health requires eating well, exercising, avoiding harmful habits, making responsible decisions about sex, learning about and recognizing the symptoms of disease, getting regular medical and dental checkups, and taking steps to prevent injuries

at home, on the road, and on the job. The habits you develop and the decisions you make today will largely determine not only how many years you will live, but the quality of your life during those years.

Emotional Wellness Optimism, trust, self-esteem, self-acceptance, self-confidence, self-control, satisfying relationships, and an ability to share feelings are just some of the qualities and aspects of emotional wellness. Emotional wellness is a dynamic state that fluctuates with your physical, intellectual, spiritual, interpersonal and social, and environmental wellness. Maintaining emotional wellness requires monitoring and exploring your thoughts and feelings, identifying obstacles to emotional well-being, and finding solutions to emotional problems, with the help of a therapist if necessary.

Intellectual Wellness The hallmarks of intellectual health include an openness to new ideas, a capacity to question and think critically, and the motivation to master new skills, as well as a sense of humor, creativity, and curiosity. An active mind is essential to wellness; it detects problems, finds solutions, and directs behavior. People who enjoy intellectual wellness never stop learning. They seek out and relish new experiences and challenges.

Spiritual Wellness To enjoy spiritual health is to possess a set of guiding beliefs, principles, or values that give meaning and purpose to your life, especially during difficult times. Spiritual wellness involves the capacity for love, compassion, forgiveness, altruism, joy, and fulfillment. It is an antidote to cynicism, anger, fear, anxiety, self-absorption, and pessimism. Spirituality transcends the individual and can be a common bond among people. Organized religions help many people develop spiritual health, while many others find meaning and purpose in their lives on their own—through nature, art, meditation, political action, or good works.

Interpersonal and Social Wellness Satisfying relationships are basic to both physical and emotional health. We

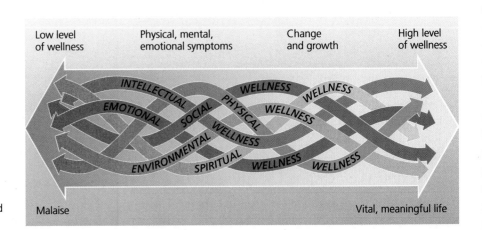

Figure 1.1 The wellness continuum.
Wellness is composed of six interrelated dimensions, all of which must be developed in order to achieve overall wellness.

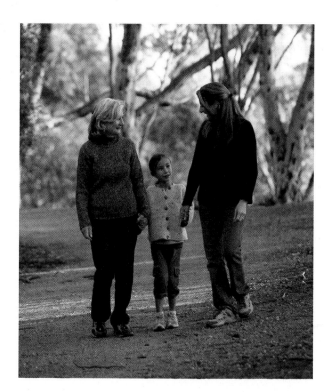
With wellness comes health and vitality throughout the life span.

need to have mutually loving, supportive people in our lives. Developing interpersonal wellness means learning good communication skills, developing the capacity for intimacy, and cultivating a support network of caring friends and/or family members. Social wellness requires participating in and contributing to your community, country, and world.

Environmental, or Planetary, Wellness Increasingly, personal health depends on the health of the planet—from the safety of the food supply to the degree of violence in a society. Other examples of environmental threats to health are ultraviolet radiation in sunlight, air and water pollution, lead in old house paint, and second-hand tobacco smoke in indoor air. Wellness requires learning about and protecting yourself against such hazards—and doing what you can to reduce or eliminate them, either on your own or with others.

The six dimensions of wellness interact continuously, influencing and being influenced by one another. For example, spiritual wellness is associated with social skills, which can help build interpersonal relationships, which are in turn linked to physical wellness and a longer life expectancy. The self-esteem that comes with emotional wellness is associated with increased physical activity and healthier eating habits, which support physical wellness. Individually and collectively, the wellness dimensions are associated with increased quality and quantity of life. Maintaining good health is a dynamic

process, and increasing your level of wellness in one area of life often influences many others. For example, regular exercise (developing the physical dimension of wellness) can increase feelings of well-being and self-esteem (emotional wellness), which in turn can increase feelings of confidence in social interactions and achievements at work or school (interpersonal and social wellness). Some of the key links among different dimensions of wellness are highlighted in this text in boxes labeled Wellness Connection.

To help discover what wellness means to you and where you currently fall on the wellness continuum, complete Lab 1.1.

New Opportunities, New Responsibilities

Wellness is a relatively recent concept. A century ago, people considered themselves lucky just to survive to adulthood (Figure 1.2, p. 4). A child born in 1900, for example, could expect to live only about 47 years. Many people died as a result of common **infectious diseases** (pneumonia, tuberculosis, diarrhea) and poor environmental conditions (unrefrigerated food, poor sanitation, air and water pollution). However, since 1900, the average life expectancy has nearly doubled, thanks largely to the development of vaccines and antibiotics to prevent and fight infectious diseases and to public health campaigns to improve environmental conditions.

But a different set of diseases has emerged as our major health threat, and heart disease, cancer, and stroke are the three leading causes of death for Americans today (Table 1.1, p. 5). Treating these and other **chronic diseases** is enormously expensive and extremely difficult. The best treatment for these diseases is prevention—people having a greater awareness about their own health and about taking care of their bodies.

The good news is that people do have some control over whether they develop cardiovascular disease (CVD), cancer, and other chronic diseases. People make choices every day that either increase or decrease their risks for these diseases—lifestyle choices involving such behaviors as exercise, diet, smoking, and drinking. When researchers look at the lifestyle factors that contribute to death in the United States (see the last column in Table 1.1), it becomes clear that individuals can profoundly influence

wellness Optimal health and vitality, encompassing physical, emotional, intellectual, spiritual, interpersonal and social, and environmental well-being.

infectious disease A disease that is communicable from one person to another; caused by invading microorganisms such as bacteria and viruses.

chronic disease A disease that develops and continues over a long period of time; usually caused by a variety of factors, including lifestyle factors.

Terms

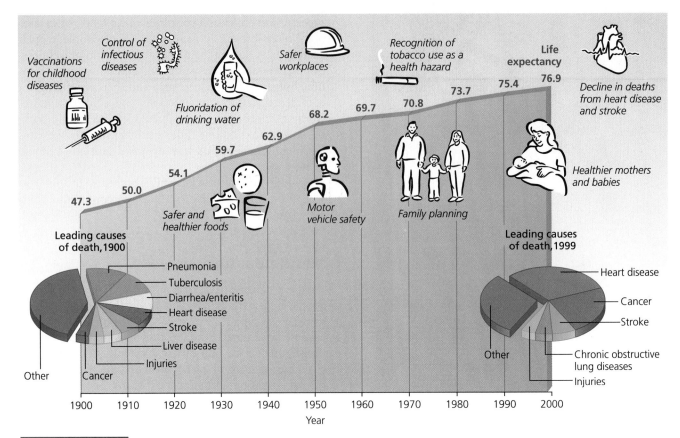

VITAL STATISTICS

Figure 1.2 Public health achievements of the twentieth century.   During the twentieth century, public health achievements greatly improved the quality of life for Americans, and life expectancy rose from 47 years to 77 years. A dramatic shift in the leading causes of death also occurred, with deaths from infectious diseases declining from more than 33% of all deaths to just 2.2%. Heart disease, cancer, and stroke are now responsible for more than 50% of all deaths among Americans.   SOURCES: National Center for Health Statistics. 2003. *Health, United States, 2003, with Chartbook on Trends in the Health of Americans.* Hyattsville, Md.: National Center for Health Statistics; Centers for Disease Control and Prevention. 1999. Ten great public health achievements—United States, 1900–1999. *Morbidity and Mortality Weekly Report* 48(50): 1141. Insel, P. M., and W. T. Roth, 2004. *Core Concepts in Health,* 9th ed. *2004 Update.* Copyright © 2004 The McGraw-Hill Companies, Inc. Reprinted with permission of The McGraw-Hill Companies, Inc.

their own health risks. Figure 1.3 (p. 6) highlights the results of just a few of the research studies that have found clear links between lifestyle behaviors and the risk of developing and dying from chronic disease. Wellness cannot be prescribed; physicians and other health care professionals can provide information, advice, and encouragement—but the rest is up to each of us.

This chapter provides an overview of a lifestyle that contributes to wellness and describes a method that can help you make lasting changes in your life to promote good health. The chapters that follow provide more detailed information about physical activity, healthy eating habits, and other components of a wellness lifestyle. The book as a whole is designed to be used to help you take charge of your behavior and improve the quality of your life—to become fit and well.

Behaviors That Contribute to Wellness

A lifestyle based on good choices and healthy behaviors maximizes the quality of life. It helps people avoid disease, remain strong and fit, and maintain their physical and mental health as long as they live. The most important behaviors and habits are described in the following sections.

Be Physically Active   The human body is designed to work best when it is active. It readily adapts to nearly any level of activity and exertion; in fact, **physical fitness** is defined as a set of physical attributes that allow the body to respond or adapt to the demands and stress of physical effort. The more we ask of our bodies—our muscles, bones, heart, lungs—the stronger and more fit they become. However, the reverse is also true: The less we ask of them, the less they can do. When our bodies are not kept active, they begin to deteriorate. Bones lose their density, joints stiffen, muscles become weak, and cellular energy systems begin to degenerate. To be truly well, human beings must be active. Unfortunately, a sedentary lifestyle is common among Americans today: More than 60% of Americans

---

Terms   **physical fitness** A set of physical attributes that allows the body to respond or adapt to the demands and stress of physical effort.

| Table 1.1 | Leading Causes of Death in the United States |

Rank	Cause of Death	Number of Deaths	Percent of Total Deaths	Female/Male Ratio[a]	Lifestyle Factors
1	Heart disease	695,754	28.4	52/48	D I S A
2	Cancer	558,847	22.8	48/52	D I S A
3	Stroke	163,010	6.7	61/39	D I S A
4	Chronic lower respiratory diseases	125,500	5.1	51/49	S
5	Unintentional injuries (accidents)	102,303	4.2	35/65	I S A
6	Diabetes mellitus	73,119	3.0	54/46	D I S
7	Influenza and pneumonia	65,984	2.6	56/44	S
8	Alzheimer's disease	58,785	2.4	71/29	
9	Kidney disease	41,018	1.7	52/48	D I S A
10	Septicemia (systemic blood infection)	33,881	1.4	56/44	A
11	Intentional self-harm (suicide)	30,646	1.3	19/81	A
12	Chronic liver disease and cirrhosis	27,045	1.1	36/64	A
13	Hypertension (high blood pressure)	20,241	0.8	62/38	D I S A
14	Pneumonia due to aspiration	17,693	0.7	50/50	
15	Assault (homicide)	17,045	0.7	23/77	A
	All causes	2,447,862			

Key
D Cause of death in which diet plays a part
I Cause of death in which an inactive lifestyle plays a part
S Cause of death in which smoking plays a part
A Cause of death in which excessive alcohol consumption plays a part

[a]Ratio of females to males who died of each cause. For example, about the same number of women and men died of heart disease, but only about half as many women as men died of unintentional injuries and four times as many men as women committed suicide.

Note: Although deaths from HIV/AIDS have declined in recent years, HIV/AIDS remains a serious public health problem, causing more than 14,000 deaths per year in the United States. It is one of the 10 leading causes of death among people between the ages of 15 and 64.

SOURCE: National Center for Health Statistics. 2004. Deaths: Preliminary data for 2002. *National Vital Statistics Report* 52(13). National Center for Health Statistics. 2003. Deaths: Final data for 2001. *National Vital Statistics Report* 52(3).

are not regularly physically active, and more than 25% are not active at all.

The benefits of physical activity are both physical and mental, immediate and long term (Figure 1.4, p. 7). In the short term, being physically fit makes it easier to do every-day tasks, such as lifting; it provides reserve strength for emergencies; and it helps people look and feel good. In the long term, being physically fit confers protection against chronic diseases and lowers the risk of dying prematurely. Physically active individuals are less likely to develop or die from heart disease, respiratory disease, high blood pressure, cancer, osteoporosis, and type 2 diabetes (the most common form of diabetes). Their cardiorespiratory systems tend to resemble those of people 10 or more years younger than themselves. As they get older, they may be able to avoid weight gain, muscle and bone loss, fatigue, and other problems associated with aging. With healthy hearts, strong muscles, lean bodies, and a repertoire of physical skills they can call on for recreation and enjoy-ment, fit people can maintain their physical and mental well-being throughout their lives.

Choose a Healthy Diet   In addition to being sedentary, many Americans have a diet that is too high in calories,

unhealthy fats, and added sugars, and too low in fiber, complex carbohydrates, fruits, and vegetables. This diet is linked to a number of chronic diseases, including heart disease, stroke, high blood pressure, type 2 diabetes, and certain kinds of cancer. It has been estimated that 15% of deaths in the United States can be attributed to poor diet combined with lack of exercise. A healthy diet promotes wellness in both the short and long term. It provides nec-essary nutrients and sufficient energy without also pro-viding too much of the dietary substances linked to diseases.

Maintain a Healthy Body Weight   Overweight and obesity are associated with a number of disabling and potentially fatal conditions and diseases, including heart disease, cancer, and type 2 diabetes. In 2004, researchers estimated that obesity kills about 400,000 Americans per year, up from 300,000 just 10 years ago; obesity may soon surpass smoking as the leading preventable cause of death in the United States. Healthy body weight is an important part of wellness—but short-term dieting is not part of a fit and well lifestyle. Maintaining a healthy body weight requires a lifelong commitment to regular exer-cise, a healthy diet, and effective stress management.

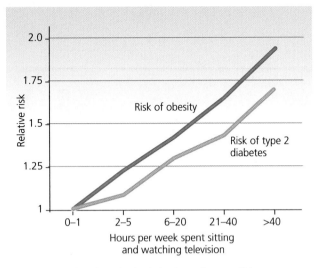

(a) Sedentary lifestyle and risk of obesity and type 2 diabetes

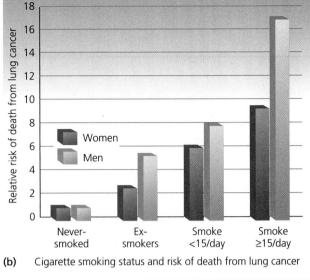

(b) Cigarette smoking status and risk of death from lung cancer

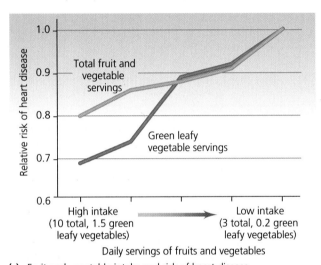

(c) Fruit and vegetable intake and risk of heart disease

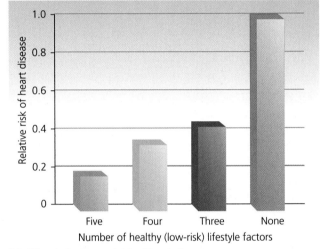

(d) Lifestyle factors and risk of heart disease

Figure 1.3 Lifestyle and risk of chronic disease. The research results shown above are just a few recent findings linking lifestyle behaviors to rates of disease and death. They indicate that (a) people who spend more time watching television are more likely to be obese and to develop type 2 diabetes; (b) people who smoke are much more likely to die of lung cancer than people who have never smoked or who have quit; (c) people who consume diets rich in fruits and vegetables, particularly green leafy vegetables, reduce their risk of heart disease; and (d) people who engage in a combination of healthy lifestyle behaviors have an 82% lower risk of heart disease than those who do not engage in such behaviors. The five lifestyle factors examined in this study were the participation in regular physical activity, the avoidance of smoking, and the maintenance of a healthy diet, body weight, and level of alcohol consumption.   SOURCES: (a) Hu, F. B., et al. 2003. Television watching and other sedentary behaviors in relation to risk of obesity and type 2 diabetes mellitus in women. *Journal of the American Medical Association* 289(14): 1785–1791. (b) Prescott, E., et al. 1998. Mortality in women and men in relation to smoking. *International Epidemiological Association* 27: 27–32. (c) Joshipura, K.J., et al. 2001. The effect of fruit and vegetable intake on risk for coronary heart disease. *Annals of Internal Medicine* 134: 1106–1114. (d) Stampfer, M. J., et al. 2000. Primary prevention of coronary heart disease in women through diet and lifestyle. *New England Journal of Medicine* 343(1): 16–22.

Manage Stress Effectively Many people cope with stress by eating, drinking, or smoking too much. Others don't deal with it at all. In the short term, inappropriate stress management can lead to fatigue, sleep disturbances, and other unpleasant symptoms. Over longer periods of time, poor management of stress can lead to less efficient functioning of the immune system and increased susceptibility to disease. There *are* effective ways to handle stress, and learning to incorporate them into daily life is an important part of a fit and well lifestyle.

Avoid Tobacco and Drug Use and Limit Alcohol Consumption Tobacco use is associated with 8 of the top 10 causes of death in the United States; it kills about 435,000 Americans each year, more than any other behavioral or environmental factor. A hundred years ago, before cigarette smoking was widespread, lung cancer was considered a rare disease. Today, with nearly 25% of the American population smoking, lung cancer is the most common cause of cancer death among both men and women and one of the leading causes of death overall.

- Increased endurance, strength, and flexibility
- Healthier muscles, bones, and joints
- Increased energy (calorie) expenditure
- Improved body composition
- More energy
- Improved ability to cope with stress
- Improved mood, greater self-esteem, and a greater sense of well-being
- Improved ability to fall asleep and sleep well

- Reduced risk of dying prematurely from all causes
- Reduced risk of developing and/or dying from heart disease, diabetes, high blood pressure, and colon cancer
- Reduced risk of becoming obese
- Reduced anxiety, tension, and depression
- Reduced risk of falls and fractures
- Reduced spending for health care

Figure 1.4   Benefits of regular physical activity.

Excessive alcohol consumption is linked to 6 of the top 10 causes of death and results in about 85,000 deaths a year in the United States. Alcohol or drug intoxication is an especially notable factor in the death and disability of young people, particularly through **unintentional injuries** (such as drownings and car crashes caused by drunken driving) and violence. Unintentional injuries, homicide, and suicide are the top three leading causes of death for 15- to 34-year-olds; in this age group, the mortality rate for males is more than twice that for females.

Protect Yourself from Disease and Injury   The most effective way of dealing with disease and injury is to prevent them. Many of the lifestyle strategies discussed here—being physically active, managing body weight, and so on—help protect you against chronic illnesses. In addition, you can take specific steps to avoid infectious diseases, particularly those that are sexually transmitted. These diseases are preventable through responsible sexual behavior, another component of a fit and well lifestyle.

Unintentional injuries are the leading cause of death for people age 45 and under, but they, too, can be prevented. Learning and adopting safe, responsible behaviors is also part of a fit and well lifestyle.

Other important behaviors in a fit and well lifestyle include developing meaningful relationships, planning ahead for successful aging, becoming knowledgeable about the health care system, and acting responsibly in relation to the environment. Lab 1.2 will help you evaluate your behaviors as they relate to wellness.

The Role of Other Factors in Wellness

Of course, behavior isn't the only factor involved in good health. Heredity, the environment, and access to adequate health care are other important influences. These factors can interact in ways that raise or lower the quality of a person's life and the risk of developing particular diseases.

For example, a sedentary lifestyle combined with a genetic predisposition for diabetes can greatly increase a person's risk for developing the disease. If this person also lacks adequate health care, he or she is much more likely to suffer dangerous complications from diabetes and to have a lower quality of life.

But in many cases, behavior can tip the balance toward health even if heredity or environment is a negative factor. Breast cancer, for example, can run in families, but it is also associated with overweight and a sedentary lifestyle. A woman with a family history of breast cancer is less likely to die from the disease if she controls her weight, exercises, performs regular breast self-exams, and consults with her physician about mammograms. By learning about her family history and taking action, this woman can influence the effects of heredity on her health.

MOTIVATION FOR CHANGE!   Do you know your family health history? Learning about the diseases and health conditions that run in your family can help you start thinking about improving your lifestyle because such knowledge helps you understand the health risks you may face in the future. For the same reason, it can also help motivate you to keep a behavior change program on track. Put together a simple family health tree by plugging key health information on your close relatives—siblings, parents, aunts and uncles, grandparents—into a family tree format. Don't focus only on causes of death. Look at all chronic conditions and key health-related behaviors that affect both quality and quantity of life; for example, record such things as alcoholism, diabetes, high blood pressure, high cholesterol, obesity, osteoporosis, and depression. What patterns do you see?

unintentional injury An injury that occurs without harm being intended.

Terms

National Wellness Goals

You may think of health and wellness as personal concerns, goals that you strive for on your own for your own benefit. But the U.S. government also has a vital interest in the health of all Americans. A healthy population is the nation's greatest resource, the source of its vigor and wealth. Poor health, in contrast, drains the nation's resources and raises national health care costs. As the embodiment of our society's values, the federal government also has a humane interest in people's health.

The U.S. government's national Healthy People initiative seeks to prevent unnecessary disease and disability and to achieve a better quality of life for all Americans. Healthy People reports, published first in 1980 and revised every decade, set national health goals based on 10-year agendas. Each report includes both broad goals and specific targets in many different areas of wellness. The latest report, *Healthy People 2010,* proposes two broad national goals:

* *Increase quality and years of healthy life.* The life expectancy of Americans has increased significantly in the past century; however, people can expect poor health to limit their activities and cause distress during the last 15% of their lives (Figure 1.5). Health-related quality of life calls for a full range of functional capacity to enable people to work, play, and maintain satisfying relationships.

* *Eliminate health disparities among Americans.* Many health problems today disproportionately affect certain American populations (see the box "Wellness Issues for Diverse Populations"). *Healthy People 2010* calls for elim-

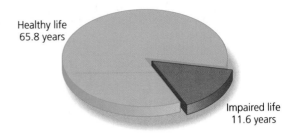

Healthy life
65.8 years

Impaired life
11.6 years

Life expectancy
77.4 years

VITAL STATISTICS

Figure 1.5 Quantity of life versus quality of life. Years of healthy life as a proportion of life expectancy in the U.S. population. SOURCES: National Center for Health Statistics. 2004. Deaths: preliminary data for 2002. *National Vital Statistics Reports* 52(13). National Center for Health Statistics. 2001. *Healthy People 2000 Final Review.* Hyattsville, Md.: Public Health Service.

inating disparities in health status, health risks, and use of preventive services among all population groups within the next decade.

Examples of individual health promotion objectives from *Healthy People 2010,* as well as estimates of how we are tracking toward the goals, appear in Table 1.2. As you can see, the objectives are tied closely to the wellness lifestyle described in this chapter. The principal topics covered in this book parallel the priority concerns of the Healthy People initiative, and the approach of *Fit and Well* is based on the initiative's premise that personal responsibility is a key to achieving wellness.

Table 1.2	Selected Healthy People 2010 Objectives		
Objective		**Estimate of Current Status (%)**	**Goal (%)**
Increase the proportion of people age 18 and older who engage regularly in moderate or vigorous physical activity.		32	50
Increase the proportion of people age 2 and older who consume at least 3 daily servings of vegetables, with at least one-third being dark-green or orange vegetables.		3	50
Increase the prevalence of healthy weight among all people age 20 and older.		34	60
Reduce the proportion of adults 18 and older who use cigarettes.		23	12
Reduce the proportion of college students reporting binge drinking during the past 2 weeks.		40	20
Increase the proportion of sexually active persons who use condoms.		23	50
Increase the proportion of adults who take protective measures to reduce the risk of skin cancer (sunscreens, sun-protective clothing, and so on).		58	75
Increase the use of safety belts by motor vehicle occupants.		75	92
Increase the number of residences with a functioning smoke alarm on every floor.		87	100
Increase the proportion of persons with health insurance.		84	100

SOURCE: National Center for Health Statistics. 2004. *DATA 2010: The Healthy People 2010 Database, January 2004 Edition* (http://wonder.cdc.gov/data2010/obj.htm; retrieved April 6, 2004).

When it comes to striving for wellness, most differences among people are insignificant. We all need to exercise, eat well, and manage stress. We need to know how to protect ourselves from heart disease, cancer, sexually transmitted diseases, and injuries.

But some of our differences—differences among us both as individuals and as members of groups—do have implications for wellness. Some of us, for example, have grown up with eating habits that increase our risk of obesity or heart disease. Some of us have inherited predispositions for certain health problems, such as osteoporosis or high cholesterol levels. These health-related differences among individuals and groups can be biological—determined genetically—or cultural—acquired as patterns of behavior through daily interactions with our family, community, and society. Many health conditions are a function of biology and culture combined.

When we talk about wellness issues as they relate to diverse populations, we face two related dangers. The first is the danger of stereotyping, of talking about people as groups rather than as individuals. The second is that of overgeneralizing, of ignoring the extensive biological and cultural diversity that exists among people who may be grouped together because of their gender, socioeconomic status, or ethnicity. Every person is an individual with her or his own unique genetic endowment as well as unique experiences in life. However, many of these influences are shared with others of similar genetic and cultural backgrounds. Information about group similarities relating to wellness issues can be useful; for example, it can alert people to areas that may be of special concern for them and their families.

Wellness-related differences among groups can be identified and described along several different dimensions, including the following:

- *Gender.* Men and women have different life expectancies and different incidences of many diseases, including heart disease, cancer, and osteoporosis. Men have higher rates of death from injuries, suicide, and homicide; women are at greater risk for Alzheimer's disease and for depression. Men and women also differ in body composition and certain aspects of physical performance.

- *Ethnicity.* A genetic predisposition for a particular health problem can be linked to ethnicity as a result of each ethnic group's relatively distinct history. Diabetes is more prevalent among individuals of Native American or Latino heritage, for example, and African Americans have higher rates of hypertension. Ethnic groups may also vary in other ways that relate to wellness: traditional diets; patterns of family and interpersonal relationships; and attitudes toward using tobacco, alcohol, and other drugs, to name just a few.

- *Income and education.* Inequalities in income and education are closely related and underlie many of the health disparities among Americans. People with low incomes and less education have higher rates of injury and many diseases, are more likely to engage in unhealthy behaviors such as smoking, and have less access to health care services. Poverty and low educational attainment are far more important predictors of poor health than any ethnic factor.

These are just some of the "dimensions of diversity"—differences among people and groups that are associated with different wellness concerns. Other factors, too, such as age, geographic location, sexual orientation, and disability, can present challenges as an individual strives for wellness. In this book, topics and issues relating to wellness that affect different American populations are given special consideration in boxes labeled Dimensions of Diversity. These discussions are designed to deepen our understanding of the concepts of wellness and vitality in the context of ever-growing diversity in the population.

REACHING WELLNESS THROUGH LIFESTYLE MANAGEMENT

Your life may not resemble the picture drawn here of a fit and well lifestyle at all. You probably have a number of healthy habits and some others that place your health at risk. Taking big steps toward a wellness lifestyle may at first seem like too much work, but as you make progress, it gets easier. At first, you'll be rewarded with a greater sense of control over your life, a feeling of empowerment, higher self-esteem, and more joy. These benefits will encourage you to make further improvements. Over time, you'll come to know what wellness feels like—more energy, greater vitality; deeper feelings of curiosity, interest, and enjoyment; and a higher quality of life.

This section introduces the general process of behavior change and highlights the decisions and challenges you'll face at each stage. For additional help and advice, work through the activities in the Behavior Change Workbook located at the end of the text and on the Online Learning Center.

Getting Serious About Your Health

Before you can start changing a wellness-related behavior, you have to know that the behavior is problematic and that you *can* change it. To make good decisions, you need information about relevant topics and issues, including what resources are available to help you change.

Examining Your Current Health Habits   Have you considered how your current lifestyle is affecting your health today and how it will affect your health in the future? Do you know which of your current habits enhance your health and which detract from it? Begin your journey toward wellness with self-assessment: Think about your own behavior, complete the self-assessment in Lab 1.2, and talk with friends and family members about what they've noticed about your lifestyle and your health.

Many people start to consider changing a behavior when they get help from others. An observation from a friend, family member, or physician can help you see yourself as others do and may get you thinking about your behavior in a new way. For example, Jason has been getting a lot of stomachaches lately. His girlfriend, Anna, notices other changes as well and suggests that the stress of classes plus a part-time job and serving as president of the school radio station might be causing some of Jason's problems. Jason never thought much about trying to control the stressors in his life, but with encouragement from Anna he starts noticing what events trigger stress for him.

Landmark events such as a birthday, the birth of a child, or the death of someone close to you, can get you thinking about behavior change. New information can also help you get started. As you read this text, you may find yourself reevaluating some of your wellness-related behaviors. This could be a great opportunity to make healthful changes that will stay with you for the rest of your life.

Choosing a Target Behavior   To maximize your chances of success, don't try to change all your problem behaviors at once—start exercising, quit smoking, give up high-fat foods, avoid drugs, get more sleep. Working on just one behavior will make high demands on your energy. Concentrate on one behavior that you want to change, your **target behavior,** and work on it systematically. Start with something simple, like snacking on candy between afternoon classes or always driving to a particular class instead of walking or biking.

Obtaining Information About Your Target Behavior
Once you've chosen a target behavior, you need to find out more about it. You need to know its risks and benefits for you—both now and in the future. How is your target behavior affecting your level of wellness today? What diseases or conditions does this behavior place you at risk for? What effect would changing your behavior have on your health? As a starting point, use material from this text and from the resources listed in the For Further Exploration section at the end of each chapter; refer to the box "Evaluating Sources of Health Information" for additional guidelines.

Finding Outside Help   Have you identified a particularly challenging target behavior, something like alcohol addiction, binge eating, or depression, that interferes with your ability to function or places you at a serious health risk? Outside help is often needed to change behaviors or conditions that may be too deeply rooted or too serious

for a self-management approach. If this is the case, don't be stopped by the seriousness of the problem—there are many resources available to help you solve it. On campus, the student health center or campus counseling center can provide assistance. To locate community resources, consult the yellow pages, your physician, your local health department, or the United Way.

Building Motivation to Change

Knowledge is a necessary ingredient for behavior change, but it isn't usually enough to make people act. Millions of people smoke or have sedentary lifestyles, for example, even though they know it's bad for their health. This is particularly true of young adults, who may not be motivated to change because they feel well despite engaging in unhealthy behaviors (see the box "Lifestyle Matters for Young Adults" on p. 12). To succeed at behavior change, you need strong motivation.

Examining the Pros and Cons of Change   Health behaviors have short-term and long-term benefits and costs. For example, in the short term, an inactive lifestyle allows more time to watch TV and hang out with friends but leaves a person less able to participate in recreational activities. In the long term, it increases risk of heart disease, cancer, stroke, and premature death. For successful behavior change, you must believe that the benefits of changing outweigh the costs.

Do a careful analysis of the short-term and long-term benefits and costs of continuing your current (target) behavior and of changing to a new, healthier behavior. Focus on the effects that are most meaningful to you, including those that are tied to your personal identity and values. For example, if you see yourself as an active person who is a good role model for others, then adopting behaviors such as regular physical activity and getting adequate sleep would support your personal identity. If you value independence and control over your life, then quitting smoking would be consistent with your values and goals. To complete your analysis, ask friends and family members about the effects of your behavior on them. For example, a younger sister may tell you that your smoking habit influenced her decision to take up smoking.

Pay special attention to the short-term benefits of behavior change, as these can be an important motivating force. Although some people are motivated by long-term goals, such as avoiding a disease that may hit them in 30 years, most are more likely to be moved to action by shorter-term, more personal goals. Feeling better, doing better in school, improving at a sport, reducing stress, and increasing self-esteem are common short-term benefits of health behavior change. Many wellness behaviors are associated with immediate improvements in quality of life. For example, surveys of Americans have found that nonsmokers feel healthy and full of energy more days each month than do smokers, and they report fewer days of sadness and troubled sleep; the same is true when

target behavior An isolated behavior selected as the object for a behavior change program.

General Strategies

A key first step in sharpening your critical thinking skills is to look carefully at your sources of wellness information. Critical thinking involves knowing where and how to find relevant information, how to separate fact from opinion, how to recognize faulty reasoning, how to evaluate information, and how to assess the credibility of sources.

- *Go to the original source.* Media reports often simplify the results of medical research. Find out for yourself what a study really reported, and determine whether it was based on good science. What type of study was it? Was it published in a recognized medical journal? Was it an animal study or did it involve people? Did the study include a large number of people? What did the authors of the study actually report in their findings? (You'll find additional strategies for evaluating research studies in Chapter 11.)

- *Watch for misleading language.* Reports that feature "breakthroughs" or "dramatic proof" are probably hype. Some studies will find that a behavior "contributes to" or is "associated with" an outcome; this does not imply a proven cause-and-effect relationship.

- *Distinguish between research reports and public health advice.* If a study finds a link between a particular vitamin and cancer, that should not necessarily lead you to change your behavior. But if the Surgeon General or the American Cancer Society advises you to eat less fat or quit smoking, you can assume that many studies point in this direction and that this is advice you should follow.

- *Remember that anecdotes are not facts.* Sometimes we do get helpful health information from our friends and family. But just because your cousin Bertha lost 10 pounds on Dr. Amazing's new protein diet doesn't mean it's a safe, effective way for you to lose weight. Before you make a big change in your lifestyle, verify the information with your physician or other reliable sources.

- *Be skeptical and use your common sense.* If a report seems too good to be true, it probably is. Be especially wary of information contained in advertisements. The goal of an ad is to sell you something, to create a feeling of need for a product where no real need exists.

- *Make choices that are right for you.* Your roommate swears by swimming; you prefer aerobics. Your sister takes a yoga class to help her manage stress; your brother unwinds by walking in the woods. Friends and family members can be a great source of ideas and inspiration, but each of us needs to find a wellness lifestyle that works for us.

Internet Resources

Evaluating health information from online sources poses special challenges; when reviewing a health-related Web site, ask the following questions:

- *What is the source of the information? Who is the author or sponsor of the Web page?* Web sites maintained by government agencies, professional associations, or established academic or medical institutions are likely to present trustworthy information. Many other groups and individuals post accurate information, but it is important to look at the qualifications of the people who are behind the site. (Check the home page or click on an "about us" or "who we are" link.)

- *How often is the site updated?* Look for sites that are updated frequently. Also check the "last modified" date of any specific Web page on a site.

- *What is the purpose of the page? Does the site promote particular products or procedures? Are there obvious reasons for bias?* Be wary of information from sites that sell specific products, use testimonials as evidence, appear to have a social or political agenda, or ask for money.

- *What do other sources say about a topic?* Be cautious of claims or information that appear at only one site or come from a chat room or bulletin board.

- *Does the site conform to any set of guidelines or criteria for quality and accuracy?* Look for sites that identify themselves as conforming to some code or set of principles, such as those set forth by the Health on the Net Foundation or the American Medical Association. These codes include criteria such as use of information from respected sources and disclosure of the site's sponsors.

---

physically active people are compared with sedentary people. Over time, these types of differences add up to a substantially greater quality of life for people who engage in healthy behaviors.

You can further strengthen your motivation by raising your consciousness about your problem behavior. This will enable you to focus on the negatives of the behavior and imagine the consequences if you don't make a change. At the same time, you can visualize the positive results of changing your behavior. Ask yourself: What do I want for myself, now and in the future?

For example, Ruby has never worried much about her smoking because the problems associated with it seem so far away. But lately she's noticed her performance on the volleyball team isn't as good as it used to be. Over the summer she visited her aunt, who has chronic emphysema from smoking and can barely leave her bed. Ruby knows she wants to have children and a career as a teacher someday, and seeing her aunt makes her wonder if her smoking habit could make it difficult for her to reach these goals. She starts to wonder whether her smoking habit is worth the short- and long-term sacrifices.

Social pressures can also increase the motivation to make changes. In Ruby's case, anti-smoking ordinances make it impossible for her to smoke in her dorm and in

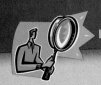
Take a good look at the next group of college students you see. Chances are, they all look pretty healthy. But if you could look inside their cells and vital organs, you would see that the external appearance of health can be deceiving. Some students would have noticeable layers of fat and scar tissue lining blood vessels, including the crucial arteries that supply blood to the heart and brain. You can safely predict that a number of these students will have heart attacks or strokes when they hit middle age. Nearly all the students would have microscopic evidence of sun damage on their skin, and a few would have the early cellular changes associated with skin cancer. If you could train your super vision on their skeletons, you would detect that some students have weaker, thinner bones—not noticeable to them now but likely to result in osteoporosis and the potential for serious fractures later in life. In some students, you would also detect something slightly amiss in the balance of sugar and insulin in their blood and tissue. Students in this group are more likely to later develop diabetes.

You might think that this group of college students—with so many impending health problems—is unusual, but unfortunately, these students are similar to the majority of young adults in the United States. Most apparently healthy young people harbor early signs of serious chronic diseases that will become obvious later in life. However, the good news is that if you make some changes now in your daily habits, you can prevent or delay the onset of nearly all of these common diseases.

What does it take to stave off the typical illnesses of middle and old age? As described in the section on behaviors that contribute to wellness, the answer is less complicated than you might have thought. Lifestyle choices you make daily throughout your life can make a tremendous difference. You can choose to be a nonsmoker, to eat a healthy diet, to keep your weight under control, to wear sunscreen and protective clothing when out in the sun, and so on. If you are successful in following the guidelines for wellness behaviors most of the time, your odds for a long and vigorous life will increase dramatically.

Unfortunately, knowing what we should do to protect our health in later years is often not enough to get us to change our habits. Most of us need a more immediate payoff to get motivated. So consider all the reasons why healthy behaviors are a plus for you today as well as for your future self. For example, if you've felt tired and blue lately, being physically active is almost certain to provide you with an infusion of energy and feelings of well-being. Keeping fit will also allow you to fully enjoy your favorite activities. If you love to ski, remember that if you are in shape when you hit the slopes, you will ski better, have more fun, experience less fatigue and soreness, and be less likely to get injured. What if you want to take a hike in the mountains or learn to windsurf? Being regularly active will make it much more likely that these experiences will be exhilarating rather than merely exhausting. Everyday chores, such as hauling your books around, cleaning, and carrying groceries or children, are much easier if you are active. Life's daily activities are more satisfying when you have the strength, energy, and confidence to handle them with ease.

Think about what might motivate you to make healthy changes in your life. Have you seen the quality of life of members of your family affected by chronic diseases? Knowing that a particular disease runs in your family can help guide your priorities and motivate you to make healthy changes. You might also find motivation from thinking about the benefits for your loved ones. Consider the examples of a pregnant smoker who is finally able to quit for good when she becomes aware that smoking is harmful to her baby, and a couch potato who becomes inspired to increase his activity level in order to keep up with his kids.

Don't feel overwhelmed by the description of a wellness lifestyle and think that you must change all your bad habits at once or overhaul your lifestyle completely. Studies show that even small improvements in your lifestyle can make a big difference in your health. Start by making a few positive changes. Your efforts will be rewarded—you'll feel better now, and you will continue to reap the benefits throughout your life.

---

many public places. The inconvenience of finding a place to smoke—and pressure from her roommate, who doesn't like the smoky smell of Ruby's clothes in their room—add to Ruby's motivation to quit.

Boosting Self-Efficacy   When you start thinking about changing a health behavior, a big factor in your eventual success is whether you have confidence in yourself and in your ability to change. **Self-efficacy** refers to your belief in your ability to successfully take action and perform a specific task. Strategies for boosting self-efficacy include developing an internal locus of control, using visualization and self-talk, and obtaining encouragement from supportive people.

Locus of Control   Who do you believe is controlling your life? Is it your parents, friends, or school? Is it "fate"? Or is it you? **Locus of control** refers to the figurative "place" a person designates as the source of responsibility for the events in his or her life. People who believe they are in control of their own lives are said to have an internal locus of control. Those who believe that factors beyond their control—heredity, friends and family, the environment, fate, luck, or other outside forces—are more important in determining the events of their lives are said to have an external locus of control.

For lifestyle management, an internal locus of control is an advantage because it reinforces motivation and commitment. An external locus of control can sabotage efforts to change behavior. For example, if you believe you are destined to die of breast cancer because your mother died from the disease, you may view monthly breast self-exams and regular checkups as a waste of time. In contrast, if you believe you can take action to reduce your hereditary risk of breast cancer, you will be motivated to follow guidelines for early detection of the disease.

If you find yourself attributing too much influence to outside forces, gather more information about your wellness-related behaviors. List all the ways that making lifestyle changes will improve your health. If you believe you'll succeed, and if you recognize and accept that you are in charge of your life, you're on your way to wellness.

VISUALIZATION AND SELF-TALK   One of the best ways to boost your confidence and self-efficacy is to visualize yourself successfully engaging in a new, healthier behavior. Imagine yourself going for a regular after-dinner walk or choosing healthier snacks. Also visualize yourself enjoying all the short-term and long-term benefits that your lifestyle change will bring. Create a new self-image: What will you and your life be like when you become a regular exerciser or a healthy eater?

You can also use self-talk, the internal dialogue you carry on with yourself, to increase your confidence in your ability to change. Counter any self-defeating patterns of thought with more positive or realistic thoughts: "I am a strong, capable person, and I can maintain my commitment to change." Refer to Chapter 10 for more on self-talk.

ROLE MODELS AND OTHER SUPPORTIVE INDIVIDUALS   Social support can make a big difference in your level of motivation and your chances of success. Perhaps you know people who have reached the goal you are striving for; they could be role models or mentors for you, providing information and support for your efforts. Gain strength from their experiences, and tell yourself, "If they can do it, so can I." In addition, find a buddy who wants to make the same changes you do and who can take an active role in your behavior change program. For example, an exercise buddy can provide companionship and encouragement for times when you might be tempted to skip your workout.

MOTIVATION FOR CHANGE!   Observation of people who are successful at what you are trying to do can suggest strategies you can try as well as boost your self-confidence and self-efficacy. For example, when you see physically active people on campus, note in what activities they are engaged and where and at what time of day they are active. Watch people who appear to be successful at weight management—what foods do they choose at the cafeteria or food court, how large are their portions, and do they finish everything? Choose people to observe who are similar to yourself in key characteristics—age, gender, level of fitness, and so on.

Identifying and Overcoming Key Barriers to Change

Don't let past failures at behavior change discourage you; they can be a great source of information you can use to boost your chances of future success. Make a list of the problems and challenges you faced in your previous behavior change attempts; to this, add the short-term costs of behavior change that you identified in your analysis of the pros and cons of change. Once you've listed these key barriers to change, develop a practical plan for overcoming each one. For example, if you always smoke when you're with certain friends, practice in advance how you will turn down the next cigarette you are offered.

Self-talk can also help overcome barriers. Make behavior change a priority in your life and plan to commit the necessary time and effort. Ask yourself: How much time and energy will behavior change *really* require? Isn't the effort worth the short- and long-term benefits?

Enhancing Your Readiness to Change

The transtheoretical, or "stages of change," model has been shown to be an effective approach to lifestyle self-management. According to this model, you move through distinct stages as you work to change your target behavior. Starting at the wrong stage or moving too quickly through the stages can reduce the likelihood that you'll succeed in changing your behavior. Read the descriptions of the stages below to determine at what stage you find yourself for the target behavior you've selected. To move forward in the cycle of change, try the techniques and strategies in the box "Tips for Moving Forward in the Cycle of Behavior Change" (p. 14). You may find it helpful to work through the strategies for all the stages. You'll find additional suggestions for successful behavior change in the next section of the chapter.

Precontemplation: No Intention of Changing Behavior
People at this stage do not intend to change their behavior. They may be unaware of the risks associated with their behavior, or they may deny that their behavior will have any serious consequences for them. They may have tried unsuccessfully to change in the past and may now feel demoralized and think the situation is hopeless. They may also blame other people or external factors for their problems. People in the precontemplation stage believe that there are more reasons or more important reasons not to change than there are reasons to change.

Contemplation: Intending to Take Action Within 6 Months   People at this stage are aware that they have a problem and have started to think and learn about it. They acknowledge the benefits that behavior change will have for them but are also very aware of the costs of changing—to be successful, people must believe that the benefits of change outweigh the costs. People in the contemplation stage wonder about possible courses of action but may feel unsure of how to proceed. There may also be specific barriers to change that appear too difficult to overcome.

---

self-efficacy The belief in one's ability to take action and perform a specific behavior.

locus of control The figurative "place" a person designates as the source of responsibility for the events in his or her life.

Terms

Precontemplation

• Raise your awareness of your target behavior and its effects on you and others. Research the ways it affects you now and how it may affect you in the future.

• Examine the defense mechanisms you use to resist change; examples include denying the consequences of your behavior and rationalizing your reasons for not changing. Develop a strategy for overcoming each of your key mental defenses. For example, "I don't exercise because I don't have time—*but* I could reduce my TV time by 30 minutes a day and go for a walk instead." Or, "I currently eat fast food every day because there are no healthier lunch options on campus—*but* I could pack up a sandwich and fruit in the morning and bring it with me for lunch." Work to recognize the difference between true barriers to your effort to change and the excuses you create to resist change.

• Talk to friends and family members about your interest in behavior change. The people around you may be very aware of your target behavior and may have insights into how you typically rationalize your choices.

• Identify relevant campus and community resources—for example, an exercise class offered by the physical education department or a stop-smoking or stress-management workshop offered by the student health center.

Contemplation

• Begin keeping a written record of your target behavior and the circumstances surrounding it to help you learn more about the behavior and to use when you begin to plan the specifics of your behavior change program.

• Complete a cost-benefit analysis of the pros and cons of your target behavior and of changing it. Examine both the present and the future in your analysis. Don't forget to include factors tied to your self-image, to how you feel about yourself, and to how your behavior affects others. Does your current behavior support your image of yourself as a responsible, healthy person? If not, can you continue to feel good about yourself if you don't change?

• Identify key barriers to change, and find options, alternatives, and strategies that can be used to overcome these barriers.

• Engage your emotions through such strategies as imagining what your life might be like if you were not to change, watching movies related to your target behavior, and reviewing certain effects of your behavior—for example, look at the residue left by cigarette smoke blown or tobacco juice spit into a white handkerchief, have someone videotape you while you are drunk or hung over and watch the tape, make a pile of the amount of candy or junk food you eat in a month, etc.

• Boost self-efficacy and begin to create a new self-image by imagining yourself and your life after you change your target behavior. Identify strategies that helped you make positive changes in the past; link your current effort to past successes.

• Think before you act, and avoid reflex behaviors. Ask yourself why you are engaging in your target behavior.

• Enlist the help of friends and family members to identify the causes and consequences of your target behavior.

Preparation

• Create a specific plan for change that includes a start date, realistic goals, rewards, and information on exactly how you will go about changing your behavior (see the section in Chapter 1 on creating a personalized plan). Make sure you have all the information and equipment called for in your plan.

• Make change a priority in your life, and commit the necessary time and effort to change. Create and sign a contract.

• Practice visualization and self-talk to prepare yourself for the change you'll be making. Imagine yourself in challenging situations—surrounded by smoking friends when you are trying to quit or invited for a late-night pizza when you are trying to cut back on snacking—and mentally prepare yourself for appropriate action.

• Try your desired behavior for a day or a week; even a brief period of success will help boost self-efficacy.

• Tell the people in your life about the change you'll be making. Ask for help, specifying both dos and don'ts.

Action

• Monitor your behavior and your program's progress.

• Make changes in your environment that will discourage your target behavior and encourage healthier responses. Plan ahead to help overcome difficult situations.

• Find alternatives for your target behavior. For example, if you typically overeat or binge drink to manage stress, substitute a walk or a relaxation technique for the target behavior. Work on developing an internal locus of control and an appropriate degree of assertiveness—believe that you can control your own behavior and help shape your environment.

• Give yourself the rewards you named in your contract as well as plenty of self-praise. Keep a positive attitude about yourself and the change you are attempting. Manage your stress level, and don't let yourself get overwhelmed. Focus on the benefits you've already obtained from your new behavior.

• Involve the people around you. Arrange with someone to join your program as a buddy and/or find a role model who has already made the change you are working toward and who can provide both inspiration and practical advice.

• Don't get discouraged if your program is difficult or if you experience brief lapses—the action stage typically lasts for at least several months. Real change is difficult.

Maintenance

• Continue with all the positive strategies you used in earlier stages—monitor your behavior with a journal, manage your environment, and practice realistic self-talk.

• Be prepared for complications and lapses, but don't let a slip set you back. As you continue on with your program, your confidence and self-efficacy will increase, and you'll be less likely to slip. But don't let continued success allow you to forget about the negative aspects of your original (target) behavior and the effort required to change it.

• Act as a role model and help someone else make a positive lifestyle change.

SOURCES: Marcus, B. H., and L. H. Forsyth. 2003. *Motivating People to Be Physically Active.* Champaign, Ill.: Human Kinetics. Sarafino, E. P. 2001. *Behavior Modification: Understanding Principles of Behavior Change.* Mountain View, Calif.: Mayfield. Centers for Disease Control and Prevention, Division of Nutrition and Physical Activity. 1999. *Promoting Physical Activity: A Guide for Community Action.* Champaign, Ill.: Human Kinetics. Prochaska, J. O., J. C. Norcross, and C. C. DiClemente. 1994. *Changing for Good: A Revolutionary Six-Stage Program for Overcoming Bad Habits and Moving Your Life Positively Forward.* New York: Avon Books.

Date _____November 5_____   Day M (TU) W TH F SA SU

Time of day	M/S	Food eaten	Cals.	H	Where did you eat?	What else were you doing?	How did someone else influence you?	What made you want to eat what you did?	Emotions and feelings?	Thoughts and concerns?
7:30	M	1 C Crispix cereal 1/2 C skim milk coffee, black 1 C orange juice	110 40 — 120	3	dorm cafeteria	reading newspaper	eating w/ friends, but I ate what I usually eat	I always eat cereal in the morning	a little keyed up & worried	thinking about quiz in class today
10:30	S	1 apple	90	1	library	studying	alone	felt tired & wanted to wake up	tired	worried about next class
12:30	M	1 C chili 1 roll 1 pat butter 1 orange 2 oatmeal cookies 1 soda	290 120 35 60 120 150	2	cafeteria terrace	talking	eating w/ friends; we decided to eat at the cafeteria	wanted to be part of group	excited and happy	interested in hearing everyone's plans for the weekend

M/S = Meal or snack   H = Hunger rating (0–3)

Figure 1.6 Sample health journal entries.

Preparation: Planning to Take Action Within a Month
People at this stage plan to take action within a month or may already have begun to make small changes in their behavior. They may be engaging in their new, healthier behavior, but not yet regularly or consistently. They may have created a plan for change but may be uncertain or anxious about the possibility of successful behavior change.

Action: Outwardly Changing Behavior During the action stage, people outwardly modify their behavior and their environment. The action stage usually requires the greatest commitment of time and energy, and people in this stage are at risk for reverting to old, unhealthy patterns of behavior.

Maintenance: Successful Behavior Change for 6 Months or More People at this stage have maintained their new, healthier lifestyle for at least 6 months. Lapses may have occurred, but people in maintenance have been successful in quickly reestablishing the desired behavior. The maintenance stage typically lasts from 6 months to about 5 years or longer.

Termination For some behaviors, such as addictions, a person may reach the sixth and final stage of termination. People at this stage have exited the cycle of change and are no longer tempted to lapse back into their old behavior. They have a new self-image and total self-efficacy with regard to their target behavior.

Lapses are a natural part of the process at all stages of change. Many people lapse and must recycle through earlier stages, although most don't go back to the first stage. If you lapse, use what you learn about yourself and the process of change to help you in your next attempt.

Developing Skills for Change: Creating a Personalized Plan

Once you are committed to making a change, it's time to put together a plan of action. Your key to success is a well-thought-out plan that sets goals, anticipates problems, and includes rewards.

1. Monitor Your Behavior and Gather Data Begin by keeping careful records of the behavior you wish to change (your target behavior) and the circumstances surrounding it. Keep these records in a health journal, or a paper or electronic notebook. Sample blank journal logs for a variety of target behaviors can be found on the Online Learning Center. Track the details of your behavior along with observations and comments. Note exactly what the activity was, when and where it happened, what you were doing, and what your feelings were at the time (see the sample journal in Figure 1.6 and Activity 3 in the Behavior Change Workbook). If your goal is to start an exercise program, use your journal to track your daily activities to determine how best to make time for your workouts. Keep your journal for a week or two to get some solid information about the behavior you want to change.

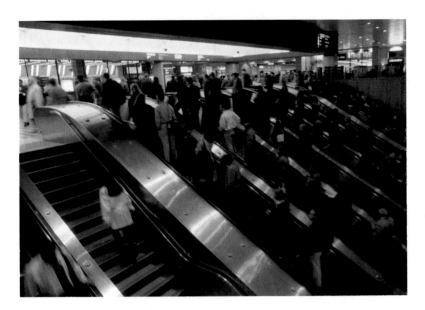

Your environment contains powerful cues for both positive and negative lifestyle choices. Identifying and using the healthier options available to you throughout the day is a key part of a successful behavior change program.

2. Analyze the Data and Identify Patterns After you have collected data on the behavior, analyze the data to identify patterns. When are you most likely to overeat? What events trigger your appetite? Perhaps you are especially hungry at midmorning or when you put off eating dinner until 9:00. Perhaps you overindulge in food and drink when you go to a particular restaurant or when you're with certain friends. Note the connections between your feelings and such external cues as time of day, location, situation, and the actions of others around you. Do you always think of having a cigarette when you read the newspaper? Do you always bite your fingernails when you're studying?

3. Set Realistic, Specific Goals Don't set an impossibly difficult overall goal for your program—going from a sedentary lifestyle to running a marathon within 2 months, for example. Working toward more realistic, achievable goals will greatly increase your chances of success. Your goal should also be specific and measurable, something you can easily track. Instead of a vague general goal such as improving eating habits or being more physically active, set a specific target—eating 5 servings of fruits and vegetables each day or walking or biking for 30 minutes at least 5 days per week.

It's a good idea to break your ultimate goal down into a few small steps. Your plan will seem less overwhelming and more manageable, increasing the chances that you'll stick to it. You'll also build in more opportunities to reward yourself (discussed in step 4), as well as milestones you can use to measure your progress. If you've been sedentary but plan to start a physical activity program, begin by taking 10- to 15-minute walks a few times a week. If you plan to increase your fruit and vegetable consumption from 3 to 7 servings per day, break your program into four steps, beginning with increasing from 3 to 4 servings per day. Take easier steps first and work up to harder steps. With each small success, you'll build your confidence and self-efficacy.

For some programs or circumstances, it may be better to focus your program on something other than outcome goals. For example, if you are in one of the early stages of change for your target behavior, setting challenging outcome goals like 60 minutes of daily physical activity or quitting smoking may be premature. The overall goal of your first change program might be to move from the precontemplation to the preparation stage of change, and your program mini-goals might be to work through specific strategies for various stages—spending 2 hours researching your target behavior or completing a detailed cost-benefit analysis, for example. Weight-loss programs can also benefit from goals that promote the development of healthy habits because specific body weight targets can take a long time to achieve and can lead to an unhealthy emphasis on weight rather than on the behaviors needed to achieve and maintain a healthy body weight. For example, a program might focus on setting weekly minutes of physical activity, or reducing portion sizes or the number of late-night snacks rather than on achieving a specific body weight.

4. Devise a Strategy or Plan of Action Next, you need to develop specific strategies and techniques that will support your day-to-day efforts at behavior change.

OBTAIN INFORMATION AND SUPPLIES Identify campus and community resources that can provide practical help—for example, a stop-smoking course or a walking club. Take any necessary preparatory steps, such as signing up for a stress-management workshop or purchasing walking shoes, nicotine replacement patches, or a special calendar to track your progress.

MODIFY YOUR ENVIRONMENT You can be more effective in changing behavior if you control the environmental cues that provoke it. This might mean not having cigarettes or certain foods or drinks in the house, not going to parties where you're tempted to overindulge, or not spending time with particular people, at least for a while. Use the data you collected in your health journal to identify patterns. If you always get a candy bar at a certain vending machine, change your route so you don't pass by it. If you always end up taking a coffee break and chatting with friends when you go to the library to study, choose a different place to study, such as your room. Finding alternatives to or substitutes for your target behavior is a key part of a successful plan for change.

It's also helpful to control other behaviors or habits that are linked to the target behavior. You may give in to an urge to eat when you have a beer (alcohol increases the appetite) or watch TV. Try substituting other activities for habits that are linked with your target behavior, such as exercising to music instead of plopping down in front of the TV. Or put an exercise bicycle in front of the set and burn calories while watching your favorite show.

You can change the cues in your environment so they trigger the new behavior you want instead of the old one. Tape a picture of a cyclist speeding down a hill on your TV screen. Leave your exercise shoes in plain view. Put a chart of your progress in a special place at home to make your goals highly visible and inspire you to keep going.

See Activity 7 in the Behavior Change Workbook for a detailed example of how to develop strategies to break the chain of events surrounding a target behavior.

REWARD YOURSELF   Another powerful way to affect your target behavior is to set up a reward system that will reinforce your efforts. Most people find it difficult to change longstanding habits for rewards they can't see right away. Giving yourself instant, real rewards for good behavior along the way will help you stick with a plan to change your behavior.

Carefully plan your reward payoffs and what they will be. In most cases, rewards should be collected when you reach specific objectives or subgoals in your plan. For example, you might treat yourself to a movie after a week of avoiding extra snacks. Don't forget to reward yourself for good behavior that is consistent and persistent—such as simply sticking with your program week after week. Decide on a reward after you reach a certain goal or mark off the sixth week or month of a valiant effort. Write it down in your health journal and remember it as you follow your plan—especially when the going gets rough. If you don't think you can successfully manage your own reward system, ask someone to help; a friend can act as your reward "bank" and administer rewards according to your plan.

Make a list of your activities and favorite events to use as rewards. They should be special, inexpensive, and preferably unrelated to food or alcohol. You might treat yourself to a concert, a ball game, a new CD, a long-distance phone call to a friend, a day off from studying, or a long hike in the woods—whatever is rewarding to you.

INVOLVE THE PEOPLE AROUND YOU   Rewards and support can also come from family and friends. Tell them about your plan and ask for their help. Encourage them to be

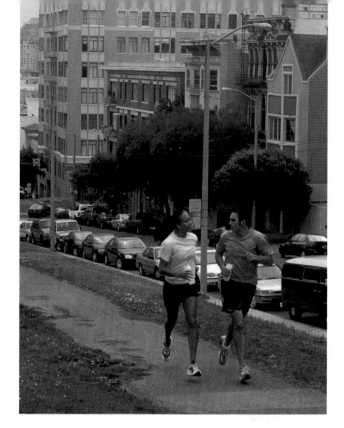

A convenient setting and a friendly companion help make exercise a satisfying and pleasurable experience. Choosing the right activity and doing it the right way are important elements in a successful behavior change program.

active, interested participants. To help friends and family members respond appropriately, you may want to create a specific list of dos and don'ts. For example, ask them to support you when you set aside time to go running or avoid second helpings at Thanksgiving dinner.

PLAN AHEAD FOR CHALLENGING SITUATIONS   Take time out now to list situations and people that have the potential to derail your program and to develop possible coping mechanisms. For example, if you think you'll have trouble exercising during finals week, schedule short bouts of physical activity as stress-reducing study breaks. If a visit to a friend who smokes is likely to tempt you to lapse, plan to bring nicotine patches and chewing gum along with you on your visit.

5. Make a Personal Contract   A serious personal contract—one that commits you to your word—can result in a higher chance of follow-through than a casual, offhand promise. Your contract can help prevent procrastination by specifying the important dates and can also serve as a reminder of your personal commitment to change. Your contract should include a statement of your goal and your commitment to reaching it. Include details of your plan: the date you'll begin, the steps you'll use to measure your progress, the concrete strategies you've developed for promoting change, and the date you expect to reach your final goal. Have someone—preferably someone who will

My Personal Contract for Eating Three Servings of Fruit per Day

I agree to increase my consumption of fruit from one serving per week to three servings per day. I will begin my program on __10/5__ and plan to reach my final goal by __12/7__. I have divided my program into three parts, with three separate goals. For each step in my program, I will give myself the reward listed.

1. I will begin to have a serving of fruit with breakfast on __10/5__.
   (Reward: __baseball game__)
2. I will begin to have a serving of fruit with lunch on __10/26__.
   (Reward: __music CD__)
3. I will begin to substitute fruit juice for soda for one snack each day on __11/16__.
   (Reward: __Concert__)

My plan for increasing fruit consumption includes the following strategies:

1. __Keeping my dorm room refrigerator stocked with easy-to-carry fruit and fruit juice.__
2. __Packing fruit in my book backpack every day.__
3. __Placing reminders to buy, carry, and eat fruit in my dorm room, backpack, and wallet.__
4. __Buying lunch at a place that serves fruit or fruit juice.__

I understand that it is important for me to make a strong personal effort to make the change in my behavior. I sign this contract as an indication of my personal commitment to reach my goal.

Michael Cook   9/28

Witness: *Katie Lim*   9/28

Figure 1.7   A sample behavior change contract.

be actively helping you with your program—sign your contract as a witness.

A Sample Behavior Change Plan   Let's take the example of Michael, who wants to improve his diet. By monitoring his eating habits in his health journal for several weeks, he gets a good sense of his typical diet—what he eats and where he eats it. Through self-assessment and investigation, he discovers that he currently consumes only about one serving of fruit per week, much less than the recommended two to four servings per day. He also finds out that fruit is a major source of fiber, vitamins, minerals, and other substances important for good health. He sets the target of eating three servings of fruit per day as the overall goal for his behavior change plan. Then Michael develops a specific plan for change that involves several changes in his behavior and his environment, which he describes in a contract that commits him to reaching his goal (Figure 1.7). Additional sample plans and contracts for other target behaviors can be found on the *Fit and Well* Online Learning Center.

Putting Your Plan into Action

The starting date has arrived, and you are ready to put your plan into action. This stage requires commitment, the resolve to stick with the plan no matter what temptations you encounter. Remember all the reasons you have to make

the change—and remember that *you* are the boss. Use all your strategies to make your plan work. Make sure your environment is change-friendly, and obtain as much support and encouragement from others as possible. Keep track of your progress in your health journal, and give yourself regular rewards. And don't forget to give yourself a pat on the back—congratulate yourself, notice how much better you look or feel, and feel good about how far you've come and how you've gained control of your behavior.

Staying with It

As you continue with your program, don't be surprised when you run up against obstacles; they're inevitable. In fact, it's a good idea to expect problems and give yourself time to step back, see how you're doing, and make some changes before going on. If your program is grinding to a halt, identify what is blocking your progress. It may come from one of these sources.

Social Influences   Take a hard look at the reactions of the people you're counting on, and see if they're really supporting you. If they come up short, connect and network with others who will be more supportive.

A related trap is trying to get your friends or family members to change *their* behaviors. The decision to make a major behavior change is something people come to only after intensive self-examination. You may be able to

- Write down the potential benefits of the change. If you want to lose weight, your list might include increased ease of movement, energy, and self-confidence.

- Now write down the costs of not changing.

- Frequently visualize yourself achieving your goal and enjoying its benefits. If you want to manage time more effectively, picture yourself as a confident, organized person who systematically tackles important tasks and sets aside time each day for relaxation, exercise, and friends.

- Discount obstacles to change. Counter thoughts such as "I'll never have time to exercise" with thoughts such as "Lots of other people have done it and so can I."

- Bombard yourself with propaganda. Take a class dealing with the change you want to make. Read books and watch talk shows on the subject. Post motivational phrases or pictures on your refrigerator or over your desk. Talk to people who have already made the change you want to make.

- Build up your confidence. Remind yourself of other goals you've achieved. At the end of each day, mentally review your good decisions and actions. See yourself as a capable person, one who is in charge of his or her health.

- Create choices. You will be more likely to exercise every day if you have two or three types of exercise to choose from and more likely to quit smoking if you've identified more than one way to distract yourself when you crave a cigarette. Get ideas from people who have been successful and adapt some of their strategies to suit you.

- If you slip, keep trying. Research suggests that four out of five people will experience some degree of backsliding when they try to change a behavior. Only one in four succeeds the first time around. If you retain your commitment to change even when you lapse, you are still farther along the path to change than before you made the commitment.

---

influence someone by tactfully providing facts or support, but that's all. Focus on yourself. If you succeed, you may become a role model for others.

Levels of Motivation and Commitment
You won't make real progress until an inner drive leads you to the stage of change at which you are ready to make a personal commitment to the goal. If commitment is your problem, you may need to wait until the behavior you're dealing with makes your life more unhappy or unhealthy; then your desire to change it will be stronger. Or you may find that changing your goal will inspire you to keep going. For more ideas, refer to the box "Motivation Boosters" and to Activity 9 in the Behavior Change Workbook at the end of the text.

Choice of Techniques and Level of Effort
If your plan is not working as well as you thought it would, make changes where you're having the most trouble. If you've lagged on your running schedule, for example, maybe it's because you don't like running. An aerobics class might suit you better. There are many ways to move toward your goal. Or you may not be trying hard enough. You do have to push toward your goal. If it were easy, you wouldn't need to have a plan.

Stress Barrier
If you've hit a wall in your program, look at the sources of stress in your life. If the stress is temporary, such as catching a cold or having a term paper due, you may want to wait until it passes before strengthening your efforts. If the stress is ongoing, find healthy ways to manage it, such as taking a half-hour walk after lunch or beginning a yoga class. You may even want to make stress management your highest priority for behavior change (see Chapter 10).

Procrastinating, Rationalizing, and Blaming
Try to detect the games you might be playing with yourself so that you can stop them. If you're procrastinating ("It's Friday already; I might as well wait until Monday to begin"), break your plan down into still smaller steps that you can accomplish one day at a time. If you're rationalizing or making excuses ("I wanted to go swimming today, but I wouldn't have had time to wash my hair afterward"), remember that when you "win" by deceiving yourself, it's not much of a victory. If you're wasting time blaming yourself or others ("Everyone in that class talks so much that I don't get a chance to speak"), recognize that blaming is a way of taking your focus off the real problem and denying responsibility for your actions. Try refocusing by taking a positive attitude and renewing your determination to succeed.

MOTIVATION FOR CHANGE!   Behavior change is like many other challenges you'll encounter at school and work—it requires that you develop certain skills. Just as when you take a course in an unfamiliar subject, you shouldn't expect that you'll master everything in your behavior change program quickly and with ease or that you'll achieve perfection. But with consistent effort, you can build your skills and achieve your goals. Think of any obstacles or difficult situations you encounter during your behavior change program as challenges to your skills that will require effort to address but that are within your ability to manage. Thinking of behavior change in this way will help you tolerate mistakes and lapses, remain motivated, and see your behavior change program as an opportunity for personal growth and improvement.

1. The persistent presence of a support network.

2. Chronic positive expectations; the tendency to frame events in a constructive light.

3. Episodic outbreaks of joyful, happy experiences.

4. A sense of spiritual involvement.

5. A tendency to adapt to changing conditions.

6. Rapid response and recovery of stress response systems to repeated challenges.

7. An increased appetite for physical activity.

8. A tendency to identify and communicate feelings.

9. Repeated episodes of gratitude and generosity.

10. A persistent sense of humor.

SOURCE: Ten warning signs of good health. 1996. *Mind/Body Health Newsletter* 5(1).

Being Fit and Well for Life

Your first attempts at making behavior changes may never go beyond the project stage. Those that do may not all succeed. But as you experience some success, you'll start to have more positive feelings about yourself. You may discover new physical activities and sports you enjoy; you may encounter new situations and meet new people. Perhaps you'll surprise yourself by accomplishing things you didn't think were possible—breaking a longstanding nicotine habit, competing in a race, climbing a mountain, developing a lean, muscular body. Most of all, you'll discover the feeling of empowerment that comes from taking charge of your health (see the box "Signs of Wellness"). Being healthy takes extra effort, but the paybacks in energy and vitality are priceless.

Once you've started, don't stop. Assume that health improvement is forever. Take on the easier problems first, and then use what you learn to tackle more difficult problems later. Periodically review what you've accomplished to make sure you don't fall into old habits. And keep informed about the latest health news and trends. Research is constantly providing new information that directly affects daily choices and habits.

This book will introduce you to the main components of a fit and well lifestyle, show you how to assess your current health status, and help you put together a program that will lead to wellness. You can't control every aspect of your health—there are too many unknowns in life for that to be possible. But you can create a lifestyle that minimizes your health risks and maximizes your enjoyment of life and well-being. You can take charge of your health in a dramatic and meaningful way. *Fit and Well* will show you how.

SUMMARY

- Wellness is the ability to live life fully, with vitality and meaning. Wellness is dynamic and multidimensional; it incorporates physical, emotional, intellectual, spiritual, interpersonal and social, and environmental dimensions.

Tips for Today

You are in charge of your health! Many of the decisions you make every day have an impact on the quality of your life, both now and in the future. By making positive choices, large and small, you help ensure a lifetime of wellness.

Right now you can

- Go for a 15-minute walk.

- Have an orange, a nectarine, or a plum for a snack.

- Call a friend and arrange for a time to catch up with each other.

- Start thinking about whether you have a health behavior you'd like to change. If you do, consider the elements of a behavior change strategy. For example,

  - Begin a mental list of the pros and cons of the behavior.

  - Create a format for a log to monitor your target behavior.

  - Think of someone who can support you in your attempts to make a behavior change and talk to that person about your plan.

- People today have greater control over and greater responsibility for their health than ever before.

- Behaviors that promote wellness include being physically active; choosing a healthy diet; maintaining a healthy body weight; managing stress effectively; avoiding use of tobacco and limiting alcohol use; and protecting oneself from disease and injury.

- Although heredity, environment, and health care all play roles in wellness and disease, behavior can mitigate their effects.

- To make lifestyle changes, you need information about yourself, your health habits, and resources available to help you change.

- You can increase your motivation for behavior change by examining the benefits and costs of change, boosting self-efficacy, and identifying and overcoming key barriers to change.

- The stages of change model describes six stages that people may move through as they try to change their behavior: precontemplation, contemplation, preparation, action, maintenance, and termination.
- A specific plan for change can be developed by (1) collecting data on your behavior and recording it in a journal; (2) analyzing the recorded data; (3) setting specific goals; (4) devising strategies for obtaining information, modifying the environment, rewarding yourself, involving others, and planning ahead; and (5) making a personal contract.
- To start and maintain a behavior change program you need commitment, a well-developed and manageable plan, social support, and strong stress management techniques. It is also important to monitor the progress of your program, revising it as necessary.

FOR FURTHER EXPLORATION

Fit and Well Online Learning Center (www.mhhe.com/fahey)

Visit the *Fit and Well* Online Learning Center and familiarize yourself with the resources available at the site. You can use the learning objectives, study guide questions, and glossary flashcards to review key terms and concepts for this chapter and prepare for exams. You can extend your knowledge of wellness and gain experience in using the Internet as a resource by completing the activities and checking out the Web links for the topics in Chapter 1 marked with the World Wide Web icon. For this chapter, there are activities relating to *Healthy People 2010* objectives, online assessments, and evaluation of online resources; there are Web links for the Vital Statistics tables and figures, the Critical Consumer box, and the chapter as a whole. Behavior change resources and tools include an online version of the Behavior Change Workbook, sample logs for a variety of target behaviors, and sample behavior change plans.

Daily Fitness and Nutrition Journal

Have you chosen a target behavior related to physical activity or diet? If so, begin reviewing the behavior change planning and monitoring tools available in the log. If you've chosen a target behavior in another area, the fitness and nutrition examples can provide a good model for the type of program plan and log you should create for your behavior change program. Visit the Online Learning Center for some blank sample logs that you can print and use.

HealthQuest

Take a closer look at your health risks and current lifestyle by completing the Wellboard activity on the HealthQuest CD-ROM. In addition to estimating your life expectancy based on your lifestyle and the health history of you and your family, this assessment will also give you scores in eight areas and provide tips for improvement. Your scores may help you identify a target behavior for behavior change. You may also want to print and save your complete Wellboard report for later comparison—you can improve your scores and your estimated life expectancy by adopting a wellness lifestyle.

Books

Beers, M. H. 2004. *The Merck Manual of Medical Information.* 2nd Home Edition. New York: Pocket Books. *Provides consumer-oriented advice for the prevention and treatment of common health concerns.*

Prochaska, J. O., J. C. Norcross, and C. C. DiClemente. 1994. *Changing for Good: The Revolutionary Program That Explains the Six Stages of Change and Teaches You How to Free Yourself from Bad Habits.* New York: Morrow. *Outlines the authors' model of behavior change and offers suggestions and advice for each stage of change.*

Smith P. B., M. MacFarlane, and E. Kalnitsky. 2002. *The Complete Idiot's Guide to Wellness.* Indianapolis, In.: Alpha Books. *A concise guide to healthy habits, including physical activity, nutrition, and stress management.*

Newsletters

Consumer Reports on Health (800-234-2188; http://www.ConsumerReports.org)

Harvard Health Letter (800-829-9045; http://www.health.harvard.edu)

Harvard Men's Health Watch (800-829-3341)

Harvard Women's Health Watch (800-829-5921)

HealthNews (781-893-3800)

Mayo Clinic Health Letter (800-333-9037)

University of California at Berkeley Wellness Letter (386-447-6328; http://www.wellnessletter.com)

Organizations, Hotlines, and Web Sites

The Internet addresses (also called uniform resource locators, or URLs) listed here were accurate at the time of publication. Up-to-date links to these and many other wellness-oriented Web sites are provided on the links page of the *Fit and Well* Online Learning Center (http://www.mhhe.com/fahey).

Centers for Disease Control and Prevention. Through phone, fax, and the Internet, the CDC provides a wide variety of health information.
   800-311-3435; 888-CDC-FAXX (CDC FAX)
   http://www.cdc.gov

Many other government Web sites provide access to health-related materials:
   Federal Trade Commission: http://www.ftc.gov
   First Gov for Consumers—Health: http://www.consumer.gov/health.htm
   National Institutes of Health: http://www.nih.gov
   National Library of Medicine, MedlinePlus: http://www.medlineplus.gov

Go Ask Alice. Sponsored by the Columbia University Health Service, this site provides answers to student questions about stress, sexuality, fitness, and many other wellness topics.
   http://www.goaskalice.columbia.edu

Healthfinder. A gateway to online publications, Web sites, support and self-help groups, and agencies and organizations that produce reliable health information.
   http://www.healthfinder.gov

Healthy People 2010. Provides information on Healthy People objectives and priority areas.
   202-205-8583
   http://www.healthypeople.gov

MedlinePlus: Evaluating Health Information. Provides background information and links to sites with guidelines for finding and evaluating health information on the Web.

    http://www.nlm.nih.gov/medlineplus/
        evaluatinghealthinformation.html

National Health Information Center (NHIC). Puts consumers in touch with the organizations that are best able to provide answers to health-related questions.

    800-336-4797

    http://www.health.gov/nhic

National Women's Health Information Center. Provides information and answers to frequently asked questions.

    800-994-WOMAN

    http://www.4woman.org

NOAH: New York Online Access to Health. Provides consumer health information in both English and Spanish.

    http://www.noah-health.org

Nutrition.Gov. Gateway to online nutrition information from the U.S. government.

    http://www.nutrition.gov

Student Counseling Virtual Pamphlet Collection. Provides links to more than 400 pamphlets produced by different student counseling centers; topics include relationships, family issues, substance abuse, anger management, and study skills.

    http://www.dr-bob.org/vpc

World Health Organization (WHO). Provides information about WHO activities and about many health topics and issues affecting people around the world.

    http://www.who.int

The following are just a few of the many sites that provide consumer-oriented information on a variety of health issues:

Family Doctor.Org: http://www.familydoctor.org

InteliHealth: http://www.intelihealth.com

Mayo Clinic: http://www.mayoclinic.com

WebMD: http://webmd.com

The following sites provide daily health news updates:

CNN Health: http://www.cnn.com/health

MedlinePlus News: http://www.nlm.nih.gov/medlineplus/
    newsbydate.html

Yahoo Health News: http://dailynews.yahoo.com/h/hl

SELECTED BIBLIOGRAPHY

American Cancer Society. 2004. *Cancer Facts and Figures 2004.* Atlanta: American Cancer Society.

American Heart Association. 2004. *2004 Heart and Stroke Statistical Update.* Dallas, Tex.: American Heart Association.

Calle, E. E., et al. 2003. Overweight, obesity, and mortality from cancer in a prospectively studied cohort of U.S. adults. *New England Journal of Medicine* 348(17): 1625–1638.

Centers for Disease Control and Prevention. 2004. Health behaviors of adults, 1999–2001. *Vital and Health Statistics* 10(219).

Centers for Disease Control and Prevention. 2003. Cigarette smoking-attributable morbidity—United States, 2000. *Morbidity and Mortality Weekly Report* 52(35): 842–844.

Centers for Disease Control and Prevention. 2003. Prevalence of diabetes and impaired fasting glucose in adults. *Morbidity and Mortality Weekly Report* 52(35): 833–837.

Centers for Disease Control and Prevention. 2003. Prevalence of physical activity, including lifestyle activities among adults. *Morbidity and Mortality Weekly Report* 52(32): 764–769.

Centers for Disease Control and Prevention. 2000. *Measuring Healthy Days: Population Assessment of Health-Related Quality of Life.* Atlanta, Ga.: Centers for Disease Control and Prevention.

Centers for Disease Control and Prevention, Division of Nutrition and Physical Activity. 1999. *Promoting Physical Activity: A Guide for Community Action.* Champaign, Ill.: Human Kinetics.

Department of Health and Human Services. 1996. *Physical Activity and Health: A Report of the Surgeon General.* Atlanta, Ga.: DHHS.

Douglas, K. A., et al. 1997. Results from the 1995 National College Health Risk Behavior Survey. *Journal of American College Health* 46(2): 55–56.

Fontaine, K. R., et al. 2003. Years of life lost due to obesity. *Journal of the American Medical Association* 289(2): 187–193.

Gallagher, K. I., and J. M. Jakicic. 2002. Overcoming barriers to effective exercise programming. *ACSM's Health and Fitness Journal,* November/December.

Glanz, K., F. M. Lewis, and B. K. Rimer, ed. 1997. *Health Behavior and Health Education: Theory, Research, and Practice,* 2nd ed. San Francisco: Jossey-Bass.

Institute of Medicine. 2001. *Health Behavior: The Interplay of Biological, Behavioral, and Societal Influences.* Washington, D.C.: National Academy Press.

Lee, C. D., and S. N. Blair. 2002. Cardiorespiratory fitness and stroke mortality in men. *Medicine and Science in Sports and Exercise* 34(4): 592–595.

Marcus, B. H., and L. H. Forsyth. 2003. *Motivating People to Be Physically Active.* Champaign, Ill.: Human Kinetics.

Mokdad, A. H., et al. 2004. Actual causes of death in the United States, 2000. *Journal of the American Medical Association* 291(10): 1238–1245.

Mokdad, A. H., et al. 2003. Prevalence of obesity, diabetes, and obesity-related health risk factors. *Journal of the American Medical Association* 289(1): 76–79.

Muller, A. 2002. Education, income inequality, and mortality: A multiple regression analysis. *British Medical Journal* 324(7328): 23–25.

National Center for Health Statistics. 2002. Leisure-time physical activity among adults: United States, 1997–1998. *Advance Data from Vital and Health Statistics,* No. 325.

National Center for Health Statistics. 2003. *Health, United States, 2003.* Hyattsville, Md.: Public Health Service.

Ortlepp, J. R., et al. 2003. Relation of body mass index, physical fitness, and the cardiovascular risk profile in 3217 young normal weight men with an apparently optimal lifestyle. *International Journal of Obesity and Related Metabolic Disorders* 27(8): 979–982.

Sesso, H. D., R. S. Paffenbarger, and I. M. Lee. 2000. Physical activity and coronary heart disease in men: The Harvard Alumni Health Study. *Circulation* 102(9): 975–980.

Slater, M. D., and D. E. Zimmerman. 2002. Characteristics of health-related Web sites identified by common Internet portals. *Journal of the American Medical Association* 288(3): 316–317.

Stampfer, M. J., et al. 2000. Primary prevention of coronary heart disease in women through diet and lifestyle. *New England Journal of Medicine* 343(1): 16–22.

Suminiski, R. R., and R. Petosa. 2002. Stages of change among ethnically diverse college students. *Journal of American College Health* 51(1): 26–31.

U.S. Department of Health and Human Services. 2000. *Healthy People 2010,* 2nd ed. Washington, D.C.: DHHS.

World Health Organization. 2002. *World Health Day 2002: Move for Health* (http://www.who.int/world-health-day; retrieved April 19, 2002).

World Health Organization. 2001. *What Is the WHO Definition of Health?* (http://www.who.int/aboutwho/en/qal.htm; retrieved July 26, 2001).

Name _____ **Section** _____ **Date** _____

LAB 1.1 *Your Wellness Profile*

Consider how your lifestyle, attitudes, and characteristics relate to each of the six dimensions of wellness. Fill in your strengths for each dimension (examples of strengths are listed with each dimension). Once you've completed your lists, choose what you believe are your five most important strengths and circle them.

Physical wellness: To maintain overall physical health and engage in appropriate physical activity (e.g., stamina, strength, flexibility, healthy body composition).

_____

_____

_____

Emotional wellness: To have a positive self-concept, deal constructively with your feelings, and develop positive qualities (e.g., optimism, trust, self-confidence, determination, persistence, dedication).

_____

_____

_____

Intellectual wellness: To pursue and retain knowledge, think critically about issues, make sound decisions, identify problems, and find solutions (e.g., common sense, creativity, curiosity).

_____

_____

_____

Spiritual wellness: To develop a set of beliefs, principles, or values that gives meaning or purpose to one's life; to develop faith in something beyond oneself (e.g., religious faith, service to others).

_____

_____

_____

Interpersonal/social wellness: To develop and maintain meaningful relationships with a network of friends and family members, and to contribute to the community (e.g., friendly, good-natured, compassionate, supportive, good listener).

_____

_____

_____

Environmental wellness: To protect yourself from environmental hazards, and to minimize the negative impact of your behavior on the environment (e.g., carpooling, recycling).

_____

_____

_____

Next, think about where you fall on the wellness continuum for each of the dimensions of wellness. Indicate your placement for each—physical, emotional, intellectual, spiritual, interpersonal/social, and environmental—by placing Xs on the continuum below.

| Low level of wellness | Physical, psychological, emotional symptoms | Change and growth | High level of wellness |

Based on both your current lifestyle and your goals for the future, what do you think your placement on the wellness continuum will be in 10 years? What new health behaviors would you have to adopt to achieve your goals? Which of your current behaviors would you need to change to maintain or improve your level of wellness in the future?

Does the description of wellness given in this chapter encompass everything you believe is part of wellness for you? Write your own definition of wellness, and include any additional dimensions that are important to you. Then rate your level of wellness based on your own definition.

Using Your Results

How did you score? Are you satisfied with your current level of wellness—overall and in each dimension? In which dimension(s) would you most like to increase your level of wellness?

What should you do next? As you consider possible target behaviors for a behavior change program, choose things that will maintain or increase your level of wellness in one of the dimensions you listed as an area of concern. Remember to consider health behaviors such as smoking or eating a high-fat diet that may threaten your level of wellness in the future. Below, list several possible target behaviors and the wellness dimensions that they influence.

For additional guidance in choosing a target behavior, complete the lifestyle self-assessment in Lab 1.2.

LAB 1.2 *Lifestyle Evaluation*

How does your current lifestyle compare with the lifestyle recommended for wellness? For each question, choose the answer that best describes your behavior; then add up your score for each section.

Exercise/Fitness

	Almost Always	Sometimes	Never
1. I engage in moderate exercise, such as brisk walking or swimming, for 20–60 minutes, three to five times a week.	4	1	0
2. I do exercises to develop muscular strength and endurance at least twice a week.	2	1	0
3. I spend some of my leisure time participating in individual, family, or team activities, such as gardening, bowling, or softball.	2	1	0
4. I maintain a healthy body weight, avoiding overweight and underweight.	2	1	0

Exercise/Fitness Score: _____

Nutrition

1. I eat a variety of foods each day, including five or more servings of fruits and/or vegetables.	3	1	0
2. I limit the amount of total fat and saturated and trans fat in my diet.	3	1	0
3. I avoid skipping meals.	2	1	0
4. I limit the amount of salt and sugar I eat.	2	1	0

Nutrition Score: _____

Tobacco Use

If you never use tobacco, enter a score of 10 for this section and go to the next section.

1. I avoid using tobacco.	2	1	0
2. I smoke only low-tar-and-nicotine cigarettes, or I smoke a pipe or cigars, or I use smokeless tobacco.	2	1	0

Tobacco Use Score: _____

Alcohol and Drugs

1. I avoid alcohol, or I drink no more than 1 (women) or 2 (men) drinks a day.	4	1	0
2. I avoid using alcohol or other drugs as a way of handling stressful situations or the problems in my life.	2	1	0
3. I am careful not to drink alcohol when taking medications (such as cold or allergy medications) or when pregnant.	2	1	0
4. I read and follow the label directions when using prescribed and over-the-counter drugs.	2	1	0

Alcohol and Drugs Score: _____

Emotional Health

1. I enjoy being a student, and I have a job or do other work that I enjoy.	2	1	0
2. I find it easy to relax and express my feelings freely.	2	1	0
3. I manage stress well.	2	1	0
4. I have close friends, relatives, or others whom I can talk to about personal matters and call on for help when needed.	2	1	0
5. I participate in group activities (such as community or church organizations) or hobbies that I enjoy.	2	1	0

Emotional Health Score: _____

Safety

1. I wear a safety belt while riding in a car.	2	1	0
2. I avoid driving while under the influence of alcohol or other drugs.	2	1	0
3. I obey traffic rules and the speed limit when driving.	2	1	0
4. I read and follow instructions on the labels of potentially harmful products or substances, such as household cleaners, poisons, and electrical appliances.	2	1	0
5. I avoid smoking in bed.	2	1	0

Safety Score: _____

Disease Prevention

1. I know the warning signs of cancer, heart attack, and stroke.	2	1	0
2. I avoid overexposure to the sun and use sunscreen.	2	1	0
3. I get recommended medical screening tests (such as blood pressure and cholesterol checks and Pap tests), immunizations, and booster shots.	2	1	0
4. I practice monthly skin and breast/testicle self-exams.	2	1	0
5. I am not sexually active *or* I have sex with only one mutually faithful, uninfected partner *or* I always engage in "safer sex" (using condoms), *and* I do not share needles to inject drugs.	2	1	0

Disease Prevention Score: _____

Scores of 9 and 10 Excellent! Your answers show that you are aware of the importance of this area to your health. More important, you are putting your knowledge to work for you by practicing good health habits. As long as you continue to do so, this area should not pose a serious health risk.

Scores of 6 to 8 Your health practices in this area are good, but there is room for improvement.

Scores of 3 to 5 Your health risks are showing!

Scores of 0 to 2 You may be taking serious and unnecessary risks with your health.

Using Your Results

How did you score? In which areas did you score the lowest? Are you satisfied with your scores in each area? In which areas would you most like to improve your scores?

What should you do next? To improve your scores, look closely at any item to which you answered "sometimes" or "never." Identify and list at least three possible targets for a health behavior change program. (If you are aware of other risky health behaviors you currently engage in, but which were not covered by this assessment, you may include those in your list.) For each item on your list, identify your current "stage of change" and one strategy you could adopt to move forward (see pp. 13–15 in Chapter 1). Possible strategies might be obtaining information about the behavior, completing an analysis of the pros and cons of change, or beginning a written record.

Behavior	**Stage**	**Strategy**
1. _____	_____	_____
2. _____	_____	_____
3. _____	_____	_____

SOURCE: Adapted from *Healthstyle: A Self-Test,* developed by the U.S. Public Health Service. The behaviors covered in this test are recommended for most Americans, but some may not apply to people with certain chronic diseases or disabilities or to pregnant women, who may require special advice from their physician.

2

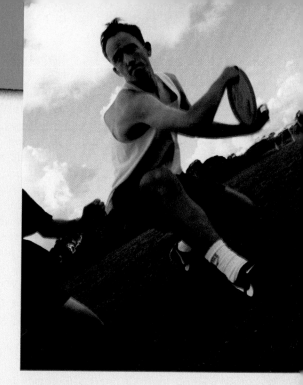

Basic Principles of Physical Fitness

LOOKING AHEAD

After reading this chapter, you should be able to

- Describe how much exercise is recommended for developing health and fitness
- Identify the components of physical fitness and how each component affects wellness
- Explain the goal of physical training and the basic principles of training
- Describe the principles involved in designing a well-rounded exercise program
- Discuss the steps that can be taken to make an exercise program safe, effective, and successful

TEST YOUR KNOWLEDGE

1. To improve your health, you must do high-intensity exercise. True or false?

2. Among American adults, about what percentage of trips of less than 1 mile long are made by walking?
   a. 15%
   b. 25%
   c. 50%

3. If all inactive American adults became physically active, the savings in direct costs for medical care would be about _____ per year.
   a. $75 million
   b. $7.5 billion
   c. $75 billion

ANSWERS

1. FALSE. Even moderate physical activity—walking the dog, taking the stairs, or doing yard work—has significant health benefits.

2. A. The vast majority of short trips are made in automobiles. On average, Americans spend 100 minutes per day driving and 170 minutes per day watching television. Most people have many opportunities to incorporate more moderate physical activity into their daily routine.

3. C. People who engage in regular physical activity make fewer physician visits, use less medication, and have fewer hospital stays than physically inactive people.

Any list of the benefits of physical activity is impressive. A physically active lifestyle helps you generate more energy, control your weight, manage stress, and boost your immune system. It provides psychological and emotional benefits, contributing to your sense of competence and well-being. It offers protection against heart disease, diabetes, high blood pressure, depression, anxiety, osteoporosis, some types of cancer, and even premature death. Exercise increases your physical capacity so that you are better able to meet the challenges of daily life with energy and vigor. Although people vary greatly in the levels of physical fitness and performance they can ultimately achieve, the benefits of regular physical activity are available to everyone. (For more on the benefits of exercise, see the box "Exercise and Total Wellness.")

This chapter provides an overview of physical fitness. It explains how lifestyle physical activity and more formal exercise programs contribute to wellness. It describes the components of fitness, the basic principles of physical training, and the essential elements of a well-rounded exercise program. Chapters 3–6 provide an in-depth look at each of the elements of a fitness program; Chapter 7 will help you put all these elements together into a complete, personalized program.

PHYSICAL ACTIVITY AND EXERCISE FOR HEALTH AND FITNESS

Despite the many benefits of an active lifestyle, levels of physical activity have declined in recent years and remain low for all populations of Americans (Figure 2.1). According to the Centers for Disease Control and Prevention (CDC), more than 55% of U.S. adults do not engage in recommended amounts of physical activity; 25% are not active at all. In the summer of 1996, the U.S. Surgeon General published *Physical Activity and Health*, a landmark report designed to reverse these trends and get Americans moving. Here is a summary of its findings:

- People of all ages benefit from regular physical activity.

- People can obtain significant health benefits by including a moderate amount of physical activity on most, if not all, days of the week. Through a modest increase in daily activity, most Americans can improve their health and quality of life.

- Additional health benefits can be gained through greater amounts of physical activity. People who can maintain a regular regimen of more vigorous or longer-duration activity are likely to obtain even greater benefits.

Why aren't more Americans active? Possible barriers include lack of time and resources, social and environmental influences, and lack of motivation and commitment (see Lab 2.3 for more on barriers). Some people also fear serious injury. Although physical activity does carry some risks, the risks of inactivity are far greater. Evidence is growing that for most Americans, simply becoming more physically active may be the single most important lifestyle change for promoting health and well-being.

> **MOTIVATION FOR CHANGE!** Habit helps us conserve mental and physical energy as we go through our daily lives, but it also blinds us to areas we could change. Make a list of ten ways you can incorporate more physical activity into your life by changing a habit, such as walking instead of riding the bus, taking the stairs in a certain building instead of the elevator, and so on. Use this list to plan strategies for your behavior change program and to counter negative self-talk about a lack of opportunities for physical activity.

Physical Activity on a Continuum

Physical activity can be defined as any body movement carried out by the skeletal muscles and requiring energy. Different types of physical activity can be arranged on a continuum based on the amount of energy they require. Quick, easy movements such as standing up or walking down a hallway require little energy or effort; more intense, sustained activities such as cycling 5 miles or running in a race require considerably more.

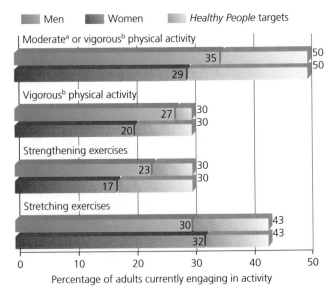

Men   Women   *Healthy People* targets

Moderate[a] or vigorous[b] physical activity: 35, 50, 50; 29
Vigorous[b] physical activity: 27, 30, 30; 20
Strengthening exercises: 23, 30, 30; 17
Stretching exercises: 30, 43, 43; 32

Percentage of adults currently engaging in activity

[a]Moderate physical activity for 30 or more minutes on 5 or more days per week
[b]Vigorous physical activity for 20 or more minutes on 3 or more days per week

VITAL STATISTICS

Figure 2.1 Current levels of physical activity among American adults. SOURCE: National Center for Health Statistics. 2004. *DATA2010: The Healthy People 2010 Database, January 2004 Edition* (http://wonder.cdc.gov/data2010; retrieved April 6, 2004).

Terms

physical activity Any body movement carried out by the skeletal muscles and requiring energy.

exercise Planned, structured, repetitive movement of the body designed to improve or maintain physical fitness.

Hundreds of studies show that exercise gives people both a longer life and a healthier life. Most of us want to live longer and avoid heart disease, cancer, and other chronic diseases, but many people choose to be active for other reasons. Some get a kick out of hitting a game-winning cross-court backhand, backpacking through a wilderness area, or completing a difficult skateboard move. Others enjoy the friends they make at the gym, on the tennis court, or on the walking trail; the way their fitness program gives them more energy; or the satisfaction they get from walking farther, running faster, or lifting more weight.

Samantha is a single 28-year-old junior executive from Boston who has a busy work and social schedule. Her fast-paced life makes it essential that she stay in shape. She attends an exercise class at a health club three times a week and lifts weights after the class. "The gym is an oasis in my incredibly busy day. I finish my exercise class refreshed and invigorated. I feel healthy, and I like the way my clothes fit. Being fit gives me the energy and self-confidence I need to compete in the business world. It's given my social life a boost, too."

Max is a 22-year-old college student who lives in Salt Lake City and loves to ski. "I came to Salt Lake because the surrounding mountains have the best snow in the world. I love the feeling of plunging down a steep chute and feeling the fresh powder surround me. The solitude and the beauty of the moun-

tains are a spiritual experience for me. I stay in shape and eat right so that I can better enjoy the high I get from skiing."

Nora is a 42-year-old mother of three children who lives in a small town outside Austin, Texas. She gets plenty of physical activity in her daily routine, which includes biking to her part-time job and helping out with after-school youth programs at the local community center. However, her passion is throwing the javelin in masters track and field competitions. "I developed a love for the sport in college. I enjoy the competition and striving to improve in a very difficult event. I have friends all over the world who share my passion. I like testing myself in competition—when I win or perform up to my personal best, the feeling is indescribable."

Bill is an 18-year-old college student at a small Midwest college who loves to run. "I run almost every day to forget my problems and relieve stress. Going away to college has been a big shock—I've gone from being part of a tight family to being on my own. Running helps me sort things out. I get lost in myself while I run through the woods and fields around the college. I do some of my best and most creative thinking when I run. I can't imagine my life without running."

The benefits of exercise go far beyond its disease-preventive effects. The enjoyment you get from physical activity enriches your life and makes you a more complete person.

Exercise refers to a subset of physical activity—planned, structured, repetitive movement of the body designed specifically to improve or maintain physical fitness. As discussed in Chapter 1, physical fitness is a set of physical attributes that allows the body to respond or adapt to the demands and stress of physical effort—to perform moderate-to-vigorous levels of physical activity without becoming overly tired. Levels of fitness depend on such physiological factors as the heart's ability to pump blood and the size of muscle fibers. To develop fitness, a person must perform enough physical activity to stress the body and cause long-term physiological changes. Only exercise will significantly improve fitness. Knowing this is important for setting goals and developing a program.

Lifestyle Physical Activity for Health Promotion   The Surgeon General's report and joint guidelines from the CDC and the American College of Sports Medicine (ACSM) recommend that all Americans include a moderate amount of physical activity on most, preferably all, days of the week. The report suggests a goal of expending 150 calories a day, or about 1000 calories a week, in physical activity. The same amount of activity can be obtained in longer sessions of moderately intense activities as in shorter sessions of more strenuous activities. Thus, 30 minutes of brisk walking or fast social dancing is equivalent to 15 minutes of running or snow shoveling. Examples of moderate physical activities are given in Figure 2.2.

Washing and waxing a car for 45–60 minutes
Washing windows or floors for 45–60 minutes
Playing volleyball for 45 minutes
Playing touch football for 30–45 minutes
Gardening for 30–45 minutes
Wheeling self in wheelchair for 30–40 minutes
Walking 1¾ miles in 35 minutes (20 min/mile)
Basketball (shooting baskets) for 30 minutes
Bicycling 5 miles in 30 minutes
Dancing fast (social) for 30 minutes
Pushing a stroller 1½ miles in 30 minutes
Raking leaves for 30 minutes
Walking 2 miles in 30 minutes (15 min/mile)
Water aerobics for 30 minutes
Swimming laps for 20 minutes
Wheelchair basketball for 20 minutes
Basketball (playing a game) for 15–20 minutes
Bicycling 4 miles in 15 minutes
Jumping rope for 15 minutes
Running 1½ miles in 15 minutes (10 min/mile)
Shoveling snow for 15 minutes
Stairwalking for 15 minutes

Less Vigorous, More Time

More Vigorous, Less Time

Figure 2.2   Examples of moderate amounts of physical activity.   A moderate amount is roughly equivalent to physical activity that uses approximately 150 calories of energy a day, or 1000 calories a week. Some activities can be performed at various intensities; the suggested durations correspond to expected intensity of effort.   SOURCE: Department of Health and Human Services. 1996. *Physical Activity and Health: A Report of the Surgeon General.* Atlanta, Ga.: DHHS.

"Too little time" is a common excuse for not being physically active. Learning to manage your time successfully is crucial if you are to maintain a wellness lifestyle. You can begin by keeping a record of how you are currently spending your time; in your health journal, use a grid broken into blocks of 15, 20, or 30 minutes to track your daily activities. Then analyze your record: List each type of activity and the total time you engaged in it on a given day—for example, sleeping, 7 hours; eating, 1.5 hours, studying, 3 hours; and so on. Take a close look at your list of activities and prioritize them according to how important they are to you, from essential to somewhat important to not important at all.

Based on the priorities you set, make changes in your daily schedule by subtracting time from some activities in order to make time for physical activity. Look particularly carefully at your leisure time activities and your methods of transportation; these are areas where it is easy to build in physical activity. Make changes using a system of tradeoffs. For example, you may choose to reduce the total amount of time you spend playing computer games, listening to the radio, and chatting on the telephone in order to make time for an after-dinner bike ride or walk with a friend. You may decide to watch 10 fewer minutes of television in the morning in order to change your 5-minute drive to class into a 15-minute walk. In making these kinds of changes in your schedule, don't feel that you have to miss out on anything you enjoy. You can get more from less time by focusing on what you are doing and by combining activities.

The following are just a few ways to become more active:

- Take the stairs instead of the elevator or escalator.
- Walk to the mailbox, post office, store, bank, or library whenever possible.
- Park your car a mile or even just a few blocks from your destination, and walk briskly.
- Do at least one chore every day that requires physical activity: wash the windows or your car, clean your room or house, mow the lawn, rake the leaves.
- Take study or work breaks to avoid sitting for more than 30 minutes at a time. Get up and walk around the library, your office, or your home or dorm; go up and down a flight of stairs.
- Stretch when you stand in line or watch TV.
- When you take public transportation, get off one stop down the line and walk to your destination.
- Go dancing instead of to a movie.
- Walk to visit a neighbor or friend rather than calling him or her on the phone. Go for a walk while you chat.
- Put your remote controls in storage; when you want to change TV or radio stations, get up and do it by hand.
- Take the dog for a walk (or an extra walk) every day.
- Play actively with children or go for a walk pushing a stroller.
- Seize every opportunity to get up and walk around. Move more and sit less.

In the lifestyle approach to physical activity, people can choose activities that they find enjoyable and that fit into their daily routine; everyday tasks at school, work, and home can be structured to contribute to the daily activity total (see the box "Becoming More Active"). The daily total of lifestyle activity can be accumulated in multiple short bouts—for example, two 10-minute bicycle rides to and from class and a brisk 15-minute walk to the post office. In addition to moderate-intensity physical activity, the Surgeon General's report recommends that people perform resistance training (exercising against an opposing force such as a weight) at least twice a week to build and maintain muscular strength.

By increasing lifestyle physical activity in accordance with the guidelines given in the Surgeon General's report, people can expect to significantly improve their health and well-being. If all the Americans who are now completely sedentary were to adopt a more active lifestyle, there would be enormous benefit to the public's health and to individual well-being. Such a program may not, however, significantly increase physical fitness. A program of 30 minutes of lifestyle activity per day may also not be enough activity for some people to achieve and maintain a healthy body weight.

Lifestyle Physical Activity for Health Promotion and Weight Management   Since the publication of the physical activity guidelines from the CDC/ACSM and Surgeon General, other organizations have released physical activity recommendations that focus on specific health concerns (Table 2.1). Because more than half of all U.S. adults are overweight, guidelines that focus on weight management are of particular interest. The guidelines from the Institute of Medicine, International Association for the Study of Obesity, and the World Health Organization/FAO Expert Report—all of which focus on weight control in addition to general health promotion—set higher daily goals for physical activity than the Surgeon General's report. These guidelines do not conflict with those from the Surgeon General, but they do have a different emphasis. They recognize that for people who need to lose weight and maintain weight loss, 30 minutes per day of physical activity may not be enough—and so they recommend 45–60 or more minutes per day of physical activity. The different recommendations may seem confusing and contradictory, but all major health organizations have the same message: People can improve their health by becoming more active.

	Summary of Physical Activity Recommendations from
Table 2.1	Selected Leading Health Organizations

Organization	Recommendation	Purpose
Centers for Disease Control and Prevention/American College of Sports Medicine	A minimum of 30 minutes per day of moderate activity on most days of the week (*The American College of Sports Medicine has separate guidelines for exercise programs to develop fitness; see pp. 35–39 and Table 2.2.*)	Health promotion and prevention of chronic disease
U.S. Surgeon General: Report on Physical Activity and Health	A minimum of 150 calories per day expended in moderate physical activity (the equivalent of about 30 minutes of brisk walking); resistance training twice a week	Health promotion and prevention of chronic disease
Institute of Medicine, National Academies	At least 60 minutes of moderate physical activity per day	Health promotion, prevention of chronic disease, and weight control
International Association for the Study of Obesity	45–60 minutes per day of moderate activity to prevent weight gain; 60–90 minutes per day of moderate physical activity to prevent weight regain in formerly obese people	Prevention of weight gain; maintenance of weight loss
World Health Organization/ FAO Expert Report	At least 60 minutes of moderate physical activity per day	Health promotion, prevention of chronic disease, and weight control
American Academy of Orthopaedic Surgeons*	30 minutes of moderate physical activity per day, appropriate for specific condition and designed by a physician; seek advice if pain is severe	Health promotion and symptom relief in people with muscle, bone, or joint pain (back pain, osteoporosis, arthritis, and so on)
American College of Obstetrics and Gynecology*	30 minutes or more of moderate exercise on most, if not all days of the week; previously inactive women or those with complications should consult with a physician before beginning activity	Promotion of a healthy pregnancy and postpartum recovery; prevention of gestational diabetes and excessive weight gain during pregnancy
American Diabetes Association*	Surgeon General's recommendations are appropriate for most people, but all levels of activity are possible if blood sugar is well-controlled; avoid exercise when blood sugar is above 250 mg/dl and ingest carbohydrates prior to exercise when blood sugar is below 100 mg/dl	Health promotion; prevention of cardiovascular disease; assistance with control of diabetes
American Heart Association*	At least 30 minutes (or 150 calories) of moderate exercise per day	Health promotion; prevention of cardiovascular disease

*See Chapter 7 for additional activity and exercise guidelines for people with special health concerns.

SOURCE: See "Selected Bibliography" for complete citations for all recommendations.

Exercise Programs to Develop Physical Fitness The Surgeon General's report also summarizes the benefits of more formal exercise programs. It concludes that people can obtain even greater health benefits by increasing the duration and intensity of activity. Thus, a person who engages in a structured, formal exercise program designed to measurably improve physical fitness will obtain even greater improvements in quality of life and greater reductions in disease and mortality risk. The American College of Sports Medicine has issued separate guidelines

for creating a formal exercise program that will develop physical fitness. These guidelines are described in detail later in this chapter.

How Much Physical Activity Is Enough?

Some experts feel that people get most of the health benefits of an exercise program simply by becoming more active over the course of the day; the amount of activity needed depends on an individual's health status and goals.

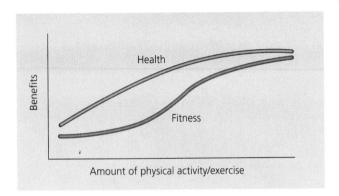

Figure 2.3   Relationship between amount of activity and health and fitness benefits.   The health benefits of physical activity and exercise exist along a continuum. A fairly low level of physical activity can provide substantial health benefits, although it does little to increase fitness. Engaging in exercise that is more intense or of longer duration leads to greater health benefits and significant increases in fitness.   SOURCE: American College of Sports Medicine. 2001. *ACSM's Resource Manual for Guidelines for Exercise Testing and Prescription*, 4th ed. Philadelphia: Williams & Wilkins, p. 452.

Other experts feel that the activity goal set by the lifestyle approach is too low; they argue that people should exercise long enough and intensely enough to improve their body's capacity for exercise—that is, to improve physical fitness. More research is needed to clarify the health effects of different amounts of lifestyle physical activity, of moderate-intensity vs. high-intensity exercise, and of continuous vs. intermittent exercise. However, there is probably truth in both of these positions.

Regular physical activity, regardless of intensity, makes you healthier and can help protect you from many chronic diseases (Figure 2.3). However, exercising at low intensities does little to improve physical fitness. Although you get many of the health benefits of exercise by simply being more active, you obtain even more benefits when you are physically fit. In addition to long-term health benefits, fitness also significantly contributes to quality of life. Fitness can give you freedom—freedom to move your body the way you want. Fit people have more energy and better body control. They can enjoy a more active lifestyle—cycling, hiking, skiing, and so on—than their more sedentary counterparts. Even if you don't like sports, you need physical energy and stamina in your daily life and for many nonsport leisure activities—visiting museums, playing with children, gardening, and so on.

Where does this leave you? Most experts agree that some physical activity is better than none, but that more—as long as it does not result in injury—is probably better than some. To set a personal goal for physical activity and exercise, consider your current activity level, your health status, and your goals. At the very least, strive to become more active and meet the goal set by the Surgeon General's report of using about 150 calories a day in physical activity. Choose to be active whenever you can. If weight management is a concern for you, begin by achieving the goal of 30 minutes of activity per day and then look to raise your activity level further, to 45–60 minutes per day or more. For even better health and well-being, participate in a structured exercise program that develops physical fitness. Any increase in physical activity will contribute to your health and well-being, now and in the future.

Next, let's take a closer look at the components of physical fitness and the basic principles of fitness training.

MOTIVATION FOR CHANGE!   Would you be more motivated to try to increase daily physical activity if you had an easy way to monitor your level of activity? If so, consider wearing a pedometer to track the number of steps you take each day—a rough but easily obtainable reflection of daily physical activity. Wear the pedometer for a week to obtain a baseline average daily number of steps, and then set an appropriate goal—for example, walking 2,000 additional steps each day or increasing daily steps to 10,000. Record your daily steps in a prominent location to monitor your progress and boost your motivation.

HEALTH-RELATED COMPONENTS OF PHYSICAL FITNESS

Physical fitness has many components, some related to general health and others related more specifically to particular sports or activities. The five components of fitness most important for health are cardiorespiratory endurance, muscular strength, muscular endurance, flexibility, and body composition. **Health-related fitness** contributes to your capacity to enjoy life, helps your body withstand physical and psychological challenges, and protects you from chronic disease.

Cardiorespiratory Endurance

Cardiorespiratory endurance is the ability to perform prolonged, large-muscle, dynamic exercise at moderate-to-high levels of intensity. It depends on such factors as the ability of the lungs to deliver oxygen from the environment to the bloodstream, the heart's capacity to pump blood, the ability of the nervous system and blood vessels to regulate blood flow, and the capability of the body's chemical systems to use oxygen and process fuels for exercise.

When levels of cardiorespiratory fitness are low, the heart has to work very hard during normal daily activities and may not be able to work hard enough to sustain high-intensity physical activity in an emergency. As cardiorespiratory fitness improves, the heart begins to function more efficiently. It doesn't have to work as hard at rest or during low levels of exercise. The heart pumps more blood per heartbeat, resting heart rate slows, blood volume increases,

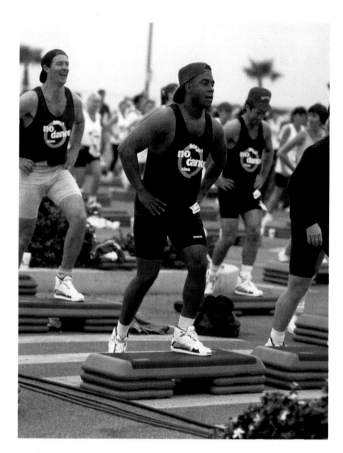

Cardiorespiratory endurance is a key component of health-related fitness. These participants in a group step aerobics class are conditioning their hearts and lungs as well as gaining many other health benefits.

blood supply to the tissues improves, the body is better able to cool itself, and resting blood pressure decreases. A healthy heart can better withstand the strains of everyday life, the stress of occasional emergencies, and the wear and tear of time. Endurance training also improves the functioning of the chemical systems, particularly in the muscles and liver, thereby enhancing the body's ability to use energy supplied by food and to do more exercise with less effort from the oxygen transport system.

Cardiorespiratory endurance is a central component of health-related fitness because the functioning of the heart and lungs is so essential to overall good health. A person can't live very long or very well without a healthy heart. Low levels of cardiorespiratory fitness are linked with heart disease, the leading cause of death in the United States. In addition to protecting against heart disease, cardiorespiratory fitness also reduces the risk of type 2 diabetes, colon cancer, stroke, depression, and anxiety. A moderate level of cardiorespiratory fitness can even help compensate for certain health risks, including excess body fat: People who are lean but who have low cardiorespiratory fitness have been found to have higher death rates than people with higher levels of body fat who are otherwise fit. Cardiorespiratory endurance exercise further benefits quality of life by improving self-image,

mood, cognitive functioning, and the ability to manage stress. Exercising to improve cardiorespiratory endurance also provides opportunities to have fun and to socialize.

Muscular Strength

Muscular strength is the amount of force a muscle can produce with a single maximum effort. It depends on such factors as the size of muscle cells and the ability of nerves to activate muscle cells. Strong muscles are important for the smooth and easy performance of everyday activities, such as carrying groceries, lifting boxes, and climbing stairs, as well as for emergency situations. They help keep the skeleton in proper alignment, preventing back and leg pain and providing the support necessary for good posture. Muscular strength has obvious importance in recreational activities. Strong people can hit a tennis ball harder, kick a soccer ball farther, and ride a bicycle uphill more easily. Muscle tissue is an important element of overall body composition. Greater muscle mass means a higher rate of **metabolism** and faster energy use. Training to build muscular strength can also help people manage stress and boost their self-confidence.

Maintaining strength and muscle mass is vital for healthy aging. Older people tend to lose both number and size of muscle cells. Many of the muscle cells that remain become slower, and some become nonfunctional because they lose their attachment to the nervous system. Strength training helps maintain muscle mass and function and possibly helps decrease the risk of osteoporosis in older people, which greatly enhances their quality of life and prevents life-threatening injuries.

Muscular Endurance

Muscular endurance is the ability to resist fatigue and sustain a given level of muscle tension—that is, to hold a muscle contraction for a long period of time or to contract a muscle over and over again. It depends on such factors as the size of muscle cells, the ability of muscles to store fuel, and the blood supply to muscles. Muscular endurance is important for good posture and for injury prevention. For example, if abdominal and back muscles can't hold

health-related fitness Physical capacities that contribute to health: cardiorespiratory endurance, muscular strength, muscular endurance, flexibility, and body composition.

cardiorespiratory endurance The ability of the body to perform prolonged, large-muscle, dynamic exercise at moderate-to-high levels of intensity.

muscular strength The amount of force a muscle can produce with a single maximum effort.

metabolism The sum of all the vital processes by which food energy and nutrients are made available to and used by the body.

muscular endurance The ability of a muscle or group of muscles to remain contracted or to contract repeatedly for a long period of time.

Terms

VW

the spine correctly, the chances of low-back pain and back injury are increased. Recent research suggests that good muscular endurance in the trunk muscles is more important than muscular strength for preventing back pain. Muscular endurance helps people cope with the physical demands of everyday life and enhances performance in sports and work. It is also important for most leisure and fitness activities.

Flexibility

Flexibility is the ability to move the joints through their full range of motion. It depends on joint structure, the length and elasticity of connective tissue, and nervous system activity. Flexible, pain-free joints are important for good health and well-being. Inactivity causes the joints to become stiffer with age. Stiffness often causes older people to assume unnatural body postures that can stress joints and muscles. Stretching exercises can help ensure a healthy range of motion for all major joints.

Body Composition

Body composition refers to the proportion of fat and **fat-free mass** (muscle, bone, and water) in the body. Healthy body composition involves a high proportion of fat-free mass and an acceptably low level of body fat, adjusted for age and gender. A person with excessive body fat—especially when excess fat is located in the abdomen—is more likely to experience a variety of health problems, including heart disease, insulin resistance, high blood pressure, stroke, joint problems, type 2 diabetes, gall-bladder disease, some types of cancer, and back pain.

The best way to lose fat is through a lifestyle that includes a sensible diet and exercise. The best way to add muscle mass is through resistance training, also known as strength training or, when weights are used, weight training. Large changes in body composition aren't necessary to improve health; even a small increase in physical activity and a small decrease in body fat can lead to substantial health improvements. As described earlier, cardiorespiratory fitness may be more important than body composition in determining overall health status.

Skill-Related Components of Fitness

In addition to the five health-related components of physical fitness, the ability to perform a particular sport or activity may depend on **skill-related fitness** components such as the following:

- *Speed:* The ability to perform a movement in a short period of time.
- *Power:* The ability to exert force rapidly, based on a combination of strength and speed.
- *Agility:* The ability to change the position of the body quickly and accurately.
- *Balance:* The ability to maintain equilibrium while moving or while stationary.
- *Coordination:* The ability to perform motor tasks accurately and smoothly using body movements and the senses.
- *Reaction time:* The ability to respond or react quickly to a stimulus.

Skill-related fitness tends to be sport-specific and is best developed through practice. For example, the speed, coordination, and agility needed to play basketball can be developed by playing basketball. Some fitness experts downplay sports participation because some sports don't contribute to all the health-related components of physical fitness. However, engaging in sports is fun and can help you build fitness and contribute to other areas of wellness. You can get immense satisfaction from hitting a well-executed cross-court backhand in tennis, climbing a challenging rock wall, hitting the green from 150 yards out in golf, or spiking a ball past an opponent in volleyball. Sports can be an important and fun part of an active wellness lifestyle.

PRINCIPLES OF PHYSICAL TRAINING: ADAPTATION TO STRESS

The human body is very adaptable. The greater the demands made on it, the more it adjusts to meet those demands. Over time, immediate, short-term adjustments translate into long-term changes and improvements. When breathing and heart rate increase during exercise, for example, the heart gradually develops the ability to pump more blood with each beat. Then, during exercise, it doesn't have to beat as fast to meet the cells' demands for oxygen. The goal of **physical training** is to produce these long-term changes and improvements in the body's functioning. Although people differ in the maximum levels of physical fitness and performance they can achieve through training, the wellness benefits of exercise are available to everyone (see the box "Fitness and Disability").

Particular types and amounts of exercise are most effective in developing the various components of fitness. To put together an effective exercise program, a person should first understand the basic principles of physical training. Important principles are specificity, progressive overload, reversibility, and individual differences. All of these rest on the larger principle of adaptation.

Specificity—Adapting to Type of Training

To develop a particular fitness component, exercises must be performed that are specifically designed for that component. This is the principle of **specificity**. Weight training, for example, develops muscular strength, but is less effective for developing cardiorespiratory endurance or flexibility. Specificity also applies to the skill-related fitness components—to improve at tennis, you must practice tennis—and to the different parts of the body—to

Physical fitness and athletic achievement are not limited to the able-bodied. People with disabilities can also attain high levels of fitness and performance, as shown by the elite athletes who compete in the Paralympics. The premier event for athletes with disabilities, the Paralympics are held in the same year and city as the Olympics. The performance of these skilled athletes makes it clear that people with disabilities can be active, healthy, and extraordinarily fit; just like able-bodied athletes, athletes with disabilities strive for excellence and can serve as role models.

Currently, some 54 million Americans are estimated to have chronic, significant disabilities. Some disabilities are the result of injury, such as spinal cord injuries sustained in car crashes. Other disabilities result from illness, such as the blindness that sometimes occurs as a complication of diabetes or the joint stiffness that accompanies arthritis. And some disabilities are present at birth, as in the case of congenital limb deformities or cerebral palsy.

Exercise and physical activity are as important for people with disabilities as for able-bodied individuals—if not *more* important. Being active helps prevent secondary conditions that may result from prolonged inactivity, such as circulatory or muscular problems. It provides an emotional boost that helps support a positive attitude as well as opportunities to make new friends, increase self-confidence, and gain a sense of accomplishment. Currently, about 21% of people with disabilities engage in regular moderate or vigorous activity.

People with disabilities don't have to be elite athletes to participate in sports and lead an active life. Some health clubs and fitness centers offer activities and events geared for people of all ages and types of disabilities. They may have modified aerobics classes, special weight training machines, classes involving mild exercise in warm water, and other activities adapted for people with disabilities. Popular sports and recreational activities include adapted horseback riding, golf, swimming, and skiing. Competitive sports are also available—for example, there are wheelchair versions of billiards, tennis, hockey, and basketball, as well as sports for people with hearing, visual, or mental impairments. For those who prefer to get their exercise at home, special videos are available geared to individuals who use wheelchairs or who have arthritis, hearing impairments, or many other disabilities.

If you have a disability and want to be more active, check with your physician about what's appropriate for you. Call your local community center, YMCA/YWCA, independent living center, or fitness center to locate potential facilities; look for a facility with experienced personnel and appropriate adaptive equipment. For specialized videos, check with hospitals and health associations that are geared to specific disabilities, such as the Arthritis Foundation. Remember that no matter what your level of ability or disability, it's possible to make physical activity an integral part of your life.

SOURCES: National Center for Health Statistics. 2004. *DATA2010: The Healthy People 2010 Database: January 2004 Edition* (http://wonder.cdc.gov/data2010; retrieved April 7, 2004). National Center on Physical Activity and Disability. 2000. *White Paper: Spinal Cord Injury and Fitness.* Chicago: National Center on Physical Activity and Disability. U.S. Department of Health and Human Services. 2000. *Healthy People 2010,* 2d ed. Washington, D.C.: DHHS. U.S. Department of Health and Human Services. 1996. *Physical Activity and Health: A Report of the Surgeon General.* Atlanta. Ga.: DHHS.

develop stronger arms, you must exercise your arms. A well-rounded exercise program includes exercises geared to each component of fitness, to different parts of the body, and to specific activities or sports.

Progressive Overload—Adapting to Amount of Training and the FITT Principle

The body adapts to the demands of exercise by improving its functioning. When the amount of exercise (also called overload or stress) is progressively increased, fitness continues to improve. This is the principle of **progressive overload.**

The amount of overload is very important. Too little exercise will have no effect on fitness (although it may improve health); too much may cause injury and problems with the body's immune system and hormone levels. The point at which exercise becomes excessive is highly individual—it occurs at a much higher level in an Olympic athlete than in a sedentary person. For every type of exercise, there is a training threshold at which fitness benefits begin to occur, a zone within which maximum fitness benefits occur, and an upper limit of safe training. The amount of exercise needed depends on the individual's current level of fitness, his or her fitness goals, and the component being developed. A novice, for example, might experience fitness benefits from jogging a mile in 10 minutes, but this level of exercise would

flexibility The range of motion in a joint or group of joints, flexibility is related to muscle length.

body composition The proportion of fat and fat-free mass (muscle, bone, and water) in the body.

fat-free mass The nonfat component of the human body, consisting of skeletal muscle, bone, and water.

skill-related fitness Physical capacities that contribute to performance in a sport or activity: speed, power, agility, balance, coordination, and reaction time.

physical training The performance of different types of activities that cause the body to adapt and improve its level of fitness.

specificity The training principle that the body adapts to the particular type and amount of stress placed on it.

progressive overload The training principle that placing increasing amounts of stress on the body causes adaptations that improve fitness.

Terms

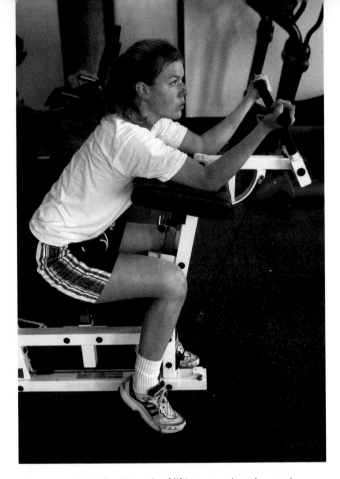

When stressed by the demands of lifting more than the usual amount of weight, the body responds by building muscular strength and endurance. To safely and effectively develop strength, this exerciser must overload her muscles with enough weight to improve her body's functioning but not so much weight that she becomes injured.

cause no physical adaptations in a trained distance runner. Beginners should start at the lower end of the fitness benefit zone; fitter individuals will make more rapid gains by exercising at the higher end of the fitness benefit zone.

The amount of overload needed to maintain or improve a particular level of fitness for a particular fitness component is determined through four dimensions, represented by the acronym FITT:

- Frequency—how often
- Intensity—how hard
- Time—how long (duration)
- Type—mode of activity

Some experts use the acronym FITTE, where the *E* stands for enjoyment—a key component of a successful, long-term fitness program.

Frequency Developing fitness requires regular exercise. Optimum exercise frequency, expressed in number of days per week, varies with the component being developed and the individual's fitness goals. For most people, a frequency

of 3–5 days per week for cardiorespiratory endurance exercise and 2–3 days per week for resistance and flexibility training is appropriate for a general fitness program.

An important consideration in determining appropriate exercise frequency is recovery time, which is also highly individual and depends on factors such as training experience, age, and intensity of training. For example, 24 hours of rest between highly intensive workouts that involve heavy weights or fast track sprints is not enough recovery time for safe and effective training; intense workouts need to be spaced out during the week to allow sufficient recovery time. On the other hand, you can exercise every day if your program consists of moderate-intensity walking or cycling. Learn to "listen to your body" to obtain a sufficient amount of rest between workouts. Chapters 3–5 provide more detailed information about training techniques and recovery periods for workouts focused on different fitness components.

Intensity Fitness benefits occur when a person exercises harder than his or her normal level of activity. The appropriate exercise intensity varies with each fitness component. To develop cardiorespiratory endurance, for example, a person must raise his or her heart rate above normal; to develop muscular strength, a person must lift a heavier weight than normal; to develop flexibility, a person must stretch muscles beyond their normal length.

Time (Duration) Fitness benefits occur when you exercise for an extended period of time. For cardiorespiratory endurance exercise, 20–60 minutes is recommended; exercise can take place in a single session or in several sessions of 10 or more minutes. The greater the intensity of exercise, the less time needed to obtain fitness benefits. For high-intensity exercise, such as running, for example, 20–30 minutes is appropriate. For more moderate-intensity exercise, such as walking, 45–60 minutes may be needed. High-intensity exercise poses a greater risk of injury than lower-intensity exercise, so if you are a nonathletic adult, it's probably best to emphasize lower-to-moderate-intensity activity of longer duration.

To build muscular strength, muscular endurance, and flexibility, similar amounts of time are advisable, but these exercises are more commonly organized in terms of a specific number of repetitions of particular exercises. For resistance training, for example, a recommended program includes 1 or more sets of 8–12 repetitions of 8–10 different exercises that work the major muscle groups.

Type (Mode of Activity) The type of exercise in which you should engage varies with each fitness component and with your personal fitness goals. To develop cardiorespiratory endurance, you need to engage in continuous activities involving large-muscle groups—walking, jogging, cycling, or swimming, for example. Resistive exercises develop muscular strength and endurance, while stretching exercises build flexibility. The frequency, intensity, and time, or duration, of the exercise will be different for each type of activity. See pp. 38–39 for more on choosing appropriate activities for your fitness program.

Reversibility—Adapting to a Reduction in Training

Fitness is a reversible adaptation. The body adjusts to lower levels of physical activity the same way it adjusts to higher levels. This is the principle of **reversibility.** When a person stops exercising, up to 50% of fitness improvements are lost within 2 months. However, not all fitness levels reverse at the same rate. Strength fitness is very resilient, so a person can maintain strength fitness by doing resistive exercise as infrequently as once a week. On the other hand, cardiovascular and cellular fitness reverse themselves more quickly—sometimes within just a few days or weeks. Thus, if a training schedule must be curtailed temporarily, fitness improvements are best maintained if exercise intensity is kept constant and frequency and/or duration is reduced.

Individual Differences—Limits on Adaptability

Anyone watching the Olympics, a professional football game, or a tennis championship match can readily see that, from a physical standpoint, we are not all created equal. There are large individual differences in our ability to improve fitness, achieve a desirable body composition, perform and learn sports skills. Some people are able to run longer distances, or lift more weight, or kick a soccer ball more skillfully than others will ever be able to, no matter how much they train. There are limits on the adaptability—the potential for improvement—of any human body. The body's ability to transport and use oxygen, for example, can be improved by only about 15–30% through training. An endurance athlete must therefore inherit a large metabolic capacity in order to reach competitive performance levels. In the past few years, scientists have identified specific genes that influence body fat, strength, and endurance.

However, a person doesn't have to be an Olympic sprinter to experience health benefits from running. Physical training improves fitness regardless of heredity. For the average person, the body's adaptability is enough to achieve reasonable fitness goals.

DESIGNING YOUR OWN EXERCISE PROGRAM

Physical training works best when you have a plan. A plan helps you make gradual but steady progress toward your goals. Once you've determined that exercise is safe for you, planning for physical fitness consists of assessing how fit you are now, determining where you want to be, and choosing the right activities to help you get there. These activities are discussed next, along with some general guidelines for training.

Medical Clearance

People of any age who are not at high risk for serious health problems can safely exercise at a moderate intensity (60% or less of maximum heart rate) without a prior medical evaluation (see Chapter 3 for a discussion of maximum heart rate). Likewise, if you are male and under 40 or female and under 50 and in good health, exercise is probably safe for you. If you do not fit into these age groups or have health problems—especially high blood pressure, heart disease, muscle or joint problems, or obesity—see your physician before starting a vigorous exercise program. The Canadian Society for Exercise Physiology has developed the Physical Activity Readiness Questionnaire (PAR-Q) to help evaluate exercise safety. This questionnaire is included in Lab 2.1. Completing it should alert you to any potential problems you may have. If a physician isn't sure whether exercise is safe for you, she or he may recommend an **exercise stress test** or a **graded exercise test (GXT)** to see whether you show symptoms of heart disease during exercise. For most people, however, it's far safer to exercise than to remain sedentary. For more information, see the box "Is Exercise Safe?" (p. 38).

Assessment

The first step in creating a successful fitness program is to assess your current level of physical activity and fitness for each of the five health-related fitness components. The results of the assessment tests will help you set specific fitness goals and plan your fitness program. Lab 2.2 gives you the opportunity to assess your current overall level of activity and determine if it is appropriate. Assessment tests in Chapters 3, 4, 5, and 6 will help you evaluate your cardiorespiratory endurance, muscular strength, muscular endurance, flexibility, and body composition.

Setting Goals

The ultimate general goal of every health-related fitness program is the same—wellness that lasts a lifetime. Whatever your specific goals, they must be important enough to you to keep you motivated. Studies have

---

reversibility The training principle that fitness improvements are lost when demands on the body are lowered.

exercise stress test A test usually administered on a treadmill or cycle ergometer that involves analysis of the changes in electrical activity in the heart from an electrocardiogram (EKG or ECG) taken during exercise. Used to determine if any heart disease is present and to assess current fitness level.

graded exercise test (GXT) An exercise test that starts at an easy intensity and progresses to maximum capacity.

Terms

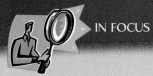

Participating in exercise and sports is usually a wonderful experience that improves wellness in both the short and long term. In rare instances, however, vigorous exertion is associated with sudden death. It may seem difficult to understand that although regular exercise protects people from heart disease, it also increases the risk of sudden death.

What causes sudden death during or immediately following exercise? In nearly all cases, coronary artery disease is responsible. In this condition, fat and other substances build up in the arteries that supply blood to the heart. Death can result if an artery becomes blocked or if the heart's rhythm and pumping action are disrupted. Exercise, particularly intense exercise, may trigger a heart attack in someone with underlying heart disease. (In the very rare cases of death among young athletes, the cause may be a congenital or genetic cardiovascular disorder rather than coronary artery disease.)

What is the risk of dying suddenly during exercise? A study of jogging deaths in Rhode Island found that there was one death per 396,000 hours of jogging, or about one death per 7620 joggers per year—an extremely low risk for each individual jogger. Another study of men involved in a variety of physical activities found one death per 1.51 million hours of exercise. This 12-year study of more than 21,000 men found that those who didn't exercise vigorously were 74 times more likely to die suddenly from cardiac arrest during or shortly after exercise. It is also important to note that people are much safer exercising than engaging in many other common activities, including driving a car.

Although quite small, the risk does exist and may lead some people to wonder why exercise is considered such an important part of a wellness lifestyle. Exercise causes many positive changes in the body—in healthy people as well as those with heart disease—that more than make up for the slightly increased short-term risk of sudden death. Training slows or reverses the fatty buildup in arteries and helps protect people from deadly heart rhythm abnormalities. People who exercise regularly have an overall risk of sudden death only about two-thirds that of nonexercisers. Active people who stop exercising can expect their heart attack risk to increase by 300%.

Who is most at risk for sudden death during exercise? Obviously, someone with underlying coronary artery disease is at greater risk than someone who is free from the condition. However, many cases of heart disease may go undiagnosed. The riskiest scenario may be when a middle-aged or older individual suddenly begins participating in a vigorous sport or activity after a long period of a sedentary lifestyle. This finding provides strong evidence for the recommendation that people increase their level of physical activity gradually and engage in regular, rather than sporadic, activity.

For the vast majority of people, exercise is a safe and effective way to increase both life expectancy and quality of life. If you decide you don't want to exercise, you might want to see your physician to determine if you can resist the deadly effects of a sedentary lifestyle.

SOURCES: Thompson, P. D. 2001. Cardiovascular risks of exercise. *Physician and Sportsmedicine* 29(4). Albert, C. M., et al. 2000. Trigger of sudden death from cardiac causes by vigorous exertion. *New England Journal of Medicine* 343(19): 1355–1361.

---

shown that exercising for yourself, rather than for the impression you think you'll make on others, is more likely to lead to long-lasting commitment. After you complete the assessment tests in Chapters 3–6, you will be able to set goals directly related to each fitness component, such as working toward a 3-mile jog or doing 20 push-ups. First, though, think carefully about your overall goals, and be clear about why you are starting a program.

Choosing Activities for a Balanced Program

An ideal fitness program combines a physically active lifestyle with a systematic exercise program to develop and maintain physical fitness. This overall program is shown in the physical activity pyramid in Figure 2.4. If you are currently sedentary, your goal is to focus on activities at the bottom of the pyramid and gradually increase the amount of moderate-intensity physical activity in your daily life. Appropriate activities include brisk walking, climbing stairs, yard work, and washing your car. You don't have to exercise vigorously, but you should experience a moderate increase in your heart and breathing rates. As described earlier, your activity time can be broken up into small blocks over the course of a day.

The next two levels of the pyramid illustrate parts of a formal exercise program. The principles of this program are consistent with those of the American College of Sports Medicine (ACSM), the professional organization for people involved in sports medicine and exercise science. The ACSM has established guidelines for creating an exercise program that will develop physical fitness (Table 2.2, p. 40). A balanced program includes activities to develop all the health-related components of fitness.

- *Cardiorespiratory endurance* is developed by continuous rhythmic movements of large-muscle groups in activities such as walking, jogging, cycling, swimming, and aerobic dance and other forms of group exercise. Choose activities that you enjoy and that are convenient. Other popular choices are in-line skating, dancing, and backpacking. Start-and-stop activities such as tennis, racquetball, and soccer can also develop endurance if one's skill level is sufficient to enable periods of continuous play. Training for cardiorespiratory endurance is discussed in Chapter 3.

- *Muscular strength and endurance* can be developed through resistance training—training with weights or

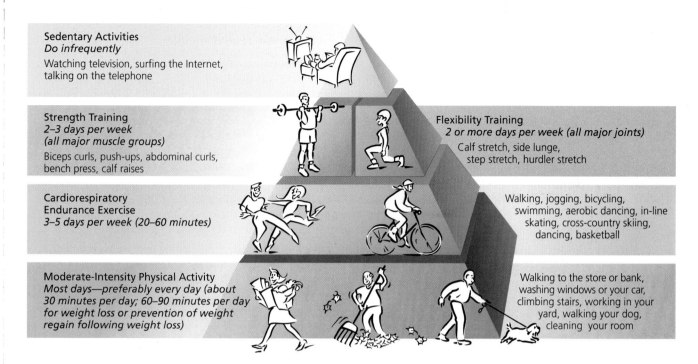

Figure 2.4 Physical activity pyramid. Similar in design to the Food Guide Pyramid, this physical activity pyramid shows the component of a balanced fitness program, and emphasizes the importance of daily moderate-intensity physical activity. If you are currently sedentary, gradually increase the amount of moderate-intensity physical activity in your life. If you are already moderately active, begin a formal exercise program that includes cardiorespiratory endurance exercise, flexibility training, and strength training to help you develop all the health-related components of fitness.

performing calisthenic exercises such as push-ups and curl-ups. Training for muscular strength and endurance is discussed in Chapter 4.

• *Flexibility* is developed by stretching the major muscle groups, regularly and with proper technique. Flexibility is discussed in Chapter 5.

• *Healthy body composition* can be developed through a sensible diet and a program of regular exercise. Endurance exercise is best for reducing body fat; resistance training builds muscle mass, which, to a small extent, helps increase metabolism. Body composition is discussed in Chapter 6.

There are as many different fitness programs as there are individuals. Consider the following examples:

• Maggie is a person whose life revolves around sports. She's been on softball teams and swim teams, and now she's on her college varsity soccer team. She follows a rigorous exercise regimen established by her soccer coach. Afternoon soccer practice begins with warm-ups, drills, and practice in specific skills, and it ends with a scrimmage and then a jog around the soccer field. Games are every Saturday. Maggie likes team sports, but she also enjoys exercising alone, so she goes on long bicycle rides whenever she can fit them in. She can't imagine what it would be like not to be active every day.

• Maria is a busy young mother of twins. To keep in shape, she joined a health club with a weight room, exercise classes, and child care. Three mornings a week, she takes the twins to the club and attends the 7:00 "wake-up"

low-impact aerobics class. The instructor leads the class through warm-ups; a 20-minute aerobic workout; exercises for the arms, abdomen, buttocks, and legs; stretches; and a relaxation exercise. Maria is exhilarated and ready for the rest of the day before 9:00 A.M.

• Tom is an engineering student with a lot of studying to do and an active social life as well. For exercise, he plays tennis three times a week. He likes to head for the courts around 6:00 P.M., when most people are eating dinner. He warms up for 10 minutes by practicing his forehand and backhand against a backboard and then plays a hard, fast game with his regular partner for 45 minutes to an hour. Afterwards, he does some stretching exercises while his muscles are still warm and then cools down with an easy 5-minute walk. Then he showers and gets ready for dinner. Twice a week he works out at the gym, with particular attention to keeping his arms strong and his shoulders limber. On Saturday nights, he goes dancing with friends.

• Ruben started a new job as a financial advisor in a large city. He spends 3 hours a day commuting on the train and has a new family, so he has no time for a structured exercise program. However, he manages to stay active during his busy work week by engaging in short bouts of physical activity. He parks some distance from the train station and walks briskly to and from his car—15 minutes each way. At work, he takes the stairs to his sixth-floor office. During several breaks during the day, he does isometric exercises and stretches; these breaks help him maintain fitness and reduce the physical and mental

Exercise to Develop and Maintain Cardiorespiratory Endurance and Body Composition

Frequency of training	3–5 days per week.
Intensity of training	55/65–90% of maximum heart rate or 40/50–85% of maximum oxygen uptake reserve.* The lower intensity values (55–64% of maximum heart rate and 40–49% of maximum oxygen uptake reserve) are most applicable to individuals who are quite unfit. For average individuals, intensities of 70–85% of maximum heart rate are appropriate.
Time (duration) of training	20–60 total minutes of continuous, or intermittent (in sessions lasting 10 or more minutes) aerobic activity. Duration is dependent on the intensity of activity; thus, lower-intensity activity should be conducted over a longer period of time (30 minutes or more). Lower-to-moderate-intensity activity of longer duration is recommended for the nonathletic adult.
Type (mode) of activity	Any activity that uses large-muscle groups, can be maintained continuously, and is rhythmic and aerobic in nature, for example, walking-hiking, running-jogging, cycling-bicycling, cross-country skiing, aerobic dance and other forms of group exercise, rope skipping, rowing, stair climbing, swimming, skating, and endurance game activities.

Exercise to Develop and Maintain Muscular Strength and Endurance, Flexibility, and Body Composition

Resistance training	One set of 8–10 exercises that condition the major muscle groups should be performed 2–3 days per week. Most people should complete 8–12 repetitions of each exercise; for older and more frail people (approximately 50–60 years of age and above), 10–15 repetitions with a lighter weight may be more appropriate. Multiple-set regimens will provide greater benefits if time allows.
Flexibility training	Stretches for the major muscle groups should be performed a minimum of 2–3 days per week; at least 4 repetitions held for 10–30 seconds should be completed.

*Instructions for calculating target heart rate intensity for cardiorespiratory endurance exercise are presented in Chapter 3.

SOURCE: American College of Sports Medicine. 1998. The recommended quantity and quality of exercise for developing and maintaining cardiorespiratory and muscular fitness, and flexibility in healthy adults. Position paper. *Medicine and Science in Sports and Exercise* 30(6): 975–991.

stress of his high-pressure, sedentary job. Twice a week, he does calisthenic exercises at home in the evening, and he goes for a 30-minute jog on Saturday mornings.

• Kadija is a paraplegic who uses a wheelchair for mobility. She considers herself a sports fanatic. She plays wheelchair basketball two nights a week and stays in shape by training on the arm ergometer and lifting weights at the gym three days a week. During the spring, she enjoys competing in track and field. Her favorite event is the 400-meter race. She also enjoys water skiing in the summertime. She has not let her disability keep her from exercising regularly or being physically fit.

Each of these people has worked an adequate or more-than-adequate fitness program into a busy daily routine. Chapter 7 contains guidelines to help you choose activities and put together a complete exercise program that suits your goals and preferences. (Refer to Figure 2.5 for a summary of the health and fitness benefits of different levels of physical activity.)

What about the tip of the activity pyramid? Although sedentary activities are often unavoidable—attending class, studying, working in an office, and so on—many people choose inactivity over activity during their leisure time. Change sedentary patterns by becoming more active whenever you can. Move more and sit less.

MOTIVATION FOR CHANGE! Your school and community may present challenges to making healthy lifestyle choices, but they also have resources that can help you. Find out what local resources are "on your side" and can support your efforts at change. For example, go to your school's physical education office and ask for a comprehensive listing of all the exercise and fitness facilities and courses available on your campus. Obtain the same information about facilities and classes in your neighborhood, including those offered by the city or county recreation department. What fitness facilities and/or courses fit your goals, schedule, preferences, and budget? If you can't find a local program or facility to fit your needs, check out the programs available through the President's Challenge (http://www.presidentschallenge.org).

Guidelines for Training

The following guidelines will make your exercise program more effective and successful.

Train the way you want your body to change. Stress your body such that it adapts in the desired direction. To have a more muscular build, lift weights. To be more

	Lifestyle physical activity	Moderate exercise program	Vigorous exercise program
Description	Moderate physical activity—an amount of activity that uses about 150 calories per day	Cardiorespiratory endurance exercise (20–60 minutes, 3–5 days per week); strength training and stretching exercises (2–3 days per week)	Cardiorespiratory endurance exercise (20–60 minutes, 3–5 days per week); interval training; strength training (3–4 days per week); and stretching exercises (3–5 days per week)
Sample activities or program	*One of the following:* • Walking briskly to and from work, 15 minutes each way • Cycling to and from class, 10 minutes each way • Yardwork for 30 minutes • Dancing (fast) for 30 minutes • Playing basketball for 20 minutes	• Jogging for 30 minutes, 3 days per week • Weight training, 1 set of 8 exercises, 2 days per week • Stretching exercises, 3 days per week	• Running for 45 minutes, 3 days per week • Intervals: running 400 m at high effort, 4 sets, 2 days per week • Weight training, 3 sets of 10 exercises, 3 days per week • Stretching exercises, 5 days per week
Health and fitness benefits	Better blood cholesterol levels, reduced body fat, better control of blood pressure, improved metabolic health, and enhanced glucose metabolism; improved quality of life; reduced risk of some chronic diseases Greater amounts of activity can help prevent weight gain and promote weight loss	All the benefits of lifestyle physical activity, plus improved physical fitness (increased cardiorespiratory endurance, muscular strength and endurance, and flexibility) and even greater improvements in health and quality of life and reductions in chronic disease risk	All the benefits of lifestyle physical activity and a moderate exercise program, with greater increases in fitness and somewhat greater reductions in chronic disease risk Participating in a vigorous exercise program may increase risk of injury and overtraining

Figure 2.5   Health and fitness benefits of different amounts of physical activity and exercise.

flexible, do stretching exercises. To improve performance in a particular sport, practice that sport or the movements used in it.

Train regularly.   Consistency is the key to improving fitness. Fitness improvements are lost if too much time is allowed to pass between exercise sessions.

Get in shape gradually.   An exercise program can be divided into three phases: the beginning phase, during which the body adjusts to the new type and level of activity; the progress phase, during which fitness is increased; and the maintenance phase, in which the targeted level of fitness is maintained over the long term (Figure 2.6, p. 42). When beginning a program, start slowly to give your body time to adapt to the stress of exercise. As you progress, increase duration and frequency before increasing intensity. If you train too much or too intensely, you are more likely to suffer injuries or become **overtrained,** a condition characterized by lack of energy, aching muscles and joints, and decreased physical performance. Injuries and overtraining slow down an exercise program and impede motivation. The goal is not to get in shape as quickly as possible but to gradually become and remain physically fit.

Warm up before exercise.   Warming up can decrease your chances of injury by helping your body gradually progress from rest to activity. A good warm-up can increase muscle temperature, reduce joint stiffness, bathe the joint surfaces in lubricating fluid, and increase blood flow to the muscles, including—very importantly—the heart. Some studies suggest that warming up may also reduce the risk of injury, enhance muscle metabolism, and mentally prepare a person for a workout.

A warm-up should include low-intensity, whole-body movements similar to those used in the activity that will follow. For example, runners may walk and jog slowly prior to running at full-speed. A tennis player might hit forehands and backhands at a low intensity before playing a vigorous set of tennis. It is important to note that a warm-up is not the same thing as a stretching workout. For safety and effectiveness, it is best to stretch *after* an endurance or strength-training workout, when muscles are warm—and not as part of a warm-up.

Cool down after exercise.   During exercise, as much as 90% of circulating blood is directed to the muscles and

overtraining A condition caused by training too much or too intensely, characterized by lack of energy, decreased physical performance, fatigue, depression, aching muscles and joints, and susceptibility to injury.

Terms

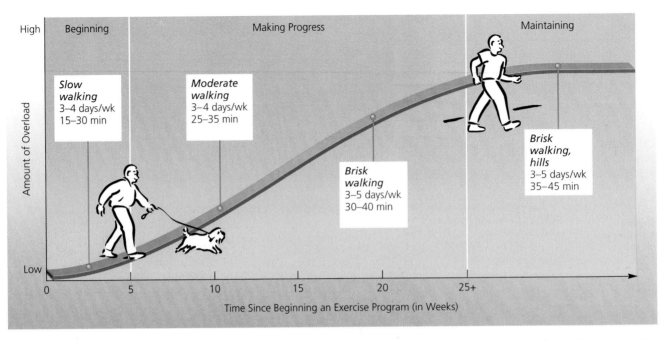

High | Beginning | Making Progress | Maintaining

Slow walking
3–4 days/wk
15–30 min

Moderate walking
3–4 days/wk
25–35 min

Brisk walking
3–5 days/wk
30–40 min

Brisk walking, hills
3–5 days/wk
35–45 min

Amount of Overload

Low

0   5   10   15   20   25+

Time Since Beginning an Exercise Program (in Weeks)

Figure 2.6   Progression of an exercise program.   This figure shows how the amount of overload is increased gradually over time in a sample walking program. Regardless of the activity chosen, it is important that an exercise program begin slowly and progress gradually. Once a person achieves the desired level of fitness, she or he can maintain it by exercising 3 to 5 days a week.   SOURCE: Progression data from American College of Sports Medicine. 2000. *ACSM's Guidelines for Exercise Testing and Prescription,* 6th ed. Baltimore, Md.: Lippincott Williams & Wilkins.

skin, up from as little as 20% during rest. If you suddenly stop moving after exercise, the amount of blood returning to your heart and brain may be insufficient, and you may experience dizziness, a drop in blood pressure, or other problems. Cooling down at the end of a workout helps safely restore circulation to its normal resting condition. So, don't sit or lie down or jump into the shower after exercise without cooling down first. Cool down by continuing to move at a slow pace—walking, for example—for 5–10 minutes, as your heart and breathing rate slowly return to normal. At the end of the cool-down period, do stretching exercises while your muscles are still warm.

Exercise safely.   Physical activity can cause injury or even death if you don't consider safety. Wear a helmet when rock climbing, skiing, or riding a bike, and wear eye protectors when playing racquetball or squash. Walk or run with a partner in a park or deserted track. Wear bright clothing when exercising on public streets. When you cycle, remember to always give cars plenty of leeway, even when you have the right of way; in a collision, a car will sustain less damage than a bicycle or your unprotected body. Train within your capacity because overloading your muscles and joints can lead to serious injury. Use good quality equipment and keep it in good repair. Report broken gym equipment to the health club manager. (See Appendix A for more information on personal safety.)

Listen to your body.   Don't exercise if it doesn't feel right. Sometimes you need a few days of rest to recover enough to train with the intensity required for improving fitness. On the other hand, you can't train sporadically

either. If you listen to your body and it always tells you to rest, you won't make any progress.

Cycle the volume and intensity of your workouts.   To add enjoyment and variety to your program, and to further improve fitness, don't train at the same intensity during every workout. Some days train very intensely and other days train more lightly. Proper management of the level of workout intensity is a key to improved physical fitness. Use cycle training, also known as periodization, to provide enough recovery for intense training. Because you trained lightly one workout, you can train harder the next. Also cycle the type of training you do during different times of the year. During the summer, you might emphasize conditioning by jogging, playing basketball, and doing high-volume strength training exercises. During the fall, you might emphasize resistance training using more weights and fewer repetitions, gradually introducing more cardiovascular exercise into your program. In the spring, you might try a variety of activities, continue weight training, and get in great shape for the summer.

Try training with a partner.   Training partners can motivate and encourage each other through hard spots and help each other develop proper exercise techniques. Training with a partner can make exercising seem easier and more fun.

Train your mind.   This is one of the most difficult skills to acquire, but it is critical for achieving and maintaining fitness. Becoming fit requires commitment, discipline, and patience. These qualities come from understanding the importance of exercise and having clear and reachable goals. Use the lifestyle management techniques discussed in Chapter 1 to keep your program on track. Believe in yourself and your potential—and you *will* achieve your goals!

Add variety and have fun. You are more likely to stick with an exercise program if it's fun. Choose a variety of activities that you enjoy. Change your exercise program occasionally to keep things fresh and help develop a higher degree of fitness. The body adapts more quickly to new activities than to familiar ones. Changing activities may also help reduce your risk of injury.

Keep your exercise program in perspective. As important as physical fitness is, it is only part of a well-rounded life. You have to have time for work and school, family and friends, relaxation and hobbies. Some people become overinvolved in exercise and neglect other parts of their lives. They think of themselves as runners, dancers, swimmers, or triathletes rather than as people who participate in those activities. Balance and moderation are the key ingredients of a fit and well life.

Tips for Today

Physical activity and exercise offer benefits in nearly every area of wellness, helping you generate energy, manage stress, improve your mood, and, of course, become physically stronger and healthier. Even a low-to-moderate level of activity provides valuable health benefits. The important thing is to get moving!

Right now you can

- Go outside and take a brisk 15-minute walk.
- Look at your calendar for the rest of the week and write in some physical activity—such as walking, running, biking, skating, swimming, hiking, or playing Frisbee—on as many days as you can. Schedule the activity for a specific time and stick to it.
- Call a friend and invite her or him to start planning a regular exercise program with you.

SUMMARY

- Exercising daily in moderation contributes substantially to good health. Even without a formal, vigorous exercise program, you can get many of the same health benefits by becoming more physically active.

- If you are already active, you benefit even more by increasing the intensity or duration of your activity.

- The five components of physical fitness most important for health are cardiorespiratory endurance, muscular strength, muscular endurance, flexibility, and body composition.

- Physical training is the process of producing long-term improvements in the body's functioning through exercise. All training is based on the fact that the body adapts to physical stress.

- According to the principle of *specificity,* bodies change specifically in response to the type of training received.

- Bodies also adapt to *progressive overload.* Therefore, when we progressively increase the frequency, intensity, and time (duration) of the right type of exercise, we become increasingly fit.

- Bodies adjust to lower levels of activity by losing fitness, a principle known as *reversibility.* To counter the effects of reversibility we should keep training at the same intensity, even if we reduce the number or length of sessions.

- According to the principle of *individual differences,* people vary in the maximum level of fitness they can achieve.

- When designing an exercise program, determine if medical clearance is needed, assess your current level of fitness, set realistic goals, and choose activities that develop all components of fitness.

- In addition, train regularly, get in shape gradually, warm up and cool down, maintain a structured but flexible program, exercise safely, consider training with a partner, train your mind, have fun, and keep exercise in perspective.

COMMON QUESTIONS ANSWERED

Where can I work out? Identify accessible and pleasant places to work out. For running, find a field or park with a soft surface. For swimming, find a pool that's open at times convenient for you. For cycling, find an area with minimal traffic and air pollution. Make sure the location is safe and convenient. If you join a health club or fitness center, follow the guidelines in the box "Choosing a Fitness Center," on p. 45.

Where can I get help and advice about exercise? Because fitness is essential to a wellness lifestyle, you need to learn as much as you can about exercise. One of the best places to get help is an exercise class. There, expert instructors can help you learn the basics of training and answer your questions. Make sure the instructor is certified by a recognized professional organization and/or has formal training in exercise physiology. Read articles by credible experts in fitness magazines. Because of competition among publications, many of these magazines include articles by leading experts in exercise science written at a layperson's level.

(continues)

A qualified personal trainer can also be helpful in getting you started in an exercise program or a new form of training. Make sure this person has proper qualifications, such as a college degree in exercise physiology or physical education or ACSM, National Strength and Conditioning Association (NSCA), or American Council on Exercise (ACE) certification. Don't seek out a person for advice simply because he or she looks fit. UCLA researchers recently found that 60% of the personal trainers in their study couldn't pass a basic exam on training methods, exercise physiology, or biomechanics. Even some trainers with more than five years experience couldn't pass the test. Trainers who performed best had college degrees in exercise physiology or physical education. So, choose your trainer carefully.

Should I follow my exercise program if I'm sick? If you have a mild head cold or feel one coming on, it is probably OK to exercise moderately. Just begin slowly and see how you feel. However, if you have symptoms of a more serious illness— fever, swollen glands, nausea, extreme tiredness, muscle aches—wait until you have fully recovered before resuming your exercise program. Continuing to exercise while suffering from an illness more serious than a cold can compromise your recovery and may even be dangerous.

How can I fit my exercise program into my day? Good time management is an important skill in creating and maintaining an exercise program. Choose a regular time to exercise, preferably the same time every day. Don't tell yourself you'll exercise "sometime during the day" when you have free time—that free time may never come. Schedule your workout, and make it a priority. Include alternative plans in your program to account for circumstances like bad weather or vacations.

You don't have to work on all fitness components in the same exercise session. The important thing is to have a regular schedule. (You'll have the chance to develop strategies for successful time management in the Behavior Change Workbook at the end of the text.)

FOR FURTHER EXPLORATION

WW *Fit and Well* Online Learning Center (www.mhhe.com/fahey)

Use the learning objectives, study guide questions, and glossary flashcards to review key terms and concepts and prepare for exams. You can extend your knowledge of physical activity and gain experience in using the Internet as a resource by completing the activities and checking out the Web links for the topics in Chapter 2 marked with the World Wide Web icon. For this chapter, Internet activities explore common fitness terms, your current level of fitness, and a variety of physical activities that you can incorporate into your life; there are Web links for the Vital Statistics figure, the Critical Consumer box on fitness centers, and the chapter as a whole.

Daily Fitness and Nutrition Journal

Start completing the fitness program planning portion of the log by beginning an analysis of the costs and benefits of increasing physical activity, setting some general fitness goals, and thinking about your current activity and exercise habits. If you need to track your daily activities in order to identify ways to incorporate more lifestyle physical activity into your daily life, visit the Online Learning Center for some blank sample logs that you can print and use; also refer to the time management section (Activity 10) in the Behavior Change Workbook at the end of the text.

HealthQuest

Are you ready to become more active? You can find out by completing the Stages of Change activity on the HealthQuest CD-ROM (select Stages of Change from the menu in the Fitness module). You'll receive an assessment of your stage plus advice on moving forward toward the action and maintenance stages.

Books

American College of Sports Medicine. 2003. *ACSM Fitness Book.* 3rd ed. Champaign, Ill.: Human Kinetics. *Provides a step-by-step approach to becoming more active and developing a fitness program.*

American College of Sports Medicine. 2000. *ACSM's Guidelines for Exercise Testing and Prescription,* 6th ed. Baltimore, Md.: Lippincott Williams & Wilkins. *Includes the ACSM guidelines for safety of exercising, a basic discussion of exercise physiology, and information about fitness testing and prescription.*

Department of Health and Human Services. 1996. *Physical Activity and Health: A Report of the Surgeon General.* Atlanta, Ga.: DHHS (also available online: http://www.cdc.gov/nccdphp/sgr/sgr.htm). *Summarizes evidence for the benefits of physical activity and makes recommendations.*

Earle, R. W., and T. R. Baechle, eds. 2004. *NSCA's Essentials of Personal Training.* Champaign, Ill.: Human Kinetics. *Comprehensive discussions of fitness testing, exercise and disease, nutrition and physical performance, and exercise prescription.*

Journals

ACSM Health and Fitness Journal (401 West Michigan Street, Indianapolis, IN 46202; http://www.acsm-healthfitness.org)

Physician and Sportsmedicine (4530 W. 77th Street, Minneapolis, MN 55435; many of the articles are also available online at http://www.physsportsmed.com)

WW Organizations, Hotlines, and Web Sites

American Alliance for Health, Physical Education, Recreation, and Dance (AAHPERD). A professional organization dedicated to promoting quality health and physical education programs.
800-213-7193
http://www.aahperd.org

Fitness centers can provide you with many benefits—motivation and companionship are among the most important. A fitness center may also offer expert instruction and supervision as well as access to better equipment than you could afford on your own. If you're thinking of joining a fitness center, here are some guidelines to help you choose a club that's right for you.

Convenience

- Look for an established facility that's within 10–15 minutes of your home or work. If it's farther away, your chances of sticking to an exercise regimen start to diminish.

- Check out the facility's hours, then visit it at the time you would normally exercise. Will you have easy access to the equipment and exercise classes you want at that time?

Atmosphere

- Look around to see if there are other members who are your age and at about your fitness level. (If everyone seems close in age or fitness level, then the club may cater to a certain age group or lifestyle—for example, hard-core bodybuilders.)

- If you like to exercise to music, make sure you like the music played there, both its type and volume.

- Observe how the members dress. Will you fit in, or will you be uncomfortable?

- Check to see that the facility is clean, including showers and lockers. Make sure the facility is climate controlled and well ventilated.

Safety

- Find out if the facility offers basic fitness testing that includes cardiovascular screening.

- Determine if there is emergency equipment on the premises and if personnel are trained in CPR.

- Ask if at least one staff member on each shift is trained in first aid.

- Find out if the club has an emergency plan in the event that a member has a heart attack or serious injury (many clubs do not).

Trained Personnel

- Determine if the personal trainers and fitness instructors are certified by a recognized professional association such as the American College of Sports Medicine (ACSM), National Strength and Conditioning Association (NSCA), or American Council on Exercise (ACE). All personal trainers are not equal—more than 100 organizations certify trainers and few of these require much formal training. Trainers with college degrees in exercise physiology or physical education are usually the most knowledgable.

- Find out if the club has a trained exercise physiologist on staff, someone with a degree in exercise physiology, kinesiology, or exercise science. If the facility offers nutritional counseling, it should employ someone who is a registered dietitian (R.D.) or who has other formal training.

- Ask how much experience the instructors have. Clubs may employ people because they were good athletes or look fit; by themselves, these are not good reasons to hire someone. Ideally, trainers should have both academic preparation and practical experience.

Cost

- Buy only what you need and can afford. If you want to use only workout equipment, you may not need a club that has racquetball courts and saunas.

- Check the contract. Choose the one that covers the shortest period of time possible, especially if it's your first fitness club experience.

- Make sure the contract permits you to extend your membership if you have a prolonged illness or go on vacation.

- Try out the club. Ask for a free trial workout, or a 1-day pass, or an inexpensive 1- or 2-week trial membership.

- Find out whether there is an extra charge for the particular services you want.

Effectiveness

- Tour the facility. Does it offer what the brochure says it does?

- Check the equipment. A good club will have treadmills, bikes, stair-climbers, resistance machines, and weights. Make sure these machines are up-to-date and well maintained.

- Make sure the facility is certified. Look for the displayed names American College of Sports Medicine (ACSM), American Council on Exercise (ACE), Aerobics and Fitness Association of America (AFAA), or International Health, Racquet, and Sportsclub Association (IHRSA).

- Don't get cheated. Check with your Better Business Bureau or Consumer Affairs office to see if others have complained.

American College of Sports Medicine (ACSM). The principal professional organization for sports medicine and exercise science. Provides brochures, publications, and audio- and videotapes.
  317-637-9200
  http://www.acsm.org

American Council on Exercise (ACE). Promotes exercise and fitness; the Web site features fact sheets on many consumer topics, including choosing shoes, cross-training, and steroids.
  800-825-3636
  http:/www.acefitness.org

American Heart Association: Just Move. Provides practical advice for people of all fitness levels plus an online fitness diary.

http://www.justmove.org

Canada's Physical Activity Guide. Offers many suggestions for incorporating physical activity into everyday life; also includes the Physical Activity Readiness Questionnaire (PAR-Q).

http://www.hc-sc.gc.ca/hppb/paguide

CDC Physical Activity Information. Provides information on the benefits of physical activity and suggestions for incorporating moderate physical activity into daily life.

http://www.cdc.gov/nccdphp/dnpa/physical

Disabled Sports USA. Provides sports and recreation services to people with physical or mobility disorders.

http://www.dsusa.org

Georgia State University: Exercise and Physical Fitness Page. Provides information about the benefits of exercise and how to get started on a fitness program.

http://www.gsu.edu/~wwwfit

International Health, Racquet, and Sportsclub Association (IHRSA): Health Clubs. Provides guidelines for choosing a health or fitness facility and links to clubs that belong to IHRSA.

http://www.healthclubs.com

MedlinePlus: Exercise and Physical Fitness. Provides links to news and reliable information about fitness and exercise from government agencies and professional associations.

http://www.nlm.nih.gov/medlineplus/
exercisephysicalfitness.html

President's Council on Physical Fitness and Sports (PCPFS). Provides information on PCPFS programs and publications, including fitness guides and fact sheets.

http://www.fitness.gov
http://www.presidentschallenge.org

Shape Up America! Provides information on the benefits of fitness, assessment tests, and tips on overcoming barriers to physical activity.

http://shapeup.org

Small Step. Gov. Provides resources for increasing activity and improving diet through small changes in daily habits.

http://www.smallstep.gov

The following provide links to sites with information on a wide variety of activities and fitness issues; evaluate commercial sites carefully.

Fitness Partner Connection Jumpsite: http//www.primusweb.
com/fitnesspartner
NetSweat: The Internet's Fitness Resource: http//www.
netsweat.com
Yahoo!Fitness: dir.yahoo.com/Health/Fitness

SELECTED BIBLIOGRAPHY

American Academy of Orthopaedic Surgeons. 2002. *Prevent Injuries America: Sports Injuries and Baby Boomers* (http://orthoinfo.aaos.org/fact/prev_report.cfm?Thread_ID=147&category=Prevention; retrieved April 7, 2004).

American College of Sports Medicine. 2000. *ACSM's Guidelines for Exercise Testing and Prescription,* 6th ed. Baltimore, Md.: Lippincott Williams and Wilkins.

American College of Sports Medicine. 1998. The recommended quantity and quality of exercise for developing and maintaining cardiorespiratory and muscular fitness, and flexibility in healthy adults. ACSM position paper. *Medicine and Science in Sports and Exercise* 30(6): 975–991.

American College of Obstetrics and Gynecology Committee on Obstetric Practice. 2002. Exercise during pregnancy and the postpartum period. Committee Opinion No. 267. *International Journal of Gynaecology and Obstetrics* 77:79–81.

American Diabetes Association. 2003. Physical activity/exercise and diabetes mellitus. *Diabetes Care* 26:S73–S77.

American Heart Association. 2003. Exercise and physical activity in the prevention and treatment of atherosclerotic cardiovascular disease. *Circulation* 107:3109–3116.

Byers, T., et al. 2002. American Cancer Society guidelines on nutrition and physical activity for cancer prevention: Reducing the risk of cancer with healthy food choices and physical activity. *CA: A Cancer Journal for Clinicians* 52(2): 92–119.

Centers for Disease Control and Prevention. 2004. Prevalence of no leisure-time physical activity. *Morbidity and Mortality Weekly Report* 53(4): 82–86.

Centers for Disease Control and Prevention. 2003. Prevalence of physical activity, including lifestyle activities among adults—United States, 2000–2001. *Morbidity and Mortality Weekly Report* 52:764–769.

Centers for Disease Control and Prevention. 2001. *Lower Direct Medical Costs Associated with Physical Activity* (http://www.cdc.gov/nccdphp/ndpa/pr-cost.htm; retrieved October 9, 2001).

Department of Health and Human Services. 1996. *Physical Activity and Health: A Report of the Surgeon General.* Atlanta, Ga.: DHHS.

Dong, L., G. Block, and S. Mandel. 2004. Activities contributing to total energy expenditure in the United States: Results from the NHAPS Study. *International Journal of Behavioral Nutrition and Physical Activity* 1(4).

Evans R. K., et al. 2002. Effects of warm-up before eccentric exercise on indirect markers of muscle damage. *Medicine and Science in Sports and Exercise* 34:1892–1899.

Exercise for health: How much exercise is enough? ACSM works with others to avoid misunderstanding. 2003. *ACSM Fit Society Page,* Winter.

Garman, J. F., et al. 2004. Occurrence of exercise dependence in a college-aged population. *Journal of American College Health* 52(5): 221–228.

Hu, F. B. 2003. Sedentary lifestyle and risk of obesity and type 2 diabetes. *Lipids* 38(2): 103–108.

Institutes of Medicine, National Academies. 2002. *Dietary, Reference Intakes for Energy, Carbohydrate, Fiber, Fat, Fatty Acids, Cholesterol, Protein, and Amino Acids.* Washington, D.C.: National Academy Press.

Is easy-does-it exercise enough? 2004. *Consumer Reports on Health,* February.

Lee, I. 2003. Physical activity in women: How much is good enough? *Journal of the American Medical Association* 290(10): 1377–1379.

Le Masurier, G. C. 2004. Walk which way? *ACSM's Health and Fitness Journal,* January/February.

Malek, M. H., et al. 2002. Importance of health science education for personal fitness trainers. *Journal of Strength and Conditioning Research* 16:19–24.

Pate, R. R., et al. 1995. Physical activity and public health: A recommendation from the Centers for Disease Control and Prevention and the American College of Sports Medicine. *Journal of the American Medical Association* 273:402–407.

President's Council on Physical Fitness and Sports. 2000. Definitions: Health, fitness, and physical activity. *Research Digest* 3(9).

Saris, W.H.M., et al. 2003. How much physical activity is enough to prevent unhealthy weight gain? Outcome of the IASO 1st Stock Conference and consensus statement. *Obesity Reviews* 4:101–114.

Takahashi T., et al. 2002. Influence of cool-down exercise on autonomic control of heart rate during recovery from dynamic exercise. *Frontiers of Medical and Biological Engineering* 11:249–259.

World Health Organization/FAO Expert Consultation. 2003. *Diet, Nutrition and the Prevention of Chronic Diseases.* WHO Technical Report Series 916. Geneva: World Health Organization.

LAB 2.1 *Safety of Exercise Participation*

VW

Physical Activity Readiness
Questionnaire - PAR-Q
(revised 2002)

PAR-Q & YOU

(A Questionnaire for People Aged 15 to 69)

Regular physical activity is fun and healthy, and increasingly more people are starting to become more active every day. Being more active is very safe for most people. However, some people should check with their doctor before they start becoming much more physically active.

If you are planning to become much more physically active than you are now, start by answering the seven questions in the box below. If you are between the ages of 15 and 69, the PAR-Q will tell you if you should check with your doctor before you start. If you are over 69 years of age, and you are not used to being very active, check with your doctor.

Common sense is your best guide when you answer these questions. Please read the questions carefully and answer each one honestly: check YES or NO.

YES	NO		
☐	☐	1.	Has your doctor ever said that you have a heart condition <u>and</u> that you should only do physical activity recommended by a doctor?
☐	☐	2.	Do you feel pain in your chest when you do physical activity?
☐	☐	3.	In the past month, have you had chest pain when you were not doing physical activity?
☐	☐	4.	Do you lose your balance because of dizziness or do you ever lose consciousness?
☐	☐	5.	Do you have a bone or joint problem (for example, back, knee or hip) that could be made worse by a change in your physical activity?
☐	☐	6.	Is your doctor currently prescribing drugs (for example, water pills) for your blood pressure or heart condition?
☐	☐	7.	Do you know of <u>any other reason</u> why you should not do physical activity?

If you answered

YES to one or more questions

Talk with your doctor by phone or in person BEFORE you start becoming much more physically active or BEFORE you have a fitness appraisal. Tell your doctor about the PAR-Q and which questions you answered YES.

• You may be able to do any activity you want — as long as you start slowly and build up gradually. Or, you may need to restrict your activities to those which are safe for you. Talk with your doctor about the kinds of activities you wish to participate in and follow his/her advice.

• Find out which community programs are safe and helpful for you.

NO to all questions

If you answered NO honestly to <u>all</u> PAR-Q questions, you can be reasonably sure that you can:

• start becoming much more physically active — begin slowly and build up gradually. This is the safest and easiest way to go.

• take part in a fitness appraisal – this is an excellent way to determine your basic fitness so that you can plan the best way for you to live actively. It is also highly recommended that you have your blood pressure evaluated. If your reading is over 144/94, talk with your doctor before you start becoming much more physically active.

→ **DELAY BECOMING MUCH MORE ACTIVE:**

• if you are not feeling well because of a temporary illness such as a cold or a fever – wait until you feel better; or

• if you are or may be pregnant – talk to your doctor before you start becoming more active.

PLEASE NOTE: If your health changes so that you then answer YES to any of the above questions, tell your fitness or health professional. Ask whether you should change your physical activity plan.

<u>Informed Use of the PAR-Q</u>: The Canadian Society for Exercise Physiology, Health Canada, and their agents assume no liability for persons who undertake physical activity, and if in doubt after completing this questionnaire, consult your doctor prior to physical activity.

No changes permitted. You are encouraged to photocopy the PAR-Q but only if you use the entire form.

NOTE: If the PAR-Q is being given to a person before he or she participates in a physical activity program or a fitness appraisal, this section may be used for legal or administrative purposes.

"I have read, understood and completed this questionnaire. Any questions I had were answered to my full satisfaction."

NAME _____

SIGNATURE _____   DATE _____

SIGNATURE OF PARENT _____   WITNESS _____
or GUARDIAN (for participants under the age of majority)

Note: This physical activity clearance is valid for a maximum of 12 months from the date it is completed and becomes invalid if your condition changes so that you would answer YES to any of the seven questions.

© Canadian Society for Exercise Physiology   Supported by: Health Santé Canada Canada   continued on other side...

Part II General Health Profile

To help further assess the safety of exercise for you, complete as much of this health profile as possible.

General Information

Age: _____

Height: _____

Weight: _____

Total cholesterol: _____

HDL: _____

LDL: _____

Blood pressure: _____ /_____

Triglycerides: _____

Blood glucose level: _____

Are you currently trying to _____ gain or _____ lose weight? (check one if appropriate)

Medical Conditions/Treatments

Check any of the following that apply to you and add any other conditions that might affect your ability to exercise safely.

_____ heart disease

_____ lung disease

_____ diabetes

_____ allergies

_____ asthma

_____ depression, anxiety, or another psychological disorder

_____ eating disorder

_____ back pain

_____ arthritis

_____ other injury or joint problem: _____

_____ substance abuse problem

_____ other: _____

_____ other: _____

_____ other: _____

_____ Do you have a family history of cardiovascular disease (CVD) (a parent, sibling, or child who had a heart attack or stroke before age 55 for men or 65 for women)?

List any medications or supplements you are taking or any medical treatments you are undergoing. Include the name of the substance or treatment and its purpose. Include both prescription and over-the-counter drugs and supplements.

_____   _____

_____   _____

Lifestyle Information

Check any of the following that is true for you, and fill in the requested information.

_____ I usually eat high-fat foods (fatty meats, cheese, fried foods, butter, full-fat dairy products) every day.

_____ I consume fewer than 5 servings of fruits and vegetables on most days.

_____ I smoke cigarettes or use other tobacco products. If true, describe your use of tobacco (type and frequency): _____

_____ I regularly drink alcohol. If true, describe your typical weekly consumption pattern: _____

_____ I often feel as if I need more sleep. (I need about _____ hours per day; I get about _____ hours per day.)

_____ I feel as though stress has adversely affected my level of wellness during the past year.

Describe your current activity pattern. What types of moderate physical activity do you engage in on a daily basis? Are you involved in a formal exercise program or do you regularly participate in sports or recreational activities?

_____

_____

Using Your Results

How did you score? Did the PAR-Q indicate that exercise is likely to be safe for you? Is there anything in your health profile that you think may affect your ability to exercise safely? Have you had any problems with exercise in the past?

What should you do next? If the assessments in this lab indicate that you should see your physician before beginning an exercise program, or if you have any questions about the safety of exercise for you, make an appointment to talk with your health care provider to address your concerns.

Name _____ Section _____ Date _____

LAB 2.2 *Your Physical Activity Profile*

Complete this lab to assess your overall level of activity on a typical day. The amount of time you spend on sleep and on light, moderate, and vigorous activity should total 24 hours. To complete the chart below, fill in your activities and the amount of time you spend on each one; in addition, keep track of the number of flights of stairs you climb. Classify each activity as light, moderate, or vigorous according to the following guidelines:

Light activities—most sitting and standing activities: Attending class; studying; using a computer; watching TV; listening to music; talking on the phone; eating meals; walking slowly; driving; most child-care activities; light housework such as ironing, cooking, dusting, vacuuming; light yard work or home repair such as pruning, weeding, plumbing; office work, sales, or another occupational activity involving sitting or standing and movement of little more than hands.

Moderate activities—breathing rate increases but comfortable conversation is possible: Walking moderately or briskly; cycling moderately; active play with children or pushing a stroller; moderate housework such as scrubbing floors, washing windows; moderate yard work or home repair such as planting, raking, painting, wallpapering; hand-washing a car; waiting tables, washing dishes, or another occupational activity involving extended periods of moderate effort; social dancing; fitness activities requiring moderate effort such as low-impact aerobic dance, Frisbee, recreational swimming, hitting a punching bag.

Vigorous activities—too out of breath to talk easily: Walking briskly uphill; heavy housework such as moving furniture or carrying heavy items upstairs; vigorous yard work or home activities such as shoveling snow, trimming trees, hand-sawing; heavy construction work or digging; fitness activities requiring vigorous effort, such as jogging or running, high-impact aerobic dance; circuit weight training, swimming laps, most competitive sports.

Activity	Duration	Classification

Number of flights of stairs: _____ flights

Physical Activity Summary (should total 24 hours)

Sleep: _____ hours

Light activity: _____ hours

Moderate activity: _____ hours

Vigorous activity: _____ hours

Number of flights of stairs: _____ flights

Using Your Results

How did you score? Are you at all surprised by the amount of time you spend in light, moderate, and vigorous activity? Do you spend at least 30 minutes each day—the recommended minimum—in moderate or vigorous activity? Are you satisfied with the amount of moderate and vigorous physical activity in your daily life? Is it appropriate for your health status and goals?

What should you do next? Enter the results of this lab in the Preprogram Assessment column in Appendix D. If you want to increase the amount of moderate or vigorous physical activity in your life, begin by analyzing the amount of time in each intensity category according to the type of activity:

	Light activity (hours)	Moderate activity (hours)	Vigorous activity (hours)
Home and child-care activities			
School- or job-related activities			
Transportation-related activities			
Leisure activities			
Exercise/sport activities			

How much of your time in transportation-related activities and leisure activities is classified as light activity? Transportation and leisure activities are often the areas where it is easiest to substitute moderate activities for light activities. Examples include walking or biking rather than driving for short errands and going for a walk with a friend rather than chatting on the phone; see p. 30 for additional suggestions. Below, identify three strategies for boosting physical activity in your daily life.

1. _____

2. _____

3. _____

Can you also identify additional opportunities to climb stairs each day?

Begin to adopt the strategies you've identified to increase physical activity. After several weeks of a program to become more physically active, do this lab again, and enter the results in the Postprogram Assessment column of Appendix D. How do the results compare?

SOURCE: Activity classifications from CDC Division of Nutrition and Physical Activity. 1999. *Promoting Physical Activity: A Guide for Community Action.* Champaign, Ill.: Human Kinetics.

LAB 2.3 *Overcoming Barriers to Being Active*

Barriers to Being Active Quiz

Directions: Listed below are reasons that people give to describe why they do not get as much physical activity as they think they should. Please read each statement and indicate how likely you are to say each of the following statements:

How likely are you to say this?	Very likely	Somewhat likely	Somewhat unlikely	Very unlikely
1. My day is so busy now, I just don't think I can make the time to include physical activity in my regular schedule.	3	2	1	0
2. None of my family members or friends like to do anything active, so I don't have a chance to exercise.	3	2	1	0
3. I'm just too tired after work to get any exercise.	3	2	1	0
4. I've been thinking about getting more exercise, but I just can't seem to get started.	3	2	1	0
5. I'm getting older so exercise can be risky.	3	2	1	0
6. I don't get enough exercise because I have never learned the skills for any sport.	3	2	1	0
7. I don't have access to jogging trails, swimming pools, bike paths, etc.	3	2	1	0
8. Physical activity takes too much time away from other commitments—like work, family, etc.	3	2	1	0
9. I'm embarrassed about how I will look when I exercise with others.	3	2	1	0
10. I don't get enough sleep as it is. I just couldn't get up early or stay up late to get some exercise.	3	2	1	0
11. It's easier for me to find excuses not to exercise than to go out and do something.	3	2	1	0
12. I know of too many people who have hurt themselves by overdoing it with exercise.	3	2	1	0
13. I really can't see learning a new sport at my age.	3	2	1	0
14. It's just too expensive. You have to take a class or join a club or buy the right equipment.	3	2	1	0
15. My free times during the day are too short to include exercise.	3	2	1	0
16. My usual social activities with family or friends do not include physical activity.	3	2	1	0
17. I'm too tired during the week and I need the weekend to catch up on my rest.	3	2	1	0

How likely are you to say this?	Very likely	Somewhat likely	Somewhat unlikely	Very unlikely
18. I want to get more exercise, but I just can't seem to make myself stick to anything.	3	2	1	0
19. I'm afraid I might injure myself or have a heart attack.	3	2	1	0
20. I'm not good enough at any physical activity to make it fun.	3	2	1	0
21. If we had exercise facilities and showers at work, then I would be more likely to exercise.	3	2	1	0

Scoring

- Enter the circled number in the spaces provided, putting the number for statement 1 on line 1, statement 2 on line 2, and so on.

- Add the three scores on each line. Your barriers to physical activity fall into one or more of seven categories: lack of time, social influence, lack of energy, lack of willpower, fear of injury, lack of skill, and lack of resources. A score of 5 or above in any category shows that this is an important barrier for you to overcome.

$$\underline{\hspace{1cm}} + \underline{\hspace{1cm}} + \underline{\hspace{1cm}} = \underline{\hspace{3cm}}$$
1   8   15   Lack of time

$$\underline{\hspace{1cm}} + \underline{\hspace{1cm}} + \underline{\hspace{1cm}} = \underline{\hspace{3cm}}$$
2   9   16   Social influence

$$\underline{\hspace{1cm}} + \underline{\hspace{1cm}} + \underline{\hspace{1cm}} = \underline{\hspace{3cm}}$$
3   10   17   Lack of energy

$$\underline{\hspace{1cm}} + \underline{\hspace{1cm}} + \underline{\hspace{1cm}} = \underline{\hspace{3cm}}$$
4   11   18   Lack of willpower

$$\underline{\hspace{1cm}} + \underline{\hspace{1cm}} + \underline{\hspace{1cm}} = \underline{\hspace{3cm}}$$
5   12   19   Fear of injury

$$\underline{\hspace{1cm}} + \underline{\hspace{1cm}} + \underline{\hspace{1cm}} = \underline{\hspace{3cm}}$$
6   13   20   Lack of skill

$$\underline{\hspace{1cm}} + \underline{\hspace{1cm}} + \underline{\hspace{1cm}} = \underline{\hspace{3cm}}$$
7   14   21   Lack of resources

Using Your Results

How did you score? How many key barriers did you identify? Are they what you expected?

What should you do next? For your key barriers, try the strategies listed on the following pages and/or develop additional strategies that work for you. Check off any strategy that you try.

Suggestions for Overcoming Physical Activity Barriers

Lack of time

_____ Identify available time slots. Monitor your daily activities for 1 week. Identify at least three 30-minute time slots you could use for physical activity.

_____ Add physical activity to your daily routine. For example, walk or ride your bike to work or shopping, organize social activities around physical activity, walk the dog, exercise while you watch TV, park farther from your destination, etc.

_____ Make time for physical activity. For example, walk, jog, or swim during your lunch hour, or take fitness breaks instead of coffee breaks.

_____ Select activities requiring minimal time, such as walking, jogging, stair climbing.

_____ Other: _____

Social influence

_____ Explain your interest in physical activity to friends and family. Ask them to support your efforts.

_____ Invite friends and family members to exercise with you. Plan social activities involving exercise.

_____ Develop new friendships with physically active people. Join a group, such as the YMCA or a hiking club.

_____ Other: _____

Lack of energy

_____ Schedule physical activity for times in the day or week when you feel energetic.

_____ Convince yourself that if you give it a chance, exercise will increase your energy level; then, try it.

_____ Other: _____

Lack of willpower

_____ Plan ahead. Make physical activity a regular part of your daily or weekly schedule and write it on your calendar.

_____ Invite a friend to exercise with you on a regular basis and write it on _both_ your calendars.

_____ Join an exercise group or class.

_____ Other: _____

Fear of injury

_____ Learn how to warm up and cool down to prevent injury.

_____ Learn how to exercise appropriately considering your age, fitness level, skill level, and health status.

_____ Choose activities involving minimal risk.

_____ Other: _____

Lack of skill

_____ Select activities requiring no new skills, such as walking, climbing stairs, or jogging.

_____ Exercise with friends who are at the same skill level as you are.

_____ Find a friend who is willing to teach you some new skills.

_____ Take a class to develop new skills.

_____ Other: _____

Lack of resources

_____ Select activities that require minimal facilities or equipment, such as walking, jogging, jumping rope, or calisthenics.

_____ Identify inexpensive, convenient resources available in your community (community education programs, park and recreation programs, worksite programs, etc.).

_____ Other: _____

Are any of the following additional barriers important for you? If so, try some of the strategies listed here or invent your own.

Weather conditions

_____ Develop a set of regular activities that are always available regardless of weather (indoor cycling, aerobic dance, indoor swimming, calisthenics, stair climbing, rope skipping, mall walking, dancing, gymnasium games, etc.).

_____ Look on outdoor activities that depend on weather conditions (cross-country skiing, outdoor swimming, outdoor tennis, etc.) as "bonuses"—extra activities possible when weather and circumstances permit.

_____ Other: _____

Travel

_____ Put a jump rope in your suitcase and jump rope.

_____ Walk the halls and climb the stairs in hotels.

_____ Stay in places with swimming pools or exercise facilities.

_____ Join the YMCA or YWCA (ask about reciprocal membership agreement).

_____ Visit the local shopping mall and walk for half an hour or more.

_____ Bring a small tape recorder and your favorite aerobic exercise tape.

_____ Other: _____

Family obligations

_____ Trade babysitting time with a friend, neighbor, or family member who also has small children.

_____ Exercise _with_ the kids—go for a walk together, play tag or other running games, get an aerobic dance or exercise tape for kids (there are several on the market) and exercise together. You can spend time together and still get your exercise.

_____ Hire a babysitter and look at the cost as a worthwhile investment in your physical and mental health.

_____ Jump rope, do calisthenics, ride a stationary bicycle, or use other home gymnasium equipment while the kids watch TV or when they are sleeping.

_____ Try to exercise when the kids are not around (e.g., during school hours or their nap time).

_____ Other: _____

Retirement years

_____ Look on your retirement as an opportunity to become more active instead of less. Spend more time gardening, walking the dog, and playing with your grandchildren. Children with short legs and grandparents with slower gaits are often great walking partners.

_____ Learn a new skill you've always been interested in, such as ballroom dancing, square dancing, or swimming.

_____ Now that you have the time, make regular physical activity a part of every day. Go for a walk every morning or every evening before dinner. Treat yourself to an exercycle and ride every day during a favorite TV show.

_____ Other: _____

SOURCE: CDC Division of Nutrition and Physical Activity. 1999. _Promoting Physical Activity: A Guide for Community Action._ Champaign, Ill.: Human Kinetics.

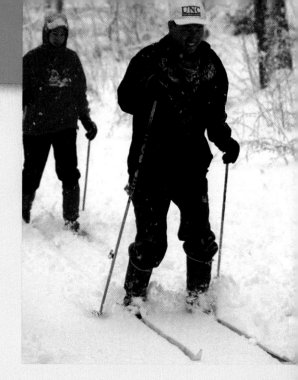

3

Cardiorespiratory Endurance

LOOKING AHEAD

After reading this chapter, you should be able to

- Describe how the body produces the energy it needs for exercise
- List the major effects and benefits of cardiorespiratory endurance exercise
- Explain how cardiorespiratory endurance is measured and assessed
- Describe how frequency, intensity, time (duration), and type of exercise affect the development of cardiorespiratory endurance
- Explain the best ways to prevent and treat common exercise injuries

TEST YOUR KNOWLEDGE

1. Compared to sedentary people, those who engage in regular moderate endurance exercise are likely to
   a. have fewer colds.
   b. be less anxious and depressed.
   c. fall asleep more quickly and sleep better.
   d. be more alert and creative.

2. About what percentage of home exercise equipment purchased in the last five years is still in use?
   a. 25%
   b. 50%
   c. 75%

3. The best treatment for a blister is to pop it and remove the overlying skin.
   True or false?

ANSWERS

1. ALL FOUR. Endurance exercise has many immediate benefits that affect all the dimensions of wellness and improve overall quality of life.

2. A. Before you buy a piece of equipment, make sure that it will help you achieve your fitness goals, that you enjoy using it regularly, and that it functions as promised.

3. FALSE. If possible, keep a blister intact to prevent infection and speed healing. If it does pop, leave the overlying skin in place and cover it with a bandage.

Ww *Fit and Well* Online Learning Center   www.mhhe.com/fahey

Visit the *Fit and Well* Online Learning Center for study aids, online labs, additional information about cardiorespiratory endurance, links, Internet activities that explore the development of cardiorespiratory fitness, consumer resources, and much more.

Cardiorespiratory endurance—the ability of the body to perform prolonged, large-muscle, dynamic exercise at moderate-to-high levels of intensity—is a key health-related component of fitness. As explained in Chapter 2, a healthy cardiorespiratory system is essential to high levels of fitness and wellness.

This chapter reviews the short- and long-term effects and benefits of cardiorespiratory endurance exercise. It then describes several tests that are commonly used to assess cardiorespiratory fitness. Finally, it provides guidelines for creating your own cardiorespiratory endurance program, one that is geared to your current level of fitness and built around activities you enjoy.

BASIC PHYSIOLOGY OF CARDIORESPIRATORY ENDURANCE EXERCISE

A basic understanding of the body processes involved in cardiorespiratory endurance exercise can help you design a safe and effective fitness program. In this section, we'll take a brief look at how the cardiorespiratory system functions and how the body produces the energy it needs to respond to the challenge of physical activity.

The Cardiorespiratory System

The cardiorespiratory system picks up and transports oxygen, nutrients, and other key substances to the organs and tissues that need them; it also picks up waste products and carries them to where they can be used or expelled. The cardiorespiratory system consists of the heart, the blood vessels, and the respiratory system (Figure 3.1).

The Heart   The heart is a four-chambered, fist-sized muscle located just beneath the ribs under the sternum (breastbone). Its role is to pump oxygen-poor blood to the lungs and oxygenated (oxygen-rich) blood to the rest of the body. Blood actually travels through two separate circulatory systems: The right side of the heart pumps blood to the lungs in what is called **pulmonary circulation,** and the left side pumps blood through the rest of the body in **systemic circulation.**

Waste-carrying, oxygen-poor blood enters the right upper chamber, or **atrium,** of the heart through the **venae cavae,** the largest veins in the body (Figure 3.2). As the right atrium fills, it contracts and pumps blood into the right lower chamber, or **ventricle,** which, when it contracts, pumps blood through the pulmonary artery into the lungs. There, blood picks up oxygen and discards carbon dioxide. Cleaned, oxygenated blood then flows from the lungs through the pulmonary veins into the left atrium. As this chamber fills, it contracts and pumps blood into the powerful left ventricle, which pumps it through the **aorta,** the body's largest artery, to be fed into the rest of the body's blood vessels.

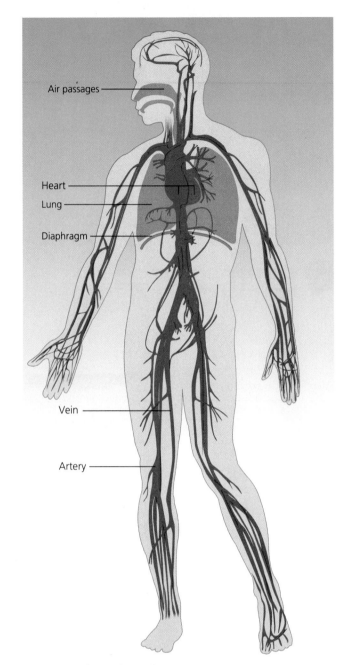

Figure 3.1   The cardiorespiratory system.

The period of the heart's contraction is called **systole;** the period of relaxation is called **diastole.** During systole, the atria contract first, pumping blood into the ventricles; a fraction of a second later, the ventricles contract, pumping blood to the lungs and the body. During diastole, blood flows into the heart. **Blood pressure,** the force exerted by blood on the walls of the blood vessels, is created by the pumping action of the heart; blood pressure is greater during systole than during diastole. A person weighing 150 pounds has about 5 quarts of blood, which are circulated about once every minute.

The heartbeat—the split-second sequence of contractions of the heart's four chambers—is controlled by nerve impulses. These signals originate in a bundle of specialized

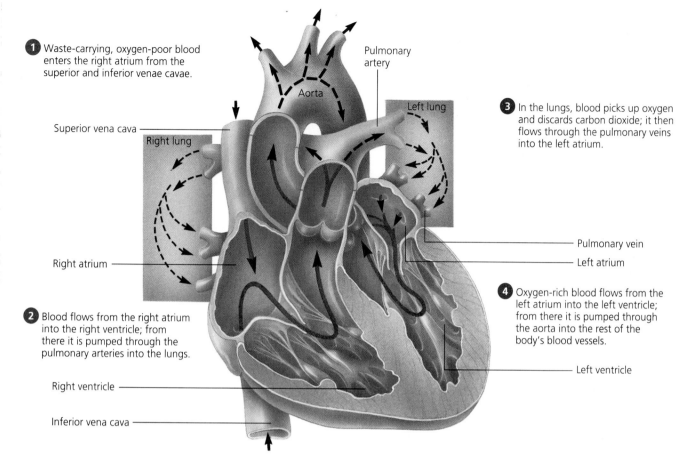

1 Waste-carrying, oxygen-poor blood enters the right atrium from the superior and inferior venae cavae.

Pulmonary artery

Aorta

Superior vena cava

Right lung

Left lung

Right atrium

2 Blood flows from the right atrium into the right ventricle; from there it is pumped through the pulmonary arteries into the lungs.

Right ventricle

Inferior vena cava

3 In the lungs, blood picks up oxygen and discards carbon dioxide; it then flows through the pulmonary veins into the left atrium.

Pulmonary vein

Left atrium

4 Oxygen-rich blood flows from the left atrium into the left ventricle; from there it is pumped through the aorta into the rest of the body's blood vessels.

Left ventricle

Figure 3.2 Circulation in the heart.

cells in the right atrium called the pacemaker or sinoatrial (SA) node. Unless it is speeded up or slowed down by the brain in response to such stimuli as danger or the tissues' need for more oxygen, the heart produces nerve impulses at a steady rate.

The Blood Vessels   Blood vessels are classified by size and function. **Veins** carry blood to the heart; **arteries** carry it away from the heart. Veins have thin walls, but arteries have thick elastic walls that enable them to expand and relax with the volume of blood being pumped through them. After leaving the heart, the aorta branches into smaller and smaller vessels. The smallest arteries branch still further into **capillaries**, tiny vessels only one cell thick. The capillaries deliver oxygen and nutrient-rich blood to the tissues and pass on oxygen-poor, waste-carrying blood. From the capillaries, this blood empties into small veins (venules) and then into larger veins that return it to the heart to repeat the cycle.

Blood pumped through the heart doesn't reach the cells of the heart, so the organ has its own network of arteries, veins, and capillaries. Two large vessels, the right and left coronary arteries, branch off the aorta and supply the heart muscle with oxygenated blood. Blockage of a coronary artery is a leading cause of heart attacks (see Chapter 11).

pulmonary circulation The part of the circulatory system that moves blood between the heart and the lungs; controlled by the right side of the heart.

systemic circulation The part of the circulatory system that moves blood between the heart and the rest of the body; controlled by the left side of the heart.

atria The two upper chambers of the heart in which blood collects before passing to the ventricles; also called *auricles*.

venae cavae The large veins through which blood is returned to the right atrium of the heart.

ventricles The two lower chambers of the heart from which blood flows through arteries to the lungs and other parts of the body.

aorta The large artery that receives blood from the left ventricle and distributes it to the body.

systole Contraction of the heart.

diastole Relaxation of the heart.

blood pressure The force exerted by the blood on the walls of the blood vessels; created by the pumping action of the heart. Blood pressure increases during systole and decreases during diastole.

veins Vessels that carry blood to the heart.

arteries Vessels that carry blood away from the heart.

capillaries Very small blood vessels that distribute blood to all parts of the body.

Terms

The Respiratory System   The **respiratory system** supplies oxygen to the body and carries off carbon dioxide, a waste product of body processes. Air passes in and out of the lungs as a result of pressure changes brought about by the contraction and relaxation of the diaphragm and rib muscles; the lungs expand and contract about 12–20 times a minute. As air is inhaled, it passes through the nasal passages, the throat, larynx, trachea (windpipe), and bronchi into the lungs. The lungs consist of many branching tubes that end in tiny, thin-walled air sacs called **alveoli.**

Carbon dioxide and oxygen are exchanged between alveoli and capillaries in the lungs. Carbon dioxide passes from blood cells into the alveoli, where it is carried up and out of the lungs (exhaled). Oxygen from inhaled air is passed from the alveoli into blood cells; these oxygen-rich blood cells then return to the heart and are pumped throughout the body. Oxygen is an important component of the body's energy-producing system, so the cardiorespiratory system's ability to pick up and deliver oxygen is critical for the functioning of the body—at rest and during exercise.

The Cardiorespiratory System at Rest and During Exercise   At rest and during light activity, the cardiorespiratory system functions at a fairly steady pace. Your heart beats at a rate of about 50–90 beats per minute, and you take about 12–20 breaths per minute. A typical resting blood pressure in a healthy adult, measured in millimeters of mercury, is 110 systolic and 70 diastolic (110/70); as described earlier, blood pressure is higher when the heart contracts (systole) than when the heart relaxes (diastole).

During exercise, the demands on the cardiorespiratory system increase. Body cells, particularly working muscles, need to obtain more oxygen and fuel and to eliminate more waste products. In order to meet this increased demand, your heart rate increases, up to 170–210 beats per minute during intense exercise; the heart also pumps out more blood with each beat (stroke volume). The combination of faster heart rate and greater stroke volume means the heart pumps and circulates more blood per minute—a **cardiac output** of 20 or more quarts per minute, compared to about 5 quarts per minute at rest. Blood flow also changes: At rest, about 15–20% of blood is distributed to the skeletal muscles; during exercise, as much as 85–90% may be delivered to working muscles. Systolic blood pressure increases, while diastolic pressure holds steady or declines slightly; a typical exercise blood pressure might be 175/65. To oxygenate this increased blood flow, you will take deeper breaths and breathe more quickly, up to 40–60 breaths per minute. All of these changes are controlled and coordinated by special centers in the brain, which use the nervous system and chemical messengers to control the process.

Later in this chapter you'll learn more about the short- and long-term effects of exercise on the body.

Energy Production

Metabolism is the sum of all the chemical processes necessary to maintain the body. Energy is required to fuel vital body functions—to build and break down tissue, contract muscles, conduct nerve impulses, regulate body temperature, and so on. The rate at which your body uses energy—its metabolic rate—depends on your level of activity. At rest, you have a low metabolic rate; if you stand up and begin to walk, your metabolic rate increases. If you jog, your metabolic rate may increase more than 800% above its resting level. Olympic-caliber distance runners can increase their metabolic rate by a whopping 2000% or more.

Energy from Food   The body converts chemical energy from food into substances that cells can use as fuel. These fuels can be used immediately or stored for later use. The body's ability to store fuel is critical, because if all the energy from food were released immediately, much of it would be wasted.

The three classes of energy-containing nutrients in food are carbohydrates, fats, and proteins. During digestion, most carbohydrates are broken down into the simple sugar **glucose.** Some glucose remains circulating in the blood ("blood sugar"), where it can be used as a quick source of fuel to produce energy. Glucose may also be converted to **glycogen** and stored in the liver, muscles, and kidneys. If glycogen stores are full and the body's immediate need for energy is met, the remaining glucose is converted to fat and stored in the body's fatty tissues. Excess energy from dietary fat is also stored as body fat. Protein in the diet is used primarily to build new tissue, but it can be broken down for energy or incorporated into fat stores. Glucose, glycogen, and fat are important fuels for the production of energy in the cells; protein is a significant energy source only when other fuels are lacking. (See Chapter 8 for more on the other roles of carbohydrate, fat, and protein in the body.)

ATP: The Energy "Currency" of Cells   The basic form of energy used by cells is **adenosine triphosphate,** or **ATP.** When a cell needs energy, it breaks down ATP, a process that releases energy in the only form the cell can use directly. Cells store a small amount of ATP; when they need more, they create it through chemical reactions that utilize the body's stored fuels—glucose, glycogen, and fat. When you exercise, your cells need to produce more energy. Consequently, your body mobilizes its stores of fuel to increase ATP production.

Exercise and the Three Energy Systems

The muscles in your body use three energy systems to create ATP and fuel cellular activity. These systems use different fuels and chemical processes and perform different, specific functions during exercise (Table 3.1).

Table 3.1 Characteristics of the Body's Energy Systems

| | ENERGY SYSTEM* | | |
	Immediate	Nonoxidatives	Oxidative
Duration of activity for which system predominates	0–10 seconds	10 seconds–2 minutes	>2 minutes
Intensity of activity for which system predominates	High	High	Low to moderately high
Rate of ATP production	Immediate, very rapid	Rapid	Slower but prolonged
Fuel	Adenosine triphosphate (ATP), creatine phosphate (CP)	Muscle stores of glycogen and glucose	Body stores of glycogen, glucose, fat, and protein
Oxygen used?	No	No	Yes
Sample activities	Weight lifting, picking up a bag of groceries	400-meter run, running up several flights of stairs	1500-meter run, 30-minute walk, standing in line for a long time

*For most activities, all three systems contribute to energy production; the duration and intensity of the activity determine which system predominates.

SOURCE: Adapted from Brooks, G. A., et. al. 2005. *Exercise Physiology. Human Bioenergetics and its Applications,* 4th ed. New York: McGraw-Hill. Copyright © 2005 The McGraw-Hill Companies. Reproduced with permission of The McGraw-Hill Companies.

The Immediate ("Explosive") Energy System The **immediate energy system** provides energy rapidly but for only a short period of time. It is used to fuel activities that last for about 10 or fewer seconds—examples in sports include weight lifting and shot-putting; examples in daily life include rising from a chair or picking up a bag of groceries. The components of this energy system include existing cellular ATP stores and creatine phosphate (CP), a chemical that cells can use to make ATP. CP levels are depleted rapidly during exercise, so the maximum capacity of this energy system is reached within a few seconds. Cells must then switch to the other energy systems to restore levels of ATP and CP. (Without adequate ATP, muscles will stiffen and become unusable.)

The Nonoxidative (Anaerobic) Energy System The **nonoxidative energy system** is used at the start of an exercise session and for high-intensity activities lasting for about 10 seconds to 2 minutes, such as the 400-meter run. During daily activities, this system may be called on to help you run to catch a bus or dash up several flights of stairs. The nonoxidative energy system creates ATP by breaking down glucose and glycogen. This system doesn't require oxygen, which is why it is sometimes referred to as the **anaerobic** system. The capacity of this system to produce energy is limited, but it can generate a great deal of ATP in a short period of time. For this reason, it is the most important energy system for very intense exercise.

There are two key limiting factors for the nonoxidative energy system. First, the body's supply of glucose and glycogen is limited. If these are depleted, a person may experience fatigue and dizziness, and judgment may be

impaired. (The brain and nervous system rely on carbohydrates as fuel and must have a continuous supply to function properly.) Second, the nonoxidative system results in the production of **lactic acid**. Although lactic acid is an

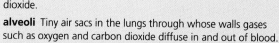

respiratory system The lungs, air passages, and breathing muscles; supplies oxygen to the body and carries off carbon dioxide.

alveoli Tiny air sacs in the lungs through whose walls gases such as oxygen and carbon dioxide diffuse in and out of blood.

cardiac output The amount of blood pumped by the heart each minute; a function of heart rate and stroke volume (the amount of blood pumped during each beat).

glucose A simple sugar that circulates in the blood and can be used by cells to fuel adenosine triphosphate (ATP) production.

glycogen A complex carbohydrate stored principally in the liver and skeletal muscles; the major fuel source during most forms of intense exercise. Glycogen is the storage form of glucose.

adenosine triphosphate (ATP) Energy source for cellular processes.

immediate ("explosive") energy system Energy system that supplies energy to muscle cells through the breakdown of cellular stores of ATP and creatine phosphate (CP).

nonoxidative (anaerobic) energy system Energy system that supplies energy to muscle cells through the breakdown of muscle stores of glucose and glycogen; also called the *anaerobic system* or the *lactic acid system* because chemical reactions take place without oxygen and produce lactic acid.

anaerobic Occurring in the absence of oxygen.

lactic acid A metabolic acid resulting from the metabolism of glucose and glycogen; an important source of fuel for many tissues of the body, its accumulation may produce fatigue.

important fuel for the body, it releases substances called hydrogen ions that are thought to interfere with metabolism and muscle contraction, thereby causing fatigue. During heavy exercise, such as sprinting, the body produces large amounts of lactic acid and hydrogen ions, and muscles become fatigued rapidly. Fortunately, exercise training increases the body's ability to cope with these substances.

The Oxidative (Aerobic) Energy System   The **oxidative energy system** is used during any physical activity that lasts longer than about 2 minutes, such as distance running, swimming, hiking, or even standing in line for a long time. The oxidative system requires oxygen to generate ATP, which is why it is considered an **aerobic** process. The oxidative system cannot produce energy as quickly as the other two systems, but it can supply energy for much longer periods of time. It provides energy during most daily activities.

In the oxidative energy system, ATP production takes place in cellular structures called **mitochondria.** Because mitochondria can use carbohydrates (glucose and glycogen) or fats to produce ATP, the body's stores of fuel for this system are much greater than those for the other two energy systems. The actual fuel used depends on the intensity and duration of exercise and on the fitness status of the individual. Carbohydrates are favored during more intense exercise (over 65% of maximum capacity); fats, for mild, low-intensity activities. During a prolonged exercise session, carbohydrates are the predominant fuel at the start of the workout, but fat utilization increases over time. Fit individuals use a greater proportion of fat as fuel because increased fitness allows people to do activities at lower intensities. This is an important adaptation because glycogen depletion is one of the limiting factors for the oxidative energy system. Thus, by being able to use more fat as fuel, a fit individual can exercise for a longer time before glycogen is depleted and muscles become fatigued.

Oxygen is another limiting factor. The oxygen requirement of this energy system is proportional to the intensity of exercise—as intensity increases, so does oxygen consumption. There is a limit to the body's ability to increase the transport and use of oxygen; this limit is referred to as **maximal oxygen consumption,** or $\dot{V}O_{2max}$. $\dot{V}O_{2max}$ is determined partly by genetics and partly by fitness status (the muscles' power-generating capacity and fatigue resistance). It depends on many factors, including the capacity of blood to carry oxygen, the rate at which oxygen is transported to the tissues, and the amount of oxygen that cells extract from the blood. $\dot{V}O_{2max}$ determines how intensely a person can perform endurance exercise and for how long, and it is considered the best overall measure of the capacity of the cardiorespiratory system. (The assessment tests described later in the chapter are designed to help you predict your $\dot{V}O_{2max}$).

The Energy Systems in Combination   Your body typically uses all three energy systems when you exercise. The intensity and duration of the activity determine which system predominates. For example, when you play tennis, you use the immediate energy system when hitting the ball, but you replenish cellular energy stores using the nonoxidative and oxidative systems. When cycling, the oxidative system predominates. However, if you must suddenly exercise very intensely—ride up a steep hill, for example—the other systems become important because the oxidative system is unable to supply ATP fast enough to sustain high-intensity effort.

Physical Fitness and Energy Production   Physically fit people can increase their metabolic rate substantially, generating the energy needed for powerful or sustained exercise. People who are not fit cannot respond to exercise in the same way. Their bodies are less capable of delivering oxygen and fuel to exercising muscles; they are also less able to cope with lactic acid and other substances produced during intense physical activity that contribute to fatigue. Because of this, they become fatigued more rapidly—their legs hurt and they breathe heavily walking up a flight of stairs, for example. Regular physical training can substantially improve the body's ability to produce energy and meet the challenges of increased physical activity.

For many sports, one energy system will be most important. For weight lifters, for example, it is the immediate energy system; for sprinters, the nonoxidative system; and for endurance runners, the oxidative system. In designing an exercise program, focus on the energy system most important to your goals. Because improving the functioning of the cardiorespiratory system is critical to overall wellness, endurance exercise that utilizes the oxidative energy system—activities performed at moderate to high intensities for a prolonged duration—is a key component of any health-related fitness program.

BENEFITS OF CARDIORESPIRATORY ENDURANCE EXERCISE

Cardiorespiratory endurance exercise helps the body become more efficient and better able to cope with physical challenges. It also lowers risk for many chronic diseases. Let's take a closer look at the physiological adaptations and long-term benefits of regular endurance exercise.

Improved Cardiorespiratory Functioning

At rest, a healthy cardiorespiratory system has little difficulty keeping pace with the body's need for oxygen, fuel, and waste removal. During exercise, however, the demands on the system increase dramatically as metabolic rate goes up. The principal cardiorespiratory responses to exercise include the following:

- Increased cardiac output and blood pressure. More blood is pumped by the heart each minute because both heart rate and stroke volume (the amount of blood pumped with each beat) go up. Increased

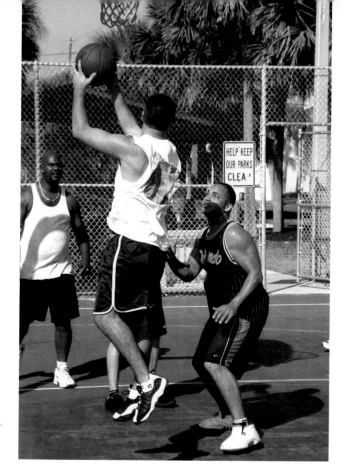

Exercise offers both long-term health benefits and immediate pleasures. Many popular sports and activities develop cardiorespiratory endurance.

cardiac output and blood pressure speed the delivery of oxygen and fuel and the removal of waste products.

- Increased ventilation (rate and depth of breathing).
- Increased blood flow to active skeletal muscles and to the heart; constant or slightly increased blood flow to the brain. The body controls blood pressure and blood flow by adjusting cardiac output and regulating the size of the blood vessels feeding different tissues.
- Increased blood flow to the skin and increased sweating. The chemical reactions that produce energy for exercise release heat, which must be dissipated to maintain a safe body temperature.
- Decreased blood flow to the stomach, intestines, liver, and kidneys, resulting in reduced activity in the gastrointestinal tract and reduced urine output.

All of these changes help the body respond to the challenge of exercise in the short term. When performed regularly, endurance exercise also causes more permanent adaptations. It improves the functioning of the heart, the ability of the cardiorespiratory system to carry oxygen to the body's tissues, and the capacity of the cells to take up and use oxygen. These improvements reduce the effort required to carry out everyday activities and make the body better able to respond to physical challenges.

Endurance training enhances the health of the heart by maintaining or increasing its blood and oxygen supply,

decreasing work and oxygen demand of the heart, and increasing the function of the heart muscle. The trained heart is more efficient and subject to less stress. It pumps more blood per beat, so heart rate is lower at rest and during exercise. The resting heart rate of a fit person is often 10–20 beats per minute lower than that of an unfit person; this translates into as many as 10 million fewer beats in the course of one year. Improved heart efficiency results because endurance training improves heart contraction strength, increases heart cavity size (in young adults), and increases blood volume so that the heart pushes more blood into the circulation system during each of its contractions. Training also tends to reduce blood pressure, so the heart does not have to work as hard when it contracts.

Improved Cellular Metabolism

Regular endurance exercise also improves metabolism at the cellular level. It increases the number of capillaries in the muscles so that they can be supplied with more oxygen and fuel and can more quickly eliminate waste products. Greater capillary density helps heal injuries more quickly and reduces muscle aches. Endurance exercise also trains the muscles to make the most of available oxygen and fuel so that they work more efficiently. Exercise increases the size and number of mitochondria in muscle cells, thereby increasing the energy capacity of the cells. Endurance training also helps in energy production by preventing glycogen depletion and increasing the muscles' ability to use lactic acid and fat as fuels.

Fitness programs that best develop metabolic efficiency include both long-duration, moderately intense endurance exercise and brief periods of more intense effort. For example, climbing a small hill while jogging or cycling introduces the kind of intense exercise that leads to more efficient use of lactic acid and fats.

Regular exercise may also help protect your cells from chemical damage. Many scientists believe that aging and some chronic diseases are linked to cellular damage caused by **free radicals.** Training activates antioxidant

oxidative (aerobic) energy system Energy system that supplies energy to cells through the breakdown of glucose, glycogen, fats, and amino acids; also called the *aerobic system* because chemical reactions require oxygen.

aerobic Dependent on the presence of oxygen.

mitochondria Intracellular structures containing enzymes used in the chemical reactions that convert the energy in food to a form the body can use.

maximal oxygen consumption ($\dot{V}O_{2max}$) The highest rate of oxygen consumption an individual is capable of during maximum physical effort, reflecting the body's ability to transport and use oxygen; measured in milliliters used per minute per kilogram of body weight.

free radicals Highly reactive compounds that can damage cells by taking electrons from key cellular components such as DNA or the cell membrane; produced by normal metabolic processes and through exposure to environmental factors, including sunlight.

Terms

Research has shown that most aspects of physiological functioning peak when people are about 30 years old and then decline at a rate of about 0.5–1.0% a year. This decline in physical capacity is characterized by a decrease in maximal oxygen consumption, cardiac output, muscular strength, fat-free mass, joint mobility, and other factors. However, regular exercise can substantially alter the rate of decline in functional status, and it is associated with both longevity and improved quality of life.

Regular endurance exercise can improve maximal oxygen consumption in older people by up to 15–30%—the same degree of improvement seen in younger individuals. In fact, studies have shown that Masters athletes in their 70s have $\dot{V}O_{2max}$ values equivalent to those of sedentary 20-year-olds: At any age, endurance training can improve cardiorespiratory functioning, cellular metabolism, body composition, and psychological and emotional well-being. Older people who exercise regularly have better balance and greater bone density and are less likely than their sedentary peers to suffer injuries as a result of falls. Regular endurance training also substantially reduces the risk of many chronic and disabling diseases including heart disease, cancer, diabetes, osteoporosis, and dementia.

Other forms of exercise training are also beneficial for older adults. Resistance training is a safe and effective way to build strength and fat-free mass and can help people remain independent as they age. Lifting weights has also been shown to boost spirits in older people, perhaps because improvements in strength appear quickly and are easily applied to everyday tasks such as climbing stairs and carrying groceries. Flexibility exercises can improve the range of motion in joints and also help people maintain functional independence as they age.

Life expectancy in the United States has increased dramatically over the past century, and about 70% of Americans now live to at least age 70. A lifetime of regular exercise is one of the best age-proofing strategies available; however, it's never too late to start. Even in people over 80, beginning an exercise program can improve physical functioning and quality of life. Most older adults are able to participate in a program that includes moderate walking and strengthening and stretching exercises, and modified programs can be created for people with chronic conditions and other special health concerns (see Chapter 7). The wellness benefits of exercise are available to people of all ages and levels of ability.

SOURCES: Brooks, G. A., et al. 2005. *Exercise Physiology: Human Bioenergetics and Its Applications,* 4th ed. New York: McGraw-Hill. American College of Sports Medicine. 2001. *ACSM's Resource Manual for Guidelines for Exercise Testing and Prescription,* 4th ed. Philadelphia: Williams and Wilkins.

---

enzymes that prevent free radical damage to cell structures, thereby enhancing health. (See Chapter 8 for more on free radicals and antioxidants.) Training also improves the functional stability of cells and tissues by improving the regulation of salts and fluids in the cells. This is particularly important in the heart, where instability can lead to cardiac arrest and death.

Reduced Risk of Chronic Disease

Regular endurance exercise lowers your risk of many chronic, disabling diseases. It can also help people with those diseases improve their health (see the box "Benefits of Exercise for Older Adults").

Cardiovascular Disease   A sedentary lifestyle is one of the six major controllable risk factors for **cardiovascular disease (CVD)** (see Chapter 11). The other primary factors are smoking, unhealthy cholesterol levels, high blood pressure, diabetes, and obesity. People who are sedentary have CVD death rates significantly higher than those of fit individuals. CVD usually begins to develop in childhood and adolescence; it progresses slowly over many years before producing any symptoms. Adopting healthy habits while young can help many people prevent or delay a heart attack or other serious form of CVD.

Endurance exercise has a positive effect on levels of fats in the blood. High concentrations of blood fats such as cholesterol and triglycerides are linked to cardiovascular disease because they contribute to the formation of fatty deposits on the lining of arteries. If one of the coronary arteries, which supply oxygenated blood to the heart, becomes blocked by such a deposit, the result is a heart attack; blockage of a cerebral artery can cause a stroke.

Cholesterol is carried in the blood by **lipoproteins,** which are classified according to size and density. Cholesterol carried by low-density lipoproteins (LDLs) tends to stick to the walls of arteries. High-density lipoproteins (HDLs), on the other hand, pick up excess cholesterol in the bloodstream and carry it back to the liver for excretion from the body. High LDL levels and low HDL levels are associated with a high risk of CVD. High levels of HDL and low levels of LDL are associated with lower risk. More information about cholesterol and heart disease is provided in Chapter 11. For our purposes in this chapter, it is important to know only that endurance exercise influences blood fat levels in a positive way—by increasing HDL and decreasing triglycerides (and possibly LDL)—thereby reducing the risk of CVD.

Regular exercise tends to reduce high blood pressure, a contributing factor in diseases such as **coronary heart disease (CHD),** stroke, kidney failure, and blindness. It further reduces the risk of CHD by enhancing the function of the cells that line the arteries (endothelial cells) and reducing inflammation. It also helps prevent obesity and type 2 diabetes, both of which contribute to CVD.

Cancer   Some studies have shown a relationship between increased physical activity and a reduction in a person's risk of all types of cancer, but these findings are not conclusive. There is strong evidence that exercise reduces the risk of colon cancer and promising data that it reduces the risk of cancer of the breast and reproductive organs in women. Exercise may decrease the risk of colon cancer by speeding the movement of food through the gastrointestinal tract (quickly eliminating potential carcinogens), enhancing immune function, and reducing blood fats. The protective mechanism in the case of reproductive system cancers is less clear, but it may be related to levels of female hormones. Physical activity during the high school and college years may be particularly important for preventing breast cancer later in life. Some preliminary evidence also suggests that regular physical activity reduces the risk of pancreatic cancer and prostate cancer.

Type 2 Diabetes   Recent studies have shown that regular exercise helps prevent the development of type 2 diabetes, the most common form of diabetes. Exercise metabolizes (burns) excess sugar and makes cells more sensitive to the hormone insulin, which is involved in the regulation of blood sugar levels. Obesity is a key risk factor for diabetes, and exercise helps keep body fat at healthy levels. But even without fat loss, exercise improves control of blood sugar levels in many people with diabetes, and physical activity is an important part of treatment. (See Chapter 6 for more on diabetes and insulin resistance.)

Osteoporosis   A special benefit of exercise, especially for women, is protection against osteoporosis, a disease that results in loss of bone density and poor bone strength. Weight-bearing exercise helps build bone during the teens and twenties. People with denser bones can better endure the bone loss that occurs with aging. With stronger bones and muscles and better balance, fit people are less likely to experience debilitating falls and bone fractures. (See Chapter 8 for more on osteoporosis.)

Deaths from All Causes   Studies of adults in the United States and Europe have found that physically fit people have a reduced risk of dying from all causes, with the greatest benefits found for people with the highest levels of fitness (see Figure 3.3 for the results of one recent study). Poor fitness is a good predictor of premature death and is as important a risk factor as smoking, high blood pressure, obesity, and diabetes.

Better Control of Body Fat

Too much body fat is linked to a variety of health problems, including CVD, cancer, and type 2 diabetes. Healthy body composition can be difficult to achieve and maintain because a diet that contains all essential nutrients can be relatively high in calories, especially for someone who is sedentary. Excess calories are stored in the body as fat. Regular exercise increases daily calorie expenditure so that a healthy diet is less likely to lead to weight gain. Endurance exercise burns calories directly and, if intense enough, continues to do so by raising resting metabolic

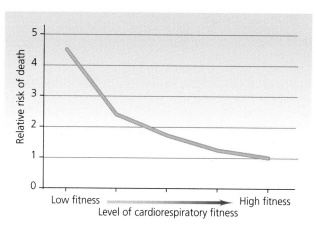

Figure 3.3   Cardiorespiratory fitness and risk of death.   People with high levels of cardiorespiratory fitness have a substantially lower risk of death than unfit individuals.   SOURCE: Myers, J., et al. 2002. Exercise capacity and mortality among men referred for exercise testing. *New England Journal of Medicine* 346 (II): 793–801.

rate for several hours following an exercise session. A higher metabolic rate means that it is easier for a person to maintain a healthy weight or to lose weight. Exercise alone cannot ensure a healthy body composition, however; as described in Chapters 6 and 9, you will lose more weight more rapidly and keep it off longer if you decrease your calorie intake as well as boost your calorie expenditure through exercise.

Endurance exercise can also help maintain or increase metabolic rate slightly by helping people maintain a high proportion of fat-free mass. Strength training, discussed in Chapter 4, is even more effective at building muscle mass than endurance training. (Energy balance and the role of exercise in improving body composition are discussed in detail in Chapter 6.) Even if regular exercise doesn't lead to significant changes in body composition, it is still extremely beneficial for wellness and has been found to help compensate for the harmful health effects of excess body fat. People with excess body fat can significantly improve health and well-being by including moderate physical activity in their daily routine.

Improved Immune Function

Exercise can have either positive or negative effects on the immune system, the physiological processes that protect us from disease. Moderate endurance exercise boosts immune function, whereas excessive training (overtraining) depresses it. Physically fit people get fewer colds and

cardiovascular disease (CVD)   Disease of the heart and blood vessels.

lipoproteins   Substances in blood, classified according to size, density, and chemical composition, that transport fats.

coronary heart disease (CHD)   Heart disease caused by the buildup of fatty deposits on the arteries that supply oxygen to the heart; also called *coronary artery disease.*

Terms

Although much of the discussion of the benefits of exercise focuses on improvements to physical wellness, many people discover that the best reason to become and stay active is the boost that regular exercise provides to the nonphysical dimensions of wellness. The following are just some of the effects of regular physical activity.

- *Reduced anxiety.* Exercise reduces symptoms of anxiety such as worry and self-doubt both in people who are anxious most of the time (trait anxiety) and in people who become anxious in response to a particular experience (state anxiety). Exercise is associated with a lower risk for panic attacks, generalized anxiety disorder, and social anxiety disorder.

- *Reduced depression and improved mood.* Exercise relieves feelings of sadness and hopelessness and can be as effective as psychotherapy in treating mild-to-moderate cases of depression. Exercise improves mood and increases feelings of well-being in both depressed and nondepressed people.

- *Improved sleep.* Regular physical activity helps people fall asleep more easily; it also improves the quality of sleep, making it more restful.

- *Reduced stress.* Exercise reduces the body's overall response to all forms of stressors and helps people deal more effectively with the stress they do experience.

- *Enhanced self-esteem, self-confidence, and self-efficacy.* Exercise can boost self-esteem and self-confidence by providing opportunities for people to succeed and excel; it also improves body image (see Chapters 6 and 9). Sticking with an

exercise program increases people's belief in their ability to be active, thereby boosting self-efficacy.

- *Enhanced creativity and intellectual functioning.* In studies of college students, physically active students score higher on tests of creativity than sedentary students. Exercise improves alertness and memory in the short term, and over time, exercise helps maintain reaction time, short-term memory, and nonverbal reasoning skills.

- *Increased opportunities for social interaction.* Exercise provides many opportunities for positive interaction with others.

How does exercise cause all these positive changes? A variety of mechanisms has been proposed. Physical activity stimulates the thought and emotion centers of the brain, producing improvements in mood and cognitive functioning. It increases alpha brain-wave activity, which is associated with a highly relaxed state. Exercise stimulates the release of chemicals such as **endorphins**, which may suppress fatigue, decrease pain, and produce euphoria; and phenylethylamine, which may boost energy, mood, and attention. Exercise decreases the secretion of hormones triggered by emotional stress and alters the levels of many other **neurotransmitters**, including serotonin, a brain chemical linked to mood.

Exercise also provides a distraction from stressful stimuli and an emotional outlet for feelings of stress, hostility and aggression. It relaxes and warms the body, which may improve both mood and sleep. And exercise is a fun way to spend time!

The message from all this research is that exercise is a critical factor in developing all the dimensions of wellness. A lifetime of physical activity can leave you with a healthier body and a sharper, happier, more creative mind.

---

upper respiratory tract infections than people who are not fit. Exercise affects immune function by influencing levels of specialized cells and chemicals involved in the immune response. In addition to regular moderate exercise, the immune system can be strengthened by eating a well-balanced diet, managing stress, and getting 7–8 hours of sleep every night.

Improved Psychological and Emotional Well-Being

Most people who participate in regular endurance exercise experience social, psychological, and emotional benefits. Performing physical activities provides proof of skill mastery and self-control, thus enhancing self-image. Recreational sports provide an opportunity to socialize, have fun, and strive to excel. Endurance exercise lessens anxiety, depression, stress, anger, and hostility, thereby improving mood and boosting cardiovascular health. Regular exercise also improves sleep. For more on the wellness benefits of regular endurance exercise, see the box "Exercise and the Mind." Refer to Figure 3.4 for a summary of specific physiological benefits of cardiorespiratory endurance exercise.

As cardiorespiratory fitness is developed, these benefits translate into both physical and emotional well-being and a much lower risk of chronic disease.

MOTIVATION FOR CHANGE!   Make a list of five benefits of endurance exercise that are particularly meaningful to you. Put the list in a prominent location—on your mirror or refrigerator, for example—and use it as a motivational tool for beginning and maintaining your fitness program.

ASSESSING CARDIORESPIRATORY FITNESS

The body's ability to maintain a level of exertion (exercise) for an extended period of time is a direct reflection of cardiorespiratory fitness. It is determined by the body's ability to take up, distribute, and use oxygen during physical activity. As explained earlier, the best quantitative measure of cardiorespiratory endurance is maximal oxygen consumption, expressed as $\dot{V}O_{2max}$, the amount of oxygen

Immediate effects

Increased levels of neurotransmitters; constant or slightly increased blood flow to the brain.

Increased heart rate and stroke volume (amount of blood pumped per beat).

Increased pulmonary ventilation (amount of air breathed into the body per minute). More air is taken into the lungs with each breath and breathing rate increases.

Reduced blood flow to the stomach, intestines, liver, and kidneys, resulting in less activity in the digestive tract and less urine output.

Increased energy (ATP) production.

Increased blood flow to the skin and increased sweating to help maintain a safe body temperature.

Increased systolic blood pressure; increased blood flow and oxygen transport to working skeletal muscles and the heart; increased oxygen consumption. As exercise intensity increases, blood levels of lactic acid increase.

Long-term effects

Improved cognitive functioning and ability to manage stress; decreased depression, anxiety, and risk for stroke.

Increased heart size and resting stroke volume; lower resting heart rate. Risk of heart disease and heart attack significantly reduced.

Improved ability to extract oxygen from air during exercise. Reduced risk of colds and upper respiratory tract infections.

Increased sweat rate and earlier onset of sweating, helping to cool the body.

Decreased body fat.

Reduced risk of colon cancer and certain other forms of cancer.

Increased number and size of mitochondria in muscle cells; increased amount of stored glycogen; increased myoglobin content; improved ability to use lactic acid and fats as fuel. All of these changes allow for greater energy production and power output. Insulin sensitivity remains constant or improves, helping to prevent type 2 diabetes. Fat-free mass may also increase somewhat.

Increased density and breaking strength of bones, ligaments, and tendons; reduced risk for osteoporosis.

Increased blood volume and capillary density; higher levels of high-density lipoproteins (HDL) and lower levels of triglycerides; lower resting blood pressure and reduced platelet stickiness (a factor in coronary artery disease).

Figure 3.4   Immediate and long-term effects of regular cardiorespiratory endurance exercise.   When endurance exercise is performed regularly, short-term changes in the body develop into more permanent adaptations; these include improved ability to exercise, reduced risk of many chronic diseases, and improved psychological and emotional well-being.

the body uses when a person reaches maximum ability to supply oxygen during exercise (measured in milliliters of oxygen used per minute for each kilogram of body weight). Maximal oxygen consumption can be measured precisely in an exercise physiology laboratory through analysis of the air a person inhales and exhales when exercising to a level of exhaustion (maximum intensity). This procedure can be expensive and time-consuming, making it impractical for the average person.

Assessment Tests

Fortunately, several simple assessment tests provide reasonably good estimates of maximal oxygen consumption (within ±10–15% of the results of a laboratory test).

Three methods are described here and presented in Lab 3.1: a 1-mile walk test, a 3-minute step test, and a 1.5-mile run-walk test. To assess yourself, choose one among these methods based on your access to equipment, your current physical condition, and your own preference. Don't take any of these tests without checking with your physician if you are ill or have any of the risk factors for exercise

endorphins Substances resembling morphine that are secreted by the brain and that decrease pain, suppress fatigue, and produce euphoria.

neurotransmitters Brain chemicals that transmit nerve impulses.

Terms

Note: The conditions for exercise safety given in Chapter 2 apply to all fitness assessment tests. If you answered yes to any question on the PAR-Q in Lab 2.1, see your physician before taking any assessment test. If you experience any unusual symptoms while taking a test, stop exercising and discuss your condition with your instructor.

Test	Fitness Prerequisites/Cautions
1-mile walk test	Recommended for anyone who meets the criteria for safe exercise. Can be used by individuals who cannot perform other tests because of low fitness level or injury.
3-minute step test	If you suffer from joint problems in your ankles, knees, or hips or you are significantly overweight, check with your physician before taking this test. People with balance problems or for whom a fall would be particularly dangerous, including older adults and pregnant women, should use special caution or avoid this test.
1.5-mile run-walk test	Recommended for people who are healthy and at least moderately active. If you have been sedentary, you should participate in a 4- to 8-week walk-run program before taking the test. Don't take this test in extremely hot or cold weather if you aren't used to exercising under those conditions.

discussed in Chapter 2 and Lab 2.1. Table 3.2 lists the fitness prerequisites and cautions recommended for each test.

• *The 1-Mile Walk Test.* The 1-mile walk test estimates your level of cardiorespiratory fitness (maximal oxygen consumption) based on the amount of time it takes you to complete 1 mile of brisk walking and your exercise heart rate at the end of your walk. A fast time and a low heart rate indicate a high level of cardiorespiratory endurance.

• *The 3-Minute Step Test.* The rate at which the pulse returns to normal after exercise is also a good measure of cardiorespiratory capacity; heart rate remains lower and recovers faster in people who are more physically fit. For the step test, you step continually at a steady rate and then monitor your heart rate during recovery.

• *The 1.5-Mile Run-Walk Test.* Oxygen consumption increases with speed in distance running, so a fast time on this test indicates high maximal oxygen consumption.

Additional assessments for cardiorespiratory fitness can be found on the *Fit and Well* Online Learning Center; these include cycle ergometer and swimming tests and a distance test for people who use wheelchairs.

Monitoring Your Heart Rate

Each time your heart beats, it pumps blood into your arteries; this surge of blood causes a pulse that you can feel by holding your fingers against an artery. Counting your pulse to determine your exercise heart rate is a key part of most assessment tests for maximal oxygen consumption. Heart rate can also be used to monitor exercise intensity during a workout. (Intensity is described in more detail in the next section.)

The two most common sites for monitoring heart rate are the carotid artery in the neck and the radial artery in the wrist. To take your pulse, press your index and middle fingers gently on the correct site. You may have to

shift position several times to find the best place to feel your pulse. Don't use your thumb to check your pulse; it has a pulse of its own that can confuse your count. Be careful not to push too hard, particularly when taking your pulse in the carotid artery (strong pressure on this artery may cause a reflex that slows the heart rate).

Heart rates are usually assessed in beats per minute (bpm). But counting your pulse for an entire minute isn't practical when you're exercising. And because heart rate slows rapidly when you stop exercising, it can give inaccurate results. It's best to do a shorter count—10 seconds—and then multiply the result by 6 to get your heart rate in beats per minute.

Interpreting Your Score

Once you've completed one or more of the assessment tests, use the table under "Rating Your Cardiovascular Fitness" at the end of Lab 3.1 to determine your current level of cardiorespiratory fitness. As you interpret your score, remember that field tests of cardiorespiratory fitness are not precise scientific measurements and do have a 10–15% margin of error.

You can use the assessment tests to monitor the progress of your fitness program by retesting yourself from time to time. Always compare scores for the *same* test: Your scores on different tests may vary considerably because of differences in skill and motivation and weaknesses in the tests themselves.

DEVELOPING A CARDIORESPIRATORY ENDURANCE PROGRAM

Cardiorespiratory endurance exercises are best for developing the type of fitness associated with good health, so they should serve as the focus of your exercise

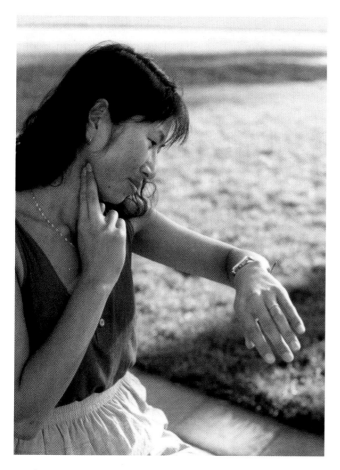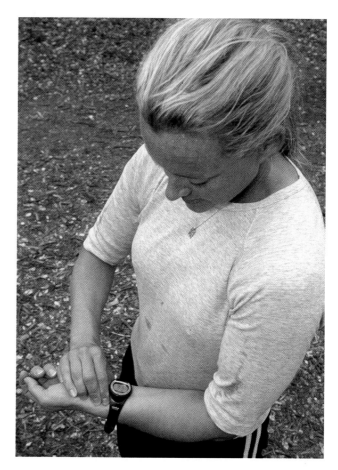

A pulse count can be used to determine exercise heart rate. The pulse can be taken at the carotid artery in the neck (left) or at the radial artery in the wrist (right).

program. To create a successful endurance exercise program, you must set realistic goals; set your starting frequency, intensity, and time (duration) of exercise at appropriate levels; choose suitable activities; remember to warm up and cool down; and adjust your program as your fitness improves.

MOTIVATION FOR CHANGE!   Are you having trouble getting started on a fitness program? Do you want to exercise more but find you just can't fit it into your day? Listen carefully to what you're telling yourself, perhaps by writing down your "self-talk" about exercise for a few days. Are you rationalizing, making excuses, procrastinating, or avoiding responsibility for your choices? For example, "I'm too busy with my classes this semester to fit exercise into my schedule," or "Right now I want to spend all my free time with my new girlfriend/boyfriend," or "I'll try to start running once the weather gets warmer." Can you think of ways to counter these statements and change your exercise habits? For example, "I see a lot of other busy people who are exercising, and I can probably do it too"; "I could ask a friend to go for a hike in the hills with me"; "I can use the exercise equipment at the gym until the weather warms up." Remember that when you make excuses, the only one who loses is you.

Setting Goals

You can use the results of cardiorespiratory fitness assessment tests to set a specific oxygen consumption goal for your cardiorespiratory endurance program. Your goal should be high enough to ensure a healthy cardiorespiratory system, but not so high that it will be impossible to achieve. Scores in the fair and good ranges for maximal oxygen consumption suggest good fitness; scores in the excellent and superior ranges indicate a high standard of physical performance.

Through endurance training, an individual may be able to improve maximal oxygen consumption ($\dot{V}O_{2max}$) by about 10–30%. The amount of improvement possible depends on age, health status, and initial fitness level; people who start at a very low fitness level can improve by a greater percentage than elite athletes because the latter are already at a much higher fitness level, a level that may approach their genetic physical limits. If you are tracking $\dot{V}O_{2max}$ using the field tests described in this chapter, you may be able to increase your score by more than 30% due to improvements in other physical factors, such as muscle power, which can affect your performance on the tests.

Another physical factor you can track to monitor progress is resting heart rate—your heart rate at complete rest, measured in the morning before you get out of bed and move around. Resting heart rate may decrease by as much as 10–15 beats per minute in response to endurance training. Changes in resting heart rate may be noticeable after only about 4–6 weeks of training.

You may want to set other types of goals for your fitness program. For example, if you walk, jog, or cycle as part of your fitness program, you may want to set a time or distance goal—working up to walking 5 miles in one session, completing a 4-mile run in 28 minutes, or cycling a total of 35 miles per week. A more modest goal might be to achieve the Surgeon General's minimum activity level of doing at least 30 minutes of moderate activity on most days. Although it's best to base your program on measurable goals, you may also want to set some more qualitative goals, such as becoming more energetic, sleeping better, and improving the fit of your clothes.

Applying the FITT Equation

As described in Chapter 2, you can use the acronym FITT to remember key parameters of your fitness program: frequency, intensity, time (duration), and type of activity.

Frequency of Training   To build cardiorespiratory endurance, you should exercise 3–5 days per week. Beginners should start with 3 and work up to 5 days per week. Training more than 5 days per week can lead to injury and isn't necessary for the typical person on an exercise program designed to promote wellness. Training fewer than 3 days per week makes it difficult to improve your fitness (unless exercise intensity is very high) or to use exercise to lose weight. In addition, you risk injury because your body never gets a chance to fully adapt to regular exercise training.

Intensity of Training   Intensity is the most important factor in achieving training effects. You must exercise intensely enough to stress your body so that fitness improves. Two methods of monitoring exercise intensity are described below; choose the method that works best for you. Be sure to make adjustments in your intensity levels for environmental or individual factors. For example, on a hot and humid day or on your first day back to your program after an illness, you should decrease your intensity level.

Target Heart Rate Zone   One of the best ways to monitor the intensity of cardiorespiratory endurance exercise is to measure your heart rate. It isn't necessary to exercise at your maximum heart rate to improve maximal oxygen consumption. Fitness adaptations occur at lower heart rates with a much lower risk of injury.

According to the American College of Sports Medicine, your **target heart rate zone**—rates at which you should exercise to experience cardiorespiratory benefits—is between 65% and 90% of your maximum heart rate. To calculate your target heart rate zone, follow these steps:

1. Estimate your maximum heart rate (MHR) by subtracting your age from 220, or have it measured precisely by

undergoing an exercise stress test in a doctor's office, hospital, or sports medicine lab. (Note: Using the formula to estimate maximum heart rate can be very inaccurate for some people, particularly older adults and young children. If your exercise heart rate seems inaccurate—that is, exercise within your target zone seems either too easy or too difficult—then used the perceived exertion method described in the next section or have your maximum heart rate measured precisely.)

2. Multiply your MHR by 65% and 90% to calculate your target heart rate zone. (Note: Very unfit people should use 55% of MHR for their training threshold.)

For example, a 19-year-old would calculate her target heart rate zone as follows:

$$MHR = 220 - 19 = 201$$
$$65\% \text{ training intensity} = 0.65 \times 201 = 131 \text{ bpm}$$
$$90\% \text{ training intensity} = 0.90 \times 201 = 181 \text{ bpm}$$

To gain fitness benefits, the young woman in our example would have to exercise at an intensity that raises her heart rate to between 131 and 181 bpm.

An alternative method for calculating target heart rate range uses **heart rate reserve**, the difference between maximum heart rate and resting heart rate. Using this method, target heart rate is equal to resting heart rate plus between 50% (40% for very unfit people) and 85% of heart rate reserve. Although some people will obtain more accurate results using this more complex method, both methods provide reasonable estimates of an appropriate target heart rate zone. Formulas for both methods of calculating target heart rate are given in Lab 3.2.

If you have been sedentary, start by exercising at the lower end of your target heart rate range (65% of maximum heart rate or 50% of heart rate reserve) for at least 4–6 weeks. Fast and significant gains in maximal oxygen consumption can be made by exercising closer to the top of the range, but you may increase your risk of injury and overtraining. You *can* achieve significant health benefits by exercising at the bottom of your target range, so don't feel pressured into exercising at an unnecessarily intense level. If you exercise at a lower intensity, you can increase the duration or frequency of training to obtain as much benefit to your health, as long as you are above the 65% training threshold. (For people with a very low initial level of fitness, a lower training intensity, 55–64% of maximum heart rate or 40–49% of heart rate reserve, may be sufficient to achieve improvements in maximal oxygen consumption, especially at the start of an exercise program. Intensities of 70–85% of maximum heart rate are appropriate for average individuals.)

By monitoring your heart rate, you will always know if you are working hard enough to improve, not hard enough, or too hard. To monitor your heart rate during exercise, count your pulse while you're still moving or immediately after you stop exercising. Count beats for 10 seconds, and then multiply that number by 6 to see if your heart rate is in your target zone. If the young woman

Table 3.3	Target Heart Rate Range and 10-Second Counts	
Age (years)	Target Heart Rate Range (bpm)*	10-Second Count (beats)*
20–24	127–180	21–30
25–29	124–176	20–29
30–34	121–171	20–28
35–59	118–167	19–27
40–44	114–162	19–27
45–49	111–158	18–26
50–54	108–153	18–25
55–59	105–149	17–24
60–64	101–144	16–24
65+	97–140	16–23

*Target heart rates lower than those shown here are appropriate for individuals with a very low initial level of fitness. Ranges are based on the following formula: Target heart rate = 0.65 to 0.90 of maximum heart rate, assuming maximum heart rate = 220 − age. The heart rate range values shown here correspond to RPE values of about 12–18.

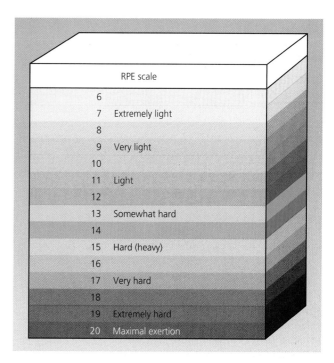

Figure 3.5 Ratings of perceived exertion (RPE). Experienced exercisers may use this subjective scale to estimate how near they are to their target heart rate zone. The scale was developed in the 1950s by Swedish exercise physiologist Gunnar Borg and is also known as the Borg scale. SOURCE: *Psychology from Research to Practice* (1978), ed. H. L. Pick. Reprinted with permission from Kluwer Academic/Plenum Publishing Corporation.

in our example were aiming for 144 bpm, she would want a 10-second count of 24 beats. Target heart rate ranges and 10-second counts based on the maximum heart rate formula are shown in Table 3.3.

RATINGS OF PERCEIVED EXERTION   Another way to monitor intensity is to monitor your perceived level of exertion. Repeated pulse counting during exercise can become a nuisance if it interferes with the activity. As your exercise program progresses, you will probably become familiar with the amount of exertion required to raise your heart rate to target levels. In other words, you will know how you feel when you have exercised intensely enough. If this is the case, you can use the scale of **ratings of perceived exertion (RPE)** shown in Figure 3.5 to monitor the intensity of your exercise session without checking your pulse.

To use the RPE scale, select a rating that corresponds to your subjective perception of how hard you are exercising when you are training in your target heart rate zone. If your target zone is about 135–155 bpm, exercise intensely enough to raise your heart rate to that level, and then associate a rating—for example, "somewhat hard" or "hard" (14 or 15)—with how hard you feel you are working. To reach and maintain intensity in future workouts, exercise hard enough to reach what you feel is the same level of exertion. You should periodically check your RPE against your target heart rate zone to make sure it's correct. Research has shown RPE to be an accurate means of monitoring exercise intensity, and you may find it easier and more convenient than pulse counting.

Time (Duration) of Training   A total duration of 20–60 minutes is recommended; exercise can take place in a single session or in multiple sessions lasting 10 or more min-

utes. The total duration of exercise depends on its intensity. To improve cardiorespiratory endurance during a low-to-moderate-intensity activity such as walking or slow swimming, you should exercise for 45–60 minutes. For high-intensity exercise performed at the top of your target heart rate zone, a duration of 20 minutes is sufficient. Some studies have shown that 5–10 minutes of extremely intense exercise (greater than 90% of maximal oxygen consumption) improves cardiorespiratory endurance. However, training at this intensity, particularly during high-impact activities, increases the risk of injury. Also, because of the discomfort of high-intensity exercise, you are more likely to discontinue your exercise program. Longer-duration, low-to-moderate-intensity activities generally result in more gradual gains in maximal oxygen consumption. In planning your program, start with less vigorous activities and gradually increase intensity.

target heart rate zone The range of heart rates that should be reached and maintained during cardiorespiratory endurance exercise to obtain training effects.

heart rate reserve The difference between maximum heart rate and resting heart rate; used in one method for calculating target heart rate range.

ratings of perceived exertion (RPE) A system of monitoring exercise intensity based on assigning a number to the subjective perception of target intensity.

Terms
VW

Cardiorespiratory endurance can be developed without special equipment or facilities, but if you choose to use fitness equipment, quality is an important factor. Good equipment can enhance your enjoyment of your fitness program and decrease your risk of injury. Before considering any piece of equipment, ask yourself the following questions:

- *Will the equipment help me achieve my fitness goals?* Make sure the piece of equipment you're considering works your target fitness components. Don't be fooled by outrageous advertising claims, and be sure to check the fine print of any advertisement. Exercise is not "easy" or "effortless," and it is impossible for any equipment to make you lose fat in a particular area (spot reduce). The Federal Trade Commission provides good general advice for people shopping for exercise equipment (http://www.ftc.gov).

- *Will I really use the equipment regularly?* Before you invest money in a piece of equipment, try it out for a time at a fitness center or health club. Make sure it is something you can use safely and comfortably over the long term.

- *Is the equipment well made?* Before you buy, do some research. Ask coaches and fitness instructors, and check consumer publications. If you intend to push the equipment to the limit, look for a heavy-duty model.

- *Is the equipment easy to use?* You will be more likely to use a piece of equipment regularly if it is easy to set up and use. Any instructions should be easy to follow.

- *Do I have room for the equipment?* A good treadmill or home gym may be large and require significant space to use and store. Make sure you have a place to use it that is pleasant and well ventilated and where any noise produced by the equipment will not be a problem.

- *Can I afford a quality piece of equipment?* Shop around to find the best deal; try discount stores, specialty shops, and catalogs. However, be aware of deals that seem too good to be

true; an exceptionally low price may indicate poor quality. In addition, get the details on warranties, guarantees, and return policies before you buy.

The following are among the most popular types of home exercise equipment:

Treadmills: Some studies of exercise equipment have found that treadmills are the best type of home exercise equipment for developing fitness and burning calories and are more likely to be used consistently. Choose a motorized treadmill with a platform or surface that is large enough to fit your stride, stable enough to accommodate your weight, and cushioned enough to absorb the impact of your feet. The handrails should be able to support your weight if you lose your balance.

Stationary cycles: Try both upright and recumbent (reclining) models to see which type suits you best. Check to make sure the seat and handlebars of the cycle can be adjusted to comfortably fit your height and leg extension. Look for a model whose resistance can be changed easily.

Cross-country ski machines: Although learning to coordinate the movements needed to use a cross-country ski machine may take time, this type of equipment typically provides a full-body workout. Look for a model that allows separate adjustment of the lower-body sliding footpads and the upper-body rope-and-pulley device.

Stair climbers and elliptical trainers: Check to be sure that you can work the pedals securely and smoothly while maintaining good posture; machines with independent foot action usually allow a more natural rhythm. For greater durability, choose a machine with hydraulic rather than air-filled shock absorbers.

Another key piece of equipment for many fitness activities and sports is proper footwear; refer to Chapter 7 for advice on shopping for athletic shoes.

Type of Activity   Cardiorespiratory endurance exercises include activities that involve the rhythmic use of large-muscle groups for an extended period of time, such as jogging, walking, cycling, aerobic dancing and other forms of group exercise, cross-country skiing, and swimming. Start-and-stop sports, such as tennis and racquetball, also qualify, as long as you have enough skill to play continuously and intensely enough to raise your heart rate to target levels.

Having fun is a strong motivator; select a physical activity that you enjoy, and it will be easier to stay with your program. Exercising with a friend can also be helpful as a motivator. Consider whether you prefer competitive or individual sports, or whether starting something

new would be best. Other important considerations are access to facilities, expense, equipment, and the time required to achieve an adequate skill level and workout (see the box "Evaluating Home Exercise Equipment").

Warming Up and Cooling Down

It's important to warm up before every session of cardiorespiratory endurance exercise and to cool down afterward. Because the body's muscles work better when their temperature is slightly above resting level, warming up enhances performance and decreases the chance of injury. It gives the body time to redirect blood to active muscles and the heart time to adapt to increased demands. Warming up also helps spread **synovial fluid** throughout the joints, which helps protect their surfaces from injury.

As mentioned in Chapter 2, a warm-up session should include low-intensity movements similar to those in the

Terms   **synovial fluid** Fluid produced within many joints that provides lubrication and nutrients for the joints.

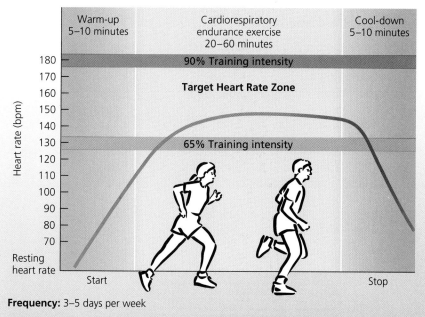

Warm-up
5–10 minutes

Cardiorespiratory
endurance exercise
20–60 minutes

Cool-down
5–10 minutes

90% Training intensity

Target Heart Rate Zone

65% Training intensity

Heart rate (bpm): 180, 170, 160, 150, 140, 130, 120, 110, 100, 90, 80, 70

Resting heart rate

Start

Stop

Frequency: 3–5 days per week

Intensity: 55/65–90% of maximum heart rate, 40/50–85% of heart rate reserve plus resting heart rate, or an RPE rating of about 12–18 (lower intensities—55–64% of maximum heart rate and 40–49% of heart rate reserve—are applicable to people who are quite unfit; for average individuals, intensities of 70–85% of maximum heart rate are appropriate)

Time (duration): 20–60 minutes (one session or multiple sessions lasting 10 or more minutes)

Type of activity: Cardiorespiratory endurance exercises, such as walking, jogging, biking, swimming, cross-country skiing, and rope skipping

Figure 3.6 The FITT principle for a cardiorespiratory endurance workout. Longer-duration exercise at lower intensities can often be as beneficial for promoting health as shorter-duration, high-intensity exercise.

activity that will follow. Low-intensity movements include walking slowly before beginning a brisk walk, hitting fore-hands and backhands before a tennis match, and running a 12-minute mile before progressing to an 8-minute one. An active warm-up of 5–10 minutes is adequate for most types of exercise. However, warm-up time will depend on your level of fitness, experience, and individual preferences.

Some people like to include stretching exercises in their warm-up. If you like to stretch before exercising, experts recommend that you stretch after the active part of your warm-up, when your body temperature has been elevated (see Chapter 5). Studies have found that stretching prior to exercise can decrease performance, so some experts even recommend that stretching be done *after* a workout.

Cooling down after exercise is important for returning the body to a nonexercising state. A cool-down helps maintain blood flow to the heart and brain and redirects blood from working muscles to other areas of the body; it helps prevent a large drop in blood pressure, dizziness, and other potential cardiovascular complications. A cool-down, consisting of 5–10 minutes of reduced activity, should follow every workout to allow heart rate, breathing, and circulation to return to normal. Decrease the intensity of exercise gradually during your cool-down. For example, following a running workout, begin your cool-down by jogging at half speed for 30 seconds to a minute; then do several minutes of walking, reducing your speed slowly. A good rule of thumb is to cool-down

at least until your heart rate drops below 100 beats per minute. Doing stretching exercises at the end of a work-out is an excellent strategy: Your muscles are warm, allowing you to stretch farther with less risk of injury; in addition, there is no danger of decreased performance.

The general pattern of a safe and successful workout for cardiorespiratory fitness is illustrated in Figure 3.6.

Building Cardiorespiratory Fitness

Building fitness is as much an art as a science. Your rate of progress will depend on your age, health status, initial level of fitness, and motivation. Your fitness improves when you overload your body. However, you must increase the intensity, frequency, and duration of exercise carefully to avoid injury and overtraining.

For the initial phase of your program, which may last anywhere from 3 to 6 weeks, exercise at the low end of your target heart rate zone. Begin with a frequency of 3–4 days per week, and choose a duration appropriate for your fitness level: 12–15 minutes if you are very unfit, 20 minutes if you are sedentary but otherwise healthy, and 30–40 minutes if you are an experienced exerciser. Use this phase of your program to allow both your body and your schedule to adjust to your new exercise routine. Once you can exercise at the upper levels of frequency (4–5 days per week) and duration (30–40 minutes) without excessive fatigue or muscle soreness, you are ready to progress.

	Table 3.4	Sample Progression for an Endurance Program		

Stage/Week	Frequency (days/week)	Intensity* (beats/minute)	Time (duration in minutes)
Initial stage			
1	3	120–135	20
2	3	120–135	25
3	4	135–150	25
4	4	135–150	30
Improvement stage			
5–7	3–4	150–160	25–30
8–10	3–4	150–160	30–35
11–13	3–4	155–170	30–35
14–16	4–5	155–170	30–35
17–20	4–5	155–170	35–40
21–24	4–5	160–180	35–40
Maintenance stage			
25+	3–5	160–180	30–45

*The target heart rates shown here are based on calculations for a healthy 20-year-old; the program progresses from an initial target heart rate of 60% to a maintenance range of 80–90% of maximum heart rate.

SOURCE: Adapted from American College of Sports Medicine. 2000. *ACSM's Guidelines for Exercise Testing and Prescription*, 6th ed. Philadelphia: Lippincott Williams and Wilkins. Reprinted with permission from the publisher.

The next phase of your program is the improvement phase, lasting from 4 to 6 months. During this phase, slowly and gradually increase the amount of overload until you reach your target level of fitness (see the sample training progression in Table 3.4). Take care not to increase overload too quickly. It is usually best to avoid increasing intensity and duration during the same session or all three training variables in one week. Increasing duration in increments of 5–10 minutes every 2–3 weeks is usually appropriate. Signs of a too rapid progression in overload include muscles aches and pains, lack of usual interest in exercise, extreme fatigue, and inability to complete a workout. Keep an exercise log or training diary to help monitor your workouts and progress.

Maintaining Cardiorespiratory Fitness

You will not improve your fitness indefinitely. The more fit you become, the harder you have to work to improve. There are limits to the level of fitness you can achieve, and if you increase intensity and duration indefinitely, you are likely to become injured or overtrained. After a progression phase of 4–6 months, you may reach your goal of an acceptable level of fitness. You can then maintain fitness by continuing to exercise at the same intensity at least 3 nonconsecutive days every week. If you stop exercising, you lose your gains in fitness fairly rapidly. If you take time off for any reason, start your program again at a lower level and rebuild your fitness in a slow and systematic way.

When you reach the maintenance phase, you may want to set new goals for your program and make some adjustments to maintain your motivation. Adding variety to your program can be a helpful strategy. Engaging in multiple types of endurance activities, an approach known as cross-training, can help boost enjoyment and prevent some types of injuries. For example, someone who has been jogging 5 days a week may change her program so that she jogs 3 days a week, plays tennis 1 day a week, and goes for a bike ride 1 day a week.

MOTIVATION FOR CHANGE! Studies of college students have found that social support is a key factor influencing whether students exercise. Do your friends and family members actively support your fitness goals and program? If not, enlist their help and encouragement—it can make a big difference.

EXERCISE SAFETY AND INJURY PREVENTION

Exercising safely in a variety of environmental conditions and preventing muscle and joint injuries are two important challenges for people who engage in cardiorespiratory endurance exercise.

Hot Weather and Heat Stress

Human beings depend on a relatively constant body temperature to survive. An increase (or decrease) of just a few degrees in body temperature can quickly lead to distress and even death. Exercise safety in a high-temperature environment depends on the body's ability to dissipate heat and maintain blood flow to active muscles. Heat from exercise is released through evaporation of sweat, which cools the skin and the blood circulating near the surface of the body. The hotter the weather, the more water the body loses through sweat; the more humid the weather, the less efficient the sweating mechanism is at lowering body temperature. If you lose too much water or if your body temperature rises too high, you may suffer from heat stress. Problems associated with heat stress can include dehydration, heat cramps, heat exhaustion, and life-threatening heat stroke.

Dehydration   Your body needs water to carry out many chemical reactions and to regulate body temperature. Sweating during exercise depletes your body's water supply and can lead to **dehydration** if fluids aren't replaced. Although dehydration is most common in hot weather, it can occur in even comfortable temperatures if fluid intake is insufficient.

Dehydration increases body temperature and decreases sweat rate, plasma volume, cardiac output, maximal oxygen consumption, exercise capacity, muscular strength, and stores of liver glycogen. You may begin to feel thirsty when you have a fluid deficit of about 1% of total body weight. In people who play sports such as football and tennis or who engage in distance running, fluid deficits of up to 5% are quite common. At this level of dehydration, people feel uncomfortable and may alternate between fatigue and restlessness. At higher levels of fluid deficit, loss of coordination, delirium, and death can occur.

Drinking fluids before and during exercise is important to prevent dehydration and enhance performance. Thirst receptors in the brain make you want to drink fluids, but during heavy or prolonged exercise or exercise in hot weather, thirst alone isn't a good indication of how much you need to drink. As a rule of thumb, drink at least 2 cups (16 ounces) of fluid 2 hours before exercise and then drink enough during exercise to match fluid loss in sweat. Drink at least 1 cup of fluid for every 20–30 minutes of exercise, more in hot weather or if you sweat heavily. To determine if you're drinking enough fluid, weigh yourself before and after an exercise session—any weight loss is due to fluid loss that needs to be replaced.

Bring a water bottle when you exercise so you can replace your fluids when they're being depleted. For exercise sessions lasting less than 60–90 minutes, cool water is an excellent fluid replacement. For longer workouts, you might want to choose a sports drink that contains water and small amounts of electrolytes (sodium, potassium, and magnesium) and simple carbohydrates ("sugar," usually in the form of sucrose or glucose). Electrolytes, which are lost from the body in sweat, are important because they help regulate the balance of fluids in body cells and the bloodstream. The carbohydrates in typical sports drinks are rapidly digestible and can thus help

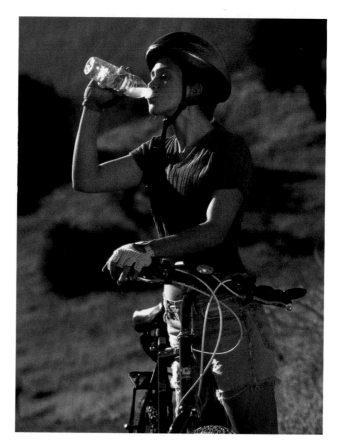

To prevent dehydration and enhance performance, consume an adequate amount of fluid before and during exercise.

maintain blood glucose levels. Choose a beverage with no more than 8 grams of simple carbohydrate per 100 ml. See Chapter 8 for more on diet and fluid recommendations for active people.

Heat Cramps   Involuntary cramping and spasms in the muscle groups used during exercise are sometimes called **heat cramps.** While depletion of sodium and potassium from the muscles are involved with the problem, the primary cause for cramps is muscle fatigue. Children are particularly susceptible to heat cramps, but the condition can also occur in adults, even those who are fit. The best treatment for heat cramps is a combination of gentle stretching, replacement of fluid and electrolytes, and rest.

Heat Exhaustion   Symptoms of **heat exhaustion** include a rapid and weak pulse, low blood pressure, faintness, profuse sweating, and, in some cases, psychological

dehydration Excessive loss of body fluid.

heat cramps Sudden development of muscle spasms and pain associated with intense exercise in hot weather.

heat exhaustion Heat illness related to dehydration resulting from exertion in hot weather.

Terms

disorientation; core body temperature may be normal or slightly elevated. Heat exhaustion occurs when an insufficient amount of blood returns to the heart because so much of the body's blood volume is being directed to working muscles (for exercise) and to the skin (for cooling). Treatment for heat exhaustion includes resting in a cool area and drinking fluids. An affected individual should rest for the remainder of the day and drink plenty of fluids for the next 24 hours.

Heat Stroke   **Heat stroke** is a major medical emergency involving the failure of the brain's temperature regulatory center. The body does not sweat enough, and body temperature rises dramatically to extremely dangerous levels. In addition to high body temperature, symptoms can include hot skin (dry or sweaty), very high or very low blood pressure, confusion, erratic behavior, and loss of consciousness. A heat stroke victim should be cooled as rapidly as possible and be immediately transported to a hospital.

Several deaths in professional sports occurred when athletes exercised intensely in hot conditions while taking supplements containing such stimulants as caffeine and ephedra. These deaths have not been positively linked to supplement use, but any supplement that can affect body temperature, fluid balance, or blood pressure is potentially risky when combined with intense exercise. (See Chapter 4 for more on supplements.)

Preventing Heat Problems   To avoid heat-related problems, use caution when exercising in hot and humid weather. Watch for the signals of heat stress, regardless of the weather, and follow the tips in the box "Exercising in Hot Weather."

Cold Weather

In extremely cold conditions, problems can result if a person's body temperature drops or if particular parts of the body are exposed. If the body's ability to warm itself through shivering or exercise can't keep pace with heat loss, the core body temperature begins to drop. This condition, known as **hypothermia,** depresses the central nervous system, resulting in sleepiness and a lower metabolic rate. As metabolic rate drops, body temperature declines even further, and coma and death can result. **Frostbite**—the freezing of body tissues—is another potential danger of exercise in extremely cold conditions. Frostbite most commonly occurs in exposed body parts like earlobes, fingers, and toes, and it can cause permanent circulatory damage. Hypothermia and frostbite both require immediate medical treatment.

What can you do to exercise safely in cold conditions? First of all, don't stay out in very cold temperatures for too long. Take both the temperature and the wind into account when planning your exercise session. Frostbite within 30 minutes is possible in calm conditions when the temperature is colder than −5°F

or in windy conditions (30 mph) if the temperature is below 10°F. **Wind chill** values that reflect both the temperature and the wind speed are available as part of a local weather forecast and from the National Weather Service (http://www.weather.gov); a complete wind chill chart is available on the *Fit and Well* Online Learning Center.

Appropriate clothing provides insulation and helps trap warm air next to the skin. Dress in layers so you can remove them as you warm up and put them back on if you get cold. A substantial amount of heat loss comes from the head and neck, so keep these areas covered. In subfreezing temperatures, protect the areas of your body most susceptible to frostbite—fingers, toes, ears, nose, and cheeks—with warm socks, mittens or gloves, and a cap, hood, or ski mask. Wear clothing that "breathes" and will wick moisture away from your skin to avoid being cooled or overheated by trapped perspiration. Many types of comfortable, lightweight clothing that provide good insulation are available. It's also important to warm up thoroughly and to drink plenty of fluids.

Poor Air Quality

Air pollution can decrease exercise performance and negatively affect health, particularly if you have respiratory problems such as asthma, bronchitis, or emphysema, or if you smoke. The effects of smog are worse during exercise than at rest because air enters the lungs faster. Polluted air may also contain carbon monoxide, which displaces oxygen in the blood and reduces the amount of oxygen available to working muscles. Symptoms of poor air quality include eye and throat irritations, difficulty breathing, and possibly headache and malaise.

Do not exercise outdoors during a smog alert or if air quality is very poor. If you have any type of cardiorespiratory difficulty, you should also avoid exertion outdoors when air quality is poor. You can avoid some smog and air pollution by exercising in indoor facilities, in parks, near water (riverbanks, lakeshores, and ocean beaches), or in residential areas with less traffic (areas with stop-and-go traffic will have lower air quality than areas where traffic moves quickly). Air quality is also usually better in the early morning and late evening, before and after the commute hours.

Exercise Injuries

Even the most careful physically active person can suffer an injury. Most injuries are annoying rather than serious or permanent. However, an injury that isn't cared for properly can escalate into a chronic problem, sometimes serious enough to permanently curtail the activity. It's important to learn how to deal with injuries so they don't derail your fitness program. Strategies for the care of common exercise injuries and discomforts appear in Table 3.5 (p. 76); some general guidelines are given below.

Following a few simple principles can minimize the problems associated with exercising in the heat. To help alert people about weather conditions that could increase the risk of heat illness, the U.S. Weather Service developed the **heat index**—a measure that incorporates both temperature and relative humidity. For example, a temperature of 95 degrees combined with a relative humidity of 50% has a heat index of 107. Prolonged exposure or physical activity when the heat index is 80–90 can cause fatigue; at a heat index of 90 or above, heat cramps, heat exhaustion, and heat stroke become more likely. Reduce and avoid exercise when the heat index is 90 or above. A complete chart of heat index values can be found on the *Fit and Well* Online Learning Center. Local heat index information is available from the National Weather Service (http://www.weather.gov). Additional strategies to help avoid the risk of heat illness include the following:

- Be in good physical condition. Exercise training can help the body adapt to heat by increasing the sweat rate.

- Use caution when exercising in extreme heat or humidity (over 80°F and/or 60% humidity).

- Slow exercise or add rest breaks to maintain your prescribed target heart rate; as you become acclimatized, you can gradually increase intensity and duration.

- Exercise in the early morning or evening, when temperatures are lowest.

- Drink 2 cups of fluids 2 hours before you begin exercising, and drink 4–8 ounces of fluid every 10–15 minutes during exercise (more frequently during high-intensity activities). Plan for regular water breaks.

- During a period of hot weather, weigh yourself every day before exercising. If your weight has decreased by 3% or more from the previous day, don't exercise without first rehydrating.

- Avoid supplements and beverages containing stimulants like ephedra and caffeine when exercising in the heat. Do not use salt pills.

- Wear clothing that "breathes," allowing air to circulate and cool the body. Wearing white or light colors will help by reflecting, rather than absorbing, heat. A hat can help keep direct sun off your face. Do not wear rubber, plastic, or other nonporous clothing. "Sauna suits" cause loss of body water, not fat, and don't improve body composition.

- Rest frequently in the shade.

- Slow down or stop if you begin to feel uncomfortable. Watch for the signs of heat disorders listed below; if they occur, act appropriately.

Problem	Symptoms	Treatment
Heat cramps	Muscle cramps, usually in the muscles most used during exercise.	Stop exercising, drink fluids, and massage or stretch cramped muscles.
Heat exhaustion	Weakness, dizziness, headache, rapid pulse, profuse sweating, pale face, normal or slightly elevated temperature.	Cool the body. Stop exercising, get out of the heat, remove excess clothing, drink cold fluids, and apply cool and/or damp towels to the body.
Heat stroke	Hot, flushed skin (may be dry or sweaty), red face, chills, shivering, disorientation, erratic behavior, high body temperature, unconsciousness, convulsions.	*Get immediate medical attention,* and try to lower body temperature. Get out of the heat, remove excess clothing, drink cold fluids, and apply cool and/or damp towels to the body or immerse it in cold water.

When to Call a Physician   Some injuries require medical attention. Consult a physician for head and eye injuries, possible ligament injuries, broken bones, and internal disorders such as chest pain, fainting, elevated body temperature, and intolerance to hot weather. Also seek medical attention for ostensibly minor injuries that do not get better within a reasonable amount of time. You may need to modify your exercise program for a few weeks to allow an injury to heal.

Managing Minor Exercise Injuries   For minor cuts and scrapes, stop the bleeding and clean the wound. Treat injuries to soft tissue (muscles and joints) with the R-I-C-E principle: rest, ice, compression, and elevation. Immediately following the injury, rest the affected area and apply ice. Elevate the affected part of the body, and

heat stroke A severe and often fatal heat illness produced by exposure to very high temperatures, especially when combined with intense exercise; characterized by significantly elevated core body temperature.

hypothermia Low body temperature due to exposure to cold conditions.

frostbite Freezing of body tissues characterized by pallor, numbness, and a loss of cold sensation.

wind chill A measure of how cold it feels based on the rate of heat loss from exposed skin caused by cold and wind; the temperature that would have the same cooling effect on a person as a given combination of temperature and wind speed.

heat index A measure of how hot it feels; the temperature that would have the same heating effect on a person as a given combination of temperature and relative humidity.

Terms
Ww

Injury	Symptoms	Treatment
Blister	Accumulation of fluid in one spot under the skin	Don't pop or drain it unless it interferes too much with your daily activities. If it does pop, clean the area with antiseptic and cover with a bandage. Do not remove the skin covering the blister.
Bruise (contusion)	Pain, swelling, and discoloration	R-I-C-E: rest, ice, compression, elevation.
Fractures and dislocations	Pain, swelling, tenderness, loss of function, and deformity	Seek medical attention, immobilize the affected area, and apply cold.
Joint sprain	Pain, tenderness, swelling, discoloration, and loss of function	R-I-C-E. Apply heat when swelling has disappeared. Stretch and strengthen affected area.
Muscle cramp	Painful, spasmodic muscle contractions	Gently stretch for 15–30 seconds at a time and/or massage the cramped area. Drink fluids and increase dietary salt intake if exercising in hot weather.
Muscle soreness or stiffness	Pain and tenderness in the affected muscle	Stretch the affected muscle gently; exercise at a low intensity; apply heat. Nonsteroidal anti-inflammatory drugs, such as ibuprofen, help some people.
Muscle strain	Pain, tenderness, swelling, and loss of strength in the affected muscle	R-I-C-E; apply heat when swelling has disappeared. Stretch and strengthen the affected area.
Shin splints	Pain and tenderness on the front of the lower leg; sometimes also pain in the calf muscle	Rest; apply ice to the affected area several times a day and before exercise; wrap with tape for support. Stretch and strengthen muscles in the lower legs. Purchase good-quality footwear and run on soft surfaces.
Side stitch	Pain on the side of the abdomen	Stretch the arm on the affected side as high as possible; if that doesn't help, try bending forward while tightening the abdominal muscles.
Tendinitis	Pain, swelling, and tenderness of the affected area	R-I-C-E; apply heat when swelling has disappeared. Stretch and strengthen the affected area.

compress it with an elastic bandage to minimize swelling. Apply ice regularly for 36–48 hours after an injury occurs or until all the swelling is gone. (Don't leave ice on one spot for more than 20 minutes.) The day after the injury, some experts also recommend taking an over-the-counter medication such as aspirin, ibuprofen, or naproxen to decrease inflammation.

Don't apply heat to an injury at first, because heat draws blood to the area and increases swelling. After the swelling has subsided, apply either moist heat (hot towels, heat packs, warm water immersion) or dry heat (heating pads) to speed up healing.

To rehabilitate your body, follow the steps listed in the box "Rehabilitation Following a Minor Athletic Injury."

Preventing Injuries   The best method for dealing with exercise injuries is to prevent them. If you choose activities for your program carefully and follow the training guidelines described here and in Chapter 2, you should be able to avoid most types of injuries. Important guidelines for preventing athletic injuries include the following:

- Train regularly and stay in condition.
- Gradually increase the intensity, duration, or frequency of your workouts.
- Avoid or minimize high-impact activities; alternate them with low-impact activities.
- Get proper rest between exercise sessions.
- Drink plenty of fluids.
- Warm up thoroughly before you exercise and cool down afterward.
- Achieve and maintain a good level of flexibility.
- Use proper body mechanics when lifting objects or executing sports skills.
- Don't exercise when you are ill or overtrained.
- Use proper equipment, particularly shoes, and choose an appropriate exercise surface. If you exercise on a grass field, soft track, or wooden floor, you are less likely to be injured than on concrete or a hard track.
- Don't return to your normal exercise program until your athletic injuries have healed. Restart your program at a lower intensity and gradually increase the amount of overload.

1. Reduce the initial inflammation using the R-I-C-E principle:

Rest: Stop using the injured area as soon as you experience pain. Avoid any activity that causes pain.

Ice: Apply ice to the injured area to reduce swelling and alleviate pain. Apply ice immediately for 10–20 minutes and repeat every few hours until the swelling disappears. Let the injured part return to normal temperature between icings, and do not apply ice to one area for more than 20 minutes. An easy method for applying ice is to freeze water in a paper cup, peel some of the paper away, and rub the exposed ice on the injured area. If the injured area is large, you can surround it with several bags of crushed ice or ice cubes, or bags of frozen vegetables. Place a thin towel between the bag and your skin. If you use a cold gel pack, limit application time to 10 minutes.

Compression: Wrap the injured area firmly with an elastic or compression bandage between icings. If the area starts throbbing or begins to change color, the bandage may be wrapped too tightly. Do not sleep with the wrap on.

Elevation: Raise the injured area above heart level to decrease the blood supply and reduce swelling. Use pillows, books, or a low chair or stool to raise the injured area.

2. After 36–48 hours, apply heat *if the swelling has completely disappeared.* Immerse the affected area in warm water or apply warm compresses, a hot water bottle, or a heating pad. As soon as it's comfortable, begin moving the affected joints slowly. If you feel pain, or if the injured area begins to swell again, reduce the amount of movement. Continue stretching and moving the affected area until you have regained normal range of motion.

3. Gradually begin exercising the injured area to build strength and endurance. Depending on the type of injury, weight training, walking, and resistance training with a partner can all be effective.

4. Gradually reintroduce the stress of an activity until you can return to full intensity. Don't progress too rapidly or you'll reinjure yourself. Before returning to full exercise participation, you should have a full range of motion in your joints, normal strength and balance among your muscles, normal coordinated patterns of movement (with no injury compensation movements, such as limping), and little or no pain.

Tips for Today

Good cardiorespiratory fitness is essential for a long and healthy life. It also provides many immediate benefits that span all the dimensions of wellness—improved mood, better sleep, greater creativity, and fewer colds, to name just a few. The good news is that you don't have to be an elite athlete to enjoy these benefits. Regular, moderate exercise, even in short bouts spread through the day, can build and maintain cardiorespiratory fitness.

Right now you can

- Do a short bout of endurance exercise: 10–15 minutes of walking, jogging, cycling, or another endurance activity.

- If you have physical activity planned for later in the day, drink some fluids now to make sure you are fully hydrated for your workout.

- Consider the exercise equipment, including shoes, you currently have on hand. If you'll need new equipment to begin your program, check the phone book, campus store, Internet, and other resources to start gathering the information you'll need to get the best equipment you can afford.

- Think of someone you know who engages in regular endurance exercise. Call or e-mail that person and ask what strategies she or he uses to find time for exercise and to stay motivated.

SUMMARY

- The cardiorespiratory system consists of the heart, blood vessels, and respiratory system; it picks up and transports oxygen, nutrients, and waste products.

- The body takes chemical energy from food and uses it to produce ATP and fuel cellular activities. ATP is stored in the body's cells as the basic form of energy.

- During exercise, the body supplies ATP and fuels cellular activities by combining three energy systems: *immediate,* for short periods of energy; *nonoxidative (anaerobic),* for intense activity; and *oxidative (aerobic),* for prolonged activity. Which energy system predominates depends on the duration and intensity of the activity.

- Cardiorespiratory endurance exercise improves cardiorespiratory functioning and cellular metabolism; it reduces the risk of chronic disease such as heart disease, cancer, type 2 diabetes, obesity, and osteoporosis; and it improves immune function and psychological and emotional well-being.

- Cardiorespiratory fitness is measured by seeing how well the cardiorespiratory system transports and uses oxygen. The upper limit of this measure is called maximal oxygen consumption, or $\dot{V}O_{2max}$.

- $\dot{V}O_{2max}$ can be measured precisely in a laboratory, or it can be estimated reasonably well through less expensive assessment tests.

What kind of clothing should I wear during exercise?
Exercise clothing should be comfortable, let you move freely, and allow your body to cool itself. Avoid clothing that constricts normal blood flow or is made from nylon or rubberized fabrics that prevent evaporation of perspiration. Cotton is an excellent material for facilitating the evaporation of sweat. If you sweat heavily when you exercise and find that too much moisture accumulates in cotton clothing, try fabrics containing synthetic materials such as polypropylene that wick moisture away from the skin. Socks made with moisture-wicking compounds may be particularly helpful for people whose feet sweat heavily.

Do I need a special diet for my endurance exercise program?
No. For most people, a nutritionally balanced diet contains all the energy and nutrients needed to sustain an exercise program. Don't waste your money on unnecessary vitamins, minerals, and protein supplements, (Chapter 8 has information about putting together a healthy diet.)

Should I use a heart rate monitor to keep track of exercise intensity?   Electronic heart rate monitors, which are relatively accurate and inexpensive, can help you stay within your target heart rate range. Heart rate monitors function by detecting the pulse in your finger or hand or by measuring the electrical activity of your heart through a belt you wear around your chest. In general, the belt models are most accurate; some of the more expensive belt models can download heart rate information to your home computer.

If very close tracking of heart rate is important in your program, you may find a monitor to be helpful. However, other measures of exercise intensity also work well, including pulse taking and RPE. An even simpler, although less accurate, method is the talk test: If you can comfortably carry on a conversation, you are probably exercising at a low to moderate intensity; if you can't finish a sentence without taking a breath, you are probably exercising at a moderate to high intensity (about 70% of maximum heart rate for most people).

Will interval training develop cardiorespiratory endurance (CRE)?   Interval training refers to short bouts of high-intensity exercise alternated with short periods of rest or light activity. An example of a workout based on interval training is a 400-meter run followed by a 200-meter walk, with the cycle repeated two to ten times. You will develop CRE more quickly doing interval training. However, intervals are also more uncomfortable and increase your risk of injury and overtraining. Don't perform interval training more than 2–3 days per week.

How can I safely increase exercise intensity to build fitness?
For both athletes and nonathletes, it is extremely important to increase intensity very gradually and to rest between exercise sessions. If you train too hard and/or don't rest enough, you are more likely to be injured—and be discouraged from continuing with your fitness program. For endurance training, overload techniques such as interval training and wind sprints can help you build fitness quickly but also pose a greater risk of injury or overtraining. Start off with a few high intensity

bouts of exercise and build up gradually. Don't practice interval training or wind sprints more than 2–3 days per week unless you have a high fitness level.

Increase intensity or duration by about 1–3% in a single workout; rest the following day and then do your typical workout. Repeat the more difficult workout after another day of rest. Adjust your progress according to how you feel. You can't increase fitness in a few days. Be patient—with gradual increases in intensity and plenty of rest between workouts, you will be able to move to a higher level of fitness without injury.

If I plan to include both cardiorespiratory endurance training and strength training in a single workout, which should I do first?   It depends on your goals. If the primary goal of your fitness program is conditioning your cardiorespiratory system, then do your endurance workout first. If your fitness program is focused on large gains in strength and you plan to lift relatively heavy weights, then do your strength training workout first. You are likely to make the most rapid gains in fitness in whichever activity you engage in first, when you are fresh.

Is it all right to participate in cardiorespiratory endurance exercise while menstruating?   Yes. There is no evidence that exercise during menstruation is unhealthy or that it has negative effects on performance. If you have headaches, backaches, and abdominal pain during menstruation, you may not feel like exercising; for some women, exercise helps relieve these symptoms. Listen to your body, and exercise at whatever intensity is comfortable for you.

What causes muscle cramps and what can I do about them?
Muscle cramps are caused by local muscle fatigue that triggers the nervous system to overstimulate the muscles. Until recently, muscle cramps were thought to be caused by dehydration or salt depletion in the muscles, but scientists have found little evidence for this. Muscle cramps can occur during or after exercise performed either in heat or in cold. You can prevent cramps by improving your fitness and making sure you consume enough fluid and electrolytes during exercise and in your diet (low intake of fluid and electrolytes contribute to fatigue). When cramps do occur, gently stretch the cramping muscle for 15–30 seconds. Do not overstretch the cramping muscle because this can lead to serious injury.

Will high altitude affect my ability to exercise?   At high altitudes (above 1500 meters or about 4900 feet) there is less oxygen available in the air than at lower altitudes. High altitude doesn't affect anaerobic exercise, such as stretching and weight lifting, but it does affect aerobic activities—that is, any type of cardiovascular endurance exercise. The reason is that the heart and lungs have to work harder, even when the body is at rest, to deliver enough oxygen to body cells. The increased cardiovascular strain of exercise reduces endurance. To play it safe when at high altitudes, avoid heavy exercise—at least for the first few days—and drink plenty of water. And don't expect to reach your normal lower altitude exercise capacity.

- To have a successful exercise program, set realistic goals; choose suitable activities; begin slowly; always warm up and cool down; and as fitness improves, exercise more often, longer, and/or harder.

- Intensity of training can be measured through target heart rate zone and ratings of perceived exertion.

- With careful attention to fluid intake, clothing, duration of exercise, and exercise intensity, endurance training can be safe in hot and cold weather conditions.

- Serious injuries require medical attention. Application of the R-I-C-E principle (rest, ice, compression, elevation) is appropriate for treating many types of muscle or joint injuries.

FOR FURTHER EXPLORATION

VW *Fit and Well* Online Learning Center (www.mhhe.com/fahey)

Use the learning objectives, study guide questions, and glossary flashcards to review key terms and concepts and prepare for exams. You can extend your knowledge of cardiorespiratory endurance and gain experience in using the Internet as a resource by completing the activities and checking out the Web links for the topics in Chapter 3 marked with the World Wide Web icon. For this chapter, Internet activities explore the benefits of endurance exercise, target heart rate zone, and activities to improve cardiorespiratory fitness; there are Web links for the Critical Consumer box on exercise equipment and the chapter as a whole.

Daily Fitness and Nutrition Journal

Complete the cardiorespiratory endurance portion of the program plan by setting goals and selecting activities that will build endurance. Also calculate and record your current resting heart rate and your target heart rate zone or RPE value.

HealthQuest

Learn more about the functioning of the cardiovascular system by completing the tutorial on the HealthQuest CD-ROM; it is found in the Cardiovascular Health module (select the tutorial in the CAD Risk Activity on the Wellness Activities menu). For further help in choosing activities for your cardiorespiratory endurance program, complete the Exercise Interest Inventory in the Fitness module (select Fitness Planner from the Wellness Activities menu). You'll receive activity suggestions based on your personal exercise preferences.

Books

American College of Sports Medicine. 2003. *ACSM Fitness Book.* 3d ed. Champaign, Ill.: Human Kinetics. *Includes fitness assessment tests and advice on creating a complete fitness program.*

Barough, N. 2004. *Walking for Fitness.* New York: DK. *Provides advice on putting together a walking program that matches your fitness goals.*

Beim, G., and R. Winter. 2003. *The Female Athlete's Body Book: How to Prevent and Treat Sports Injuries in Women and Girls.* New York: McGraw-Hill/Contemporary. *Provides detailed information on the prevention and treatment of athletic injuries in women and girls.*

Bingham, J. 2002. *No Need for Speed: A Beginner's Guide to the Joy of Running.* Emmaus, Pa.: Rodale Press. *A practical, nonintimidating, and inspirational guide for the beginning runner.*

Brennfleck, J. 2002. *Sports Injuries Sourcebook.* Detroit, Mich.: Omnigraphics. *Provides information about the prevention and care of exercise injuries, with specific sections on different age groups and popular activities.*

Heyward, V. 2002. *Advanced Fitness Assessment and Exercise Prescription.* 4th ed. Champaign, Ill.: Human Kinetics. *Provides information and ratings for a large number of fitness tests as well as guidelines for putting together a successful program.*

Juba, K. 2002. *Swimming for Fitness.* New York: Lyons Press. *Provides step-by-step instructions for setting up a swimming fitness program, including advice on technique and avoiding injury and overtraining.*

Ledeboer, S. 2001. *A Basic Guide to Cycling.* Torrance, Calif.: Griffin Pub. *Includes information on buying and caring for a bicycle as well as increasing fitness.*

National Institute on Aging. 2003. *Fitness Over Fifty: An Exercise Guide from the National Institute on Aging.* Long Island City, N.Y.: Hatherleigh Press. *Includes information on a safe and effective fitness program.*

Nieman, D. C. 2003. *Exercise Testing and Prescription: A Health-Related Approach,* 5th ed. New York: McGraw-Hill. *A comprehensive discussion of the effect of exercise and exercise testing and prescription.*

Noakes, T. 2003. *Lore of Running.* 4th ed. Champaign, Ill.: Human Kinetics. *Provides detailed information on physiology, training, racing, and injury prevention.*

Pryor, E., and M. Kraines. 2000. *Keep Moving! Fitness through Aerobics and Step,* 4th ed. Mountain View, Calif.: Mayfield. *The fitness principles and techniques every aerobic dancer should know.*

VW Organizations and Web Sites

American Academy of Orthopaedic Surgeons. Provides fact sheets on many fitness and sports topics, including how to begin a program, how to choose equipment, and how to prevent and treat many types of injuries.
http://orthinfo.aaos.org

American Heart Association. Provides information on cardiovascular health and disease, including the role of exercise in maintaining heart health and exercise tips for people of all ages.
800-AHA-USA1
http://www.americanheart.org
http://www.justmove.org

Dr. Pribut's Running Injuries Page. Provides information about running and many types of running injuries.
http://www.drpribut.com/sports/spsport.html

Federal Trade Commission: Consumer Protection—Diet, Health, and Fitness. Provides several brochures with consumer advice about purchasing exercise equipment.
http://www.ftc.gov/bcp/menu-health.htm

Franklin Institute Science Museum/The Heart: An Online Exploration. An online museum exhibit with information on the structure and function of the heart, blood vessels, and respiratory system.
http://www.fi.edu/biosci/heart.html

Georgia State University: Exercise and Physical Fitness Page. Provides information about the benefits of exercise and how to get started on a fitness program.
http://www.gsu.edu/~wwwfit

MedlinePlus: Exercise and Physical Fitness. Provides links to news and reliable information about fitness from government agencies and professional associations.

http://www.nlm.nih.gov/medlineplus/
exercisephysicalfitness.html

Physician and Sportsmedicine. Provides many articles with easy-to-understand advice about exercise injuries.

http://www.physsportsmed.com

Runner's World Online. Contains a wide variety of information about running, including tips for beginning runners, advice about training, and a shoe buyer's guide.

http://www.runnersworld.com

University of Florida: Keeping Fit. Provides useful information about fitness in a question-and-answer format; an extensive set of links is also provided.

http://www.hhp.ufl.edu/keepingfit
http://www.hhp.ufl.edu/personalfitness.htm

Women's Sports Foundation. Provides information and links about training and about many specific sports activities.

http://www.womenssportsfoundation.org/cgi-bin/iowa/

Yahoo/Recreation. Contains links to many sites with practical advice on many sports and activities.

http://dir.yahoo.com/recreation/sports

See also the listings in Chapters 2 and 11.

SELECTED BIBLIOGRAPHY

Achten, J., and A. E. Jeukendrup. 2003. Heart rate monitoring: Applications and limitations. *Sports Medicine* 33:517–538.

American Academy of Orthopaedic Surgeons. 2001. *Selecting Home Exercise Equipment* (http://orthoinfo.aaos.org/fact/thr_report.cfm; retrieved October 17, 2001).

American College of Sports Medicine. 1998. The recommended quantity and quality of exercise for developing and maintaining cardiorespiratory and muscular fitness, flexibility in healthy adults. ACSM position paper. *Medicine and Science in Sports and Exercise* 30(6): 975–991.

American College of Sports Medicine. 2001. *ACSM's Resource Manual for Guidelines for Exercise Testing and Prescription*, 4th ed. Philadelphia: Williams and Wilkins.

Brooks, G. A., et al. 2005. *Exercise Physiology: Human Bioenergetics and Its Applications*, 4th ed. New York: McGraw-Hill.

Carroll, J. F., and C. K. Kyser. 2002. Exercise training in obesity lowers blood pressure independent of weight change. *Medicine and Science in Sports and Exercise* 34(4): 596–601.

Cheuvront, S. N., I. R. Carter, and M. N. Sawka. 2003. Fluid balance and endurance exercise performance. *Current Sports Medicine Reports* 2:202–208.

Colcombe, S. J., et al. 2004. Cardiovascular fitness, cortical plasticity, and aging. *Proceedings of the National Academy of Sciences* 101(9): 3316–3321.

Coris, E. E., A. M. Ramirez, and D. J. Van Durme. 2004. Heat illness in athletes: A dangerous combination of heat, humidity, and exercise. *Sports Medicine* 34(1): 9–16.

Friedenreich, C. M., et al. 2004. Case-control study of lifetime total physical activity and prostate cancer risk. *American Journal of Epidemiology* 159(8): 740–749.

Garcin, M., M. Wolff, and T. Bejma. 2003. Reliability of rating scales of perceived exertion and heart rate during progressive and maximal constant load exercises till exhaustion in physical education students. *International Journal of Sports Medicine* 24:285–290.

Gleeson, M., D. C. Nieman, and B. K. Pedersen. 2004. Exercise, nutrition, and immune function. *Journal of Sports Science* 22(1): 115–125.

Goodwin, R. D. 2003. Association between physical activity and mental disorders among adults in the United States. *Preventive Medicine* 36(6): 698–703.

Humpel, N., N. Owen, and E. Leslie. 2002. Environmental factors associated with adults' participation in physical activity. A review. *American Journal of Preventive Medicine* 22(3): 188–199.

John, E. M., P. L. Horn-Ross, and J. Koo. 2004. Lifetime physical activity and breast cancer risk in a multiethnic population. *Cancer Epidemiology, Biomarkers, and Prevention* 12(11 Pt 1): 1143–1152.

Ketelhut, R. G., I. W. Franz, and J. Scholze. 2004. Regular exercise as an effective approach in antihypertensive therapy. *Medicine and Science in Sports and Exercise* 36(1): 4–8.

Keteyian, S. J., and I. Kolokouri. 2001. Guidelines for selecting home exercise equipment. *ACSM's Fit Society Page*, January/February.

Kriska, A. M., et al. 2003. Physical activity, obesity, and the incidence of Type 2 diabetes in a high-risk population. *American Journal of Epidemiology* 158(7): 669–675.

Lakka, T. A., et al. 2003. Sedentary lifestyle, poor cardiorespiratory fitness, and the metabolic syndrome. *Medicine and Science in Sports and Exercise* 35(8): 1279–1286.

Lee, C. D., A. R. Folsom, and S. N. Blair. 2003. Physical activity and stroke risk: A meta-analysis. *Stroke* 34(10): 2475–2481.

Mora, S., et al. 2003. Ability of exercise testing to predict cardiovascular and all-cause death in asymptomatic women. *Journal of the American Medical Association* 290(12): 1600–1607.

National Weather Service. 2003. *Extreme Heat: Heat Index* (http://www.crh.noaa.gov/arx/heatindex.html; retrieved October 31, 2003).

Noakes, T. D. 2003. Over consumption of fluids by athletes. *British Medical Journal* 327:113–114.

Nurmi-Lawton, J. A., et al. 2004. Evidence of sustained skeletal benefits from impact-loading exercise in young females. *Journal of Bone and Mineral Research* 19(2): 314–322.

Oh, R. C., and J. S. Henning. 2003. Exertional heatstroke in an infantry soldier taking ephedra-containing dietary supplements. *Military Medicine* 168:429–430.

PBS Healthweek. 2001. *Home Exercise Equipment* (http://www.pbs.org/healthweek/featurep4_339.htm; retrieved October 18, 2001).

Pope, S. K., V. M. Shue, and C. Beck. 2003. Will a healthy lifestyle help prevent Alzheimer's disease? *Annual Review of Public Health* 24:111–132.

Slattery, M. L. 2004. Physical activity and colorectal cancer. *Sports Medicine* 34(4): 239–252.

Thompson, P. D., et al. 2003. Exercise and physical activity in the prevention and treatment of atherosclerotic cardiovascular disease. *Arteriosclerosis, Thrombosis, and Vascular Biology* 23:E42–49.

Thompson, P. D., et al. 2001. The acute versus the chronic response to exercise. *Medicine and Science in Sports and Exercise* 33(6 Suppl): S438–S445.

Uusi-Rasi, K., et al. 2002. Associations of calcium intake and physical activity with bone density and size in premenopausal and postmenopausal women. *Journal of Bone Mineral Research* 17(3): 544–552.

Verghese, J., et al. 2003. Leisure activities and the risk of dementia in the elderly. *New England Journal of Medicine* 348(25): 2508–2516.

Whelton, S. P., et al. 2002. Effect of aerobic exercise on blood pressure: A meta-analysis of randomized, controlled trials. *Annals of Internal Medicine* 136(7): 493–503.

Williams, P. T. 2001. Health effects resulting from exercise versus those from body fat loss. *Medicine and Science in Sports and Exercise* 33(6 Suppl): S611–S621.

LAB 3.1 *Assessing Your Current Level of Cardiorespiratory Endurance* W↓w

Before taking any of the cardiorespiratory endurance assessment tests, refer to the fitness prerequisites and cautions given in Table 3.2. Choose one of the following three tests presented in this lab:

- 1-mile walk test
- 3-minute step test
- 1.5-mile run-walk test

For best results, don't exercise strenuously or consume caffeine the day of the test, and don't smoke or eat a heavy meal within about 3 hours of the test.

The 1-Mile Walk Test

Equipment

1. A track or course that provides a measurement of 1 mile
2. A stopwatch, clock, or watch with a second hand
3. A weight scale

Preparation

Measure your body weight (in pounds) before taking the test.

Body weight: _____ lb

Instructions

1. Warm up before taking the test. Do some walking, easy jogging, or calisthenics and some stretching exercises.
2. Cover the 1-mile course as quickly as possible. Walk at a pace that is brisk but comfortable. You must raise your heart rate above 120 beats per minute (bpm).
3. As soon as you complete the distance, note your time and take your pulse for 10 seconds.

   Walking time: _____ min _____ sec

   10-second pulse count: _____ beats

4. Cool down after the test by walking slowly for several minutes.

Determining Maximal Oxygen Consumption

1. Convert your 10-second pulse count into a value for exercise heart rate by multiplying it by 6.

   Exercise heart rate: _____ × 6 = _____ bpm

  ‎ ‎ ‎ ‎ ‎ ‎ ‎ ‎ ‎ ‎ ‎ ‎ ‎ 10-sec pulse count

2. Convert your walking time from minutes and seconds to a decimal figure. For example, a time of 14 minutes and 45 seconds would be 14 + (45/60), or 14.75 minutes.

   Walking time: _____ min + (_____ sec ÷ 60 sec/min) = _____ min

3. Insert values for your age, gender, weight, walking time, and exercise heart rate in the following equation, where

   W = your weight (in pounds)

   A = your age (in years)

   G = your gender (male = 1; female = 0)

   T = your time to complete the 1-mile course (in minutes)

   H = your exercise heart rate (in beats per minute)

   $\dot{V}O_{2max} = 132.853 - (0.0769 \times W) - (0.3877 \times A) + (6.315 \times G) - (3.2649 \times T) - (0.1565 \times H)$

For example, a 20-year-old, 190-pound male with a time of 14.75 minutes and an exercise heart rate of 152 bpm would calculate maximal oxygen consumption as follows:

$$\dot{V}O_{2max} = 132.853 - (0.0769 \times 190) - (0.3877 \times 20) + (6.315 \times 1) - (3.2649 \times 14.75) - (0.1565 \times 152)$$
$$= 45 \ ml/kg/min$$

$$\dot{V}O_{2max} = 132.853 - (0.0769 \times \underline{\hspace{2cm}}) - (0.3877 \times \underline{\hspace{2cm}}) + (6.315 \times \underline{\hspace{2cm}})$$
$$\text{weight (lb)} \qquad\qquad \text{age (years)} \qquad\qquad \text{gender}$$

$$- (3.2649 \times \underline{\hspace{2cm}}) - (0.1565 \times \underline{\hspace{2cm}}) = \underline{\hspace{1.5cm}} ml/kg/min$$
$$\text{walking time (min)} \qquad\qquad \text{exercise heart rate (bpm)}$$

4. Copy this value for $\dot{V}O_{2max}$ into the appropriate place in the chart on the final page of this lab.

The 3-Minute Step Test

Equipment

1. A step, bench, or bleacher step that is 16.25 inches from ground level
2. A stopwatch, clock, or watch with a second hand
3. A metronome

Preparation

Practice stepping up onto and down from the step before you begin the test. Each step has four beats: up-up-down-down. Males should perform the test with the metronome set for a rate of 96 beats per minute, or 24 steps per minute. Females should set the metronome at 88 beats per minute, or 22 steps per minute.

Instructions

1. Warm up before taking the test. Do some walking, easy jogging, and stretching exercises.
2. Set the metronome at the proper rate. Your instructor or a partner can call out starting and stopping times; otherwise, have a clock or watch within easy viewing during the test.
3. Begin the test and continue to step at the correct pace for 3 minutes.
4. Stop after 3 minutes. Remain standing and count your pulse for the 15-second period from 5 to 20 seconds into recovery.
   15-second pulse count: _____ beats
5. Cool down after the test by walking slowly for several minutes.

Determining Maximal Oxygen Consumption

1. Convert your 15-second pulse count to a value for recovery heart rate by multiplying by 4.
   Recovery heart rate: $\underline{\hspace{3cm}} \times 4 = \underline{\hspace{2cm}}$ bpm
   $\qquad\qquad\quad$ 15-sec pulse count

2. Insert your recovery heart rate in the equation below, where

   H = recovery heart rate (in beats per minute)
   Males: $\dot{V}O_{2max} = 111.33 - (0.42 \times H)$
   Females: $\dot{V}O_{2max} = 65.81 - (0.1847 \times H)$

   For example, a man with a recovery heart rate of 162 bpm would calculate maximal oxygen consumption as follows:

   $$\dot{V}O_{2max} = 111.33 - (0.42 \times 162) = 43 \ ml/kg/min$$

   Males: $\dot{V}O_{2max} = 111.33 - (0.42 \times \underline{\hspace{3cm}}) = \underline{\hspace{2cm}}$ ml/kg/min
   $\qquad\qquad\qquad\qquad\qquad\qquad$ recovery heart rate (bpm)

   Females: $\dot{V}O_{2max} = 65.81 - (0.1847 \times \underline{\hspace{3cm}}) = \underline{\hspace{2cm}}$ ml/kg/min
   $\qquad\qquad\qquad\qquad\qquad\qquad$ recovery heart rate (bpm)

3. Copy this value for $\dot{V}O_{2max}$ into the appropriate place in the chart on the final page of this lab.

The 1.5-Mile Run-Walk Test

Equipment

1. A running track or course that is flat and provides exact measurements of up to 1.5 miles
2. A stopwatch, clock, or watch with a second hand

Preparation

You may want to practice pacing yourself prior to taking the test to avoid going too fast at the start and becoming prematurely fatigued. Allow yourself a day or two to recover from your practice run before taking the test.

Instructions

1. Warm up before taking the test. Do some walking, easy jogging, and stretching exercises.
2. Try to cover the distance as fast as possible without overexerting yourself. If possible, monitor your own time, or have someone call out your time at various intervals of the test to determine whether your pace is correct.
3. Record the amount of time, in minutes and seconds, it takes you to complete the 1.5-mile distance.

   Running-walking time: _____ min _____ sec
4. Cool down after the test by walking or jogging slowly for about 5 minutes.

Determining Maximal Oxygen Consumption

1. Convert your running time from minutes and seconds to a decimal figure. For example, a time of 14 minutes and 25 seconds would be $14 + (25/60)$, or 14.4 minutes.

   Running-walking time: _____ min + (_____ sec ÷ 60 sec/min) = _____ min
2. Insert your running time in the equation below, where

   T = running time (in minutes)
   $\dot{V}O_{2max} = (483 \div T) + 3.5$

   For example, a person who completes 1.5 miles in 14.4 minutes would calculate maximal oxygen consumption as follows:
   $\dot{V}O_{2max} = (483 \div 14.4) + 3.5 = 37$ ml/kg/min

   $\dot{V}O_{2max} = (483 \div \underset{\text{run-walk time (min)}}{\underline{\hspace{2cm}}}) + 3.5 = $ _____ **ml/kg/min**
3. Copy this value for $\dot{V}O_{2max}$ into the appropriate place in the chart on the final page of this lab.

Rating Your Cardiovascular Fitness

Record your $\dot{V}O_{2max}$ score(s) and the corresponding fitness rating from the table below.

Women	Very Poor	Poor	Fair	Good	Excellent	Superior
Age: 18–29	Below 31.6	31.6–35.4	35.5–39.4	39.5–43.9	44.0–50.1	Above 50.1
30–39	Below 29.9	29.9–33.7	33.8–36.7	36.8–40.9	41.0–46.8	Above 46.8
40–49	Below 28.0	28.0–31.5	31.6–35.0	35.1–38.8	38.9–45.1	Above 45.1
50–59	Below 25.5	25.5–28.6	28.7–31.3	31.4–35.1	35.2–39.8	Above 39.8
60–69	Below 23.7	23.7–26.5	26.6–29.0	29.1–32.2	32.3–36.8	Above 36.8
Men						
Age: 18–29	Below 38.1	38.1–42.1	42.2–45.6	45.7–51.0	51.1–56.1	Above 56.1
30–39	Below 36.7	36.7–40.9	41.0–44.3	44.4–48.8	48.9–54.2	Above 54.2
40–49	Below 34.6	34.6–38.3	38.4–42.3	42.4–46.7	46.8–52.8	Above 52.8
50–59	Below 31.1	31.1–35.1	35.2–38.2	38.3–43.2	43.3–49.6	Above 49.6
60–69	Below 27.4	27.4–31.3	31.4–34.9	35.0–39.4	39.5–46.0	Above 46.0

SOURCE: Ratings based on norms from the Cooper Institute for Aerobics Research, Dallas, Texas, *The Physical Fitness Specialist Manual,* Revised 2002. Used with permission.

	$\dot{V}O_{2max}$	Cardiovascular Fitness Rating
1-mile walk test		
3-minute step test		
1.5-mile run-walk test		

Using Your Results

How did you score? Are you surprised by your rating for cardiovascular fitness? Are you satisfied with your current rating?

If you're not satisfied, set a realistic goal for improvement:_____

Are you satisfied with your current level of cardiovascular fitness as evidenced in your daily life—your ability to walk, run, bicycle, climb stairs, do yardwork, engage in recreational activities?

If you're not satisfied, set some realistic goals for improvement, such as completing a 5K run or 25-mile bike ride:

What should you do next? Enter the results of this lab in the Preprogram Assessment column in Appendix D. If you've set goals for improvement, begin planning your cardiorespiratory endurance exercise program by completing the plan in Lab 3.2. After several weeks of your program, complete this lab again, and enter the results in the Postprogram Assessment column of Appendix D. How do the results compare? (Remember, it's best to compare $\dot{V}O_{2max}$ scores for the same test.)

SOURCES: Kline, G. M., et al. 1987. Estimation of $\dot{V}O_{2max}$ from a one-mile track walk, gender, age, and body weight. *Medicine and Science in Sports and Exercise* 19(3): 253–259. McArdle, W. D., F. I. Katch, and V. L. Katch. 1991. *Exercise Physiology: Energy, Nutrition, and Human Performance.* Philadelphia: Lea and Febiger, pp. 225–226. Brooks, G. A., and T. D. Fahey. 1987. *Fundamentals of Human Performance.* New York: Macmillan.

LABORATORY ACTIVITIES

LAB 3.2 *Developing an Exercise Program for Cardiorespiratory Endurance* **WW**

1. **Goals.** List goals for your cardiorespiratory endurance exercise program. Your goals can be specific or general, short or long term. In the first section, include specific, measurable goals that you can use to track the progress of your fitness program. These goals might be things like raising your cardiorespiratory fitness rating from fair to good or swimming laps for 30 minutes without resting. In the second section, include long-term and more qualitative goals, such as improving self-confidence and reducing your risk for chronic disease.

Specific Goals: Current Status	Final Goal
_____	_____
_____	_____
_____	_____

Other goals: _____

_____

2. **Type of Activities.** Choose one or more endurance activities for your program. These can include any activity that uses large-muscle groups, can be maintained continuously, and is rhythmic and aerobic in nature. Examples include walking, jogging, cycling, group exercise such as aerobic dance, rowing, rope skipping, stair climbing, cross-country skiing, swimming, skating, and endurance game activities such as soccer and tennis. Choose activities that are both convenient and enjoyable. Fill in the activity names on the program plan.

3. **Frequency.** On the program plan on the following page, fill in how often you plan to participate in each activity; the ACSM recommends participating in cardiorespiratory endurance exercise 3–5 days per week.

Program Plan

Type of Activity	Frequency (check ✓) M | T | W | Th | F | Sa | Su	Intensity (bpm or RPE)	Time (min)

4. **Intensity.** Determine your exercise intensity using one of the following methods, and enter it on the program plan on the following page. You should begin your program at a lower intensity and slowly increase intensity as your fitness improves, so select a range of intensities for your program.

   a. Target heart rate zone: Calculate target heart rate zone in beats per minute and then calculate the corresponding 10-second exercise count by dividing the total count by 6. For example, the 10-second exercise counts corresponding to a target heart rate zone of 122–180 bpm would be 20–30 beats.

   Maximum heart rate: 220 − _____ = _____ bpm
    age (years)

   Maximum Heart Rate Method

   65% training intensity = _____ bpm × 0.65 = _____ bpm
    maximum heart rate

   90% training intensity = _____ bpm × 0.90 = _____ bpm
    maximum heart rate

   Target heart rate zone = _____ to _____ bpm   10-second count = _____ to _____

Heart Rate Reserve Method

Resting heart rate: _____ bpm (taken after 10 minutes of complete rest)

Heart rate reserve = _____ bpm − _____ bpm = _____ bpm
                     maximum heart rate   resting heart rate

50% training intensity = (_____ bpm × 0.50) + _____ bpm = _____ bpm
                          heart rate reserve   resting heart rate

85% training intensity = (_____ bpm × 0.85) + _____ bpm = _____ bpm
                          heart rate reserve   resting heart rate

Target heart rate zone = _____ to _____ bpm   **10-second count = _____ to _____**

b. Ratings of perceived exertion (RPE): If you prefer, determine an RPE value that corresponds to your target heart rate range (see p. 69 and Figure 3.5).

5. *Time (Duration).* A total time of 20–60 minutes is recommended; your duration of exercise will vary with intensity. For developing cardiorespiratory endurance, higher-intensity activities can be performed for a shorter duration; lower intensities require a longer duration. Enter a duration (or a range of duration) on the program plan.

6. *Monitoring your program.* Complete a log like the one below to monitor your program and track your progress. Note the date on top, and fill in the intensity and time (duration) for each workout. If you prefer, you can also track other variables such as distance. For example, if your cardiorespiratory endurance program includes walking and swimming, you may want to track miles walked and yards swum in addition to the duration of each exercise session. For more extensive sets of logs, refer to the Daily Fitness and Nutrition Journal that accompanies your text.

Activity/Date														
1	Intensity													
	Time													
	Distance													
2	Intensity													
	Time													
	Distance													
3	Intensity													
	Time													
	Distance													
4	Intensity													
	Time													
	Distance													

7. *Making progress.* Follow the guidelines in the chapter and Table 3.4 to slowly increase the amount of overload in your program. Continue keeping a log, and periodically evaluate your progress.

Progress Check-Up: Week _____ of program

Goals: Original Status   Current Status

_____   _____

_____   _____

_____   _____

List each activity in your program and describe how satisfied you are with the activity and with your overall progress. List any problems you've encountered or any unexpected costs or benefits of your fitness program so far.

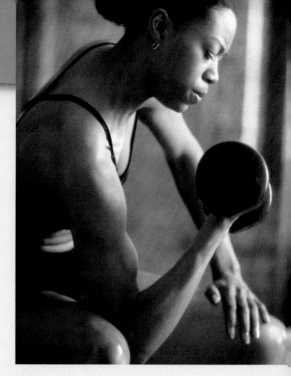

4

Muscular Strength and Endurance

LOOKING AHEAD

After reading this chapter, you should be able to

- Describe the basic physiology of muscles and how strength training affects muscles
- Define muscular strength and endurance and describe how they relate to wellness
- Explain how muscular strength and endurance can be assessed
- Apply the FITT principle to create a safe and successful strength training program
- Describe the effects of supplements and drugs that are marketed to active people and athletes
- Explain how to safely perform common strength training exercises using free weights and weight machines

TEST YOUR KNOWLEDGE

1. For women, weight training typically results in which of the following?
   a. bulky muscles
   b. significant increases in body weight
   c. improved body image

2. To maximize strength gains, it is a good idea to hold your breath as you lift a weight.
   True or false?

3. Regular strength training is associated with which of the following benefits?
   a. denser bones
   b. reduced risk of heart disease
   c. improved body composition
   d. higher grades

ANSWERS

1. C. Because the vast majority of women have low levels of testosterone, they do not develop large muscles or gain significant amounts of weight in response to a moderate weight training program. Men have higher levels of testosterone, so they can build large muscles more easily.

2. FALSE. Holding one's breath while lifting weights, called the Valsalva maneuver, can significantly (and possibly dangerously) elevate blood pressure; it also reduces blood flow to the heart and may cause faintness. You should breathe smoothly and normally while weight training.

3. ALL FOUR. Regular strength training has many benefits for lifetime wellness.

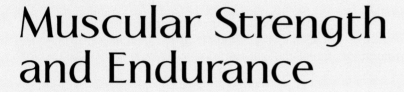 **Fit and Well Online Learning Center**   www.mhhe.com/fahey

Visit the *Fit and Well* Online Learning Center for study aids, online labs, additional information about muscular strength and endurance, links, Internet activities that explore the development of a strength training program, consumer resources, and much more.

Exercise experts have long emphasized the importance of cardiovascular fitness. Other physical fitness factors, such as muscle strength and flexibility, were mentioned almost as an afterthought. As more was learned about how the body responds to exercise, however, it became obvious that these other factors are vital to health, wellness, and overall quality of life. Muscles make up more than 40% of your body mass. You depend on them for movement, and, because of their mass, they are the site of a large portion of the energy reactions (metabolism) that take place in your body. Strong, well-developed muscles help you perform daily activities with greater ease, protect you from injury, and enhance your well-being in other ways.

As described in Chapter 2, **muscular strength** is the ability to generate force during a maximal effort; **muscular endurance** is the ability to resist fatigue while holding or repeating a muscular contraction. This chapter explains the benefits of strength training (also called resistance training) and describes methods of assessing muscular strength and endurance. It then explains the basics of weight training and provides guidelines for setting up your own strength training program.

BASIC MUSCLE PHYSIOLOGY AND THE EFFECTS OF STRENGTH TRAINING

Muscles move the body and enable it to exert force because they move the skeleton. When a muscle contracts (shortens), it moves a bone by pulling on the tendon that attaches the muscle to the bone. Muscles consist of individual muscle cells, or **muscle fibers,** connected in bundles (Figure 4.1). A single muscle is made up of many bundles of muscle fibers and is covered by layers of connective tissue that hold the fibers together. Muscle fibers, in turn, are made up of smaller units called **myofibrils.** When your muscles are given the signal to contract, protein filaments (*actin* and *myosin*) within the myofibrils slide across one another, causing the muscle fiber to shorten.

Strength training causes the size of individual muscle fibers to increase by increasing the number of myofibrils. Larger muscle fibers mean a larger and stronger muscle. The development of large muscle fibers is called **hypertrophy;** inactivity causes **atrophy,** the reversal of this process. In some species, muscles can increase in size through a separate process called **hyperplasia,** which involves an increase in the number of muscle fibers rather than the size of muscle fibers. In humans, hyperplasia is not thought to play a significant role in determining muscle size.

Muscle fibers are classified as fast-twitch or slow-twitch fibers according to their strength, speed of contraction, and energy source. **Slow-twitch fibers** are relatively fatigue resistant, but they don't contract as rapidly or strongly as fast-twitch fibers. The principal energy system that fuels slow-twitch fibers is aerobic (oxidative). **Fast-twitch fibers** contract more rapidly and forcefully than slow-twitch fibers but fatigue more quickly. Although oxygen is important in the energy system that fuels fast-twitch fibers, they rely more on anaerobic (nonoxidative) metabolism than do slow-twitch fibers (see Chapter 3 for a discussion of energy systems).

Most muscles contain a mixture of slow-twitch and fast-twitch fibers. The proportion of the types of fibers varies significantly among different muscles and different individuals, and that proportion is largely fixed at birth. The type of fiber that acts depends on the type of work required. Endurance activities like jogging tend to use slow-twitch fibers, whereas strength and **power** activities like sprinting use fast-twitch fibers. Strength training can

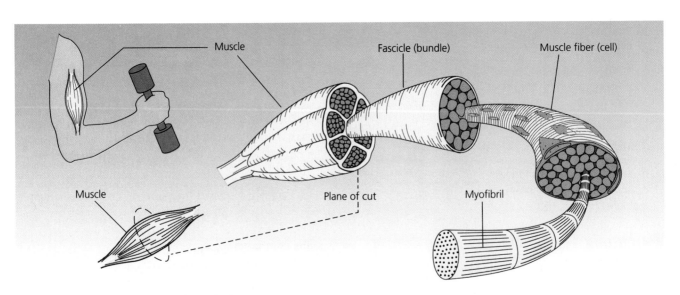

Figure 4.1 Components of skeletal muscle tissue.

Table 4.1   *Physiological Changes and Benefits from Strength Training*

Change	Benefits
Increased muscle mass*	Increased muscular strength Improved body composition Higher rate of metabolism Toned, healthy-looking muscles
Increased utilization of motor units during muscle contractions	Increased muscular strength and power
Improved coordination of motor units	Increased muscular strength and power
Increased strength of tendons, ligaments, and bones	Lower risk of injury to these tissues
Increased storage of fuel in muscles	Increased resistance to muscle fatigue
Increased size of fast-twitch muscle fibers (from a high-resistance program)	Increased muscular strength and power
Increased size of slow-twitch muscle fibers (from a high-repetition program)	Increased muscular endurance
Increased blood supply to muscles (from a high-repetition program)	Increased delivery of oxygen and nutrients Increased elimination of wastes
Biochemical improvements (for example, increased sensitivity to insulin)	Enhanced metabolic health
Improved blood fat levels	Reduced risk of heart disease

*Due to genetic and hormonal differences, men will build more muscle mass than women, but both genders make about the same percent gains in strength through a good program.

increase the size and strength of both fast-twitch and slow-twitch fibers, although fast-twitch fibers are preferentially increased.

To exert force, the body recruits one or more motor units to contract. A **motor unit** is made up of a nerve connected to a number of muscle fibers. The number of muscle fibers in a motor unit varies from two to hundreds. When a motor nerve calls on its fibers to contract, all fibers contract to their full capacity. The number of motor units recruited depends on the amount of strength required: When a person picks up a small weight, he or she uses fewer motor units than when picking up a large weight. Strength training improves the body's ability to recruit motor units—a phenomenon called muscle learning—which increases strength even before muscle size increases.

In summary, strength training increases muscle strength because it increases the size of muscle fibers and improves the body's ability to call on motor units to exert force. The physiological changes and benefits that result from strength training are summarized in Table 4.1.

BENEFITS OF MUSCULAR STRENGTH AND ENDURANCE

Enhanced muscular strength and endurance can lead to improvements in the areas of performance, injury prevention, body composition, self-image, lifetime muscle and bone health, and chronic disease prevention.

Improved Performance of Physical Activities

A person with a moderate-to-high level of muscular strength and endurance can perform everyday tasks—such as climbing stairs and carrying books or groceries—with ease. Muscular strength and endurance are also

muscular strength The amount of force a muscle can produce with a single maximum effort.

muscular endurance The ability of a muscle or group of muscles to remain contracted (sustain a level of muscular force) or to contract repeatedly.

muscle fiber A single muscle cell, usually classified according to strength, speed of contraction, and energy source.

myofibrils Protein structures that make up muscle fibers.

hypertrophy An increase in the size of a muscle fiber, usually stimulated by muscular overload.

atrophy A decrease in the size of muscle cells.

hyperplasia An increase in the number of muscle cells.

slow-twitch fibers Red muscle fibers that are fatigue-resistant but have a slow contraction speed and a lower capacity for tension; usually recruited for endurance activities.

fast-twitch fibers White muscle fibers that contract rapidly and forcefully but fatigue quickly; usually recruited for actions requiring strength and power.

power The ability to exert force rapidly.

motor unit A motor nerve (one that initiates movement) connected to one or more muscle fibers.

Terms

important in recreational activities: People with poor muscle strength tire more easily and are less effective in activities like hiking, skiing, and playing tennis. Increased strength can enhance your enjoyment of recreational sports by making it possible to achieve high levels of performance and to handle advanced techniques. Strength training also results in modest improvements in maximal oxygen consumption.

Injury Prevention

Increased muscle strength and endurance provides protection against injury because it helps people maintain good posture and appropriate body mechanics when carrying out everyday activities like walking, lifting, and carrying. Good muscle strength and, particularly, endurance in the abdomen, hips, lower back, and legs support the back in proper alignment and help prevent low-back pain, which afflicts more than 85% of all Americans at some time in their lives. (Prevention of low-back pain is discussed in Chapter 5.) Training for muscular strength and endurance also makes the **tendons, ligaments,** and cartilage cells stronger and less susceptible to injury.

Improved Body Composition

As Chapter 2 explained, healthy body composition means that the body has a high proportion of fat-free mass (primarily composed of muscle) and a relatively small proportion of fat. Strength training improves body composition by increasing muscle mass, thereby tipping the body composition ratio toward fat-free mass and away from fat. Building muscle mass through strength training also helps with losing fat because metabolic rate is related to muscle mass: The more muscle mass, the higher the metabolic rate. A high metabolic rate means that a nutritionally sound diet coupled with regular exercise will not lead to an increase in body fat. Strength training can boost resting metabolic rate by 0–15%, depending on how hard you train.

Enhanced Self-Image and Quality of Life

Strength training leads to an enhanced self-image by providing stronger, firmer-looking muscles and a toned, healthy-looking body. Men tend to build larger, stronger muscles. Women tend to lose inches, increase strength, and develop greater muscle definition. The larger muscles in men combine with high levels of the hormone **testosterone,** the principal androgen, for a strong tissue-building effect; see the box "Gender Differences in Muscular Strength." Strength training improves body image in both men and women.

Because strength training involves measurable objectives (pounds lifted, repetitions accomplished), a person can easily recognize improved performance, leading to greater self-confidence and self-esteem. It's especially satisfying to work on improving one's personal record. Strength training also improves quality of life by increasing energy, preventing injuries, and making daily activities easier and more enjoyable.

Improved Muscle and Bone Health with Aging

Research has shown that good muscle strength helps people live healthier lives. A lifelong program of regular strength training prevents muscle and nerve degeneration that can compromise the quality of life and increase the risk of hip fractures and other potentially life-threatening injuries. In the general population people begin to lose muscle mass after age 30, a condition called *sarcopenia.* At first they may notice that they can't play sports as well as they could in high school. After more years of inactivity and strength loss, people may have trouble performing even the simple movements of daily life—getting out of a bathtub or automobile, walking up a flight of stairs, or doing yard work. By age 75 about 25% of men and 75% of women can't lift more than 10 pounds. Although aging contributes to decreased strength, inactivity causes most of the loss. Poor strength makes it much more likely that a person will be injured during everyday activities.

As a person ages, motor nerves can become disconnected from the portion of muscle they control. Muscle physiologists estimate that by age 70, 15% of the motor nerves in most people are no longer connected to muscle tissue. Aging and inactivity also cause muscles to become slower and therefore less able to perform quick, powerful movements. Strength training helps maintain motor nerve connections and the quickness of muscles.

Osteoporosis is common in people over age 55, particularly postmenopausal women. Osteoporosis leads to fractures that can be life-threatening. Hormonal changes from aging account for much of the bone loss that occurs, but lack of bone stress due to inactivity and a poor diet are contributing factors. Strength training can lessen bone loss even if it is taken up later in life, and if practiced regularly, strength training can even build bone mass in postmenopausal women. Increased muscle strength can also help prevent falls, which are a major cause of injury in people with osteoporosis. (Additional strategies for preventing osteoporosis are described in Chapter 8.)

Prevention and Management of Chronic Disease

Strength training helps in the prevention and management of several major chronic diseases. Strength training improves glucose metabolism, an important factor in the prevention of the most common form of diabetes (type 2 diabetes). It also modifies risk factors for cardiovascular disease. Regular strength training is associated with

Men are generally stronger than women because they typically have larger bodies overall and a larger proportion of their total body mass is made up of muscle. But when strength is expressed per unit of cross-sectional area of muscle tissue, men are only 1–2% stronger than women in the upper body and about equal to women in the lower body. (Men have a larger proportion of muscle tissue in the upper body, so it's easier for them to build upper-body strength than it is for women.) Individual muscle fibers are larger in men, but the metabolism of cells within those fibers is the same in both sexes.

Two factors that help explain these disparities between the sexes are testosterone levels and the speed of nervous control of muscle. Testosterone is responsible for the development of secondary sex characteristics in males (facial hair, deep voice, and so forth). Testosterone also promotes the growth of muscle tissue in both males and females. Testosterone levels are about 6–10 times higher in men than in women, so men tend to have larger muscles. Also, because the male nervous system can activate muscles faster, men tend to have more power.

Some women are concerned that they will develop large muscles from strength training. Because of hormonal differences, most women do not develop big muscles unless they train intensely over many years or take anabolic steroids. Women do gain muscle and improve body composition through strength training, but they don't develop bulky muscles or gain significant amounts of weight: A study of average women who weight trained 2–3 days per week for 8 weeks found that the women gained about 1.75 pounds of muscle and lost about 3.5 pounds of fat.

Losing muscle over time is a much greater health concern for women than small gains in muscle weight in response to strength training, especially since any gains in muscle weight are typically more than balanced with loss of fat weight. Both men and women lose muscle mass and power as they age, but because men start out with more muscle when they are young and don't lose power as quickly, older women tend to have greater impairment of muscle function than older men. This may partially account for the higher incidence of life-threatening falls in older women.

The bottom line is that both men and women can increase strength through strength training. Women may not be able to lift as much weight as men, but pound for pound of muscle, they have nearly the same capacity to gain strength as men. The lifetime wellness benefits of strength training are available to everyone. Strength training is particularly beneficial for women because it helps prevent bone and muscle loss with aging and maintains fat-free weight during weight control programs.

SOURCE: Fahey, T. D. 2004. *Weight Training for Men and Women*, 5th ed. New York: McGraw-Hill. IDEA. 2001. *Fitness Tip—Why Women Need Weight Training* (http://www.ideafit.com/ftwomen.htm; retrieved October 22, 2002). Krivickas, L. S., et al. 2001. Age and gender-related differences in maximum shortening velocity of skeletal muscle fibers. *American Journal of Physical Medicine and Rehabilitation* 80:447–455.

increased maximal oxygen consumption, decreased diastolic blood pressure, and, in some people, positive changes in blood fat levels (increased HDL cholesterol and decreased LDL cholesterol). Improvements in body composition and glucose metabolism are also beneficial for cardiovascular health. As described earlier, strength training also boosts bone mineral density, helping to prevent osteoporosis and associated bone fractures.

MOTIVATION FOR CHANGE!   Make a list of five benefits of muscular strength and endurance that are particularly meaningful to you. Post the list in a prominent location and use it as a motivational tool for beginning and maintaining your strength training program.

ASSESSING MUSCULAR STRENGTH AND ENDURANCE

Muscular strength and muscular endurance are distinct but related components of fitness. Muscular strength, the maximum amount of force a muscle can produce in a single effort, is usually assessed by measuring the maximum amount of weight a person can lift one time. This single maximal movement is referred to as a **repetition maximum (RM).** You can assess the strength of your major muscle groups by taking the one-repetition maximum (1 RM) tests for the bench press and the leg press. You can measure 1 RM directly or estimate it by doing multiple repetitions with a submaximal (lighter) weight. Refer to Lab 4.1 for guidelines on taking these tests. Instructions for assessing grip strength using a dynamometer are also

tendon A tough band of fibrous tissue that connects a muscle to a bone or other body part and transmits the force exerted by the muscle.

ligament A tough band of tissue that connects the ends of bones to other bones or supports organs in place.

testosterone The principal male hormone, responsible for the development of secondary sex characteristics and important in increasing muscle size.

repetition maximum (RM) The maximum amount of resistance that can be moved a specified number of times; 1 RM is the maximum weight that can be lifted once. 5 RM is the maximum weight that can be lifted five times.

Terms

included in Lab 4.1. For more accurate results, avoid any strenuous weight training for 48 hours beforehand.

Muscular endurance is the ability of a muscle to exert a submaximal force repeatedly or continuously over time. This ability depends on muscular strength because a certain amount of strength is required for any muscle movement. Muscular endurance is usually assessed by counting the maximum number of **repetitions** of a muscular contraction a person can do (such as in push-ups) or the maximum amount of time a person can hold a muscular contraction (such as in the flexed-arm hang). You can test the muscular endurance of major muscle groups in your body by taking the curl-up test and the push-up test. Refer to Lab 4.2 for complete instructions on taking these assessment tests.

Record your results and your fitness rating from the assessment tests in Labs 4.1 and 4.2. If the results show that improvement is needed, a weight training program will enable you to make rapid gains in muscular strength and endurance.

CREATING A SUCCESSFUL STRENGTH TRAINING PROGRAM

Strength training develops muscular strength and endurance in the same way that endurance exercise develops cardiovascular fitness: When the muscles are stressed by a greater load than they are used to, they adapt and improve their function. The type of adaptation that occurs depends on the type of stress applied. To get the most out of your strength training program, you must design it to achieve maximum fitness benefits with a low risk of injury. Before you begin, seriously consider the type and amount of training that's right for you.

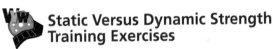 ### Static Versus Dynamic Strength Training Exercises

Strength training exercises are generally classified as static or dynamic. Each involves a different way of using and strengthening muscles.

Static Exercise Also called **isometric** exercise, **static exercise** involves a muscle contraction without a change in the length of the muscle or the angle in the joint on which the muscle acts. To perform an isometric exercise, a person can use an immovable object like a wall to provide resistance, or just tighten a muscle while remaining still (for example, tightening the abdominal muscles while sitting at a desk). In isometrics, the muscle contracts, but there is no movement.

Isometric exercises aren't as widely used as isotonic exercises because they don't develop strength throughout a joint's entire range of motion. However, static exercises are useful in strengthening muscles after an injury or sur-

gery, when movement of the affected joint could delay healing. Isometrics are also used to overcome weak points in an individual's range of motion. Statically strengthening a muscle at its weakest point will allow more weight to be lifted with that muscle during dynamic exercise. For maximum strength gains, hold the isometric contraction maximally for 6 seconds; do 5–10 repetitions.

Dynamic Exercise Also called **isotonic** exercise, **dynamic exercise** involves a muscle contraction with a change in the length of the muscle. Dynamic exercises are the most popular type of exercises for increasing muscle strength and seem to be most valuable for developing strength that can be transferred to other forms of physical activity. They can be performed with weight machines, free weights, or a person's own body weight (as in sit-ups or push-ups).

There are two kinds of dynamic muscle contractions: concentric and eccentric. A **concentric muscle contraction** occurs when the muscle applies enough force to overcome resistance and shortens as it contracts. An **eccentric muscle contraction** (also called a pliometric contraction) occurs when the resistance is greater than the force applied by the muscle and the muscle lengthens as it contracts. For example, in an arm curl, the biceps muscle works concentrically as the weight is raised toward the shoulder and eccentrically as the weight is lowered.

Two of the most common dynamic exercise techniques are constant resistance exercise and variable resistance exercise. Constant resistance exercise uses a constant load (weight) throughout a joint's entire range of motion. Training with free weights is a form of constant resistance exercise. A problem with this technique is that, because of differences in leverage, there are points in a joint's range of motion where the muscle controlling the movement is stronger and points where it is weaker. The amount of weight a person can lift is limited by the weakest point in the range. In variable resistance exercise, the load is changed to provide maximum load throughout the entire range of motion. This form of exercise uses machines that place more stress on muscles at the end of the range of motion, where a person has better leverage and is capable of exerting more force. The Nautilus pull-over machine is an example of a variable resistance exercise machine. Constant and variable resistance exercises are both extremely effective for building strength and endurance.

Four other kinds of isotonic techniques, used mainly by athletes for training and rehabilitation, are eccentric loading, plyometrics, speed loading, and isokinetics.

• **Eccentric (pliometric) loading** involves placing a load on a muscle as it lengthens. The muscle contracts eccentrically in order to control the weight. Eccentric loading is practiced during most types of resistance training. For example, you are performing an eccentric

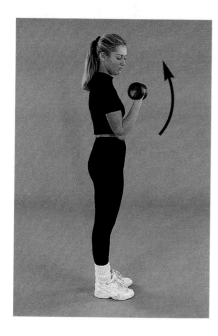 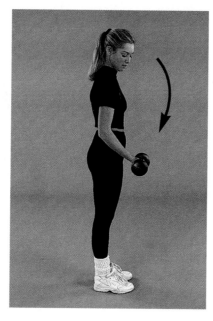

Left: A concentric contraction: The biceps muscle shortens as the arm lifts a weight toward the shoulder. **Right:** An eccentric contraction: The biceps muscle lengthens as the arm lowers a weight toward the thigh.

movement as you lower the weight to your chest during a bench press in preparation for the active movement. You can also perform exercises designed specifically to overload muscle eccentrically, a technique called negatives.

• **Plyometrics** is the sudden eccentric loading and stretching of muscles followed by a forceful concentric contraction. An example would be the action of the lower-body muscles when jumping from a bench to the ground and then jumping back onto the bench. This type of exercise is used to develop explosive strength; it also helps build and maintain bone density.

• **Speed loading** involves moving a weight as rapidly as possible in an attempt to approach the speeds used in movements like throwing a softball or sprinting. In the bench press, for example, speed loading might involve doing 5 repetitions as fast as possible using a weight that is half the maximum load you can lift. You can gauge your progress by timing how fast you can perform the repetitions.

• **Isokinetic** exercise involves exerting force at a constant speed against an equal force exerted by a special strength training machine. The isokinetic machine provides variable resistance at different points in the joint's range of motion, matching the effort applied by the individual, while keeping the speed of the movement constant. In other words, the force exerted by the individual at any point in the range of motion is resisted by an equal force from the isokinetic machine. Isokinetic exercises are excellent for building strength and endurance, but the equipment is expensive and less commonly available than other kinds of weight machines.

Comparing the Different Types of Exercise Static exercises require no equipment, so they can be done vir-

tually anywhere. They build strength rapidly and are useful for rehabilitating injured joints. On the other hand, they have to be performed at several different angles for each joint to improve strength throughout the joint's entire range of motion. Dynamic exercises can be performed without equipment (calisthenics) or with equipment (weight lifting). They are excellent for building strength and endurance, and they tend to build strength through a joint's full range of motion.

Most people develop muscular strength and endurance using dynamic exercises. Ultimately, the type of exercise a person chooses depends on individual goals, preferences, and access to equipment.

repetitions The number of times an exercise is performed during one set. **Terms**

static (isometric) exercise Exercise involving a muscle contraction without a change in the length of the muscle.

dynamic (isotonic) exercise Exercise involving a muscle contraction with a change in the length of the muscle.

concentric muscle contraction An isotonic contraction in which the muscle gets shorter as it contracts.

eccentric muscle contraction An isotonic contraction in which the muscle lengthens as it contracts; also called a pliometric contraction.

eccentric (pliometric) loading Loading the muscle while it is lengthening; sometimes called *negatives*.

plyometrics Rapid stretching of a muscle group that is undergoing eccentric stress (the muscle is exerting force while it lengthens), followed by a rapid concentric contraction.

speed loading Moving a load as rapidly as possible.

isokinetic The application of force at a constant speed against an equal force.

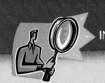
Exercise Machines

Advantages

- Safe and convenient
- Don't require spotters
- Don't require lifter to balance bar
- Provide variable resistance
- Require less skill
- Make it easy to move from one exercise to the next
- Allow easy isolation of muscles and muscle groups
- Support back (on many machines)

Disadvantages

- Limited availability
- Inappropriate for performing dynamic movements
- Allow a limited number of exercises

Free Weights

Advantages

- Allow dynamic movements
- Allow the user to develop control of the weights
- Allow a greater variety of exercises
- Widely available
- Truer to real-life situations; strength transfers to daily activities

Disadvantages

- Not as safe
- Require spotters
- Require more skill
- Cause more blisters and calluses

Weight Machines Versus Free Weights

Your muscles will get stronger if you make them work against a resistance. Resistance can be provided by free weights, by your own body weight, or by sophisticated exercise machines. Weight machines are preferred by many people because they are safe, convenient, and easy to use. You just set the resistance (usually by placing a pin in the weight stack), sit down at the machine, and start working. Machines make it easy to isolate and work specific muscles. You don't need a **spotter**, someone who stands by to assist when free weights are used, and you don't have to worry about dropping a weight on yourself.

Free weights require more care, balance, and coordination to use, but they strengthen your body in ways that are more adaptable to real life. They are also more popular with athletes for developing explosive strength for sports. Unless you are training seriously for a sport that requires a great deal of strength, training on machines is probably safer, more convenient, and just as effective as training with free weights. However, you can increase strength with either weight machines or free weights. Information listed in the box "Exercise Machines Versus Free Weights" can help you make a decision about which equipment you may prefer.

Don't forget that you don't need a fitness center or expensive equipment to strength train. Resistance can be provided by your own body weight—as in sit-ups, push-ups, chair dips, lunges, and so on—or by using such inexpensive home equipment as resistance bands or exercise balls. Examples of strength training programs that can be done at home without equipment can be found on the *Fit and Well* Online Learning Center.

Applying the FITT Principle: Selecting Exercises and Putting Together a Program

A complete weight training program works all the major muscle groups. It usually takes about 8–10 different exercises to get a complete workout. Use the FITT principle—frequency, intensity, time, and type—to set the parameters of your program.

Frequency of Exercise   For general fitness, the American College of Sports Medicine recommends a frequency of 2–3 days per week for weight training. Allow your muscles at least 1 day of rest between workouts; if you train too often, your muscles won't be able to work at a high enough intensity to improve their fitness, and soreness and injury are more likely to result. If you enjoy weight training and would like to train more often, try working different muscle groups on alternate days—a training plan called a split routine. For example, work your arms and upper body one day, work your lower body the next day, and then return to upper-body exercises on the third day.

Intensity of Exercise: Amount of Resistance   The amount of weight (resistance) you lift in weight training exercises is equivalent to intensity in cardiorespiratory endurance training. It determines the way your body will adapt to weight training and how quickly these adaptations will occur. Choose weights based on your current level of muscular fitness and your fitness goals. To build strength rapidly, you should lift weights as heavy as 80% of your maximum capacity (1 RM). If you're more interested in building endurance, choose a lighter weight (perhaps 40–60% of 1 RM) and do more repetitions. For example, if your maximum capacity for the leg press is 160 pounds, you might lift 130 pounds to build strength and 80 pounds to build endurance. For a general fitness program to develop both strength and endurance, choose a weight in the middle of this range, perhaps 70% of 1 RM.

Because it can be tedious and time-consuming to continually reassess your maximum capacity for each exercise, you might find it easier to choose a weight based on the number of repetitions of an exercise you can perform with a given resistance.

Time of Exercise: Repetitions and Sets   To improve fitness, you must do enough repetitions of each exercise to fatigue your muscles. The number of repetitions needed to cause fatigue depends on the amount of resistance: the heavier the weight, the fewer repetitions to reach fatigue. In general, a heavy weight and a low number of repetitions (1–5) build strength, whereas a light weight and a high number of repetitions (15–20) build endurance (Figure 4.2). For a general fitness program to build both strength and endurance, try to do about 8–12 repetitions of each exercise; a few exercises, such as abdominal crunches and calf raises, may require

more. Choose a weight heavy enough to fatigue your muscles but light enough for you to complete the repetitions with good form. To avoid risk of injury, older (approximately 50–60 years of age and above) and more frail people should perform more repetitions (10–15) using a lighter weight.

In weight training, a **set** refers to a group of repetitions of an exercise followed by a rest period. For developing strength and endurance for general fitness, you can make gains doing a single set of each exercise, provided you use enough resistance to fatigue your muscles. (You should just barely be able to complete the 8–12 repetitions—using good form—for each exercise.) Doing more than 1 set of each exercise will increase strength development, and most serious weight trainers do at least 3 sets of each exercise (see the section "More Advanced Strength Training Programs" for guidelines on more advanced programs).

If you perform more than 1 set of an exercise, you need to rest long enough between sets to allow your muscles to work at a high enough intensity to increase fitness. The length of the rest interval depends on the amount of resistance. In a program to develop a combination of strength and endurance for wellness, a rest period of 1–3 minutes between sets is appropriate; if you are lifting heavier loads to build maximum strength, rest 3–5 minutes between sets. You can save time in your workouts if you alternate sets of different exercises. Each muscle group can rest between sets while you work on other muscles.

Overtraining—doing more exercise than your body can recover from—can occur in response to heavy resistance training. Possible signs of overtraining include lack of progress or decreased performance, chronic fatigue, decreased coordination, and chronic muscle soreness. The best remedy for overtraining is rest: Add more days of recovery between workouts. With extra rest, chances are you'll be refreshed and ready to train again. Adding variety to your program, discussed later in the chapter, can also help with overtraining from resistance exercise.

Type or Mode of Exercise   For overall fitness, you need to include exercises for your neck, upper back, shoulders, arms, chest, abdomen, lower back, thighs, buttocks, and calves—about 8–10 exercises in all. If you are also training for a particular sport, include exercises to strengthen the muscles important for optimal performance and the muscles most likely to be injured. A weight training program for general fitness is presented later in this chapter, on pp. 107–119.

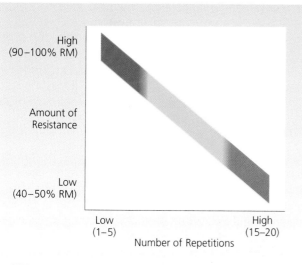

Training results in a large gain in strength but little or no gain in endurance.

Training results in moderate gains in both strength and endurance.

Training results in a large gain in endurance but little or no gain in strength.

Figure 4.2   Training for strength versus training for endurance.

spotter A person who assists with a weight training exercise done with free weights.

set A group of repetitions followed by a rest period.

Terms

Warm-up 5–10 minutes	Strength training exercises for major muscle groups (8–10 exercises)		Cool-down 5–10 minutes
	Sample program		
	Exercise	*Muscle group developed*	
	Bench press	Chest, shoulders, triceps	
	Pull-ups	Lats, biceps	
	Shoulder press	Shoulders, trapezius, triceps	
	Upright rowing	Deltoids, trapezius	
	Biceps curls	Biceps	
	Lateral raises	Shoulders	
	Squats	Gluteals, quadriceps	
	Heel raises	Calves	
	Abdominal curls	Abdominals	
	Spine extensions	Low- and mid-back spine extensors	
Start	Side bridges	Obliques, quadratus lumborum	*Stop*

Frequency: 2–3 days per week

Intensity/Resistance: Weights heavy enough to cause muscle fatigue when exercises are performed with good form for the selected number of repetitions

Time: Repetitions: 8–12 of each exercise (10–15 with a lower weight for people over age 50–60); **Sets:** 1 (doing more than 1 set per exercise may result in faster and greater strength gains)

Type of activity: 8–10 strength training exercises that focus on major muscle groups

Figure 4.3 The FITT principle for a strength training workout.

It is important to balance exercises between **agonist** and **antagonist** muscle groups. (When a muscle contracts, it is known as the agonist; the opposing muscle, which must relax and stretch to allow contraction by the agonist, is known as the antagonist.) Whenever you do an exercise that moves a joint in one direction, also select an exercise that works the joint in the opposite direction. For example, if you do knee extensions to develop the muscles on the front of your thighs, also do leg curls to develop the antagonistic muscles on the back of your thighs.

The order of exercises can also be important. Do exercises for large-muscle groups or for more than one joint before you do exercises that use small-muscle groups or single joints. This allows for more effective overload of the larger, more powerful muscle groups. Small-muscle groups fatigue more easily than larger ones, and small-muscle fatigue limits your capacity to overload larger-muscle groups. For example, lateral raises, which work the shoulder muscles, should be performed after bench presses, which work the chest and arms in addition to the shoulders. If you fatigue your shoulder muscles by doing lateral raises first, you won't be able to lift as much weight and effectively fatigue all the key muscle groups used during the bench press. Also, order exercises so that you work agonist and antagonist muscle groups in sequence, one after the other. For example, follow biceps curls, which work the biceps, with triceps extensions, which exercise the triceps—the antagonist muscle to the biceps.

The Warm-Up and Cool-Down

As with cardiorespiratory endurance exercise, you should warm up before every weight training session and cool down afterward (Figure 4.3). You should do both a general warm-up—several minutes of walking or easy jogging—and a warm-up for the weight training exercises you plan to perform. For example, if you plan to do 1 or more sets of 10 repetitions of bench presses with 125 pounds, you might do 1 set of 10 repetitions with 50 pounds as a warm-up. Do similar warm-up exercises for each exercise in your program.

To cool down after weight training, relax for 5–10 minutes after your workout. Although this is controversial, a few studies have suggested that including a period of post-exercise stretching may help prevent muscle soreness;

Terms

agonist A muscle in a state of contraction, opposed by the action of another muscle, its *antagonist*.

antagonist A muscle that opposes the action of another muscle, its *agonist*.

warmed-up muscles and joints make this a particularly good time to work on flexibility.

Making Progress The first few sessions of weight training should be devoted to learning the exercises. You need to learn the movements, and your nervous system needs to practice communicating with your muscles so you can develop strength effectively. To start, choose a weight that you can move easily through 8–12 repetitions, and do only 1 set of each exercise. Gradually add weight and (if you want) sets to your program over the first few weeks until you are doing 1–3 sets of 8–12 repetitions of each exercise.

As you progress, add weight when you can do more than 12 repetitions of an exercise. If adding weight means you can do only 7 or 8 repetitions, stay with that weight until you can again complete 12 repetitions per set. If you can do only 4–6 repetitions after adding weight, or if you can't maintain good form, you've added too much and should take some off. Knowing how much resistance to add and when to add it is as much an art as a science. You can add more resistance in large muscle exercises, such as squats and bench presses, than you can in smaller muscle exercises, such as curls. For example, when you can complete 12 repetitions of squats with good form, you may be able to add 10–20 pounds of additional resistance; for curls, on the other hand, you might add only 3–5 pounds. As a general guideline, try increases of approximately 5%, half a pound of additional weight for each 10 pounds you are currently lifting.

You can expect to improve rapidly during the first 6–10 weeks of training: a 10–30% increase in the amount of weight lifted. Gains will then come more slowly. Your rate of improvement will depend on how hard you work and how your body responds to resistance training. There will be individual differences in the rate of improvement. Factors such as age, motivation, and heredity will affect your progress.

Your ultimate goal depends on you. After you have achieved the level of strength and muscularity that you want, you can maintain your gains by training 2–3 days per week. You can monitor the progress of your program by recording the amount of resistance and the number of repetitions and sets you perform on a workout card like the one shown in Figure 4.4.

WORKOUT CARD FOR Sara Lopez

Exercise/Date		9/14	9/16	9/18	9/21	9/23	9/25	9/28	9/30	10/2	10/5	10/7	10/9	10/12	10/14	10/16									
Bench press	Wt.	45	45	45	50	50	50	60	60	60	65	65	65	70	70	70									
	Sets	1	1	1	1	1	1	1	1	1	1	1	1	1	1	1									
	Reps.	10	10	12	10	12	12	10	9	12	10	12	12	9	9	10									
Pull-ups (assisted)	Wt.	–	–	–	–	–	–	–	–	–	–	–	–	–	–	–									
	Sets	1	1	1	1	1	1	1	1	1	1	1	1	1	1	1									
	Reps.	5	5	5	6	6	6	7	7	7	8	8	8	9	9	10									
Shoulder press	Wt.	20	20	20	25	25	25	30	30	30	30	30	30	35	35	35									
	Sets	1	1	1	1	1	1	1	1	1	1	1	1	1	1	1									
	Reps.	10	10	12	10	12	12	8	10	9	10	12	12	10	10	10									
Upright rowing	Wt.	5	5	10	10	10	10	12	12	12	12	15	15	15	15	15									
	Sets	1	1	1	1	1	1	1	1	1	1	1	1	1	1	1									
	Reps.	12	12	8	10	11	12	9	10	10	12	8	8	8	9	10									
Biceps curls	Wt.	15	15	15	20	20	20	25	25	25	25	25	25	30	30	30									
	Sets	1	1	1	1	1	1	1	1	1	1	1	1	1	1	1									
	Reps.	10	10	10	10	12	12	8	10	10	10	12	12	9	10	12									
Lateral raise	Wt.	5	5	5	5	5	5	7.5	7.5	7.5	7.5	7.5	7.5	10	10	10									
	Sets	1	1	1	1	1	1	1	1	1	1	1	1	1	1	1									
	Reps.	8	8	10	10	12	12	8	10	10	10	12	12	8	8	9									
Squats	Wt.	–	–	–	45	45	45	55	55	55	65	65	65	75	75	75									
	Sets	1	1	1	1	1	1	1	1	1	1	1	1	1	1	1									
	Reps.	10	12	15	8	12	12	8	12	12	10	10	12	8	10	10									
Heel raises	Wt.	–	–	–	45	45	45	55	55	55	65	65	65	75	75	75									
	Sets	1	1	1	1	1	1	1	1	1	1	1	1	1	1	1									
	Reps.	15	15	15	8	12	12	10	12	12	10	12	12	10	12	12									
Abdominal curls	Wt.	–	–	–	–	–	–	–	–	–	–	–	–	–	–	–									
	Sets	1	1	1	1	1	1	1	1	1	1	1	1	1	1	1									
	Reps.	20	20	20	20	20	20	25	25	25	25	25	25	25	25	25									
Spine extensions	Wt.	–	–	–	–	–	–	–	–	–	–	–	–	–	–	–									
	Sets	1	1	1	1	1	1	1	1	1	1	1	1	1	1	1									
	Reps.	5	5	5	8	8	8	10	10	10	10	10	10	11	12	12									
Side bridge	Wt.	–	–	–	–	–	–	–	–	–	–	–	–	–	–	–									
	Sets	1	1	1	1	1	1	1	1	1	1	1	1	1	1	1									
	Seconds	60	60	60	65	65	70	70	70	70	76	75	80	80	80	80									

Figure 4.4 A sample workout card for a general fitness strength training program.

More Advanced Strength Training Programs

The weight training program described in this section—at least 1 set of 8–12 repetitions of 8–10 exercises, performed 2–3 days per week—is sufficient to develop and maintain muscular strength and endurance for general fitness. If you have a different goal, you may need to adjust your program accordingly. As described above, performing more sets of a smaller number of repetitions with a heavier load will cause greater increases in strength. A program designed to build strength might include 3–5 sets of 4–6 repetitions each; the load used should be heavy enough to cause fatigue with the smaller number of repetitions. Rest long enough after a set to allow your muscles to recover and to work intensely during the next set.

Experienced weight trainers often engage in some form of cycle training, also called periodization, in which the exercises, number of sets and repetitions, and intensity are varied within a workout and/or between workouts. For example, you might do a particular exercise more intensely during some sets or on some days than others; you might also vary the exercises you perform for particular muscle groups. Several sample cycle training programs can be found on the *Fit and Well* Online Learning Center. For more detailed information on these more advanced training techniques, consult a strength coach certified by the National Strength and Conditioning Association or another reliable source. If you decide to adopt a more advanced training regimen, start off slowly to give your body a chance to adjust and to minimize the risk of injury.

Weight Training Safety

Injuries do happen in weight training. Maximum physical effort, elaborate machinery, rapid movements, and heavy weights can combine to make the weight room a dangerous place if proper precautions aren't taken. To help ensure that your workouts are safe and productive, follow the guidelines in the box "Safe Weight Training" and the suggestions given below.

Use Proper Lifting Technique Every exercise has a proper technique that is important for obtaining maximum benefits and preventing injury. Your instructor or weight room attendant can help explain the specific techniques for performing different exercises and using different weight machines. Perform exercises smoothly and with good form. Lift or push the weight forcefully during the active phase of the lift and then lower it slowly with control. Perform all lifts through the full range of motion.

Use Spotters and Collars with Free Weights Spotters are necessary when an exercise has potential for danger: A weight that is out of control or falls can cause a serious injury. A spotter can assist you if you cannot complete a lift or if the weight tilts. A spotter can also help you move a weight into position before a lift and provide help or additional resistance during a lift. Spotting requires practice and coordination between the lifter and the spotter(s).

Collars are devices that secure weights to a barbell or dumbbell. Although people lift weights without collars, doing so is dangerous. It is easy to lose your balance or to raise one side of the weight faster than the other. Without collars, the weights on one side of the bar will slip off, and the weights on the opposite side will crash to the floor.

Be Alert for Injuries Report any obvious muscle or joint injuries to your instructor or physician, and stop exercising the affected area. Training with an injured joint or muscle can lead to a more serious injury. Make sure you get the necessary first aid. Even minor injuries heal faster if you use the R-I-C-E principle of treating injuries described in Chapter 3.

Consult a physician if you're having any unusual symptoms during exercise or if you're uncertain whether weight training is a proper activity for you. Conditions

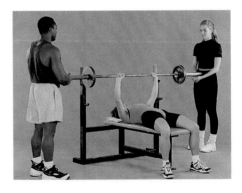

Spotters should be present when a person trains with free weights. If two spotters are used, one spotter should stand at each end of the barbell. If one spotter is present, he or she should stand behind the lifter.

General Guidelines

- When beginning a program or trying new exercises or equipment, ask an instructor for help doing exercises safely and with correct technique.

- Lift weights from a stabilized body position; keep weights as close to your body as possible.

- Protect your back by maintaining control of your spine and avoiding dangerous positions. Don't twist your body while lifting.

- Observe proper lifting techniques and good form at all times. If you have to alter your technique to complete a repetition, you are probably lifting too much weight. Don't lift beyond the limits of your strength.

- Don't hold your breath while doing weight training exercises. Holding your breath, called the Valsalva maneuver, causes a decrease in blood returning to the heart and can make you become dizzy and faint. It can also increase blood pressure to dangerous levels. Exhale when exerting the greatest force, and inhale when moving the weight into position for the active phase of the lift. Breathe smoothly and steadily.

- Rest between sets if you perform more than 1 set of each exercise. Fatigue hampers your ability to obtain maximum benefits from your program and is a prime cause of injury. Also allow muscles a full day of rest (48 hours) between workouts.

- Do exercises through a full range of motion, and do stretching exercises after your workout to help prevent tightness.

- Be aware of what's going on around you. Stay away from other people when they're doing exercises, and don't get distracted. If you bump into someone, you could cause an injury.

- Gloves are not mandatory but may prevent calluses on your hands.

- Don't use defective equipment. Be aware of broken collars or bolts, frayed cables, broken chains, or loose cushions. Report equipment damage or malfunctions immediately.

- Don't chew gum when exercising; you could choke on the gum or bite your tongue.

- Always warm up before training and cool down afterward.

- Don't exercise if you're ill, injured, or overtrained. Do not try to work through the pain.

- When returning to training after an illness or layoff, start with lighter weights than you were using before the break in training.

- Don't take dangerous and/or illegal drugs or supplements, such as anabolic steroids, in an attempt to speed the progress of your program. (See pp. 100–104 for more on supplements.)

Free Weights

- Make sure the bar is loaded evenly on both sides.

- When you pick a weight up from the ground, keep your back straight and your head level or up. Don't bend at the waist with straight legs.

- Lift weights smoothly and slowly; don't jerk them. Control the weight through the entire range of motion. Lifting a weight too fast can increase the force output to dangerous levels.

- Do most of your lifting with your legs. Keep your hips and buttocks tucked in. When doing standing lifts, maintain a good posture so that you protect your back.

- Don't bounce weights against your body during an exercise.

- When lifting barbells and dumbbells, wrap your thumbs around the bar when gripping it. You can easily drop a weight when using a "thumbless" grip.

Spotting

- Use spotters for free-weight exercises in which the bar crosses the face or head (e.g., the bench press), is placed on the back (e.g., squats), or is racked in front of the chest (e.g., overhead press from the rack).

- Spotters should be at least as tall and as strong as the lifter.

- If one spotter is used, the spotter should stand behind the lifter; if two spotters are used, one spotter should stand at each end of the barbell.

- For squats with heavy resistance, use at least three spotters— one behind the lifter (hands near lifter's hips, waist, or torso) and one on each side of the bar.

- Spot dumbbell exercises at the forearms, as close to the weights as possible.

- For over-the-face and over-the-head lifts, the spotter should hold the bar with an alternate grip (one palm up and one palm down) inside the lifter's grip.

- When providing a handoff, the spotter should make sure that the lifter has control of the weight before moving away.

- Ensure good communication between spotter and lifter by agreeing on verbal signals before the exercise.

- Spotters should pay attention and be ready to act quickly to assist a person who is having trouble. Lifters should tell spotters to "take it" if they can no longer contribute to making the lift.

Weight Machines

- Keep away from moving weight stacks. Pay attention when you're changing weights. Someone may jump on the machine ahead of you and begin an exercise while your fingers are close to the weight stack.

- Adjust each machine for your body so that you don't have to work in an awkward position. Lock everything in place before you begin.

- Stay away from moving parts of the machine that could pinch your skin.

- Make sure the machines are clean. Dirty vinyl is a breeding ground for germs that can cause skin diseases. Carry a towel around with you, and place it on the machine where you will sit or lie down.

such as heart disease and high blood pressure can be aggravated during weight training. Symptoms such as headaches; dizziness; labored breathing; numbness; vision disturbances; and chest, neck, or arm pains should be reported immediately.

A Caution About Supplements and Drugs

Many active people use a wide variety of nutritional supplements and drugs in the quest for improved performance and appearance. Most of these substances are ineffective and expensive and many are dangerous. A balanced diet should be your primary nutritional strategy. A selective summary of "performance aids" is given in Table 4.2, along with their potential side effects.

Supplements Taken to Increase Muscle Growth   The most popular category of supplements are those taken to increase muscle growth. Most of the supplements in this group are controlled substances that require a prescription to obtain through legal means. In addition to health risks, there are serious legal consequences for using them to enhance performance or appearance.

• **Anabolic steroids** are a group of synthetic derivatives of testosterone. People take them in hope of gaining weight and muscle size and improving strength, power, speed, endurance, aggressiveness, and appearance. Despite drug testing, anabolic steroids are taken by some athletes in sports such as bodybuilding, track and field, and football. Some world class athletes play a cat-and-mouse game with athletic drug testing agencies by disguising samples against drug tests or using drugs that can't be detected with current methods. In 2003–2004, a number of world class and professional athletes tested positive for a new anabolic steroid called tetrahydrogestrinone (THG) that was specifically formulated to beat the drug tests. The discovery of this drug led to a U.S. congressional investigation and more stringent anti-doping rules in many sports. Use of anabolic steroids has filtered down to high school students, and about 6% of all high school students have used them.

Anabolic steroids increase protein synthesis, which enhances fat-free weight, muscle mass, and strength. Side effects include liver damage and tumors, decreased levels of high-density lipoprotein (good cholesterol), heart disease, depressed sperm and testosterone production, high blood pressure, increased risk of AIDS (through shared needles), depressed immune function, problems with sugar metabolism, psychological disturbances, masculinization in women and children, premature

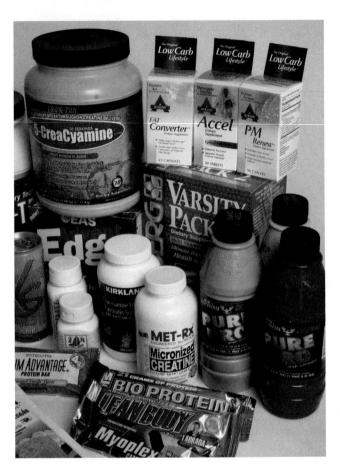

Many dietary supplements are marketed to athletes and other active people. Few have been proven safe and/or effective, many are expensive, and some are dangerous, illegal, and/or banned by major sports organizations.

closure of bone growth centers, and an increased risk of cancer. Side effects are greatest in people who take high doses of drugs for prolonged periods.

• Human chorionic gonadotrophin (HCG) is sometimes taken by anabolic steroid users to boost natural testosterone production, which is suppressed by steroids, and to prevent the muscle atrophy common during withdrawal from steroids. Although HCG tends to increase testosterone levels, it sometimes interferes with normal testosterone regulation, which causes additional deterioration in health and well-being. Use of HCG is not recommended and is banned in most sports.

• Growth hormone is used to increase muscle mass and strength. Reports in the news media suggest that, as with anabolic steroids, its general use has filtered down to high school students. Although advances in genetics have made human growth hormone more widely available, it is extremely expensive and has serious side effects. Growth hormone builds muscles, but the few studies on the hormone in humans have shown no beneficial effects on muscle or exercise performance. Prolonged growth hormone administration may result in

Terms   **anabolic steroids** Synthetic male hormones taken to enhance athletic performance and body composition.

| Table 4.2 | Performance Aids Marketed to Weight Trainers |

Substance	Supposed Effects	Actual Effects	Selected Potential Side Effects
Adrenal androgens: DHEA, androstenedione	Increased testosterone, muscle mass, and strength; decreased body fat	Increased testosterone, strength, and fat-free mass and decreased fat in older subjects (more studies needed in younger people)	Gonadal suppression, prostate hypertrophy, breast development in males, masculinization in women and children. Long-term effects unknown
Amino acids	Increased muscle mass	No effects if dietary protein intake is adequate	Minimal side effects; unbalanced amino acid intake can cause problems with protein metabolism
Anabolic steroids	Increased muscle mass, strength, power, psychological aggressiveness, and endurance	Increased strength, power, fat-free mass, and aggression; no effects on endurance	Minor to severe: gonadal suppression, liver disease, acne, breast development in males, masculinization in women and children, heart disease, cancer. Steroids are controlled substances[a]
Chromium picolinate	Increased muscle mass; decreased body fat, improved blood sugar control	Well-controlled studies show no significant effect on fat-free mass or on body fat	Moderate doses (50–200 μg) appear safe; higher doses may cause DNA damage and other serious effects. Long-term effects unknown
Creatine monohydrate	Increased muscle creatine phosphate, muscle mass, and capacity for high-intensity exercise	Increased muscle mass and performance in some types of high-intensity exercise	Minimal side effects; some reports of muscle cramping and exacerbation of existing kidney problems. Long-term effects unknown
Ephedra	Decreased body fat; increased training intensity due to stimulant effect	Decreased appetite, particularly when taken with caffeine; some evidence for increased training intensity	Abnormal heart rhythms, nervousness, headache, gastrointestinal distress, and heatstroke; banned by the FDA in 2004
Ginseng	Decreased effects of physical and emotional stress; increased oxygen consumption	Most well-controlled studies show no effect on performance	No serious side effects; high doses can cause high blood pressure, nervousness, and insomnia
Growth hormone	Increased muscle mass, strength, and power; decreased body fat	Increased muscle mass and strength	Diabetes, acromegaly (disease characterized by increased growth of bones in hands and face), enlarged heart and other organs. An extremely expensive controlled substance[a]
HMB (beta-hydroxy-beta-methylbutyrate)	Increased strength and muscle mass; decreased body fat	Some studies show increased fat-free mass and decreased fat; more research needed	No reported side effects. Long-term effects unknown
"Metabolic-optimizing" meals for athletes	Increased muscle mass; energy supply; decreased body fat	No proven effects beyond those of balanced meals	No reported side effects; extremely expensive
Protein	Increased muscle mass	No effects if dietary protein intake is adequate	Can be dangerous for people with liver or kidney disease

[a]Possession of a controlled substance is illegal without a prescription, and physicians are not allowed to prescribe controlled substances for the improvement of athletic performance. In addition, the use of anabolic steroids, growth hormone, or any of several other substances listed in this table is banned for athletic competition.

SOURCES: Brooks, G. A., et al. 2005. *Exercise Physiology: Human Bioenergetics and Its Applications,* 4th ed. New York: McGraw-Hill. Sports-supplement dangers. 2001. *Consumer Reports,* June. Williams, M. H. 1998. *The Ergogenics Edge: Pushing the Limits of Sports Performance.* Champaign, Ill.: Human Kinetics.

elevated blood sugar, high insulin levels, carpal tunnel syndrome, heart enlargement, and increased blood fat levels. Prolonged use could also lead to acromegaly, characterized by enlarged bones in the head, face, and hands, as well as diseases of the heart, nerves, bones, and joints.

• Dehydroepiandrosterone (DHEA) and androstenedione are two relatively weak male hormones produced in the adrenal glands of both men and women. Both are broken down into testosterone. People take these drugs to stimulate muscle growth and aid in weight control. Because they were classified as supplements, they have been widely available in health food stores and supermarkets (see the box "Dietary Supplements: A Consumer Dilemma"). The few studies in humans show that they are of little value in improving athletic performance. These substances have side effects similar to those of anabolic steroids, particularly when taken in high doses. In 2004, the FDA acted to remove androstenedione from the supplement market.

• Insulin is used by the body to help control carbohydrate, fat, and protein metabolism. Some athletes take insulin injections to promote muscle hypertrophy, but its effectiveness in stimulating muscle growth is not known. Insulin supplementation is an extremely dangerous practice because it can cause insulin shock (characterized by extremely low blood sugar), which can lead to unconsciousness and death.

• Insulin-like growth factor (IGF-1) is produced by the pituitary gland and is stimulated by growth hormone. Although IGF-1 is a powerful anabolic agent, its effects in healthy, active people are unknown. Side effects are thought to be similar to those of growth hormone. Long-term use is known to promote cancer.

• Beta-agonists are a type of medication used to treat asthma, including exercise-induced asthma; this family of drugs includes clenbuterol, salmeterol, and terbutaline. Some athletes who do not have asthma take beta-agonists in an attempt to enhance performance. They hope to prevent muscle atrophy, increase fat-free weight, and decrease body fat. Potential side effects include insomnia, heart arrhythmias, anxiety, anorexia, and nausea. More serious effects include heart enlargement, heart attack (particularly if used with steroids), and heart failure.

• Protein, amino acid, and polypeptide supplements are taken to accelerate muscle development, decrease body fat, and stimulate the release of growth hormone. By a wide margin, these products are the most popular supplements taken by active people. Still, there is little scientific proof to support their use, even in athletes on extremely heavy training routines. The protein requirements of these athletes are not much higher than those of sedentary individuals. Also, most athletes take in more than enough protein in their diets. Although there appear to be few side effects from using these products, substituting amino acid or polypeptide supplements for protein-rich food can cause deficiencies in important nutrients, such as iron and the B vitamins.

• So-called metabolic-optimizing meals contain a wide variety of individual supplemental components and are widely used by athletes and active people. Some studies suggest that these meals may increase the hormone concentrations necessary for the development of fitness, but their effects on muscle growth and performance have not been demonstrated.

Supplements Taken to Speed Recovery from Training
The primary purpose of taking these agents is to replenish depleted body fuel supplies that are important during exercise and recovery.

• Creatine monohydrate is used in an effort to enhance recovery, power, strength, and muscle size. Creatine monohydrate supplements increase creatine phosphate levels in muscle. As discussed in Chapter 3, creatine phosphate is a critical fuel source in the body. Physicians have used it successfully to treat muscle-wasting diseases. It may also help improve mental function. Several, but not all, studies have shown that creatine monohydrate supplementation improves performance in short-term, high-intensity, repetitive exercise. It may help to enlarge muscles in people who lift weights by allowing them to train harder. On the other hand, a panel of ACSM experts found no evidence that creatine supplements increase the aerobic power of muscle. Creatine may increase water retention in muscles, giving the feeling of increased muscularity without an actual increase in muscle size. Although this supplement appears safe, its long-term effects are unknown, so people should take this substance with caution.

• Chromium picolinate is used to enhance the action of insulin and to improve carbohydrate metabolism. Although a few studies have shown benefits, the efficacy of this supplement is extremely controversial.

• Other substances in this category include carbohydrate beverages that athletes use during and immediately following exercise to help them recover from intense training; these beverages may speed the replenishment of liver and muscle glycogen.

Substances Taken to Increase Training Intensity and Overcome Fatigue
Active people often spend many hours a day training, and monotony and fatigue sometimes impede significant improvement. Some people use stimulants to help them increase training intensity and overcome fatigue.

• Amphetamines are sometimes used by athletes to prevent fatigue and to increase confidence and training intensity. These drugs stimulate the nervous system, causing increased arousal, wakefulness, confidence, and the feeling of an enhanced capability to make decisions; they mask fatigue, so users feel energized, but once the drug wears off, depression or fatigue sets in. Because amphetamines can cause extreme confusion, they are of

"Builds lean muscle fast!" "Burns fat and gives you super energy!"
"The most effective muscle-building product ever!" It's only human
nature to want to feel, perform, and look as good as possible.
But wading through advertising hype can be tricky when you
are considering taking a dietary supplement. While drugs and
food products undergo stringent government testing, dietary
supplements can be freely marketed without testing for safety
or effectiveness. There is no guarantee that advertising claims
about dietary supplements are accurate or true.

What's the difference between a drug—which must be
approved by the Food and Drug Administration (FDA)—and a
dietary supplement? In some cases, the only real difference is in
how the product is marketed. Some dietary supplements are as
potentially dangerous as potent prescription drugs. But because
they have a different classification, dietary supplements do not
have to prove they are safe and effective before being sold; the
FDA can, however, take action against any unsafe supplement
product after it reaches the market. This is what occurred in two
high-profile cases in 2004 when the FDA acted against popular
dietary supplements—androstenedione and ephedra.

The male hormone testosterone is a powerful drug with many
adverse effects; it is closely regulated by the FDA. Androstenedione, a hormone converted into the body to testosterone (and
estrogen), was widely available without a prescription as a dietary
supplement. Andro disrupts the hormonal balance of its users
and can increase the risk of heart disease. Teens who take andro
are at risk for early closure of bone growth centers, which could
limit their adult height. Other potential adverse effects of andro
include acne, psychological disturbances, male breast development, baldness, and kidney and liver dysfunction. Advertisements for andro claimed that it will increase muscle size,
strength, and performance, but there are actually very few good
studies of andro's effects on humans; the two best studies showed
no significant difference in muscle growth and strength in andro
users compared with nonusers. Most medical experts believe that
andro is neither safe nor effective—yet it has been used by thousands of athletes, most of whom are unaware of the risks. In
2004, the FDA stated that androstenedione was potentially dangerous and should not be marketed as a supplement; it asked
manufacturers to stop selling supplements containing andro.

The controversy over another compound, ephedra, continues
despite an FDA ban that went into effect in April 2004. Ephedra
was a common ingredient of dietary supplements, often touted
as an "energy booster" and a "fat burner." Marketed as a natural
herbal product and available without a prescription, consumers
might assume that ephedra is free from serious side effects. However, the drug can cause severe high blood pressure, heart
attacks, strokes, seizures, and heat illness, and it has been linked
to a number of deaths. It may be especially risky in users who are
dehydrated and/or fatigued or when it is combined with other
stimulants such as caffeine. Many sports organizations banned
the use of ephedra because of safety concerns, and following the
publication of additional studies and reports, the FDA acted
to remove ephedra-containing products from the market. It is
likely that some people will continue to use the drug by obtaining it illegally, and new formulations of supplements are likely to
appear containing combinations of other stimulants. Chapter 9
has more information about ephedra and other dietary supplements marketed for weight loss.

Glowing reports about the supposed effects of dietary supplements may sound very enticing, but how can you determine
if a particular supplement might be helpful? Ask yourself the
following questions:

- *Do you really need a supplement at all?* Nutritional authorities
  agree that most athletes and young adults can obtain all the
  necessary ingredients for health and top athletic performance
  by eating a well-balanced diet and training appropriately.
  There is no dietary supplement that outperforms wholesome
  real food and a good training regimen. Remember, too, that
  athletic performance and appearance are not life and death
  issues. It's one thing to take a cancer chemotherapy drug with
  many known adverse effects if there is a reasonable chance
  that it will save your life. It's another to take a potentially
  dangerous dietary supplement that may not even work for
  you when your goal is to increase your sports performance.

- *Is the product safe and effective?* The fact that a dietary supplement is available in your local store is no guarantee of safety.
  As described above, the FDA doesn't regulate supplements
  in the same way as drugs. The only way to determine if a
  supplement really works is to perform carefully controlled
  research on human subjects. Testimonials from individuals
  who claim to have benefited from the product don't count.
  Few dietary supplements have undergone careful human
  testing, so it is difficult to tell which of them may actually
  work. Reliable resources for information on dietary supplements include the FDA Center for Food Safety and Applied
  Nutrition (http://www.cfsan.fda.gov/~dms/supplmnt.html)
  and the Nutritional Supplements for Athletes Web site from
  Kansas State University (http://www.oznet.ksu.edu/nutrition/
  supplements.htm).

- *Can you be sure that the specific product is of high quality?*
  There is no official agency that ensures the quality of dietary
  supplements. There is no guarantee that a supplement contains the desired ingredient, that dosages are appropriate,
  that potency is standardized, or that the product is free from
  contaminants (see Chapter 8 for more information on dietary supplement labeling).

A recent study of 12 over-the-counter brands of supplements
containing androstenedione and related steroids found that one
brand contained more and eleven brands contained less than the
amount stated on the label; in addition, one brand contained a
significant amount of a controlled steriod. The International
Olympic Committee recently issued a warning to athletes based
on a test of 634 different nutritional supplements; researchers
found that 15% of the supplements tested contained unlabled
substances that would cause an athlete to fail a drug test.

Many dietary supplements are ineffective and/or unsafe, but
it is extremely difficult for consumers to get the information
they need to make an informed decision. Once you have
gathered the best information you can find, consider whether
the potential benefits of the supplement appear to outweigh the
risks and the cost. When in doubt, it's best not to buy or take
the product. Remember that no supplement eliminates the need
for proper training, and no supplement has been shown to be
safe and effective in long-term weight loss. A product that is
marginally effective, not proven safe, and expensive to boot is
probably not worth the money or the risk.

little use in sports requiring rapid decisions. Amphetamines can cause severe neural and psychological effects that include aggressiveness, paranoia, hallucinations, compulsive behavior, restlessness, irritability, heart arrhythmias, high blood pressure, and chest pains (see Chapter 13).

• Caffeine, found naturally in many plant species, is a favorite stimulant among many active people. Caffeine stimulates the nervous system and helps increase fat levels in the blood. Although there is some evidence that caffeine may improve endurance, the drug does not appear to enhance short-term maximal exercise capacity. Caffeine increases the incidence of abnormal heart rhythms and insomnia and is addictive. Ephedra, another naturally occurring stimulant, is described in more detail below and in the box on dietary supplements.

Substances Taken to Increase Endurance Erythropoietin and darbepoetin are related drugs that stimulate the growth of oxygen-carrying red blood cells. These drugs are used to help treat anemia in patients with cancer and kidney disease. Some athletes have taken these drugs in an effort to boost their performance in endurance events. By increasing the production of red blood cells, erythropoietin and darbepoetin enhance oxygen uptake and endurance. However, these supplements are extremely dangerous because they increase blood viscosity (thickness) and can cause potentially fatal blood clots.

Substances Taken to Aid Weight Control Substances used in weight control include drugs that suppress appetite, drugs that affect metabolic rate, and diuretics to control weight and increase muscle definition.

• Prescription appetite suppressants include diethylpropion and phentermine; these and related drugs can have serious side effects and are not approved for long-term use. Over-the-counter stimulants, including caffeine, phenylpropanolamine (PPA), and ephedra, have sometimes been used for weight control. However, there have been reports of adverse effects from PPA and ephedra, including an increased risk of heart attack or stroke in some people. Because of these risks, the FDA banned PPA in 2000 and ephedra in 2004. An additional concern with over-the-counter supplements is that due to lack of standardization, labels may not correctly indicate the amount of stimulant in a product. See Chapter 9 for more on diet pills.

• Dinitrophenol (DPN) is a drug that was prescribed in the 1920s and 1930s for weight loss; it works by releasing food energy as heat. The drug was banned in 1938 because it can cause a dangerous increase in body temperature, leading to heat injury and death. The use of DPN has been reported among some athletes (who obtain it illegally), but the drug is no safer now than it was in the past.

• Diuretics (drugs that promote loss of body fluid) and potassium supplements are sometimes taken by people in an attempt to accentuate muscle definition. Others take potassium supplements to promote fluid retention in their muscle cells, thus increasing muscle size. Athletes may combine these practices with very-low-calorie diets and dehydration in the quest for weight loss and leanness. There is no evidence that these unhealthy practices improve appearance or muscle size. Serious complications have developed from these practices, including muscle cell destruction, low blood pressure, blood chemistry abnormalities, and heart problems.

Supplement and Drug Use by Active People The variety and combinations of supplements and drugs used by physically active people make it extremely difficult to determine the efficacy of these practices or to predict their side effects. Many medical studies describe catastrophic side effects from use of unsafe drugs and nutritional supplements. Most supplements simply don't work.

Keep in mind that no nutritional supplement or drug will change a weak, untrained person into a strong, fit person. Those changes require regular training that stresses the muscles, heart, lungs, and metabolism and causes the body to adapt. They also require a healthy, balanced diet, as described in Chapter 8. The next section describes weight training exercises that can help you reach your goals.

WEIGHT TRAINING EXERCISES

A general book on fitness and wellness cannot include a detailed description of all weight training exercises. Here we present a basic program for developing muscular strength and endurance for general fitness using free weights and weight machines. Instructions for each exercise are accompanied by photographs and a listing of the muscles being trained. (Figure 4.5 is a diagram of the muscular system.) Table 4.3 on p. 106 lists alternative and additional exercises that can be performed on various machines or with free weights. If you are interested in learning how to do these exercises, ask your instructor or coach for assistance.

If you want to develop strength for a particular activity, your program should contain exercises for general fitness, exercises for the muscle groups most important for the activity, and exercises for muscle groups most often injured. Labs 4.2 and 4.3 will help you assess your current level of muscular endurance and design your own weight training program. Regardless of the goals of your program or the type of equipment you use, your program should be structured so that you obtain maximum results without risking injury. You should train at least 2 days per week, and each exercise session should contain a warm-up, 1 or more sets of 8–12 repetitions of 8–10 exercises, and a period of rest.

Weight training exercises begin on p. 107.

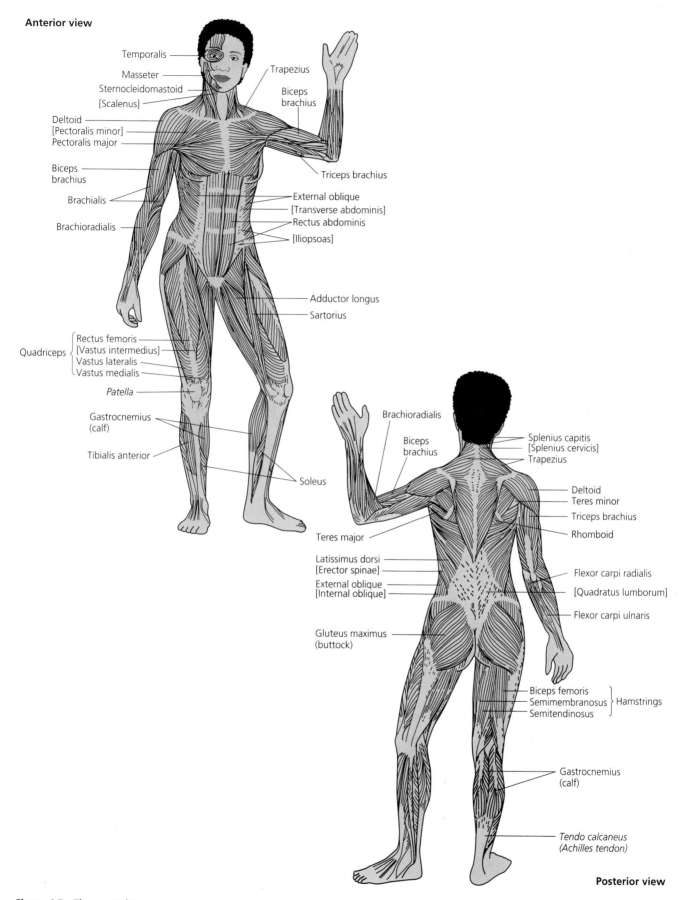

Anterior view

Temporalis
Masseter
Sternocleidomastoid
[Scalenus]
Deltoid
[Pectoralis minor]
Pectoralis major
Biceps brachius
Brachialis
Brachioradialis

Trapezius
Biceps brachius
Triceps brachius
External oblique
[Transverse abdominis]
Rectus abdominis
[Iliopsoas]
Adductor longus
Sartorius

Quadriceps
Rectus femoris
[Vastus intermedius]
Vastus lateralis
Vastus medialis
Patella
Gastrocnemius (calf)
Tibialis anterior
Soleus

Brachioradialis
Biceps brachius
Teres major
Latissimus dorsi
[Erector spinae]
External oblique
[Internal oblique]
Gluteus maximus (buttock)

Splenius capitis
[Splenius cervicis]
Trapezius
Deltoid
Teres minor
Triceps brachius
Rhomboid
Flexor carpi radialis
[Quadratus lumborum]
Flexor carpi ulnaris

Biceps femoris
Semimembranosus
Semitendinosus
} Hamstrings

Gastrocnemius (calf)

Tendo calcaneus (Achilles tendon)

Posterior view

Figure 4.5 The muscular system. The muscle names enclosed in brackets refer to deep muscles.

Company	Legs	Arms	Shoulders and Chest	Torso
Cybex	Hip abduction Hip adduction Leg extension Leg press Prone leg curl Rotary calf Seated leg curl	Arm curl Triceps extension	Chest press Incline press Overhead press	Ab crunch Pull-down Torso rotation
Hammer	Abductor Adductor Calf H squat Iso leg curl Iso leg extension Iso lateral leg press Leg curl Leg extension Leg press Seated calf raise Seated leg curl	Behind-neck press Bench press Flat back chest Front military press Incline press Iso behind-neck press Iso incline press Iso wide chest Seated bicep Seated triceps	Bench press Flat back chest Iso wide chest Lateral raise Rear deltoid Rotator cuff Seated dip	Behind-neck pull-down Bilateral row Dead lift Front pull-down High row Iso pullover Low row Pullover Row Shrug
Life Machines	Calf raise Leg abduction Leg adduction Leg curl Leg extension Leg press Seated leg curl	Bicep curl Triceps extension	Chest press Incline press lateral raise Pec fly Seated raise Shoulder press	Ab crunch Lat pull-down Low back extension Seated row Shoulder pullover
Nautilus	Calf raise Leg curl Leg extension Leg press	Biceps curl Preacher curl Triceps extension	10-degree chest 50-degree chest Bench press Incline press Lateral raise Military press Seated dip	Abdominal Compound row Hip and back Hip flexion Lat pull-down Pullover Rotary torso
Magnum	Glute/ham Leg abduction Leg adduction Leg curl Leg extension Leg press Multi-hip Seated calf	Arm curl Biangular arm curl Triceps extension Triceps pushdown	Bench press Bilateral chest Lateral raise Pec real delt Shoulder press Vertical bench press	Biangular lat row Cable cross over Lat pull-down Rogers row Rotary back Upper back
Universal Gym	Abductor kick Adductor kick Calf raises (leg press) Knee extension Knee flexion Leg press	Biceps curl Dips Lat pull	Bench press Front raise Incline press Rip-up Shoulder press Upright row	Bent-over row Crunch Lat pull Pullover Pull-up Side bend
Free weights	Back squat Front squat Hack squat Leg curl Leg extension Leg press Lunges Seated calf Smith machine Step-ups	Barbell curl Dumbbell curl French curl Preacher curl	Bench press Decline press Dumbbell back raise Dumbbell flys Dumbbell front raise Dumbbell lateral raise Incline press Incline press Overhead press	Abdominal crunch Abdominal sit-ups Bent-over row Dead lift Incline lever row Lat pull-down Pullover Seated row Shrug Upright row

SOURCE: Fahey., T. D., 2004. *Basic Weight Training for Men and Women*, 5th ed., New York: McGraw-Hill. Copyright © 2004 The McGraw-Hill Companies, Inc. Reprinted with permission of The McGraw-Hill Companies, Inc.

WEIGHT TRAINING EXERCISES
Free Weights

EXERCISE 1

BENCH PRESS

Muscles developed: Pectoralis major, triceps, deltoids

Instructions: (a) Lying on a bench on your back with your feet on the floor, grasp the bar with palms upward and hands shoulder-width apart. If the weight is on a rack, move the bar carefully from the supports to a point over the middle of your chest. **(b)** Lower the bar to your chest. Then press it to the starting position. If your back arches too much, try doing this exercise with your feet on the bench.

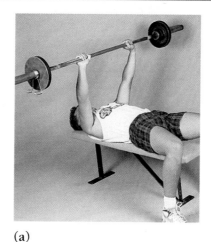

(a)

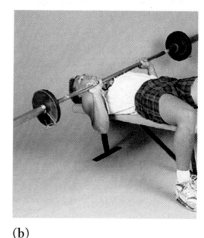

(b)

EXERCISE 2

PULL-UP

Muscles developed: Latissimus dorsi, biceps

Instructions: (a) Begin by grasping the pull-up bar with both hands, palms facing forward and elbows extended fully. **(b)** Pull yourself upward until your chin goes above the bar. Then return to the starting position.

Assisted pull-up: (c) This is done as described above for a pull-up, except that a spotter assists the person by pushing upward at the waist, hips, or legs during exercise.

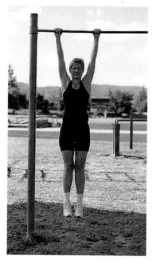

(a)

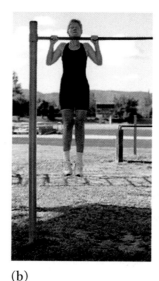

(b)

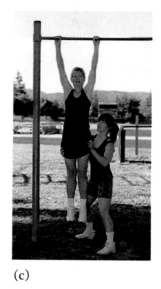

(c)

To allow an optimal view of exercise technique, a spotter does not appear in these demonstration photographs; however, spotters should be used for most exercises with free weights. Video clips illustrating spotting technique can be found on the *Fit and Well* Online Learning Center.

Weight Training Exercises **107**

SHOULDER PRESS (Overhead or Military Press)

Muscles developed: Deltoids, triceps, trapezius

Instructions: This exercise can be done standing or seated, with dumbbells or a barbell. The shoulder press begins with the weight at your chest, preferably on a rack. (**a**) Grasp the weight with your palms facing away from you. (**b**) Push the weight overhead until your arms are extended. Then return to the starting position (weight at chest). Be careful not to arch your back excessively.

If you are a more advanced weight trainer, you can "clean" the weight to your chest (lift it from the floor to your chest). The clean should be attempted only after instruction from a knowledgeable coach; otherwise, it can lead to injury.

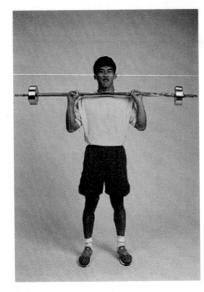
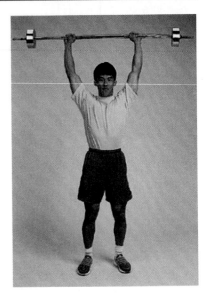

(a) (b)

UPRIGHT ROWING

Muscles developed: trapezius, deltoids, and biceps brachius

Instructions: From a standing position with arms extended fully, grasp a barbell with a close grip (hands about 6–12 inches apart) and palms toward the body. Raise the bar to about the level of your collarbones, keeping your elbows above bar level at all times. Return to the starting position.

This exercise can be done using dumbbells, a weighted bar (shown), or a barbell.

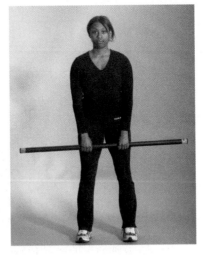
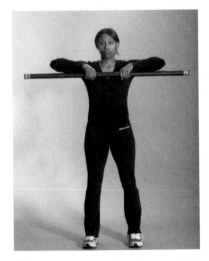

(a) (b)

To allow an optimal view of exercise technique, a spotter does not appear in these demonstration photographs; however, spotters should be used for most exercises with free weights. Video clips illustrating spotting technique can be found on the *Fit and Well* Online Learning Center.

BICEPS CURL

Muscles developed: Biceps, brachialis

Instructions: **(a)** From a standing position, grasp the bar with your palms upward and your hands shoulder-width apart. **(b)** Keeping your upper body rigid, flex (bend) your elbows until the bar reaches a level slightly below the collarbone. Return the bar to the starting position.

The exercise can be done using dumbbells, a curl bar (shown), or a barbell; some people find that using a curl bar places less stress on the wrists.

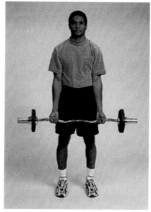
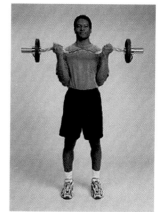

(a)   **(b)**

LATERAL RAISE

Muscles developed: Deltoids

Instructions: **(a)** Stand with feet shoulder-width apart and a dumbbell in each hand. Hold the dumbbells parallel to each other. **(b)** With elbows slightly bent, slowly lift both weights until they reach shoulder level. Keep your wrists in a neutral position, in line with your forearms. Return to the starting position.

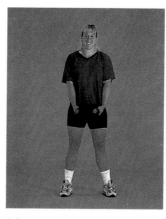
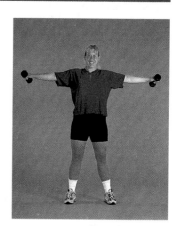

(a)   **(b)**

SQUAT

Muscles developed: Quadriceps, gluteus maximus, hamstrings, gastrocnemius

Instructions: If the bar is racked, place the bar on the fleshy part of your upper back and grasp the bar at shoulder width. Keeping your back straight and head level, remove the bar from the rack and take a step back. Stand with feet shoulder-width apart and toes pointed slightly outward. **(a)** Rest the bar on the back of your shoulders, holding it there with hands facing forward. **(b)** Keeping your head up and lower back straight, squat down until your thighs are almost parallel with the floor, your back starts to round, *or* your heels come off the floor. Drive upward toward the starting position, keeping your back in a fixed position throughout the exercise.

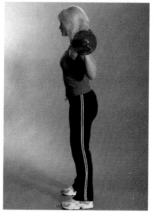
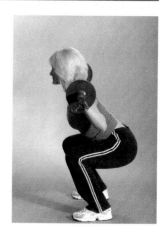

(a)   **(b)**

HEEL RAISE

Muscles developed: Gastrocnemius, soleus

Instructions: Stand with feet shoulder-width apart and toes pointed straight ahead. (**a**) Rest the bar on the back of your shoulders, holding it there with hands facing forward. (**b**) Press down with your toes while lifting your heels. Return to the starting position.

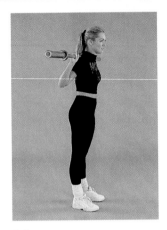
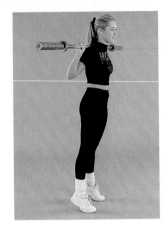

(a)　　　　　　　　　　　　(b)

CURL-UP OR CRUNCH

Muscles developed: Rectus abdominis, obliques, transverse abdominis

Instructions: (**a**) Lie on your back on the floor with your arms folded across your chest and your feet on the floor or on a bench. (**b**) Curl your trunk up and forward by raising your head and shoulders from the ground. Lower to the starting position. Focus on using your abdominal muscles rather than the muscles in your shoulders, chest, and neck.

This exercise can also be done using an exercise ball (see p. 153).

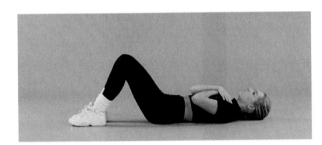
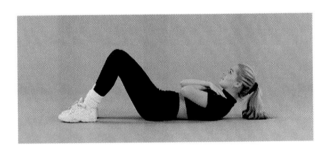

(a)　　　　　　　　　　　　(b)

To allow an optimal view of exercise technique, a spotter does not appear in these demonstration photographs; however, spotters should be used for most exercises with free weights. Video clips illustrating spotting technique can be found on the *Fit and Well* Online Learning Center.

SPINE EXTENSION (Isometric Exercises)

Muscles developed: Erector spinae, gluteus maximus, hamstrings, deltoids

Instructions: Begin on all fours with your knees below your hips and your hands below your shoulders.

Unilateral spine extension: (a) Extend your right leg to the rear and reach forward with your right arm. Keep your neck neutral and your raised arm and leg in line with your torso. Don't arch your back or let your hip or shoulder sag. Hold this position for 10–30 seconds. Repeat with your left leg and left arm.

Bilateral spine extension: (b) Extend your left leg to the rear and reach forward with your right arm. Keep your neck neutral and your raised leg in line with your torso. Don't arch your back or let your hip or shoulder sag. Hold this position for 10–30 seconds. Repeat with your right leg and left arm.

You can make this exercise more difficult by attaching weights to your ankles and wrists.

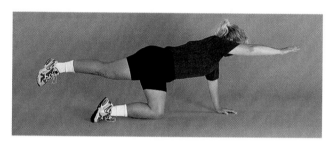 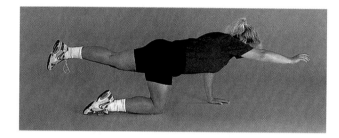

(a)

(b)

ISOMETRIC SIDE BRIDGE

Muscles developed: Obliques, quadratus lumborum

Instructions: Lie on the ground on your side with your knees bent and your top arm lying alongside your body. Lift your hips so that your weight is supported by your forearm and knee. Hold this position for 10 seconds, breathing normally. Repeat on the other side. Work up to a 60-second hold; perform one or more repetitions on each side.

Variation: You can make the exercise more difficult by keeping your legs straight and supporting yourself with your feet and forearm (see Lab 5.3) or with your feet and hand (with elbow straight). You can also do this exercise on an exercise ball.

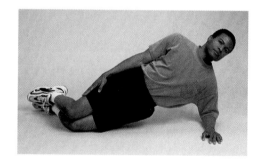

Weight Machines

BENCH PRESS (Chest or Vertical Press)

Muscles developed: Pectoralis major, anterior deltoids, triceps

Instructions: Sit or lie on the seat or bench, depending on the type of machine and the manufacturer's instructions. Your back, hips, and buttocks should be pressed against the machine pads. Place your feet on the floor or the foot supports. **(a)** Grasp the handles with your palms facing away from you; the handles should be aligned with your armpits. **(b)** Push the bars until your arms are fully extended, but don't lock your elbows. Return to the starting position.

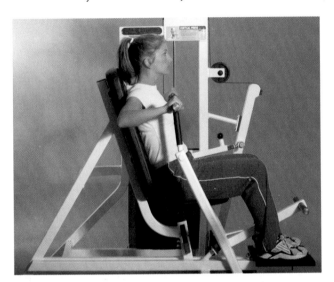

(a)

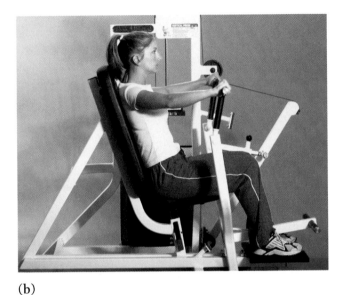

(b)

 EXERCISE 2

LAT PULL

Muscles developed: Latissimus dorsi, biceps

Instructions: Begin in a seated or kneeling position, depending on the type of lat machine and the manufacturer's instructions. **(a)** Grasp the bar of the machine with arms fully extended. **(b)** Slowly pull the weight down until it reaches the top of your chest. Slowly return to the starting position.

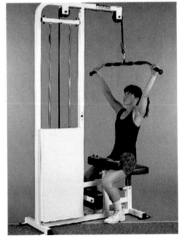

(a)

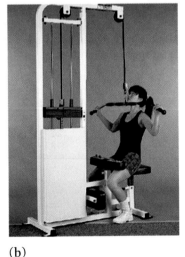

(b)

ASSISTED PULL-UP

Note: This exercise focuses on the same major muscles as the lat pull; choose an appropriate exercise for your program based on your preferences and equipment availability.

Muscles developed: Latissimus dorsi, biceps

Instructions: Set the weight according to the amount of assistance you need to complete a set of pull-ups—the heavier the weight, the more assistance provided. **(a)** Stand or kneel on the assist platform, and grasp the pull-up bar with your elbows fully extended and your palms facing away. **(b)** Pull up until your chin goes above the bar and then return to the starting position.

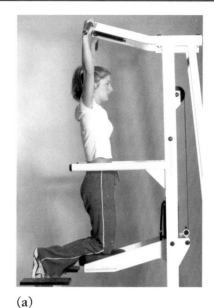

(a)

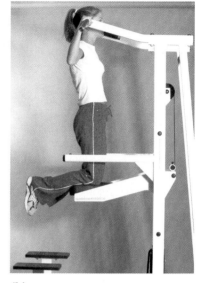

(b)

OVERHEAD PRESS (Shoulder Press)

Muscles developed: Deltoids, trapezius, triceps

Instructions: Adjust the seat so that your feet are flat on the ground and the hand grips are slightly above your shoulders. **(a)** Sit down, facing away from the machine, and grasp the hand grips with your palms facing forward. **(b)** Press the weight upward until your arms are extended. Return to the starting position.

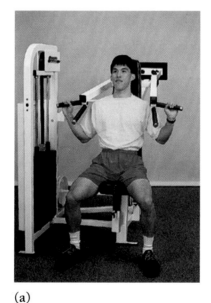

(a)

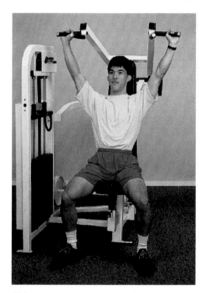

(b)

BICEPS CURL

Muscles developed: Biceps, brachialis

Instructions: (a) Adjust the seat so that your back is straight and your arms rest comfortably against the top and side pads. Place your arms on the support cushions and grasp the hand grips with your palms facing up.
(b) Keeping your upper body still, flex (bend) your elbows until the hand grips almost reach your collarbone. Return to the starting position.

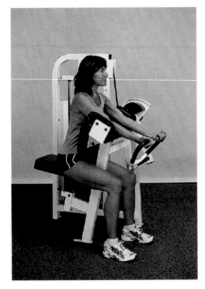

(a)

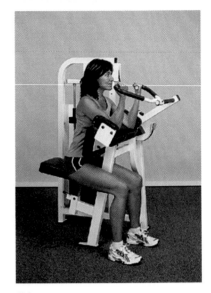

(b)

PULLOVER

Muscles developed: Latissimus dorsi, pectoralis major and minor, triceps, abdominals

Instructions: Adjust the seat so your shoulders are aligned with the cams. Push down on the foot pads with your feet to bring the bar forward until you can place your elbows on the pads. Rest your hands lightly on the bar. If possible, place your feet flat on the floor. (a) To get into the starting position, let your arms go backward as far as possible.
(b) Pull your elbows forward until the bar almost touches your abdomen. Return to the starting position.

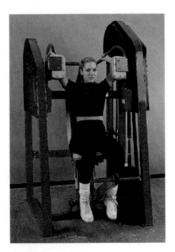

(a)

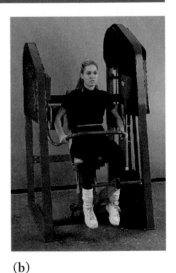

(b)

LATERAL RAISE

Muscles developed: Deltoids, trapezius

Instructions: (**a**) Adjust the seat so the pads rest just above your elbows when your upper arms are at your sides, your elbows are bent, and your forearms are parallel to the floor. Lightly grasp the handles. (**b**) Push outward and up with your arms until the pads are shoulder height. Lead with your elbows rather than trying to lift the bars with your hands. Return to the starting position.

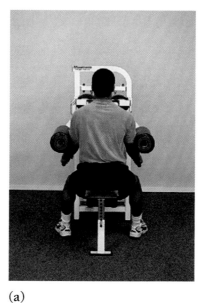
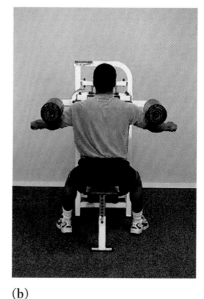

(**a**)   (**b**)

TRICEPS EXTENSION

Muscles developed: Triceps

Instructions: (**a**) Adjust the seat so that your back is straight and your arms rest comfortably against the top and side pads. Place your arms on the support cushions and grasp the hand grips with palms facing inward.
(**b**) Keeping your upper body still, extend your elbows as much as possible. Return to the starting position.

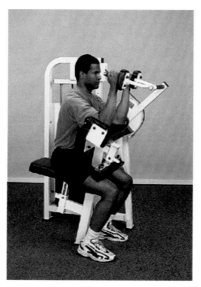
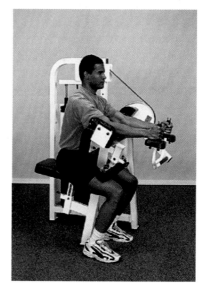

(**a**)   (**b**)

ASSISTED DIP

Note: This exercise focuses on the same major muscles as the triceps extension; choose an appropriate exercise for your program based on your preferences and equipment availability.

Muscles developed: Triceps, deltoid, pectoralis major

Instructions: Set the weight according to the amount of assistance you need to complete a set of dips—the heavier the weight, the more assistance provided. **(a)** Stand or kneel on the assist platform with your body between the dip bar. With your elbows fully extended and palms facing your body, support your weight on your hands. **(b)** Lower your body until your upper arms are approximately parallel with the bars. Then push up until you reach the starting position.

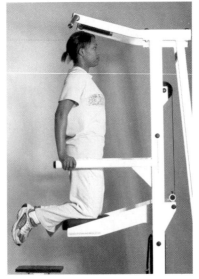

(a)

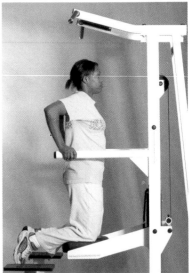

(b)

LEG PRESS

Muscles developed: Gluteus maximus, quadriceps, hamstrings

Instructions: Sit or lie on the seat or bench, depending on the type of machine and the manufacturer's instructions. Your head, back, hips, and buttocks should be pressed against the machine pads. Loosely grasp the handles at the side of the machine. **(a)** Begin with your feet flat on the foot platform about shoulder width apart. Your legs should be fully extended, but do not forcefully lock your knees. **(b)** Slowly lower the weight by bending your knees and flexing your hips until your knees are bent at about a 90-degree angle or your heels start to lift off the foot platform. Then extend your knees and return to the starting position.

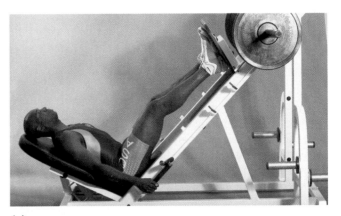

(a)

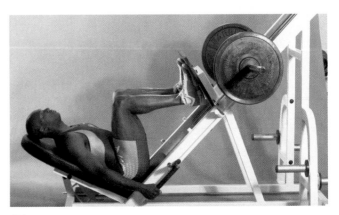

(b)

ABDOMINAL CURL

Muscles developed: Rectus abdominis, internal and external obliques, hip flexors (rectus femoris and iliopsoas muscle group) as stabilizers

Instructions: (a) Adjust the seat so the machine rotates at the level of your navel, the pad rests on your upper chest, and your feet can rest comfortably on the floor. **(b)** Move your trunk forward as far as possible. Return to the starting position.

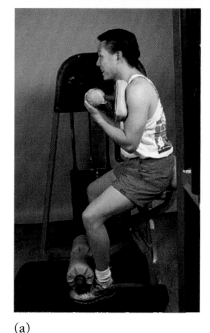

(a)

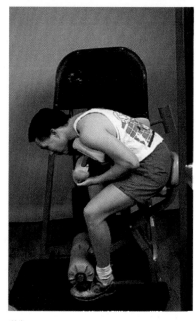

(b)

LEG EXTENSION (Knee Extension)

Muscles developed: Quadriceps

Instructions: (a) Adjust the seat so that the pads rest comfortably on top of your lower shins. Loosely grasp the handles. **(b)** Extend your knees until they are almost straight. Return to the starting position.

Knee extensions cause kneecap pain in some people. If you have kneecap pain during this exercise, check with an orthopedic specialist before repeating it.

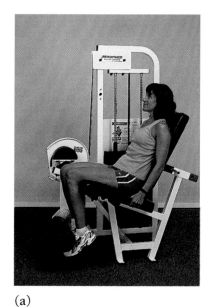

(a)

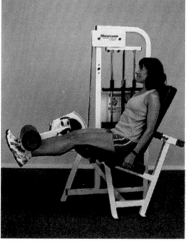

(b)

PRONE LEG CURL (Knee Flexion)

Muscles developed: Hamstrings, gastrocnemius

Instructions: (a) Lie on the front of your body, resting the pads of the machine just below your calf muscles and with your knees just off the edge of the bench. **(b)** Flex your knees until they approach your buttocks. Return to the starting position.

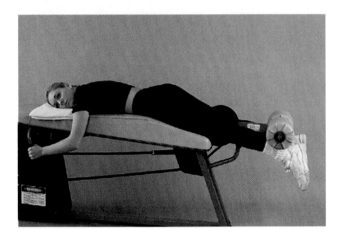

(a)

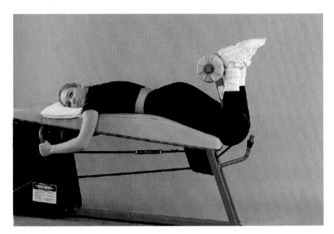

(b)

 EXERCISE 14

HEEL RAISE

Muscles developed: Gastrocnemius, soleus

Instructions: (a) Stand with your head between the pads and one pad on each shoulder. The balls of your feet should be on the platform. Lightly grasp the handles. **(b)** Press down with your toes while lifting your heels. Return to the starting position. Changing the direction your feet are pointing (straight ahead, inward, and outward) will work different portions of your calf muscles.

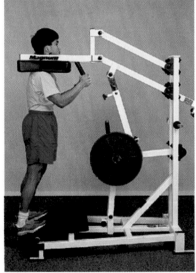

(a)

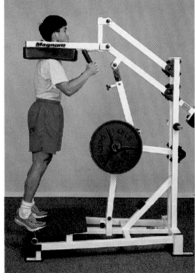

(b)

LOW-BACK MACHINE

(Back Extensions)

Muscles developed: Erector spinae, quadratus lumborum

Instructions: (a) Sit on the seat with your upper legs under the thigh-support pads, your back on the back roller pad, and your feet on the platform. (b) Extend backward until your back is straight. Return to the starting position. Try to keep your spine rigid.

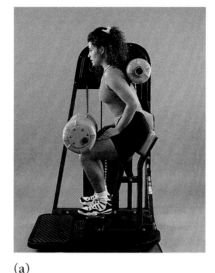
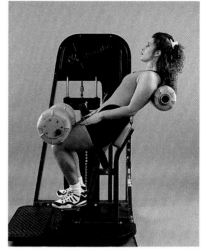

(a) (b)

Tips for Today

Good muscular strength and endurance will enhance your quality of life—both now and in the future. You don't need a complicated or heavy training program to improve strength: Just 1 set of 8–12 repetitions of 8–10 exercises, done 2–3 days per week, is enough for general fitness.

Right now you can

- Think of three things you've done in the past 24 hours that would have been easier or more enjoyable if you increased your level of muscular strength and endurance. Examples might be carrying your books, climbing stairs, or playing recreational sports. Begin to visualize improvements in your quality of life that could come from increased muscular strength and endurance.

- Do a set of static (isometric) exercises. If you're sitting, try tightening your abdominal muscles as you press your lower back into the seat or work your arms by placing the palms of your hands on top of your thighs and pressing down. Hold the contraction for 6 seconds and do 5–10 repetitions; don't hold your breath.

- Make an appointment with a trainer at your campus or neighborhood fitness facility. A trainer can help you put together an appropriate weight training program and introduce you to the equipment at the facility.

- Invest in an inexpensive set of free weights.

SUMMARY

- Hypertrophy, or increased muscle fiber size, occurs when weight training causes the number of myofibrils to increase; total muscle size thereby increases. Strength also increases through muscle learning.

- Improvements in muscular strength and endurance lead to enhanced physical performance, protection against injury, improved body composition, better self-image, improved muscle and bone health with aging, and reduced risk of chronic disease.

- Muscular strength can be assessed by determining the amount of weight that can be lifted in one repetition of an exercise; muscular endurance can be assessed by determining the number of repetitions of a particular exercise that can be performed.

- Static (isometric) exercises (contraction without movement) are most useful when a person is recovering from an injury or surgery or needs to overcome weak points in a range of motion.

- Dynamic (isotonic) exercises involve contraction that results in movement. The two most common types are constant resistance (free weights) and variable resistance (many weight machines).

- Free weights and weight machines are basically equally effective in producing fitness, although machines tend to be safer.

- Lifting heavy weights for only a few repetitions helps develop strength. Lifting lighter weights for more repetitions helps develop muscular endurance.

- A strength training program for general fitness includes at least 1 set of 8–12 repetitions (enough to cause fatigue) of 8–10 exercises, along with warm-up

COMMON QUESTIONS ANSWERED

How long must I weight train before I begin to see changes in my body? You will increase strength very rapidly during the early stages of a strength training program, primarily the result of muscle learning (the increased ability of the nervous system to recruit muscle fibers to exert force). Actual changes in muscle size usually begin after about 6–8 weeks of training.

I am concerned about my body composition. Will I gain weight if I do resistance exercises? Your weight probably will not change significantly as a result of a general fitness program: 1 set of 8–12 repetitions of 8–10 exercises. You will tend to increase muscle mass and lose body fat, so your weight will stay about the same. You may notice a change in how your clothes fit, however, because muscle is more dense than fat. Men will tend to build larger muscles than women because of the tissue-building effects of testosterone. Increased muscle mass will help you control body fat. Muscle increases your metabolism, which means you burn more calories every day. If you combine resistance exercises with endurance exercises, you will be on your way to developing a healthier body composition. Concentrate on fat loss rather than weight loss.

Do I need more protein in my diet when I train with weights? No. Although there is some evidence that power athletes involved in heavy training have a higher-than-normal protein requirement, there is no reason for most people to consume extra protein. Most Americans take in more protein than they need, so even if there is an increased protein need during heavy training, it is probably supplied by the average diet. (See Chapter 8 for more on dietary needs of athletes and specific recommendations for protein intake.)

What causes muscle soreness the day or two following a weight training workout? The muscle pain you feel a day or two after a heavy weight training workout is caused by injury to the muscle fibers and surrounding connective tissue. Contrary to popular belief, delayed-onset muscle soreness is not caused by lactic acid buildup. Scientists believe that injury to muscle fibers causes inflammation, which in turn causes the release of chemicals that break down part of the muscle tissue and cause pain. After a bout of intense exercise that causes muscle injury and delayed-onset muscle soreness, the muscles produce protective proteins that prevent soreness during future workouts. If you don't work out regularly, you lose these protective proteins and become susceptible to muscle soreness again.

Will strength training improve my sports performance? Strength developed in the weight room does not automatically increase your power in sports such as skiing, tennis, or cycling. Hitting a forehand in tennis and making a turn on skis are precise skills that require coordination between your nervous system and muscles. In skilled people, movements become reflex—you don't think about them when you do them. Increasing strength can disturb this coordination. Only by simultaneously practicing a sport and improving fitness can you expect to become more powerful in the skill. Practice helps you integrate your new strength with your skills, which makes you more powerful. Consequently, you can hit the ball harder in tennis or make more graceful turns on the ski slopes. (Refer to Chapter 2 for more on the concept of specificity of physical training.)

Will I improve faster if I train every day? No. Your muscles need time to recover between training sessions. Doing resistance exercises every day will cause you to become overtrained, which will increase your chance of injury and impede your progress. If you find that your strength training program has reached a plateau, try one of these strategies:

- Train less frequently. If you are currently training the same muscle groups three or more times per week, you may not be allowing your muscles to fully recover from intense workouts.

- Change exercises. Using different exercises for a particular muscle group may stimulate further strength development.

- Vary the load and number of repetitions. Try increasing or decreasing the loads you are using and changing the number of repetitions accordingly.

- Vary the number of sets. If you have been performing 1 set of each exercise, add sets.

- If you are training alone, find a motivated training partner. A partner can encourage you and assist you with difficult lifts, forcing you to work harder.

If I stop weight training, will my muscles turn to fat? No. Fat and muscle are two different kinds of tissue, and one cannot turn into the other. Muscles that aren't used become smaller (atrophy), and body fat may increase if caloric intake exceeds calories burned. Although the result of inactivity may be smaller muscles and more fat, the change is caused by two separate processes.

Should I wear a weight belt when I lift? Until recently, most experts advised people to wear weight belts. However, several studies have shown that weight belts do not prevent back injuries and may, in fact, increase the risk of injury by encouraging people to lift more weight than they are capable of lifting with

and cool-down periods; the program should be carried out 2–3 times a week.

- Safety guidelines for strength training include using proper technique, using spotters and collars when necessary, and taking care of injuries.

- Supplements or drugs that are promoted as instant or quick "cures" usually don't work and are either dangerous or expensive or both.

ⅤⅤ *Fit and Well* **Online Learning Center** (www.mhhe.com/fahey)

Use the learning objectives, study guide questions, and glossary flashcards to review key terms and concepts and prepare for exams. You can extend your knowledge of muscular strength and endurance and gain experience in using the Internet as a resource by completing the activities and checking out the Web

good form. Although wearing a belt may allow you to lift more weight in some lifts, you may not get the full benefit of your program because use of a weight belt reduces the effectiveness of the workout on the muscles that help support your spine.

Do abdominal machines advertised on television really work?
Studies comparing major types of abdominal exercises have found that "ab" machines are less effective than curl-ups and sit-ups for developing the abdominal muscles. There is no advantage to using an abdominal machine as compared to performing crunches—and a machine may cost $50 or more. A 2004 review of abdominal machines by *Consumer Reports* concluded that no infomercial machine was worth the money and suggested that consumers stick to crunches, possibly with an exercise ball for added difficulty.

Can activities such as yoga, tai chi chuan, and Pilates be used to build muscular strength and endurance? Each of these forms of exercise involve carefully controlled body movements and precise body positions, so they can help build muscular strength and endurance—although probably not to the degree of traditional weight training exercises.

- Yoga involves a series of physical postures that stretch, strengthen, and relax different parts of the body. Some forms of yoga are much more vigorous than others but most emphasize breathing, stretching, body awareness, and balance.

- Taijíquan (pronounced *tie jee choo-en*), commonly referred to as "tai chi chuan" or simply "tai chi," is a martial art consisting of a series of slow, fluid, elegant movements that promote relaxation and concentration as well as the development of body awareness, balance, and muscular strength.

- Pilates (*pil LAH teez*) was developed by German gymnast and boxer George Pilates early in the twentieth century. It typically involves the use of specially designed resistance training devices, although some classes feature just mat or floor work. Pilates focuses on working the core muscles in the back, abdomen, and buttocks; the emphasis is on concentration, control, movement flow, and breathing.

To obtain the greatest benefit from these techniques with the least risk of injury, it's best to begin by finding a qualified instructor. See Chapter 10 for more on the use of yoga and tai chi specifically for stress management.

What is core strength training? Most body movements involve several joints and many muscles, either as prime movers, assist muscles, stabilizers, or antagonists. The link and coordination among these movements in called the kinetic chain. The key to most linked movements is the core, also called the trunk or midsection, consisting of the abdominal muscles, deep lateral stabilizing muscles, and the spinal extensor muscles. The core is critical because it transmits forces between the lower and upper body and helps stabilize the spine. Building strength and endurance in these muscle groups is key to most sports movements, to many activities of daily living, and to a healthy lower back.

What exercises build core strength and endurance? You can build core strength by forcing the trunk muscles to stabilize the spine while standing, sitting, or lying down. Examples of simple, low-tech core strengthening exercises include sitting on an exercise ball and keeping it from falling over and holding a push-up position on your forearms for 15 seconds. Whole body exercises are particularly effective; examples include curl-ups on an exercise ball, side bridges, spine extensions, squats, and standing bench presses on a crossover pulley. Pilates, a form of exercise discussed in this section, often focuses on the core muscles. The program of strength and stretching exercises for low-back health presented in Chapter 5 also features many exercises that help build core strength.

What is circuit training? Circuit training is a system of organizing a series of exercises that are performed consecutively. Exercises for different muscle groups follow each other, providing a well-rounded workout and helping to delay the onset of fatigue. By moving directly from one exercise to the next, you can keep your heart rate in your training zone and so train both your muscles and your cardiorespiratory system.

Circuit training can be done at home using calisthenic exercises and/or exercises with free weights, or circuits can be put together at a fitness center. A circuit may include just strength training exercises or may alternate between weight training machines and cardiorespiratory endurance stations. For example, you may perform a set of bench presses followed by 3 minutes on a treadmill and then a set of shoulder presses. Circuit training can be an effective method for building cardiorespiratory endurance and muscular strength during the same workout. It is important to warm up thoroughly before a circuit training workout and to cool down after. Other safety tips include maintaining proper form for each exercise (not rushing), not lifting beyond the limits of your strength, and keeping your heart rate within your target zone. A sample calisthenics circuit-training program is included on the *Fit and Well* Online Learning Center.

links for the topics in Chapter 4 marked with the World Wide Web icon. For this chapter, Internet activities explore the benefits of muscular strength and endurance, different exercises that build strength, and strategies for evaluating supplements; there are Web links for the Critical Consumer box on dietary supplements and the chapter as a whole.

Daily Fitness and Nutrition Journal

Complete the muscular strength and endurance portion of the program plan by setting goals and selecting exercises. Fill in the information for the specific exercises you will perform, including which muscles they develop, how much resistance you plan to start with, and the number of reps and sets you plan to perform.

HealthQuest

If you haven't already done so, complete the How Fit Are You? section of the Wellness Activities in the fitness module of HealthQuest. This section provides an overview of your muscular strength and endurance status based on your current level of strength and endurance and your strength training habits.

Books

Bahrke, M., and C. Yesalis. 2002. *Performance-Enhancing Substances in Sport and Exercise.* Champaign, Ill.: Human Kinetics. *Provides up-to-date coverage of the issues surrounding supplements as well as the current state of research on major types of supplements and their effects on athletic performance.*

Delavier, F. 2001. *Strength Training Anatomy.* Champaign, Ill.: Human Kinetics. *Includes exercises for all major muscle groups as well as full anatomical pictures of the muscular system. A matching volume for women (Women's Strength Training Anatomy) was published in 2003.*

Fahey, T. D. 2004. *Basic Weight Training for Men and Women,* 5th ed. New York: McGraw-Hill. *A practical guide to developing training programs, using free weights, tailored to individual needs.*

Graves, J. E., and B. A. Franklin. 2001. *Resistance Training for Health and Rehabilitation.* Champaign, Ill.: Human Kinetics. *Provides detailed information on resistance training for a variety of goals.*

Nelson, M. 2000. *Strong Women Stay Young.* Rev. ed. New York: Bantam Books. *A program of strengthening exercises geared toward first-time exercisers, written by a Tufts University professor.*

▼▲▼ Organizations and Web Sites

American College of Sports Medicine Position Stand: Progression Models in Resistance Training for Healthy Adults. Provides an in-depth look at strategies for setting up a strength training program and making progress based on individual program goals; look for the February 2002 Position Stand.

  http://www.acsm-msse.org

Exercise: A Guide from the National Institute on Aging. Provides practical advice on fitness for seniors; includes animated instructions for specific weight training exercises.

  http://www.nia.nih.gov/exercisebook

Georgia State University: Strength Training. Provides information about the benefits of strength training and how to develop a safe and effective program; also includes illustrations of a variety of exercises.

  http://www.gsu.edu/~wwwfit/strength.html

Human Anatomy On-line. Provides text, illustrations, and animation about the muscular system, nerve-muscle connections, muscular contraction, and other topics.

  http://www.innerbody.com/htm/body.html

Kansas State University: Nutritional Supplements for Athletes. Provides information and links to recent research findings about specific supplements.

  http://www.oznet.ksu.edu/nutrition/supplements.htm

National Strength and Conditioning Association. Professional organization that focuses on strength development for fitness and athletic performance.

  http://www.nsca-lift.org

University of California, San Diego/Muscle Physiology Home Page. Provides an introduction to muscle physiology, including information about types of muscle fibers and energy cycles.

  http://muscle.ucsd.edu

University of Michigan/Muscles in Action. Interactive descriptions of muscle movements.

  http://www.med.umich.edu/lrc/Hypermuscle/Hyper.html

See also the listings in Chapter 2.

SELECTED BIBLIOGRAPHY

Acacio, B. D., et al. 2004. Pharmacokinetics of dehydroepiandrosterone and its metabolites after long-term daily oral administration to healthy young men. *Fertility and Sterility* 81(3): 595–604.

American College of Sports Medicine. 2002. Position Stand: Progression models in resistance training for healthy adults. *Medicine and Science in Sports and Exercise* 34(2): 364–380.

American College of Sports Medicine. 2001. *ACSM's Resource Manual for Guidelines for Exercise Testing and Prescription,* 4th ed. Philadelphia: Lippincott Williams and Wilkins.

American College of Sports Medicine. 2001. Overtraining with resistance exercise. *Current Comment,* January.

American College of Sports Medicine. 2001. Rest during resistance exercise. *Current Comment,* May.

Bhasin, S., L. Woodhouse, and T. W. Storer. 2001. Proof of the effect of testosterone on skeletal muscle. *Journal of Endocrinology* 170(1): 27–38.

Brooks, G. A., et al. 2005. *Exercise Physiology: Human Bioenergetics and Its Applications.*

Centers for Disease Control and Prevention. 2004. Strength training among adults aged ≥65 years. *Morbidity and Mortality Weekly Report* 53(2): 25–28.

Cronin, J. B., P. J. McNair, and R. N. Marshall. 2003. Force-velocity analysis of strength-training techniques and load: implications for training strategy and research. *Journal of Strength and Conditioning Research* 17:148–155.

Cussler E. C., et al. 2003. Weight lifted in strength training predicts bone change in postmenopausal women. *Medicine and Science in Sports and Exercise* 35:10–17.

Durell, D. L., T. J. Pujol, and J. T. Barnes. 2003. A survey of the scientific data and training methods utilized by collegiate strength and conditioning coaches. *Journal of Strength and Conditioning Research* 17:368–373.

Earle, R. W., and T. R. Baechle, eds. 2004. *NSCA's Essentials of Personal Training.* Champaign, Ill: Human Kinetics.

Folland, J. P., et al. 2001. Acute muscle damage as a stimulus for training-induced gains in strength. *Medicine and Science in Sports and Exercise* 33(7): 1200–1205.

Food and Drug Administration. 2004. *Questions and Answers: Androstenedione* (http://cfsan.fda.gov/~androqa.html; retrieved April 8, 2004).

Green, G. A., D. H. Catlin, and B. Starcevic. 2001. Analysis of over-the-counter dietary supplements. *Clinical Journal of Sports Medicine* 11(4): 254–259.

Izquierdo, M., et al. 2002. Effects of creatine supplementation on muscle power, endurance, and sprint performance. *Medicine and Science in Sports and Exercise* 34(2): 332–343.

Kraemer W. J., et al. 2002. Detraining produces minimal changes in physical performance and hormonal variables in recreationally strength-trained men. *Journal of Strength and Conditioning Research* 16:373–382.

Liemohn, W., and G. Pariser. 2002. Core strength: Implications for fitness and low back pain. *ACSM's Health & Fitness Journal,* September/October.

McCarthy, J. P., M. A. Pozniak, and J. C. Agre. 2002. Neuromuscular adaptations to concurrent strength and endurance training. *Medicine and Science in Sports and Exercise* 34(3): 511–519.

Millar, L. 2004. Training your abs. *ACSM Fit Society Page,* Spring.

Namdar, M. 2003. Caffeine decreases coronary flow reserve at exercise in healthy volunteers. *Journal of the American College of Cardiology* 19; 41(6 Suppl B): 460.

Pollock, M. L., et al. 2000. AHA Science Advisory: Resistance exercise in individuals with and without cardiovascular disease. *Circulation* 101:828–833.

Rhea M. R., et al. 2002. Three sets of weight training superior to 1 set with equal intensity for eliciting strength. *Journal of Strength and Conditioning Research* 16:525–529.

Ryan, A. S., et al. 2000. Changes in plasma leptin and insulin action with resistive training in postmenopausal women. *International Journal of Obesity and Related Metabolic Disorders* 24(1): 27–32.

Shekelle, P. G., et al. 2003. Efficacy and safety of ephedra and ephedrine for weight loss and athletic performance: A meta-analysis. *Journal of the American Medical Association* 289(12): 1537–1545.

Trockel, M. T., M. D. Barnes, and D. L. Eggert. 2000. Health-related variables and academic performance among college students: Implications for sleep and other behaviors. *Journal of American College Health* 49(3): 125–131.

TV exercise devices. 2004. *Consumer Reports,* January.

LAB 4.1 *Assessing Your Current Level of Muscular Strength*

  WW

For best results, don't do any strenuous weight training within 48 hours of any test. Use great caution when completing 1 RM tests; do not take the maximum bench press or leg press test if you have any injuries to your shoulders, elbows, back, hips, or knees. In addition, do not take these tests until you have had at least one month of weight training experience.

The Maximum Bench Press Test

Equipment

1. Universal Gym Dynamic Variable Resistance machine
2. Weight scale

If free weights are used, the following equipment is needed:

1. Flat bench (with or without racks)
2. Barbell
3. Assorted weight plates, with collars to hold them in place
4. One or two spotters
5. Weight scale

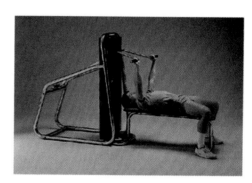

Maximum bench press test.

Preparation

Try a few bench presses with a small amount of weight so you can practice your technique, warm up your muscles, and, if you use free weights, coordinate your movements with those of your spotters. Weigh yourself and record the results.

Body weight: _____ lb

Instructions

1. Set the machine for a weight that is lower than the amount you believe you can lift. For free weights, men should begin with a weight about 2/3 of their body weight; women should begin with the weight of just the bar (45 lb).

2. Lie on the bench with your feet firmly on the floor. If you are using a weight machine, grasp the handles with palms away from you; the tops of the handles should be aligned with the tops of your armpits.

   If you are using free weights, grasp the bar slightly wider than shoulder width with your palms away from you. If you have one spotter, she or he should stand directly behind the bench; if you have two spotters, they should stand to the side, one at each end of the barbell. Lower the bar to your chest in preparation for the lift.

3. Push the bars or barbell until your arms are fully extended. Exhale as you lift. If you are using free weights, the weight moves from a low point at the chest to a high point over the chin. Keep your feet firmly on the floor, don't arch your back, and push the weight evenly with your right and left arms. Don't bounce the weight on your chest.

4. Rest for several minutes, then repeat the lift with a heavier weight. It will probably take several attempts to determine the maximum amount of weight you can lift (1 RM).

   1 RM: _____ lb   Check one : _____ Universal _____ Free weights _____ Other

5. If you used free weights, convert your free weights bench press score to an estimated value for 1 RM on the Universal bench press using the appropriate formula:

   Males: Estimated Universal 1 RM = (1.016 × free weights 1 RM _____ lb) + 18.41 = _____ lb

   Females: Estimated Universal 1 RM = (0.848 × free weights 1 RM _____ lb) + 21.37 = _____ lb

Rating Your Bench Press Result

1. Divide your Universal 1 RM value by your body weight.

   1 RM _____ lb ÷ body weight _____ lb = _____

2. Find this ratio in the table below to determine your bench press strength rating. Record the rating here and in the chart at the end of this lab.

   Bench press strength rating: _____

Strength Ratings for the Maximum Bench Press Test

Pounds Lifted/Body Weight (lb)

Men	Very Poor	Poor	Fair	Good	Excellent	Superior
Age: Under 20	Below 0.89	0.89–1.05	1.06–1.18	1.19–1.33	1.34–1.75	Above 1.75
20–29	Below 0.88	0.88–0.98	0.99–1.13	1.14–1.31	1.32–1.62	Above 1.62
30–39	Below 0.78	0.78–0.87	0.88–0.97	0.98–1.11	1.12–1.34	Above 1.34
40–49	Below 0.72	0.72–0.79	0.80–0.87	0.88–0.99	1.00–1.19	Above 1.19
50–59	Below 0.63	0.63–0.70	0.71–0.78	0.79–0.89	0.90–1.04	Above 1.04
60 and over	Below 0.57	0.57–0.65	0.66–0.71	0.72–0.81	0.82–0.93	Above 0.93
Women						
Age: Under 20	Below 0.53	0.53–0.57	0.58–0.64	0.65–0.76	0.77–0.87	Above 0.87
20–29	Below 0.51	0.51–0.58	0.59–0.69	0.70–0.79	0.80–1.00	Above 1.00
30–39	Below 0.47	0.47–0.52	0.53–0.59	0.60–0.69	0.70–0.81	Above 0.81
40–49	Below 0.43	0.43–0.49	0.50–0.53	0.54–0.61	0.62–0.76	Above 0.76
50–59	Below 0.39	0.39–0.43	0.44–0.47	0.48–0.54	0.55–0.67	Above 0.67
60 and over	Below 0.38	0.38–0.42	0.43–0.46	0.47–0.53	0.54–0.71	Above 0.71

SOURCE: Based on norms from the Cooper Institute for Aerobics Research, Dallas, Texas; from *The Physical Fitness Specialist Manual*, Revised 2002. Used with permission.

The Maximum Leg Press Test

Equipment

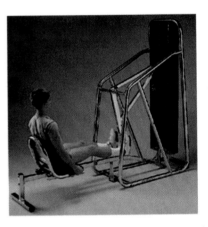

1. Universal Gym Dynamic Variable Resistance leg press machine. (If you're using a Universal Gym leg press with two sets of pedals, use the lower pedals.)
2. Weight scale

The ratings for this test were developed using the Universal Gym Dynamic Variable Resistance machine; results will be somewhat less accurate if the test is performed on another type of machine.

Preparation

Try a few leg presses with the machine set for a small amount of weight so you can practice your technique and warm up your muscles. Weigh yourself and record the results.

Maximum leg press test.

Body weight: _____ lb

Instructions

1. Set the machine for a weight that is lower than the amount you believe you can press.
2. Adjust the seat so that your knees are bent at a 70-degree angle to start.
3. Grasp the side handlebars and push with your legs until your knees are fully extended.
4. Rest for several minutes, then repeat the press with a higher weight setting. It will probably take several attempts to determine the maximum amount of weight you can press.

   1 RM: _____ lb

Rating Your Leg Press Result

1. Divide your 1 RM value by your body weight.

   1 RM _____ lb ÷ body weight _____ lb = _____

2. Find this ratio in the table below to determine your leg press strength rating. Record the rating below and in the chart at the end of this lab.

   Leg press strength rating: _____

Strength Ratings for the Maximum Leg Press Test

Pounds Lifted/Body Weight (lb)

Men	Very Poor	Poor	Fair	Good	Excellent	Superior
Age: Under 20	Below 1.70	1.70–1.89	1.90–2.03	2.04–2.27	2.28–2.81	Above 2.81
20–29	Below 1.63	1.63–1.82	1.83–1.96	1.97–2.12	2.13–2.39	Above 2.39
30–39	Below 1.52	1.52–1.64	1.65–1.76	1.77–1.92	1.93–2.19	Above 2.19
40–49	Below 1.44	1.44–1.56	1.57–1.67	1.68–1.81	1.82–2.01	Above 2.01
50–59	Below 1.32	1.32–1.45	1.46–1.57	1.58–1.70	1.71–1.89	Above 1.89
60 and over	Below 1.25	1.25–1.37	1.38–1.48	1.49–1.61	1.62–1.79	Above 1.79
Women						
Age: Under 20	Below 1.22	1.22–1.37	1.38–1.58	1.59–1.70	1.71–1.87	Above 1.87
20–29	Below 1.22	1.22–1.36	1.37–1.49	1.50–1.67	1.68–1.97	Above 1.97
30–39	Below 1.09	1.09–1.20	1.21–1.32	1.33–1.46	1.47–1.67	Above 1.67
40–49	Below 1.02	1.02–1.12	1.13–1.22	1.23–1.36	1.37–1.56	Above 1.56
50–59	Below 0.88	0.88–0.98	0.99–1.09	1.10–1.24	1.25–1.42	Above 1.42
60 and over	Below 0.85	0.85–0.92	0.93–1.03	1.04–1.17	1.18–1.42	Above 1.42

SOURCE: Based on norms from the Cooper Institute for Aerobics Research, Dallas, Texas; from *The Physical Fitness Specialist Manual*, Revised 2002. Used with permission.

Predicting 1 RM from Submaximal Lifts

Values for 1 RM can be predicted by performing multiple repetitions using a submaximal weight. Although less accurate than direct measurement of 1 RM, this method may be safer for some people. To calculate 1 RM using this method, choose a weight with which you can perform about 5 repetitions. Follow the instructions given in the maximum bench press and maximum leg press test descriptions for warming up and performing the lifts—but do as many repetitions as you can using the amount of resistance you have chosen. Enter your resistance and number of repetitions into the formula below to predict your 1 RM on these tests. Then, enter your 1 RM values into the appropriate formula in the maximum bench press and maximum leg press tests to obtain your rating.

Bench press: 1 RM = (resistance _____ lb ÷ 2.2 lb/kg) ÷ (1.0278 − (0.0278 × number of repetitions _____))
= _____ kg × 2.2 lb/kg = _____ lb

Leg press: 1 RM = (resistance _____ lb ÷ 2.2 lb/kg) ÷ (1.0278 − (0.0278 × number of repetitions _____))
= _____ kg × 2.2 lb/kg = _____ lb

SOURCE: Brzycki, M. 1993. Strength testing: Predicting a one-rep max from a reps-to-fatigue. *Journal of Physical Education, Recreation, and Dance* 64:88–90.

Hand Grip Strength Test

Equipment   Grip strength dynamometer

Preparation   If necessary, adjust the hand grip size on the dynamometer into a position that is comfortable for you; then lock the grip in place. The second joint of your fingers should fit snugly under the handle of the dynamometer.

Instructions

1. Stand with the hand to be tested first at your side, away from your body. The dynamometer should be in line with your forearm and held at the level of your thigh. Squeeze the dynamometer as hard as possible without moving your arm; exhale as you squeeze. During the test, don't let the dynamometer touch your body or any other object.

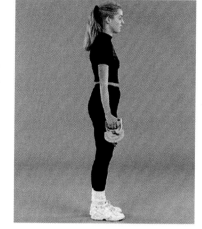

Hand grip strength test.

2. Perform two trials with each hand. Rest for about a minute between trials. Record the scores for each hand to the nearest kilogram.

Right hand: Trial 1: _____ kg   Trial 2: _____ kg   Right hand best trial _____ kg

Left hand: Trial 1: _____ kg   Trial 2: _____ kg   Left hand best trial _____ kg

(Scores on the dynamometer should be given in kilograms. If the dynamometer you are using gives scores in pounds, convert pounds to kilograms by dividing your score by 2.2.)

Rating Your Hand Grip Strength

Refer to the table for a rating of your grip strength. Record the rating below and in the chart at the end of this lab.

Total score (sum of the best trial for each hand) _____ kg   Rating for hand grip strength: _____

Grip Strength* (kg)

Men	Needs Improvement	Fair	Good	Very Good	Excellent
Age: 15–19	Below 84	84–94	95–102	103–112	Above 112
20–29	Below 97	97–105	106–112	113–123	Above 123
30–39	Below 97	97–104	105–112	113–122	Above 122
40–49	Below 94	94–101	102–109	110–118	Above 118
50–59	Below 87	87–95	96–101	102–109	Above 109
60–69	Below 79	79–85	86–92	93–101	Above 101
Women					
Age: 15–19	Below 54	54–58	59–63	64–70	Above 70
20–29	Below 55	55–60	61–64	65–70	Above 70
30–39	Below 56	56–60	61–65	66–72	Above 72
40–49	Below 55	55–58	59–64	65–72	Above 72
50–59	Below 51	51–54	55–58	59–64	Above 64
60–69	Below 48	48–50	51–53	54–59	Above 59

*Combined right and left hand grip strength.

SOURCE: *The Canadian Physical Activity, Fitness and Lifestyle Appraisal: CSEP's Plan for Healthy Active Living,* 2d ed., 1998. Reprinted by permission from the Canadian Society for Exercise Physiology.

Summary of Results

Maximum bench press test: Weight pressed: _____ lb   Rating: _____

Maximum leg press test: Weight pressed: _____ lb   Rating: _____

Hand grip strength test: Total score: _____ kg   Rating: _____

Remember that muscular strength is specific: Your ratings may vary considerably for different parts of your body.

Using Your Results

How did you score? Are you at all surprised by your rating for muscular strength? Are you satisfied with your current rating?

If you're not satisfied, set a realistic goal for improvement: _____

Are you satisfied with your current level of muscular strength as evidenced in your daily life—for example, your ability to lift objects, climb stairs, and engage in sports and recreational activities?

If you're not satisfied, set some realistic goals for improvement:

What should you do next? Enter the results of this lab in the Preprogram Assessment column in Appendix D. If you've set goals for improvement, begin planning your strength training program by completing the plan in Lab 4.3. After several weeks of your program, complete this lab again and enter the results in the Postprogram Assessment column of Appendix D. How do the results compare?

LAB 4.2 *Assessing Your Current Level of Muscular Endurance*   V̄iW

For best results, don't do any strenuous weight training within 48 hours of any test. To assess endurance of the abdominal muscles, perform the curl-up test. To assess endurance of muscles in the upper body, perform the push-up test.

 The Curl-Up Test

Equipment

1. Four 6-inch strips of self-stick Velcro or heavy tape
2. Ruler
3. Partner
4. Mat (optional)

Preparation

Affix the strips of Velcro or long strips of tape on the mat or testing surface. Place the strips 3 inches apart.

Instructions

1. Start by lying on your back on the floor or mat, arms straight and by your sides, shoulders relaxed, palms down and on the floor, and fingers straight. Adjust your position so that the longest fingertip of each hand touches the end of the near strip of Velcro or tape. Your knees should be bent about 90 degrees, with your feet about 12–18 inches from your buttocks.

2. To perform a curl-up, flex your spine while sliding your fingers across the floor until the fingertips of each hand reach the second strip of Velcro or tape. Then, return to the starting position; the shoulders must be returned to touch the mat between curl-ups, but the head need not touch. Shoulders must remain relaxed throughout the curl-up, and feet and buttocks must stay on the floor. Breathe easily, exhaling during the lift phase of the curl-up; do not hold your breath.

3. Once your partner says "go," perform as many curl-ups as you can at a steady pace with correct form. Your partner counts the curl-ups you perform and calls a stop to the test if she or he notices any incorrect form or drop in your pace.

   Number of curl-ups: _____

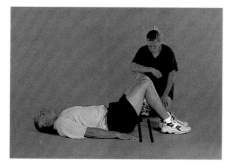

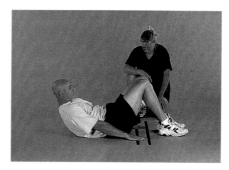

Curl-up test: (a) starting position.   (b) Curl-up.

Rating Your Curl-Up Test Result

Your score is the number of completed curl-ups. Refer to the appropriate portion of the table below for a rating of your abdominal muscular endurance. Record your rating below and in the chart at the end of this lab.

Rating: _____

Ratings for the Curl-Up Test

Number of Curl-Ups

Men	Very Poor	Poor	Average	Good	Excellent	Superior
Age: 16–19	Below 48	48–57	58–64	65–74	75–93	Above 93
20–29	Below 46	46–54	55–63	64–74	75–93	Above 93
30–39	Below 40	40–47	48–55	56–64	65–81	Above 81
40–49	Below 38	38–45	46–53	54–62	63–79	Above 79
50–59	Below 36	36–43	44–51	52–60	61–77	Above 77
60–69	Below 33	33–40	41–48	49–57	58–74	Above 74
Women						
Age: 16–19	Below 42	42–50	51–58	59–67	68–84	Above 84
20–29	Below 41	41–51	52–57	58–66	67–83	Above 83
30–39	Below 38	38–47	48–56	57–66	67–85	Above 85
40–49	Below 36	36–45	46–54	55–64	65–83	Above 83
50–59	Below 34	34–43	44–52	53–62	63–81	Above 81
60–69	Below 31	31–40	41–49	50–59	60–78	Above 78

SOURCE: Ratings based on norms calculated from data collected by Robert Lualhati on 4545 college students, 16–80 years of age, at Skyline College, San Bruno, California. Used with permission.

The Push-Up Test

Equipment: Mat or towel (optional)

Preparation

In this test, you will perform either standard push-ups or modified push-ups, in which you support yourself with your knees. The Cooper Institute developed the ratings for this test with men performing push-ups and women performing modified push-ups. (Biologically, males tend to be stronger than females; the modified technique reduces the need for upper-body strength in a test of muscular endurance.) Therefore, for an accurate assessment of upper-body endurance, men should perform standard push-ups and women should perform modified push-ups. (However, in using push-ups as part of a strength training program, individuals should choose the technique most appropriate for increasing their level of strength and endurance—regardless of gender.)

Instructions

1. *For push-ups:* Start in the push-up position with your body supported by your hands and feet. *For modified push-ups:* Start in the modified push-up position with your body supported by your hands and knees. *For both positions,* your arms and your back should be straight and your fingers pointed forward.

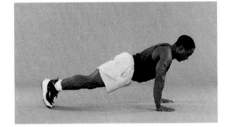
(a) Push-up.

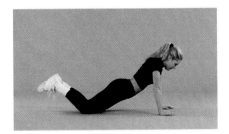
(b) Modified push-up.

2. Lower your chest to the floor with your back straight, and then return to the starting position.

3. Perform as many push-ups or modified push-ups as you can without stopping.

    Number of push-ups: _____ or number of modified push-ups: _____

Rating Your Push-Up Test Result

Your score is the number of completed push-ups or modified push-ups. Refer to the appropriate portion of the table below for a rating of your upper-body endurance. Record your rating below and in the chart at the end of this lab.

Rating: _____

Ratings for the Push-Up and Modified Push-Up Tests

Men	Very Poor	Poor	Fair	Good	Excellent	Superior
			Number of Push-Ups			
Age: 18–29	Below 22	22–28	29–36	37–46	47–61	Above 61
30–39	Below 17	17–23	24–29	30–38	39–51	Above 51
40–49	Below 11	11–17	18–23	24–29	30–39	Above 39
50–59	Below 9	9–12	13–18	19–24	25–38	Above 38
60 and over	Below 6	6–9	10–17	18–22	23–27	Above 27

Women	Very Poor	Poor	Fair	Good	Excellent	Superior
			Number of Modified Push-Ups			
Age: 18–29	Below 17	17–22	23–29	30–35	36–44	Above 44
30–39	Below 11	11–18	19–23	24–30	31–38	Above 38
40–49	Below 6	6–12	13–17	18–23	24–32	Above 32
50–59	Below 6	6–11	12–16	17–20	21–27	Above 27
60 and over	Below 2	2–4	5–11	12–14	15–19	Above 19

SOURCE: Based on norms from the Cooper Institute for Aerobics Research, Dallas, Texas; from *The Physical Fitness Specialist Manual*, Revised 2002. Used with permission.

Summary of Results

Curl-up test: Number of curl-ups: _____ Rating: _____

Push-up test: Number of push-ups: _____ Rating: _____

Remember that muscular endurance is specific: Your ratings may vary considerably for different parts of your body.

Using Your Results

How did you score? Are you at all surprised by your ratings for muscular endurance? Are you satisfied with your current ratings?

If you're not satisfied, set realistic goals for improvement: _____
Are you satisfied with your current level of muscular endurance as evidenced in your daily life—for example, your ability to carry groceries or your books, hike, and do yardwork?

If you're not satisfied, set some realistic goals for improvement:

What should you do next? Enter the results of this lab in the Preprogram Assessment column in Appendix D. If you've set goals for improvement, begin planning your strength training program by completing the plan in Lab 4.3. After several weeks of your program, complete this lab again and enter the results in the Postprogram Assessment column of Appendix D. How do the results compare?

LAB 4.3 *Designing and Monitoring a Strength Training Program*   Viw

1. *Set goals.* List goals for your strength training program. Your goals can be specific or general, short or long term. In the first section, include specific, measurable goals that you can use to track the progress of your fitness program. These goals might be things like raising your upper body muscular strength rating from fair to good or being able to complete 10 repetitions of a lat pull with 125 pounds of resistance. In the second section, include long-term and more qualitative goals, such as improving self-confidence and reducing your risk for back pain.

   Specific Goals: Current Status   Final Goal

   _____   _____

   _____   _____

   _____   _____

   Other goals:

   _____

   _____

2. *Choose exercises.* Based on your goals, choose 8–10 exercises to perform during each weight training session. If your goal is general training for wellness, use one of the sample programs in Figure 4.3 (p. 96) and on pp. 107–119. List your exercises and the muscles they develop in the program plan below.

3. *Frequency: Choose the number of training sessions per week.* Work out at least 2 days per week. Indicate the days you will train on your program plan; be sure to include days of rest to allow your body to recover.

4. *Intensity: Choose starting weights.* Experiment with different amounts of weight until you settle on a good starting weight, one that you can lift easily for 10–12 repetitions. As you progress in your program, you can add more weight. Fill in the starting weight for each exercise on the program plan.

5. *Time: Choose a starting number of sets and repetitions.* Include at least 1 set of 8–12 repetitions of each exercise. (As you add weight, you may have to decrease the number of repetitions slightly until your muscles adapt to the heavier load.) If your program is focusing on strength alone, your sets can contain fewer repetitions using a heavier load. If you are over approximately 50–60 years of age, your sets should contain more repetitions (10–15) using a lighter load. Fill in the starting number of sets and repetitions of each exercise on the program plan.

6. *Monitor your progress.* Use the workout card on the next page to monitor your progress and keep track of exercises, weights, sets, and repetitions. (A more extensive series of logs is included in the Daily Fitness and Nutrition Journal.)

Program Plan for Weight Training

Exercise	Muscle(s) Developed	Frequency (check ✓)							Intensity: Weight (lb)	Time Repetitions	Sets
		M	T	W	Th	F	Sa	Su			

WORKOUT CARD FOR _____

Exercise/Date	Wt	Sets	Reps	Wt	Sets	Reps	Wt	Sets	Reps	Wt	Sets	Reps	Wt	Sets	Reps	Wt	Sets	Reps	Wt	Sets	Reps	Wt	Sets	Reps	Wt	Sets	Reps	Wt	Sets	Reps	Wt	Sets	Reps	Wt	Sets	Reps

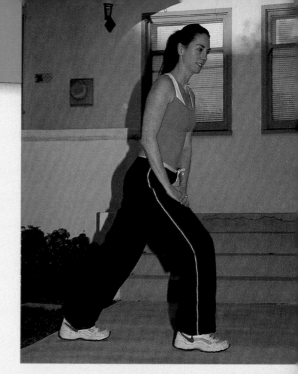

5

Flexibility and Low-Back Health

LOOKING AHEAD

After reading this chapter, you should be able to

- Describe the potential benefits of flexibility and stretching exercises
- List the factors that affect the flexibility in a joint
- Explain the different types of stretching exercises and how they affect muscles
- Describe the intensity, duration, and frequency of stretching exercises that will develop the most flexibility with the lowest risk of injury
- List safe stretching exercises for major joints
- Describe how low-back pain can be prevented and managed

TEST YOUR KNOWLEDGE

1. Stretching exercises should be performed
   a. at the start of a warm-up.
   b. following the active part of a warm-up.
   c. after endurance exercise or strength training.

2. If you injure your back, it's usually best to rest in bed for several days.
   True or false?

3. To gain flexibility, you should stretch until you feel pain.
   True or false?

ANSWERS

1. **B and/or C.** It's best to do stretching exercises when your muscles are warm, after either the active part of a warm-up (5–10 minutes of an activity such as walking or easy jogging) or an endurance or strength training workout. If a high-performance workout is your goal, it is best to stretch after exercise because stretching muscles may temporarily reduce their explosive strength.

2. **FALSE.** Prolonged bed rest may actually worsen back pain. Limit bed rest to a day or less, treat pain and inflammation with cold and then heat, and begin moderate physical activity as soon as possible.

3. **FALSE.** Stretch to the point of slight tension or mild discomfort, not pain. If you are very sore or sore for more than 24 hours following a stretching workout, you have stretched too intensely.

WW *Fit and Well* **Online Learning Center**   www.mhhe.com/fahey

Visit the *Fit and Well* Online Learning Center for study aids, online labs, additional information about flexibility and low-back health, links, Internet activities that explore the development of flexibility, and much more.

Flexibility—the ability of a joint to move through its full **range of motion**—is extremely important for general fitness and wellness. The smooth and easy performance of everyday and recreational activities is impossible if flexibility is poor. Flexibility is a highly adaptable physical fitness component. It increases in response to a regular program of stretching exercises and decreases with inactivity. Flexibility is also specific: Good flexibility in one joint doesn't necessarily mean good flexibility in another. Flexibility can be increased through stretching exercises for all major joints.

There are two basic types of flexibility: static and dynamic. Static flexibility refers to the ability to assume and maintain an extended position at one end or point in a joint's range of motion; it is what most people mean by the term *flexibility*. Dynamic flexibility, unlike static flexibility, involves movement; it is the ability to move a joint through its range of motion with little resistance. For example, static shoulder flexibility would determine how far you could extend your arm across the front of your body or out to the side. Dynamic shoulder flexibility would affect your ability to pitch a softball, swing a golf club, or swim the crawl stroke. When gymnasts perform a split on the balance beam, they must have good static flexibility in their legs and hips; to perform a split leap, they must have good dynamic flexibility.

Static flexibility depends on many factors, including the ability to tolerate stretched muscles, the structure of a joint, and the tightness of muscles, tendons, and ligaments that are attached to the joint. Dynamic flexibility depends on static flexibility, but it also involves such factors as strength, coordination, and resistance to movement. Dynamic flexibility can be important for both daily activities and sports. However, because static flexibility is easier to measure and better researched, most assessment tests and stretching programs—including those presented in this chapter—target static flexibility.

This chapter describes the factors that affect flexibility and the benefits of maintaining good flexibility. It provides guidelines for assessing your current level of flexibility and putting together a successful stretching program. It also examines the common problem of low-back pain.

WHAT DETERMINES FLEXIBILITY?

The flexibility of a joint is affected by its structure, by muscle elasticity and length, and by nervous system activity. Some factors—joint structure, for example—can't be changed. Other factors, such as the length of resting muscle fibers, can be changed through exercise; these factors should be the focus of a program to develop flexibility.

Joint Structure

The amount of flexibility in a joint is determined in part by the nature and structure of the joint. Hinge joints such as those in your fingers and knees allow only limited forward and backward movement; they lock when fully extended. Ball-and-socket joints like the hip enable movement in many different directions and have a greater range of motion. Major joints are surrounded by **joint capsules,** semielastic structures that give joints strength and stability but limit movement. Heredity also plays a part in joint structure and flexibility; for example, although everyone has a broad range of motion in the ball-and-socket hip joint, not everyone can do a split.

Muscle Elasticity and Length

Soft tissues, including skin, muscles, tendons, and ligaments, also limit the flexibility of a joint. Muscle tissue is the key to developing flexibility because it can be lengthened if it is regularly stretched. As described in Chapter 4, muscles contain proteins that create movement by causing muscles to contract. These contractile proteins can also stretch, and they are involved in the development of flexibility. However, the most important component of muscle tissue related to flexibility is the connective tissue that surrounds and envelops every part of muscle tissue, from individual muscle fibers to entire muscles. Connective tissue provides structure, elasticity, and bulk and makes up about 30% of muscle mass. Two principal types of connective tissue are **collagen,** white fibers that provide structure and support, and **elastin,** yellow fibers that are elastic and flexible. Muscles contain both collagen and elastin, closely intertwined, so muscle tissue exhibits the properties of both types of fibers. A recently discovered structural protein in muscles called **titin** also has elastic properties and contributes to flexibility.

When a muscle is stretched, the wavelike elastin fibers straighten; when the stretch is relieved, they rapidly snap back to their resting position. If gently and regularly stretched, connective tissues may lengthen and flexibility may improve. Without regular stretching, the process

---

Terms

WW

flexibility The range of motion in a joint or group of joints.

range of motion The full motion possible in a joint.

joint capsules Semielastic structures, composed primarily of connective tissue, that surround major joints.

soft tissues Tissues of the human body that include skin, fat, linings of internal organs and blood vessels, connective tissues, tendons, ligaments, muscles, and nerves.

collagen White fibers that provide structure and support in connective tissue.

elastin Yellow fibers that make connective tissue flexible.

titin A filament in muscle that helps align proteins that cause muscle contraction; titin has elastic properties and also plays a role in flexibility.

stretch receptors Sense organs in skeletal muscles that initiate a nerve signal to the spinal cord in response to a stretch; a contraction follows.

proprioceptive neuromuscular facilitation (PNF) A technique for stretching and strengthening muscles; PNF relies on neuromuscular reflexes to stimulate training effects.

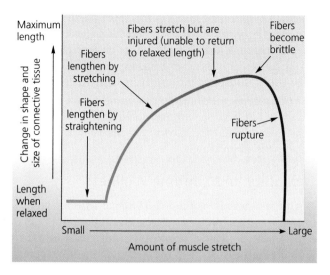

Figure 5.1 The effect of stretch on connective tissue.

reverses: These tissues shorten, resulting in decreased flexibility. Regular stretching may contribute to flexibility by lengthening muscle fibers through the addition of contractile units called sarcomeres.

The stretch characteristics of connective tissue in muscle are important considerations for a stretching program. The amount of stretch a muscle will tolerate is limited, and as the limits of its flexibility are reached, connective tissue becomes more brittle and may rupture if overstretched (Figure 5.1). A safe and effective program stretches muscles enough to slightly elongate the tissues but not so much that they are damaged. Research has shown that flexibility is improved best by stretching when muscles are warm (following exercise or the application of heat) and the stretch is applied gradually and conservatively. Sudden, high-stress stretching is less effective and can lead to muscle damage.

Nervous System Activity

Muscles contain **stretch receptors** that control their length. If a muscle is stretched suddenly, stretch receptors send signals to the spinal cord, which then sends a signal back to the same muscle, causing it to contract. These reflexes occur frequently in active muscles. They help the body know what the muscles are doing and allow for fine control of muscle length.

Small movements that only slightly stimulate these receptors cause small reflex actions. Rapid, powerful, and sudden movements that strongly stimulate the receptors cause large, powerful reflex muscle contractions. Stretches that involve rapid, bouncy movements are considered dangerous because they may stimulate a reflex muscle contraction during a stretch. A muscle that contracts at the same time it's being stretched can be easily injured, so slow, gradual stretches are always safest. Holding a stretch allows the stretch receptor to adjust to the new muscle length and to reduce the signals it sends to the spine, thereby allowing muscles to lengthen and, over time, improving flexibility.

Strong muscle contractions produce a reflex of the opposite type—one that causes muscles to relax and keeps them from contracting too hard. This inverse stretch reflex can be used as an aid to improving flexibility: Contracting a muscle prior to stretching it causes it to relax, allowing it to stretch farther. The contraction-stretch technique for developing flexibility is called **proprioceptive neuromuscular facilitation (PNF)**.

Doing each stretching exercise several times in a row can "reset" the sensitivity of muscle stretch receptors. Stretching a muscle, relaxing, and then stretching it again cause the stretch receptors to become slightly less sensitive, thereby enabling the muscle to stretch farther. It is not known if stretch receptor sensitivity continues to change following prolonged flexibility training, but it's likely that neural changes do occur to help increase flexibility.

BENEFITS OF FLEXIBILITY AND STRETCHING EXERCISES

Good flexibility provides benefits for the entire musculoskeletal system; it may also prevent injuries and soreness and improve performance in all physical activities.

Joint Health

Good flexibility is essential to good joint health. When the muscles and other tissues that support a joint are tight, the joint is subject to abnormal stresses that can cause joint deterioration. For example, tight thigh muscles cause excessive pressure on the kneecap, leading to pain in the knee joint. Tight shoulder muscles can compress sensitive soft tissues in the shoulder, leading to pain and disability in the joint. Poor joint flexibility can also cause abnormalities in joint lubrication, leading to deterioration of the sensitive cartilage cells lining the joint; pain and further joint injury can result.

Improved flexibility can greatly improve your quality of life, particularly as you get older. Aging decreases the natural elasticity of muscles, tendons, and joints, resulting in stiffness. The problem is compounded if you have arthritis. Good joint flexibility may prevent arthritis, and stretching may lessen pain in people who have the disease. Flexibility exercises also improve the elasticity in your tissues, making it easier to move your body. When you're flexible, everything from tying your shoes to reaching for a jar on an upper shelf becomes easier.

Prevention of Low-Back Pain and Injuries

Low-back pain can be related to poor spinal alignment, which puts pressure on the nerves leading out from the spinal column. Strength and flexibility in the back, pelvis, and thighs may help prevent this type of back pain. Unfortunately, research studies have not yet clearly defined the relationship between back pain and lack of flexibility. Few studies have found that trunk flexibility improves back health or reduces the risk of injury; in some people, greater spinal mobility may actually increase the risk of low-back problems. However, good hip and knee flexibility has been found to protect the spine from excessive motion during the tasks of daily living. Maintaining normal levels of flexibility helps maintain healthy joints and is probably necessary for good back health.

Poor flexibility does increase one's risk for injury. A general stretching program has been shown to be effective in reducing the frequency of injuries as well as their severity. When injuries do occur, flexibility exercises can be used in treatment: They reduce symptoms and help restore normal range of motion in affected joints.

Overstretching—stretching muscles to extreme ranges of motion—may actually decrease the stability of a joint. Although some activities, such as gymnastics and ballet, require extreme joint movements, such flexibility is not recommended for the average person. In fact, extreme flexibility may increase the risk of injury in activities such as skiing, basketball, and volleyball. Again, as with other types of exercise, moderation is the key to safe training.

Additional Potential Benefits

• *Temporary reduction of postexercise muscle soreness.* **Delayed-onset muscle soreness,** occurring 1–2 days after exercise, is thought to be caused by damage to the muscle fibers and supporting connective tissue. Some studies have shown that stretching after exercise decreases the degree of muscle soreness—but this improvement appears to be temporary. Postexercise stretching does not appear to relieve muscle soreness for an extended period of time.

• *Relief of aches and pains.* Stretching helps relieve pain that develops from stress or prolonged sitting. Studying or working in one place for a long time can make your muscles tense. Stretching helps relieve tension, so you can go back to work refreshed and effective.

• *Relief of muscle cramps.* Recent research suggests that exercise-related muscle cramps are caused by increased electrical activity within the affected muscle. The best treatment for muscle cramps is gentle stretching, which reduces the electrical activity and allows the muscle to relax.

• *Improved body position and strength for sports (and life).* Good flexibility lets a person assume more efficient body positions and exert force through a greater range of motion. For example, swimmers with more flexible shoulders have stronger strokes because they can pull their arms through the water in the optimal position. Flexible joints and muscles let you move more fluidly. Some studies also suggest that flexibility training enhances strength development.

• *Maintenance of good posture and balance.* Good flexibility also contributes to body symmetry and good posture. Bad posture can gradually change your body structures. Sitting in a slumped position, for example, can lead to tightness in the muscles in the front of your chest and

overstretching and looseness in the upper spine, causing a rounding of the upper back. This condition, called kyphosis, is common in older people. It may be prevented by stretching regularly. Another benefit of good flexibility to older adults is that it increases balance and stability.

• *Relaxation.* Flexibility exercises are a great way to relax. Studies have shown that doing flexibility exercises reduces mental tension, slows your breathing rate, and reduces blood pressure.

Flexibility and Lifetime Wellness

Part of wellness is being able to move without pain or hindrance. Flexibility exercises are an important part of this process. Sedentary people often effectively lose their mobility at an early age. Even relatively young people are often handicapped by back, shoulder, knee, and ankle pain. As they age, the pain can become debilitating, leading to injuries and a lower quality of life. Good flexibility helps keep your joints and muscles moving without pain so that you can do all the things you enjoy.

MOTIVATION FOR CHANGE! Make a list of five benefits of flexibility that are particularly meaningful to you. Put the list in a prominent location and use it as a motivational tool for beginning and maintaining your stretching program.

ASSESSING FLEXIBILITY

Because flexibility is specific to each joint, there are no tests of general flexibility. The most commonly used flexibility test is the sit-and-reach test, which rates the flexibility of the muscles in the lower back and hamstrings. To assess your flexibility and identify inflexible joints, complete Lab 5.1.

CREATING A SUCCESSFUL PROGRAM TO DEVELOP FLEXIBILITY

A successful program for developing flexibility contains safe exercises executed with the most effective techniques.

Applying the FITT Principle

As with the programs described for developing other health-related components of fitness, the acronym FITT can be used to remember key components of a stretching program: frequency, intensity, time, and type of exercise.

Frequency The ACSM recommends that stretching exercises be performed a minimum of 2–3 days a week. Many people do flexibility training more often—3–5 days a week—for even greater benefits. It's best to stretch when your muscles are warm, so try incorporating stretching into your cool-down after cardiorespiratory endurance exercise or weight training.

Stretching can also be part of a warm-up, as long as the active part of the warm-up (for example, 5–10 minutes of walking) comes first. Never stretch when your muscles are "cold"; doing so can increase your risk of injury as well as limit the amount of flexibility you can develop. Although stretching before exercise is a time-honored ritual practiced by athletes in many sports, several recent studies found that pre-exercise stretching decreases muscle strength and performance in explosive muscle activities like jumping for about 15–30 minutes after stretching. So, if your workout involves participation in a sport or high-performance activity, you may be better off stretching after your workout; for moderate-intensity activities like walking or cycling, stretching before your workout is unlikely to affect performance.

Intensity and Time (Duration)   For each exercise, slowly apply stretch to your muscles to the point of slight tension or mild discomfort. Hold the stretch for 10–30 seconds. As you hold the stretch, the feeling of slight tension should slowly subside; at that point, try to stretch a bit farther. Throughout the stretch, try to relax and breathe easily. Rest for about 30–60 seconds between each stretch, and do at least 4 repetitions of each stretch. A complete flexibility workout usually takes about 20–30 minutes (Figure 5.2).

Types of Stretching Techniques   Stretching techniques vary from simply stretching the muscles during the course of normal activities to sophisticated methods based on patterns of muscle reflexes. Improper stretching techniques can do more harm than good, so it's important to understand the different types of stretching exercises and how they affect the muscles. Three common techniques are static stretches, ballistic stretches, and PNF. These techniques can be performed passively or actively.

STATIC STRETCHING   In **static stretching**, each muscle is gradually stretched, and the stretch is held for 10–30 seconds. (Holding the stretch longer than 30 seconds will not further improve flexibility, whereas stretching for less than 10 seconds will provide little benefit.) A slow stretch prompts less reaction from stretch receptors, and the muscles can safely stretch farther than usual. Static stretching is the type most often recommended by fitness experts because it's safe and effective. The key to this technique is to stretch the muscles and joints to the point where a pull is felt, but not to the point of pain. Most experts consider static stretching the best and safest stretching technique.

BALLISTIC STRETCHING   In **ballistic stretching**, the muscles are stretched suddenly in a bouncing movement. For example, touching the toes repeatedly in rapid succession is a ballistic stretch for the hamstrings. A problem with this technique is that the heightened activity of stretch receptors caused by the rapid stretches can continue for some time, possibly causing injuries during any physical activities that follow. Another concern is that triggering strong responses from the stretch receptors can cause a reflex muscle contraction that makes it harder to stretch. For these reasons, ballistic stretching is usually not recommended.

PROPRIOCEPTIVE NEUROMUSCULAR FACILITATION (PNF)   PNF techniques use reflexes initiated by both muscle and joint receptors to cause greater training effects. The most popular PNF stretching technique is the contract-relax stretching method, in which a muscle is contracted before it is stretched. For example, in a seated stretch of calf muscles, the first step in PNF is to contract the calf muscles. The individual or a partner can provide resistance for an isometric contraction. Following a brief period of relaxation, the next step is to stretch the calf muscles by pulling the tops of the feet toward the body. A duration of 6 seconds for the contraction and 10–30 seconds for the stretch is recommended. PNF appears to be most effective if the individual pushes hard during the isometric contraction.

Another example of a PNF stretch is the contract-relax-contract pattern. In this technique, begin by contracting

Warm-up 5–10 minutes or following an endurance or strength training workout	Stretching exercises for major joints **Sample program**	
	Exercise	*Areas stretched*
	Head turns and tilts	Neck
	Towel stretch	Triceps, shoulders, chest
	Across-the-body and overhead stretches	Shoulders, upper back, back of arm
	Upper back stretch	Upper back
	Lateral stretch	Trunk muscles
	Step stretch	Hip, front of thigh
	Side lunge	Inner thigh, hip, calf
	Inner thigh stretch	Inner thigh, hip
	Hip and trunk stretch	Trunk, outer thigh, hip, buttocks, lower back
	Modified hurdler stretch	Back of thigh, lower back
	Alternate leg stretcher	Back of thigh, hip, knee, ankle, buttocks
	Lower-leg stretch	Calf, soleus, Achilles tendon

Frequency: 2–3 days per week or more

Intensity: Stretch to the point of mild discomfort, not pain

Time (duration): All stretches should be held for 10–30 seconds and performed at least 4 times

Type of activity: Stretching exercises that focus on major joints

Figure 5.2   A flexibility workout.

delayed-onset muscle soreness   Soreness that occurs 1–2 days after exercising, probably caused by tissue damage and inflammation that leads to further tissue damage.

static stretching   A technique in which a muscle is slowly and gently stretched and then held in the stretched position.

ballistic stretching   A technique in which muscles are stretched by the force generated as a body part is repeatedly bounced, swung, or jerked.

Terms

- Do stretching exercises statically. Stretch to the point of mild discomfort, hold the position for 10–30 seconds, rest for 30–60 seconds, and repeat, trying to stretch a bit farther.

- Do not stretch to the point of pain. Any soreness after a stretching workout should be mild and last no more than 24 hours. If you are sore for a longer period, you stretched too intensely.

- Relax and breathe easily as you stretch. Inhale through the nose and exhale through pursed lips during the stretch. Try to relax the muscles being stretched.

- Perform all exercises on both sides of your body.

- Increase intensity and duration gradually over time. Improved flexibility takes many months to develop.

- Stretch when your muscles are warm. Do gentle warm-up exercises such as easy jogging or calisthenics before doing a pre-exercise stretching routine.

- There are large individual differences in joint flexibility. Don't feel you have to compete with others during stretching workouts.

the muscle to be stretched and then relaxing it. Next, contract the opposing muscle (the antagonist). Finally, stretch the first muscle. For example, using this technique to stretch the hamstrings (the muscles in the back of the thigh) would require the following steps: contract the hamstrings, relax the hamstrings, contract the quadriceps (the muscles in the front of the thigh), stretch the hamstrings.

PNF appears to allow more effective stretching, and greater increases in flexibility than static stretching, but it tends to cause more muscle stiffness and soreness. It also usually requires a partner and takes more time.

PASSIVE VERSUS ACTIVE STRETCHING   Stretches can be done either passively or actively. In **passive stretching,** an outside force or resistance provided by yourself, a partner, gravity, or a weight helps your joints move through their range of motion. For example, a seated stretch of the hamstring and back muscles can be done by reaching the hands toward the feet until a "pull" is felt in those muscles. You can achieve a greater range of motion (a more intense stretch) using passive stretching. However, because the stretch is not controlled by the muscles themselves, there is a greater risk of injury. Communication between partners in passive stretching is very important so joints aren't forced outside their normal functional range of motion.

In **active stretching,** a muscle is stretched by a contraction of the opposing muscle (the muscle on the opposite side of the limb). For example, an active seated stretch of the calf muscles occurs when a person actively contracts the muscles on the top of the shin. The contraction of this opposing muscle produces a reflex that relaxes the muscles to be stretched. The muscle can be stretched farther with a low risk of injury.

The only disadvantage of active stretching is that a person may not be able to produce enough stress (enough stretch) to increase flexibility using only the contraction

of opposing muscle groups. The safest and most convenient technique is active static stretching, with an occasional passive assist. For example, you might stretch your calves both by contracting the muscles on the top of your shin and by pulling your feet toward you. This way you combine the advantages of active stretching—safety and the relaxation reflex—with those of passive stretching—greater range of motion.

Putting Exercises Together in a Complete Program

Your program should include stretches for all major joints; a complete sample program is found on pp. 139–144. Refer to Figure 5.2 and the box "Safe Stretching" for a summary of guidelines for creating a safe and successful stretching program. Complete Lab 5.2 when you're ready to start your own program.

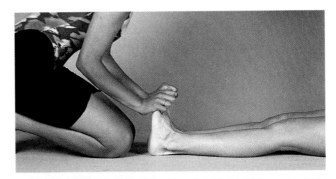
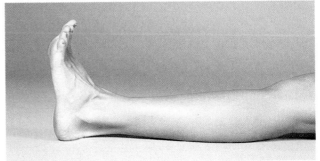

In passive stretching (top), an outside force—such as pressure exerted by another person—helps move the joint and stretch the muscles. In active stretching (bottom), the force to move the joint and stretch the muscles is provided by a contraction of the opposing muscles.

Terms

passive stretching A technique in which muscles are stretched by force applied by an outside source.

active stretching A technique in which muscles are stretched by the contraction of the opposing muscles.

Making Progress

As with any type of training, you will make progress and improve your flexibility if you stick with your program. Follow the guidelines outlined in this chapter and train at least 2–3 days per week. The best way to judge your progress is to note your body position while stretching. For example, note how far you can lean forward during a modified hurdler stretch. If you wish, you can repeat the assessment tests that appear in Lab 5.1 periodically; be sure to take the test at the same time of day each time. You will likely notice some improvement after only 2–3 weeks of a stretching program; however, attaining significant improvements will take at least 2 months. By then, you can expect flexibility increases of about 10–20% in many joints.

Exercises to Improve Flexibility

There are hundreds of exercises that can improve flexibility. Your program should include exercises that work all the major joints of the body by stretching their associated muscles. The exercises illustrated here are simple to do and pose a minimum risk of injury. Use the exercises on p. 139–143, or substitute your favorite stretches, to create a well-rounded program for developing flexibility. Be sure to perform each stretch using the proper technique. Hold each position for 10–30 seconds and perform at least 4 repetitions of each exercise. Avoid exercises that put excessive pressure on your joints (see the box "Stretches to Avoid", on p. 144).

FLEXIBILITY EXERCISES

EXERCISE 1

HEAD TURNS AND TILTS

Areas stretched: Neck

Instructions

Head turns: Turn your head to the right and hold the stretch. Repeat to the left.

Head tilts: Tilt your head to the left and hold the stretch. Repeat to the right.

Variation: Place your right palm on your right cheek; try to turn your head to the right as you resist with your hand. Repeat on the left side.

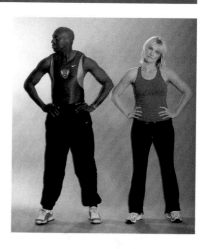

EXERCISE 2

TOWEL STRETCH

Areas stretched: Triceps, shoulders, chest

Instructions: Roll up a towel and grasp it with both hands, palms down. With your arms straight, slowly lift it back over your head as far as possible. The closer together your hands are, the greater the stretch.

Variation: Repeat the stretch with your arms down and the towel behind your back. Grasp the towel with your palms forward and thumbs pointing out. Gently raise your arms behind your back.

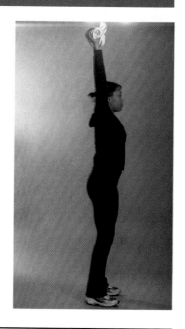

ACROSS-THE-BODY AND OVERHEAD STRETCHES

Areas stretched: Shoulders, upper back, back of the arm (triceps)

Instructions: **(a)** Keeping your back straight, cross your right arm in front of your body and grasp it with your left hand. Stretch your arm, shoulders, and back by gently pulling your arm as close to your body as possible. Hold. **(b)** Bend your right arm over your head, placing your right elbow as close to your right ear as possible. Grasp your right elbow with your left hand over your head. Stretch the back of your arm by gently pulling your right elbow back and toward your head. Hold. Repeat both stretches on your left side.

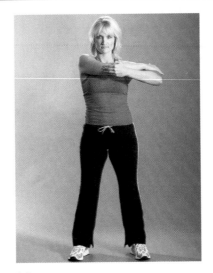

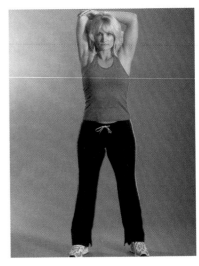

(a)   **(b)**

UPPER-BACK STRETCH

Areas stretched: Upper back

Instructions: Stand with your feet shoulder-width apart, knees slightly bent, and pelvis tucked under. Clasp your hands in front of your body and press your palms forward.

Variation: In the same position, wrap your arms around your body as if you were giving yourself a hug.

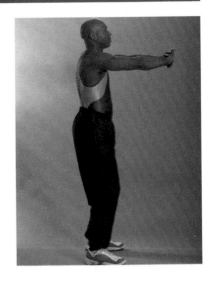

EXERCISE 5

LATERAL STRETCH

Areas stretched: Trunk muscles

Instructions: Stand with your feet shoulder-width apart, knees slightly bent, and pelvis tucked under. Raise one arm over your head and bend sideways from the waist. Support your trunk by placing the hand or forearm of your other arm on your thigh or hip for support. Be sure you bend directly sideways and don't move your body below the waist. Repeat on the other side.

Variation: Perform the same exercise in a seated position.

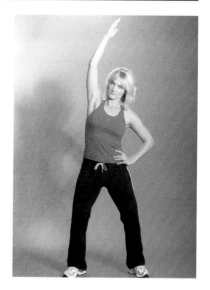

EXERCISE 6

STEP STRETCH

Areas stretched: Hip, front of thigh (quadriceps)

Instructions: Step forward and flex your forward knee, keeping your knee directly above your ankle. Stretch your other leg back so that it is parallel to the floor. Press your hips forward and down to stretch. Your arms can be at your sides, on top of your knee, or on the ground for balance. Repeat on the other side.

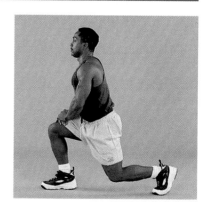

EXERCISE 7

SIDE LUNGE

Areas stretched: Inner thigh, hip, calf

Instructions: Stand in a wide straddle with your legs turned out from your hip joints and your hands on your thighs. Lunge to one side by bending one knee and keeping the other leg straight. Keep your knee directly over your ankle; do not bend it more than 90 degrees. Repeat on the other side.

Variation: In the same position, lift the heel of the bent knee to provide additional stretch. The exercise may also be performed with your hands on the floor for balance.

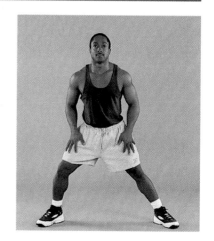

INNER THIGH STRETCH

Areas stretched: Inner thigh, hip

Instructions: Sit with the soles of your feet together. Push your knees toward the floor using your hands or forearms.

Variation: When you first begin to push your knees toward the floor, use your legs to resist the movement. Then relax and press your knees down as far as they will go.

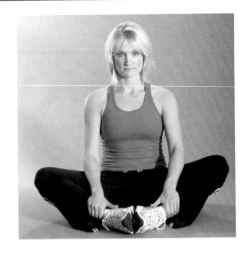

HIP AND TRUNK STRETCH

Areas stretched: Trunk, outer thigh and hip, buttocks, lower back

Instructions: Sit with your left leg straight, right leg bent and crossed over the left knee, and right hand on the floor next to your right hip. Turn your trunk as far as possible to the right by pushing against your right leg with your left forearm or elbow. Keep your right foot on the floor. Repeat on the other side.

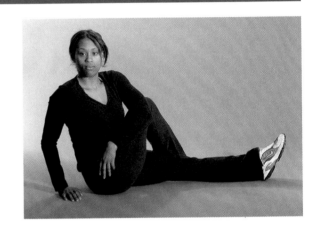

MODIFIED HURDLER STRETCH
(Seated Single-Toe Touch)

Areas stretched: Back of the thigh (hamstring), lower back

Instructions: Sit with your left leg straight and your right leg tucked close to your body. Reach toward your left foot as far as possible. Repeat for the other leg.

Variation: As you stretch forward, alternately flex and point the foot of your extended leg.

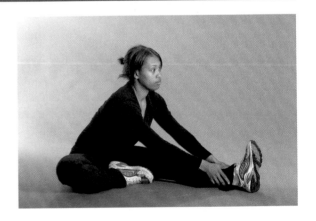

ALTERNATE LEG STRETCHER

Areas stretched: Back of the thigh (hamstring), hip, knee, ankle, buttocks

Instructions: Lie flat on your back with both legs straight. **(a)** Grasp your left leg behind the thigh, and pull in to your chest. **(b)** Hold this position, and then extend your left leg toward the ceiling. **(c)** Hold this position, and then bring your left knee back to your chest and pull your toes toward your shin with your left hand. Stretch the back of the leg by attempting to straighten your knee. Repeat for the other leg.

Variation: Perform the stretch on both legs at the same time.

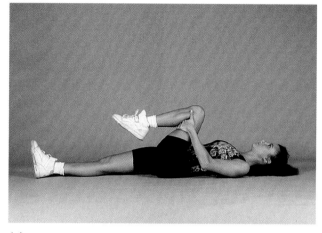

(a)

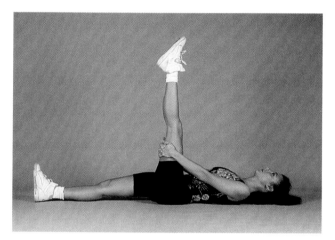

(b)

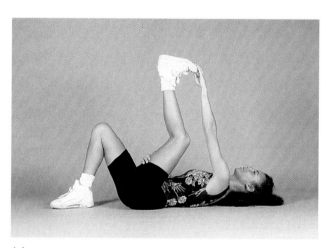

(c)

LOWER-LEG STRETCH

Areas stretched: Back of the lower leg (calf, soleus, Achilles tendon)

Instructions: Stand with one foot about 1–2 feet in front of the other, with both feet pointing forward. **(a)** Keeping your back leg straight, lunge forward by bending your front knee and pushing your rear heel backward. Hold. **(b)** Then pull your back foot in slightly, and bend your back knee. Shift your weight to your back leg. Hold. Repeat on the other side.

Variation: Place your hands on a wall and extend one foot back, pressing your heel down to stretch; or stand with the balls of your feet on a step or bench and allow your heels to drop below the level of your toes.

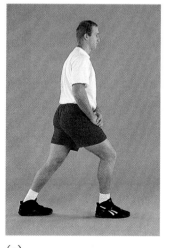

(a)

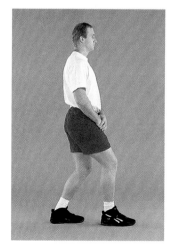

(b)

The safe alternatives listed here are described and illustrated on pages 139–143 as part of the complete program of safe flexibility exercises presented in this chapter.

Standing Toe Touch

Problem: Puts excessive strain on the spine.

Alternatives: Alternate leg stretcher (Exercise 11), modified hurdler stretch (Exercise 10), and lower leg stretch (Exercise 12).

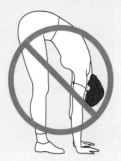

Standing Hamstring Stretch

Problem: Puts excessive strain on the knee and lower back.

Alternatives: Alternate leg stretcher (Exercise 11) and modified hurdler stretch (Exercise 10).

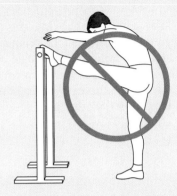

Standing Ankle-to-Buttocks Quadriceps Stretch

Problem: Puts excessive strain on the ligaments of the knee.

Alternative: Step stretch (Exercise 6).

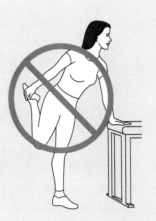

Yoga Plow

Problem: Puts excessive strain on the neck, shoulders and back.

Alternatives: Head turns and tilts (Exercise 1), across-the-body and overhead stretches (Exercise 3), and upper-back stretch (Exercise 4).

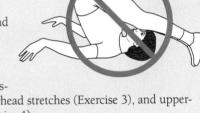

Full Squat

Problem: Puts excessive strain on the ankles, knees, and spine.

Alternatives: Alternate leg stretcher (Exercise 11) and lower leg stretch (Exercise 12).

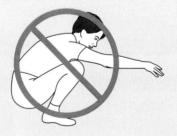

Hurdler Stretch

Problem: Turning out the bent leg can put excessive strain on the ligaments of the knee.

Alternatives: Modified hurdler stretch (Exercise 10).

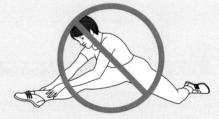

Neck Circles

Problem: Puts excessive strain on the neck and cervical disks.

Alternatives: Head turns and tilts (Exercise 1).

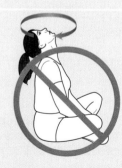

Prone Arch

Problem: Puts excessive strain on the spine, knees, and shoulders.

Alternatives: Towel stretch (Exercise 2) and step stretch (Exercise 6).

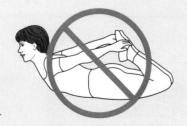

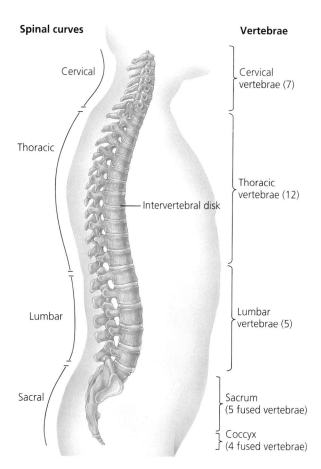

Figure 5.3   The spinal column.   The spine is made up of five separate regions and has four distinct curves. An intervertebral disk is located between vertebrae.

PREVENTING AND MANAGING LOW-BACK PAIN

More than 85% of Americans experience back pain at some time in their lives. Low-back pain is the second most common ailment in the United States—headache tops the list—and the second most common reason for absences from work and visits to a physician. Low-back pain is estimated to cost as much as $50 billion a year in lost productivity, medical and legal fees, and disability insurance and compensation.

Back pain can result from sudden traumatic injuries, but it is more often the long-term result of weak and inflexible muscles, poor posture, or poor body mechanics during activities like lifting and carrying. Any abnormal strain on the back can result in pain. Most cases of low-back pain clear up within a few weeks or months, but some people have recurrences or suffer from chronic pain.

Function and Structure of the Spine

The spinal column performs many important functions in the body.

- It provides structural support for the body, especially the thorax (upper-body cavity).
- It surrounds and protects the spinal cord.
- It supports much of the body's weight and transmits it to the lower body.
- It serves as an attachment site for a large number of muscles, tendons, and ligaments.
- It allows movement of the neck and back in all directions.

The spinal column is made up of bones called **vertebrae** (Figure 5.3). The spine consists of 7 cervical vertebrae in the neck, 12 thoracic vertebrae in the upper back, and 5 lumbar vertebrae in the lower back. The 9 vertebrae at the base of the spine are fused into two sections and form the sacrum and the coccyx (tailbone). The spine has four curves: the cervical, thoracic, lumbar, and sacral curves.

These curves help bring the body weight supported by the spine in line with the axis of the body.

Although the structure of vertebrae depends on their location on the spine, the different types of vertebrae do share common characteristics. Each consists of a body, an arch, and several bony processes (Figure 5.4, p. 146). The vertebral body is cylindrical, with flattened surfaces where **intervertebral disks** are attached. The vertebral body is designed to carry the stress of body weight and physical activity. The vertebral arch surrounds and protects the spinal cord. The bony processes serve as joints for adjacent vertebrae and attachment sites for muscles and ligaments. **Nerve roots** from the spinal cord pass through notches in the vertebral arch.

vertebrae Bony segments composing the spinal column that provide structural support for the body and protect the spinal cord.

intervertebral disk An elastic disk located between adjoining vertebrae consisting of a gel- and water-filled nucleus surrounded by fibrous rings; it serves as a shock absorber for the spinal column.

nerve root Base of one of the 31 pairs of spinal nerves that branch off the spinal cord through spaces between vertebrae.

Terms

Intervertebral disks, which absorb and disperse the stresses placed on the spine, separate vertebrae from each other. Disks are made up of a gel- and water-filled nucleus surrounded by a series of fibrous rings. The liquid nucleus can change shape when it is compressed, allowing the disk to absorb shock. The intervertebral disks also help maintain the spaces between vertebrae where the spinal nerve roots are located.

Causes of Back Pain

Back pain can occur at any point along your spine; the lumbar area, because it bears the majority of your weight, is the most common site. Any movement that causes excessive stress on the spinal column can cause injury and pain. The spine is well equipped to bear body weight and the force or stress of body movements along its long axis. However, it is less capable of bearing loads at an angle to its long axis. You do not have to carry a heavy load or participate in a vigorous contact sport to injure your back. Picking a pencil up from the floor using poor body mechanics—reaching too far out in front of you or bending over with your knees straight, for example—can also result in back pain.

Risk factors associated with low-back pain include age greater than 34 years, degenerative diseases such as arthritis or osteoporosis, a family or personal history of back pain or trauma, a sedentary lifestyle, low job satisfaction, and low socioeconomic status. Smoking increases risk because smoking appears to increase degenerative changes in the spine. Excess body weight also increases strain on the back, and psychological stress or depression can cause muscle tension and back pain. Occupations and activities associated with low-back pain are those involving physically hard work, such as frequent lifting, twisting, bending, standing up, or straining in forced positions; those requiring high concentration demands (such as computer programming); and those involving vibrations affecting the entire body (such as truck driving).

Underlying causes of back pain include poor muscle endurance and strength in the muscles of the abdomen, back, hips, and legs; excess body weight; poor posture or body position when standing, sitting, or sleeping; and poor body mechanics when performing actions like lifting and carrying, or sports movements. Abnormal spinal loading resulting from any of these causes can have short-term or long-term direct and indirect effects on the spine. Strained muscles, tendons, or ligaments can cause pain and can, over time, lead to injuries to vertebrae or the intervertebral disks.

Stress can cause disks to break down and lose some of their ability to absorb shock. A damaged disk may bulge out between vertebrae and put pressure on a nerve root, a condition commonly referred to as a slipped disk. Painful pressure on nerves can also occur if damage to a disk narrows the space between two vertebrae. With age, you lose fluid from the disks, making them more likely to bulge and put pressure on nerve roots. Depending on the amount of pres-

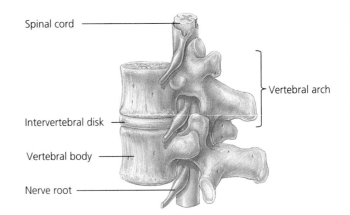

Figure 5.4   Vertebrae and an intervertebral disk.

sure on a nerve, symptoms may include numbness in the back, hip, leg, or foot; radiating pain; loss of muscle function; depressed reflexes; and muscle spasm. If the pressure is severe enough, loss of function can be permanent.

Preventing Low-Back Pain

Incorrect posture when standing, sitting, lying, and lifting is responsible for many back injuries. In general, think about moving your spine as a unit, with the force directed through its long axis. Strategies for maintaining good posture during daily activities are presented in the box "Good Posture and Low-Back Health." Follow the same guidelines for posture and movement when you engage in sports or recreational activities. Maintain control over your body movements and warm up thoroughly before you exercise. Take special care when lifting weights as part of a resistance training program (see Chapter 4).

The role of exercise in preventing and treating back pain is still being investigated. However, many experts do recommend exercise, especially for people who have already experienced an episode of low-back pain. Regular exercise aimed at increasing muscle endurance and strength in the back and abdomen is often recommended to prevent back pain, as is lifestyle physical activity such as walking. Movement helps lubricate your spinal disks and increases muscle fitness in your trunk and legs. Other lifestyle recommendations for preventing back pain include:

- Lose weight, stop smoking, and reduce emotional stress.
- Avoid sitting, standing, or working in the same position for too long.
- Use a supportive seat and a medium-firm mattress. Use lumbar support when driving, particularly for long distances, to prevent back muscle fatigue and pain.
- Warm up thoroughly before engaging in vigorous exercise or sports.
- Progress gradually when attempting to improve strength or fitness.

Changes in everyday posture and behavior can help prevent and alleviate low-back pain.

- *Lying down.* When resting or sleeping, lie on your side with your knees and hips bent. If you lie on your back place a pillow under your knees. Don't lie on your stomach. Use a medium-firm mattress.

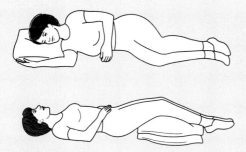

- *Sitting.* Sit with your lower back slightly rounded, knees bent, and feet flat on the floor. Alternate crossing your legs, or use a footrest to keep your knees higher than your hips. If this position is uncomfortable or if your back flattens when you sit, try using a lumbar roll pillow behind your lower back.

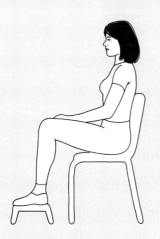

- *Lifting.* If you need to lower yourself to grasp an object, bend at the knees and hips rather than at the waist. Your feet should be about shoulder-width apart. Lift gradually, keeping your arms straight, by standing up or by pushing with your leg muscles. Keep the object close to your body. Don't twist, if you have to turn with the object, change the position of your feet.

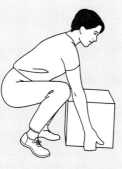

- *Standing.* When you are standing, a straight line should run from the top of your ear through the center of your shoulder, the center of your hip, the back of your kneecap, and the front of your ankle bone. Support your weight mainly on your heels, with one or both knees slightly bent. Try to keep your lower back flat by placing one foot on a stool. Don't let your pelvis tip forward or your back arch. Shift your weight back and forth from foot to foot. Avoid prolonged standing. (To check your posture, stand in a normal way with your back to a wall. Your upper back and buttocks should touch the wall; your heels may be a few inches away. Slide one hand into the space between your lower back and the wall. It should slide in easily but should almost touch both your back and the wall. Adjust your posture as needed, and try to hold this position as you walk away from the wall.)

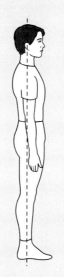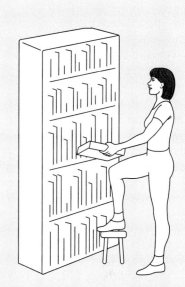

- *Walking.* Walk with your toes pointed straight ahead. Keep your back flat, head up and centered over your body, and chin in. Swing your arms freely. Don't wear high-heeled shoes.

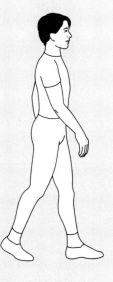

The act of writing down feelings and thoughts about stressful life events has been shown to help people with chronic conditions improve their health. In one recent study, people with asthma or rheumatoid arthritis were asked to write down their feelings about the most stressful event in their lives; they wrote for 20 minutes a day over a three-day period. In follow-up exams four months later, nearly half of the patients who engaged in expressive writing experienced positive changes in their condition such as reduced joint pain. Only about a quarter of the control group, who wrote about their daily plans, experienced a positive change in health.

Investigators remain unsure why writing about one's feelings has beneficial effects. It is possible that expressing feelings about a traumatic event helps people work through the event and put it behind them. The resulting sense of release and control may reduce stress levels and have positive physical effects. Alternatively, expressive writing may change the way people think about previous stressful events in their lives and help them cope with new stressors. Whatever the cause, it's clear that expressive writing can be a safe, inexpensive, and effective supplement to standard treatment of certain chronic conditions.

What about the effects of expressive writing on otherwise healthy individuals? Other studies have, in fact, found such a benefit: People who wrote about traumatic experiences reported fewer symptoms, fewer days off work, fewer visits to the doctor, improved mood, and a more positive outlook.

If you'd like to try expressive writing to help you deal with a traumatic event, set aside a special time—15 minutes a day for four consecutive days, for example, or one day a week for four weeks. Write in a place where you won't be interrupted or distracted. Explore your very deepest thoughts and feelings and why you feel the way you do. Don't worry about grammar or coherence or about what someone else might think about what you're writing; you are writing just for yourself. You may find the writing exercise to be distressing in the short term—sadness and depression are common when dealing with feelings about a stressful event—but most people report relief and contentment soon after writing for several days.

SOURCES: Smyth, J. M., et al. 1999. Effects of writing about stressful experiences on symptom reduction in patients with asthma or rheumatoid arthritis: A randomized trial. *Journal of the American Medical Association* 281(14): 1304–1309. Spiegel, D. 1999. Healing words: Emotional expression and disease outcome. *Journal of the American Medical Association* 281(14): 1328–1329. Pennebaker, J. 1997. *Opening Up: The Healthy Power of Expressing Emotions.* New York: Guilford Press.

Managing Acute Back Pain

Sudden back pain usually involves tissue injury. Symptoms may include pain, muscles spasms, stiffness, and inflammation. Many cases of acute back pain go away by themselves within a few days or weeks. You may be able to reduce pain and inflammation by applying cold and then heat. Begin with a cold treatment: Apply ice several times a day; once inflammation and spasms subside, you can apply heat using a heating pad or a warm bath. (See Chapter 3 for more on injury treatment and the use of ice.) If the pain is bothersome, an over-the-counter, non-steroidal anti-inflammatory medication such as ibuprofen or naproxen may be helpful; stronger pain medications and muscle relaxants are available by prescription.

Bed rest immediately following the onset of back pain may make you feel better, but it should be of very short duration. Prolonged bed rest—5 days or more—was once thought to be an effective treatment for back pain, but most physicians now advise against it because it may weaken muscles and actually worsen pain. Limit bed rest to one day and begin moderate physical activity as soon as possible. Exercise can increase muscular endurance and flexibility and protect your disks from loss of fluid. Three of the back exercises discussed later in the chapter may be particularly helpful following an episode of acute back pain: curl-ups, side bridges, and back extensions.

See your physician if acute back pain doesn't resolve within a short time. Other warning signals of a more severe problem that requires a professional evaluation include the following: severe pain, numbness, pain that radiates down one or both legs, problems with bladder or bowel control, fever, or rapid weight loss.

Managing Chronic Back Pain

Low-back pain is considered chronic if it persists for more than 3 months. Symptoms vary—some people experience stabbing or shooting pain, others a steady ache accompanied by stiffness. Sometimes pain is localized; in other cases, it radiates to another part of the body. Psychological symptoms may also occur. Underlying causes of chronic back pain include injuries, infection, muscle or ligament strains, and disk herniations.

Because symptoms and causes are so varied, different people benefit from different treatment strategies, and researchers have found that many treatments have only limited benefits. Potential treatments may include over-the-counter or prescription medications; exercise; physical therapy, massage, or chiropractic care; acupuncture; percutaneous electrical nerve stimulation (PENS), in which acupuncture-like needles are used to deliver an electrical current; education and advice about posture, exercise, and body mechanics; and surgery.

Psychological therapy may also be beneficial in some cases. Reducing emotional stress that causes muscle tension can provide direct benefits, and other therapies can help people deal better with chronic pain and its effects on their daily lives. Support groups and expressive writing are strategies that have been found beneficial for people with chronic pain and other conditions (see the box "Expressive Writing and Chronic Conditions.").

Exercises for the Prevention and Management of Low-Back Pain

The tests in Labs 5.3 and 5.4 can help you assess low-back muscular endurance and posture. The exercises that follow are designed to help you maintain a healthy back by stretching and strengthening the major muscle groups that affect the back—the abdominal muscles, the muscles along your spine and sides, and the muscles of your hips and thighs. If you have back problems, check with your physician before beginning any exercise program. Perform the exercises slowly and progress very gradually. Stop and consult your physician if any exercise causes back pain. General guidelines for back exercise programs include the following:

• Do low-back exercises at least 3 days per week; many experts recommend that back exercises be done daily.

• Emphasize muscular endurance rather than muscular strength—endurance may be more protective. Many back injuries are caused by problems with motor control: If you attempt complex trunk movements (such as picking up a book from the floor) when your muscles are tired, you are more likely to strain muscles and/or put pressure on nerves, thereby causing pain.

• Don't do spine exercises involving a full range of motion early in the morning because your disks have a high fluid content early in the day and injuries may occur as a result.

• Engage in regular endurance exercise such as cycling or walking in addition to performing exercises that specifically build muscular endurance and flexibility.

• Be patient and stick with your program. Increased back fitness and pain relief may require as long as 3 months of regular exercise.

LOW-BACK EXERCISES

EXERCISE 1

CAT STRETCH

Target: Improved flexibility, relaxation, and reduced stiffness in the spine

Instructions: Begin on all fours with your knees below your hips and your hands below your shoulders. Slowly and deliberately move through a cycle of extension and flexion of your spine. **(a)** Begin by slowly pushing your back up and dropping your head slightly until your spine is extended (rounded). **(b)** Then, slowly lower your back and lift your chin slightly until your spine is flexed (relaxed and slightly arched). *Do not press at the ends of the range of motion.* Stop if you feel pain. Do 10 slow, continuous cycles of the movement.

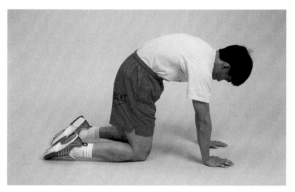

(a)

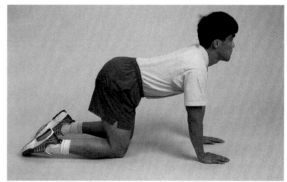

(b)

EXERCISE 2

STEP STRETCH
(see Exercise 6 in the flexibility program, p. 141)

Target: Improved flexibility, strength, and endurance in the muscles of the hip and the front of the thigh

Instructions: Hold each stretch for 10–30 seconds and do at least 4 repetitions on each side.

EXERCISE 3

ALTERNATE LEG STRETCHER
(see Exercise 11 in the flexibility program, p. 143)
Target: Improved flexibility in the back of the thigh, hip, knee, and buttocks
Instructions: Hold each stretch for 10–30 seconds and do at least 4 repetitions on each side.

 EXERCISE 4

TRUNK TWIST
Target: Improved flexibility in the lower back and sides
Instructions: Lie on your side with top knee bent, lower leg straight, lower arm extended out in front of you on the floor, and upper arm at your side. Push down with your upper knee while you twist your trunk backward. Try to get your shoulders and upper body flat on the floor, turning your head as well. Return to the starting position, and then repeat on the other side. Hold the stretch for 10–30 seconds and do at least 4 repetitions on each side.

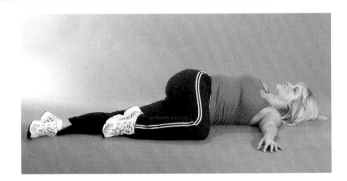

 EXERCISE 5

CURL-UP
Target: Improved strength and endurance in the abdomen
Instructions: Lie on your back with one or two knees bent and arms crossed on your chest or hands under your lower back. Tilt your pelvis under, flattening your back. Tuck your chin in and slowly curl up, one vertebra at a time, as you use your abdominal muscles to lift your head first and then your shoulders. Stop when you can see your knees and hold for 5–10 seconds before returning to the starting position. Do 10 or more repetitions.

Variation: Add a twist to develop other abdominal muscles. When you have curled up so that your shoulder blades are off the floor, twist your upper body so that one shoulder is higher than the other; reach past your knee with your upper arm. Hold and then return to the starting position. Repeat on the opposite side. Curl-ups can also be done using an exercise ball (see p. 153).

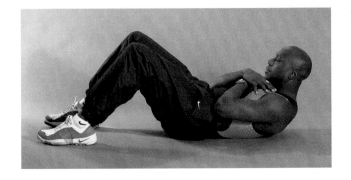

 EXERCISE 6

ISOMETRIC SIDE BRIDGE
(See Exercise 11 in the free weights program in Chapter 4, p. 111)
Target: Increased strength and endurance in the muscles along the sides of the abdomen
Instructions: Hold the bridge position for 10 seconds, breathing normally. Work up to a 60-second hold. Perform one or more repetitions on each side.
Variation: You can make the exercise more difficult by keeping your legs straight and supporting yourself with your feet and forearm (see Lab 5.3) or with your feet and hand (with elbow straight).

EXERCISE 7

SPINE EXTENSIONS

(see Exercise 10 in the free weights program in Chapter 4, p. 111)

Target: Increased strength and endurance in the back, buttocks, and back of the thighs

Instructions: Hold each position for 10–30 seconds. Begin with one repetition on each side and work up to several repetitions.

Variation: If you have experienced back pain in the past or if this exercise is very difficult for you, do the exercise with both hands on the ground rather than with one arm lifted. You can make this exercise more difficult by doing it balancing on an exercise ball. Find a balance point on your chest while lying face down on the ball with one arm and the opposite leg on the ground. Tense your abdominal muscles while reaching and extending with one arm and reaching and extending with the opposite leg. Repeat this exercise using the other arm and leg.

EXERCISE 8

WALL SQUAT (Phantom Chair)

Target: Increased strength and endurance in the lower back, thighs, and abdomen

Instructions: Lean against a wall and bend your knees as though you are sitting in a chair. Support your weight with your legs. Begin by holding the position for 5–10 seconds. Build up to 1 minute or more. Perform one or more repetitions.

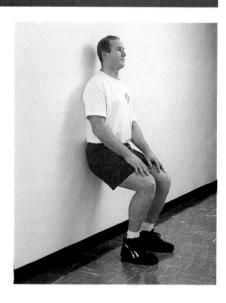

EXERCISE 9

PELVIC TILT

Target: Increased strength and endurance in the abdomen and buttocks

Instructions: Lie on your back with knees bent and arms extended to the side. Tilt your pelvis under and try to flatten your lower back against the floor. Tighten your buttock and abdominal muscles while you hold this position for 5–10 seconds. Don't hold your breath. Work up to 10 repetitions of the exercise. Pelvic tilts can also be done standing or leaning against a wall. (Note: Although this is a popular exercise with many therapists, some experts question the safety of pelvic tilts. Stop if you feel pain in your back at any time during the exercise.)

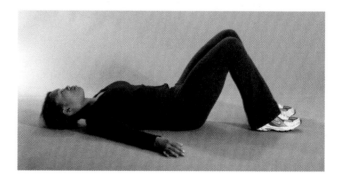

BACK BRIDGE

Target: Increased strength and endurance in the hips and buttocks

Instructions: Lie on your back with knees bent and arms extended to the side. Tuck your pelvis under, and then lift your tailbone, buttocks, and lower back from the floor. Hold this position for 5–10 seconds with your weight resting on your feet, arms, and shoulders, and then return to the starting position. Work up to 10 repetitions of the exercise. (Note: Although this is a popular exercise with many therapists, some experts question the safety of back bridges. Stop if you feel pain in your back at any time during the exercise.)

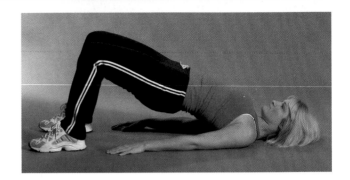

Tips for Today

Good flexibility and proper posture improve the health of your joints and muscles and may prevent injuries and low-back pain, contributing to long-term quality of life. Stretching exercises are also a great way to relax and relieve aches and pains. To improve and maintain your flexibility, perform stretches that work the major joints at least twice a week.

Right now you can

- Stand up and stretch—do either the upper-back stretch or the across-the-body stretch shown in the chapter.

- Practice the recommended sitting and standing postures suggested in the chapter. If needed, adjust your chair or find something to use as a footrest.

- If you frequently work at a computer, check the position in which you typically sit and make any needed adjustments to improve your posture. Your back should be flat or slightly rounded, feet flat on the floor (or a footrest), and knees at or slightly above hip level. When your hands are on the keyboard, your shoulders should be relaxed, your forearms and hands should be in a straight line, and the top of the monitor screen should be at or slightly below eye level. Your eyes should be about 18–30 inches from the screen.

SUMMARY

- Flexibility, the ability of joints to move through their full range of motion, is highly adaptable and specific to each joint.

- Range of motion can be limited by joint structure, muscle inelasticity, and stretch receptor activity.

- Developing flexibility depends on stretching the elastic tissues within muscles regularly and gently until they lengthen. Overstretching can make connective tissue brittle and lead to rupture.

- Signals sent between stretch receptors and the spinal cord can enhance flexibility because contracting a muscle stimulates a relaxation response, thereby allowing a longer muscle stretch, and because stretch receptors become less sensitive after repeated stretches, initiating fewer contractions.

- The benefits of flexibility include preventing abnormal stresses that lead to joint deterioration and possibly reducing the risk of injuries and low-back pain.

- Stretches should be held for 10–30 seconds; perform at least 4 repetitions. Flexibility training should be done 2 or more days a week, preferably following activity, when muscles are warm.

- Static stretching is done slowly and held to the point of mild tension; ballistic stretching consists of bouncing stretches and can lead to injury. Proprioceptive neuromuscular facilitation uses muscle receptors in contracting and relaxing a muscle.

- Passive stretching, using an outside force in moving muscles and joints, achieves a greater range of motion (and has a higher injury risk) than active stretching, which uses opposing muscles to initiate a stretch.

- The spinal column consists of vertebrae separated by intervertebral disks. It provides structure and support for the body and protects the spinal cord.

- Acute back pain can be treated as a soft tissue injury, with cold treatment followed by application of heat (once swelling subsides); prolonged bed rest is not recommended. A variety of treatments have been suggested for chronic back pain, including regular exercise, physical therapy, acupuncture, education, and psychological therapy.

- In addition to good posture, proper body mechanics, and regular physical activity, a program for preventing low-back pain includes exercises that stretch and strengthen major muscle groups that affect the lower back.

COMMON QUESTIONS ANSWERED

Is stretching the same as warming up? No. People often confuse stretching with a pre-exercise warm-up. Although they are complementary, they are two distinct activities. A warm-up involves light exercise that increases body temperature so your metabolism works better when you're exercising at high intensity. Stretching increases the movement capability of your joints, so you can move more easily with less risk of injury. Stretching may also induce cellular changes that protect muscles from injury.

Whenever you stretch, first spend 5–10 minutes engaged in some form of low-intensity exercise, such as walking, jogging, or low-intensity calisthenics. When your muscles are warmed, begin your stretching routine. Warmed muscles stretch better than cold ones and are less prone to injury.

How much flexibility do I need? This question is not always easy to answer. If you're involved in a sport such as gymnastics, figure skating, or ballet, you are often required to reach extreme joint motions to achieve success. However, nonathletes do not need to reach these extreme joint positions. In fact, too much flexibility may, in some cases, increase your risk of injury. As with other types of fitness, moderation is the key. You should regularly stretch your major joints and muscle groups but not aspire to reach extreme flexibility.

Can I stretch too far? Yes. As muscle tissue is progressively stretched, it reaches a point where it becomes damaged and may rupture. The greatest danger occurs during passive stretching when a partner is doing the stretching for you. It is critical that your stretching partner not force your joint outside its normal functional range of motion.

Can physical training limit flexibility? Weight training, jogging, or any physical activity will decrease flexibility if the exercises are not performed through a full range of motion. When done properly, weight training increases flexibility. However, because of the limited range of motion used during the running stride, jogging tends to compromise flexibility. It is very important for runners to practice flexibility exercises for the hamstrings and quadriceps regularly.

Does stretching affect muscular strength? Several recent studies have found that stretching decreases strength and power for about 5 minutes following the stretch. This is one reason why some experts suggest that people not stretch as part of their exercise warm-up. However, the effects of stretching on muscle strength and athletic performance are still being investigated. Regardless of when you choose to stretch, it is still important to warm up before any workout by engaging in 5–10 minutes of light exercise such as walking or slow jogging.

Can a workout with an exercise ball be useful in preventing and managing low-back pain? Yes. The exercise or stability ball is an extra-large inflatable ball. It was originally developed for use in physical therapy but has recently become a popular piece of exercise equipment for use in the home or gym. The exercise ball is particularly effective for working the so-called stability muscles in the abdomen, chest, and back—muscles that are important for preventing back problems. The ball's instability forces an exerciser to use the stability muscles to balance the body. Moves such as crunches have been found to be more effective when they are performed with an exercise ball. Beginners should use caution (and choose a larger-sized ball) until they feel comfortable with the movements.

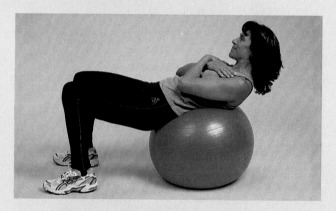

Using an exercise ball for curl-ups works the muscles in the chest, back, buttocks, and legs in addition to those in the abdomen.

FOR FURTHER EXPLORATION

W W *Fit and Well* **Online Learning Center** (www.mhhe.com/fahey)

Use the learning objectives, study guide questions, and glossary flashcards to review key terms and concepts and prepare for exams. You can extend your knowledge of flexibility and low-back health and gain experience in using the Internet as a resource by completing the activities and checking out the Web links for the topics in Chapter 5 marked with the World Wide Web icon. For this chapter, Internet activities explore the types of stretching techniques, different exercises that build flexibility, and techniques for preventing and managing back pain; there is also a helpful set of Web links.

Daily Fitness and Nutrition Journal

Complete the flexibility portion of the program plan by setting goals and selecting exercises. Fill in the information for the specific exercises you will perform, including which joints they work.

HealthQuest

If you haven't already done so, complete the How Fit Are You? section of the Wellness Activities in the fitness module of HealthQuest. This section provides an overview of your flexibility status based on your current level of flexibility and your stretching habits.

Books

Alter, M. J. 2004. *Science of Flexibility,* 3d ed. Champaign, Ill.: Human Kinetics. *An extremely well-researched book that discusses the scientific basis of stretching exercises and flexibility.*

Anderson, B., and J. Anderson. 2003. *Stretching*, 20th anniv. ed. Bolinas, Calif.: Shelter Publications. *A best-selling exercise book, updated with more than 200 stretches for 60 sports and activities.*

Blahnik, J. 2004. *Full-Body Flexibility.* Champaign, Ill.: Human Kinetics. *Presents a blend of stretching techniques derived from sports training, martial arts, yoga, and Pilates.*

Gallagher-Mundy, C. 2001. *Stretching for Health and Fitness.* Alexandria, Va.: Time Life. *A brief guide to safe and effective stretching exercises.*

Hochschuler, S., and B. Reznik. 2002. *Treat Your Back without Surgery.* 2nd ed. Alameda, Calif.: Hunter House. *Provides information about exercises and other nonsurgical techniques for treating back problems.*

Jemmet, M. 2001. *Spinal Stabilization: The New Science of Back Pain.* Halifax, Nova Scotia: RMJ Fitness and Rehabilitation Consultants. *Provides information on anatomy, biomechanics, common back problems, and helpful exercises.*

ᐺᐺ Organizations and Web Sites

American Academy of Orthopaedic Surgeons: Public Information. Provides information about a variety of joint problems, including back, neck, and shoulder pain.

   http://orthoinfo.aaos.org

CUErgo: Cornell University Ergonomics Web Site. Provides information about how to arrange a computer workstation to prevent back pain and repetitive strain injuries as well as other topics related to ergonomics.

   http://ergo.human.cornell.edu

Exercise: A Guide from the National Institute on Aging. Practical advice on fitness for seniors; includes animated instructions for specific flexibility exercises.

   http://www.nia.nih.gov/exercisebook

Georgia State University: Flexibility. Provides information about the benefits of stretching and how to develop a safe and effective program; includes illustrations of stretches.

   http://www.gsu.edu/~wwwfit/flexibility.html

MedlinePlus Back Pain Tutorial. An interactive, illustrated tutorial of the causes and prevention of back pain.

   http://www.nlm.nih.gov/medlineplus/tutorials/backpain.html

NIH Back Pain Fact Sheet. Basic information on the prevention and treatment of back pain.

   http://www.ninds.nih.gov/health_and_medical/disorders/backpain_doc.htm

Southern California Orthopedic Institute. Provides information about a variety of orthopedic problems, including back injuries; also has illustrations of spinal anatomy.

   http://www.scoi.com

Stretching and Flexibility. Provides information about the physiology of stretching and different types of stretching exercises.

   http://www.ifafitness.com/stretch/index.html

See also the listings for Chapters 2 and 4.

SELECTED BIBLIOGRAPHY

Amako, M., et al. 2003. Effect of static stretching on prevention of injuries for military recruits. *Military Medicine* 168:442–446.

American College of Sports Medicine. 2001. *ACSM's Resource Manual for Guidelines for Exercise Testing and Prescription*, 4th ed. Philadelphia: Lippincott Williams and Wilkins.

Back pain: Does anything work? 2000. *Consumer Reports on Health,* May.

Buchbinder, R., and J. Hoving. 2002. Specific spinal exercise substantially reduces the risk of low back pain recurrence. *Australian Journal of Physiotherapy* 48:55.

Fatouros, I. G., et al. 2002. The effects of strength training, cardiovascular training, and their combination on flexibility of inactive older adults. *International Journal of Sports Medicine* 23(20): 112–119.

Funk, D. C., et al. 2003. Impact of prior exercise on hamstring flexibility: A comparison of proprioceptive neuromuscular facilitation and static stretching. *Journal of Strength and Conditioning Research* 17:489–492.

Grenier, S. G., C. Russell, and S. M. McGill. 2003. Relationships between lumbar flexibility, sit-and-reach test, and a previous history of low back discomfort in industrial workers. *Canadian Journal of Applied Physiology* 28:165–177.

Harwood, M. I., and S. I. Chang. 2002. What is the most effective treatment for acute low back pain? *Journal of Family Practice* 51:118.

Herbert, R. D., and M. Gabriel. 2002. Effects of stretching before and after exercising on muscle soreness and risk of injury: Systematic review. *British Medical Journal* 325:468–472.

Hodges, P., and G. Jull. 2000. Does strengthening the abdominal muscles prevent low back pain? *Journal of Rheumatology* 27(9): 2286–2288.

Hodges, P. W. 2003. Core stability exercise in chronic low back pain. *Orthopedic Clinics of North America* 34:245–254.

Kovacs, F. M., et al. 2003. Effect of firmness of mattress on chronic nonspecific low-back pain: Randomised, double-blind, controlled, multicentre trial. *Lancet* 362(9396): 1594–1595.

Knudson, D. V. 2000. Current issues in flexibility fitness. *President's Council on Physical Fitness and Sports: Research Digest* 3(1).

Luebbers, P. 2002. Enhancing your flexibility. *ACSM Fit Society Page,* Spring, pp. 5, 8.

McGill, S. M. 1998. Low back exercises: Evidence for improving exercise regimens. *Physical Therapy* 78(7): 754–765.

Nieman, D. C. 2004. You asked for it: Low back pain. *ACSM's Health and Fitness Journal,* January/February.

Nieman, D. C. 2003. *Exercise Testing and Prescription: A Health-Related Approach,* 5th ed. New York: McGraw-Hill.

Palmer, K. T., et al. 2003. Smoking and musculoskeletal disorders: Findings from a British national survey. *Annals of Rheumatoid Diseases* 62:33–36.

Parente, D. 2000. Influence of aerobic and stretching exercise on anxiety and sensation-seeking mood state. *Perceptual and Motor Skills* 90(1): 347–348.

Parks, K. A., et al. 2003. A comparison of lumbar range of motion and functional ability scores in patients with low back pain: Assessment for range of motion validity. *Spine* 28:380–384.

Patel, A. T., and A. A. Ogle. 2000. Diagnosis and management of acute low back pain. *American Family Physician* 61(6): 1779–1786, 1789–1790.

Power, C., et al. 2001. Predictors of low back pain onset in a prospective British study. *American Journal of Public Health* 91(10): 1671–1678.

Rainville, J., et al. 2004. Exercise as treatment for chronic low back pain. *Spine Journal* 4(1): 106–115.

Rowlands, A. V., V. F. Marginson, and J. Lee. 2003. Chronic flexibility gains: Effect of isometric contraction duration during proprioceptive neuromuscular facilitation stretching techniques. *Research Quarterly for Exercise and Sport* 74:47–51.

Schur, P. E. 2001. Effectiveness of stretching to reduce injury. *British Journal of Sports Medicine* 35:138.

Ten nice-to-know facts about flexibility and stretching. 2003. *ACSM's Health & Fitness Journal,* July/August.

Thacker, S. B., et al. 2004. The impact of stretching on sports injury risk: A systematic review of the literature. *Medicine and Science in Sports and Exercise* 36(3): 371–378.

Underwood, M. R. 2000. Exercise and the prevention of back pain disability. *British Journal of Sports Medicine* 34(1): 5.

Name _____ Section _____ Date _____

LAB 5.1 *Assessing Your Current Level of Flexibility*

 Part I Sit-and-Reach Test

Equipment

Use a modified Wells and Dillon flexometer or construct your own measuring device using a firm box or two pieces of wood about 30 centimeters (12 inches) high attached at right angles to each other. Attach a metric ruler to measure the extent of reach. With the low numbers of the ruler toward the person being tested, set the 26-centimeter mark of the ruler at the footline of the box. (Individuals who cannot reach as far as the footline will have scores below 26 centimeters; those who can reach past their feet will have scores above 26 centimeters.)

Preparation

Warm up your muscles with a low-intensity activity such as walking or easy jogging. Then perform slow stretching movements.

Instructions

1. Remove your shoes and sit facing the flexibility measuring device with your knees fully extended and your feet flat against the device about 10 centimeters (4 inches) apart.
2. Reach as far forward as you can, with palms down, arms evenly stretched, and knees fully extended; hold the position of maximum reach for about 2 seconds.
3. Perform the stretch 2 times, recording the distance of maximum reach to the nearest 0.5 centimeters: _____ cm

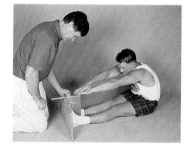

Rating Your Flexibility

Find the score in the table below to determine your flexibility rating. Record it here and on the final page of this lab.

Rating: _____

Ratings for Sit-and-Reach Test

Rating/Score (cm)*

Men	Needs Improvement	Fair	Good	Very Good	Excellent
Age: 15–19	Below 24	24–28	29–33	34–38	Above 38
20–29	Below 25	25–29	30–33	34–39	Above 39
30–39	Below 23	23–27	28–32	33–37	Above 37
40–49	Below 18	18–23	24–28	29–34	Above 34
50–59	Below 16	16–23	24–27	28–34	Above 34
60–69	Below 15	15–19	20–24	25–32	Above 32
Women					
Age: 15–19	Below 29	29–33	34–37	38–42	Above 42
20–29	Below 28	28–32	33–36	37–40	Above 40
30–39	Below 27	27–31	32–35	36–40	Above 40
40–49	Below 25	25–29	30–33	34–37	Above 37
50–59	Below 25	25–29	30–32	33–38	Above 38
60–69	Below 23	23–26	27–30	31–34	Above 34

*Footline is set at 26 cm.

SOURCE: Ratings from Canadian Society for Exercise Physiology. 1998. *The Canadian Physical Activity, Fitness and Lifestyle Appraisal: CSEP's Plan for Healthy Active Living*, 2d ed. Ottawa: Canadian Society for Exercise Physiology. Adapted with permission from the Canadian Society for Exercise Physiology.

Part II Range-of-Motion Assessment

This portion of the lab can be completed by doing visual comparisons or by measuring joint range of motion with a goniometer or other instrument.

Equipment

1. A partner to do visual comparisons or to measure the range of motion of your joints. (You can also use a mirror to perform your own visual comparisons.)
2. For the measurement method, you need a goniometer, flexometer, or other instrument to measure range of motion.

Preparation

Warm up your muscles with some low-intensity activity such as walking or easy jogging.

Instructions

On the following pages, the average range of motion is illustrated and listed quantitatively for some of the major joints. Visually assess the range of motion in your joints and compare it to that shown in the illustrations. For each joint, note (with a check mark) whether your range of motion is above average, average, or below average and in need of improvement. Average values for range of motion are given in degrees for each joint in the assessment. You can also complete the assessment by measuring your range of motion with a goniometer, flexometer, or other instrument. If you are using this measurement method, identify your rating (above average, average, or below average) and record your range of motion in degrees next to the appropriate category. Although the measurement method is more time-consuming, it allows you to track the progress of your stretching program more precisely and to note changes within the broader ratings categories (below average, above average).

Record your ratings on the following pages and on the chart on the final page of this lab. (Ratings were derived from several published sources.)

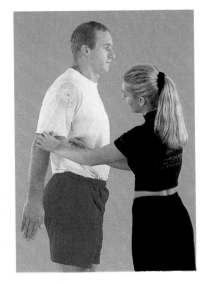

Assessment of range of motion using a goniometer.

1. Shoulder Abduction and Adduction

For each position and arm, check one of the following; also fill in degrees if using the measurement method.

Shoulder abduction—raise arm up to the side

Right   *Left*

_____ _____   Below average/needs improvement

_____ _____   Average (92–95°)

_____ _____   Above average

Shoulder adduction—move arm down and in front of body

Right   *Left*

_____ _____   Below average/needs improvement

_____ _____   Average (124–127°)

_____ _____   Above average

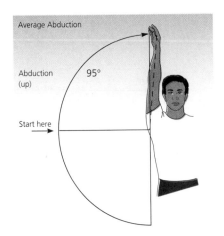

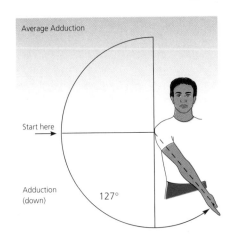

2. Shoulder Flexion and Extension

For each position and arm, check one of the following; also fill in degrees if using the measurement method.

Shoulder flexion—raise arm up in front of the body

Right   *Left*

_____   _____   Below average/needs improvement

_____   _____   Average (92–95°)

_____   _____   Above average

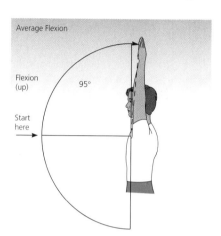

Shoulder extension—move arm down and behind the body

Right   *Left*

_____   _____   Below average/needs improvement

_____   _____   Average (145–150°)

_____   _____   Above average

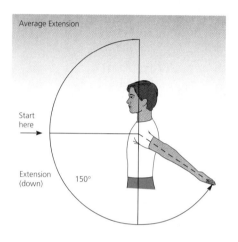

3. Trunk/Low Back Lateral Flexion

Bend directly sideways at your waist. To prevent injury, keep your knees slightly bent, and support your trunk by placing your hand or forearm on your thigh. Check one of the following for each side; fill in degrees if using the measurement method.

Right   *Left*

_____   _____   Below average/needs improvement

_____   _____   Average (36–40°)

_____   _____   Above average

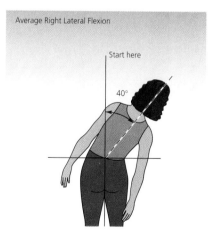

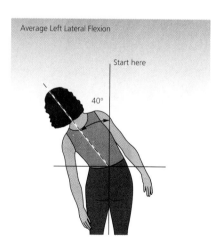

4. Hip Abduction

Raise your leg to the side at the hip. Check one of the following for each leg; fill in degrees if using the measurement method.

Right   Left

_____   _____   Below average/needs improvement

_____   _____   Average (40–45°)

_____   _____   Above average

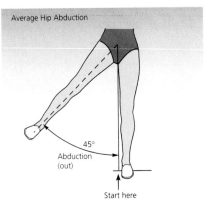

5. Hip Flexion (Bent Knee)

With one leg flat on the floor, bend the other knee and lift the leg up at the hip. Check one of the following for each leg; fill in degrees if using the measurement method.

Right   Left

_____   _____   Below average/needs improvement

_____   _____   Average (121–125°)

_____   _____   Above average

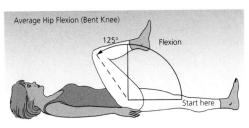

6. Hip Flexion (Straight Leg)

With one leg flat on the floor, raise the other leg at the hip, keeping both legs straight. Take care not to put excess strain on your back. Check one of the following for each leg; fill in degrees if using the measurement method.

Right   Left

_____   _____   Below average/needs improvement

_____   _____   Average (79–81°)

_____   _____   Above average

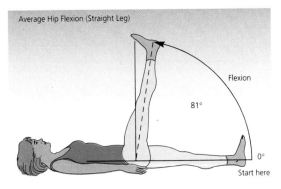

7. Ankle Dorsiflexion and Plantar Flexion

For each position and foot, check one of the following; also fill in degrees if using the measurement method.

Ankle dorsiflexion—pull your toes toward your shin

Right   Left

_____ _____   Below average/needs improvement

_____ _____   Average (9–13°)

_____ _____   Above average

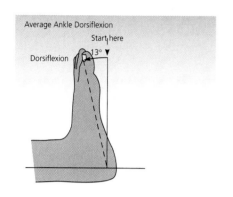

Plantar flexion—point your toes

Right   Left

_____ _____   Below average/needs improvement

_____ _____   Average (50–55°)

_____ _____   Above average

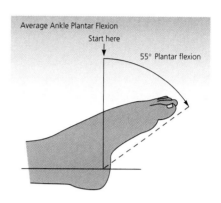

Rating Your Flexibility

Sit-and-Reach Test: Score: _____ cm.   Rating: _____

Range of Motion Assessment

Identify your rating for each joint on each side of the body. If you used the comparison method, put check marks in the appropriate categories; if you measured range of motion, enter the degrees for each joint in the appropriate category.

Joint/Assessment		Right			Left		
		Below Average	Average	Above Average	Below Average	Average	Above Average
1. Shoulder abduction and adduction	Abduction						
	Adduction						
2. Shoulder flexion and extension	Flexion						
	Extension						
3. Trunk/low back lateral flexion	Flexion						
4. Hip abduction	Abduction						
5. Hip flexion (bent knee)	Flexion						
6. Hip flexion (straight leg)	Flexion						
7. Ankle dorsiflexion and plantar flexion	Dorsiflexion						
	Plantar flexion						

Using Your Results

How did you score? Are you at all surprised by your ratings for flexibility? Are you satisfied with your current ratings?

If you're not satisfied, set a realistic goal for improvement: _____

Are you satisfied with your current level of flexibility as expressed in your daily life—for example, your ability to maintain good posture and move easily and without pain?

If you're not satisfied, set some realistic goals for improvement:

What should you do next? Enter the results of this lab in the Preprogram Assessment column in Appendix D. If you've set goals for improvement, begin planning your flexibility program by completing the plan in Lab 5.2. After several weeks of your program, complete this lab again and enter the results in the Postprogram Assessment column of Appendix D. How do the results compare?

LAB 5.2 *Creating a Personalized Program for Developing Flexibility*   WW

Goals: List goals for your flexibility program. On the left, include specific, measurable goals that you can use to track the progress of your fitness program. These goals might be things like raising your sit-and-reach score from fair to good or your bent-leg hip flexion rating from below average to average. On the right, include long-term and more qualitative goals, such as reducing your risk for back pain.

Specific Goals: Current Status

_____

_____

_____

Final Goals

_____

_____

_____

Other goals: _____

_____

Exercises: The exercises in the program plan below are from the general stretching program presented in Chapter 5. You can add or delete exercises depending on your needs, goals, and preferences. For any exercises you add, fill in the areas of the body affected.

Frequency: A minimum frequency of 2–3 days per week is recommended. You may want to do your stretching exercises the same days you plan to do cardiorespiratory endurance exercise or weight training, because muscles stretch better following exercise, when they are warm.

Intensity: All stretches should be done to the point of mild discomfort, not pain.

Time/duration: All stretches should be held for 10–30 seconds. (PNF techniques should include a 6-second contraction followed by a 10–30-second assisted stretch.) All stretches should be performed at least 4 times.

Program Plan for Flexibility

Exercise	Areas Stretched	Frequency (check ✔)						
		M	T	W	Th	F	Sa	Su
Head turns and tilts	Neck							
Towel stretch	Triceps, shoulders, chest							
Across-the-body and overhead stretches	Shoulders, upper back, back of the arm							
Upper-back stretch	Upper back							
Lateral stretch	Trunk muscles							
Step stretch	Hip, front of thigh							
Side lunge	Inner thigh, hip, calf							
Inner Thigh stretch	Inner thigh, hip							
Trunk rotation	Trunk, outer thigh and hip, lower back							
Modified hurdler stretch	Back of the thigh, lower back							
Alternate leg stretcher	Back of the thigh, hip, knee, ankle, buttocks							
Lower-leg stretch	Back of the lower leg							

You can monitor your program using a chart like the one on the next page.

LABORATORY ACTIVITIES

Flexibility Program Chart

Fill in the dates you perform each stretch, the number of seconds you hold each stretch (should be 10–30), and the number of repetitions of each (should be at least 4). For an easy check on the duration of your stretches, count "one thousand one, one thousand two," and so on. You will probably find that over time you'll be able to hold each stretch longer (in addition to being able to stretch farther).

Exercise/Date																			
	Duration																		
	Reps																		
	Duration																		
	Reps																		
	Duration																		
	Reps																		
	Duration																		
	Reps																		
	Duration																		
	Reps																		
	Duration																		
	Reps																		
	Duration																		
	Reps																		
	Duration																		
	Reps																		
	Duration																		
	Reps																		
	Duration																		
	Reps																		
	Duration																		
	Reps																		
	Duration																		
	Reps																		
	Duration																		
	Reps																		
	Duration																		
	Reps																		
	Duration																		
	Reps																		
	Duration																		
	Reps																		
	Duration																		
	Reps																		

LAB 5.3   *Assessing Muscular Endurance for Low-Back Health*

The three tests in this lab evaluate the muscular endurance of major spine stabilizing muscles.

 Side Bridge Endurance Test

Equipment

1. Stopwatch or clock with a second hand
2. Exercise mat
3. Partner

Preparation

Warm up your muscles with some low-intensity activity such as walking or easy jogging. Practice assuming the side bridge position described below.

Instructions

1. Lie on the mat on your side with your legs extended. Place your top foot in front of your lower foot for support. Lift your hips off the mat so that you are supporting yourself on one elbow and your feet (see photo). Your body should maintain a straight line. Breathe normally; don't hold your breath.
2. Hold the position as long as possible. Your partner should keep track of the time and make sure that you maintain the correct position. Your final score is the total time you are able to hold the side bridge with correct form—from the time you lift your hips until your hips return to the mat.
3. Rest for 5 minutes and then repeat the test on the other side. Record your times here and on the chart at the end of the lab. Right side bridge time: _____ sec   Left side bridge time: _____ sec

 Trunk Flexors Endurance Test

Equipment

1. Stopwatch or clock with a second hand
2. Exercise mat or padded exercise table
3. Two helpers
4. Jig angled at 60° from the floor or padded bench (optional)

Preparation

Warm up with some low-intensity activity such as walking or easy jogging.

Instructions

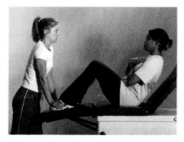

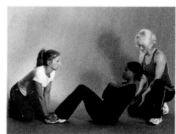

1. To start, assume a sit-up posture with your back supported at an angle of 60° from the floor; support can be provided by a jig, a padded bench, or a spotter (see photos). Your knees and hips should both be flexed at 90°, and your arms should be folded across your chest with your hands placed on the opposite shoulders. Your toes should be secured under a toe strap or held by a partner.
2. Your goal is to hold the starting position (isometric contraction) as long as possible after the support is pulled away. To begin the test, a helper should pull the jig or other support back about 10 cm (4 inches). A helper should keep track of the time; if a spotter is acting as your support, she or he should be ready to support your weight as soon as your torso begins to move back. Your final score is the total time you are able to hold the contraction—from the time the support is removed until any part of your back touches the support. Remember to breathe normally throughout the test.
3. Record your time here and on the chart at the end of the lab. Trunk flexors endurance time: _____ sec

Back Extensors Endurance Test

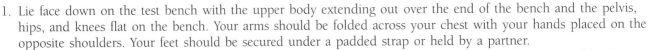

Equipment

1. Stopwatch or clock with a second hand
2. Extension bench with padded ankle support or any padded bench
3. Partner

Preparation

Warm up with some low-intensity activity such as walking or easy jogging.

Instructions

1. Lie face down on the test bench with the upper body extending out over the end of the bench and the pelvis, hips, and knees flat on the bench. Your arms should be folded across your chest with your hands placed on the opposite shoulders. Your feet should be secured under a padded strap or held by a partner.
2. Your goal is to hold your upper body in a straight horizontal line with your lower body as long as possible. Keep your neck straight and neutral; don't raise your head and don't arch your back. Breathe normally. Your partner should keep track of the time and watch your form. Your final score is the total time you are able to hold the horizontal position—from the time you assume the position until your upper body drops from the horizontal position.
3. Record your time here and on the chart below. Back extensors endurance time: _____ sec

Rating Your Test Results for Muscular Endurance for Low-Back Health

The table below shows mean endurance test times for healthy young college students with a mean age of 21 years. Compare your scores with the times shown in the table. (If you are older or have suffered from low-back pain in the past, these ratings are less accurate; however, your time scores can be used as a point of comparison.)

Mean Endurance Times (sec)

	Right side bridge	Left side bridge	Trunk flexors	Back extensors
Men	95	99	136	161
Women	75	78	134	185

SOURCE: McGill, S. M. 2002. *Low Back Disorders: Evidence Based Prevention and Rehabilitation.* Champaign, Ill.: Human Kinetics.

Right side bridge: _____ sec   Rating (above mean, at mean, below mean): _____
Left side bridge: _____ sec   Rating (above mean, at mean, below mean): _____
Trunk flexors: _____ sec   Rating (above mean, at mean, below mean): _____
Back extensors: _____ sec   Rating (above mean, at mean, below mean): _____

Using Your Results

How did you score? Are you at all surprised by your scores for the low-back tests? Are you satisfied with your current ratings?

If you're not satisfied, set a realistic goal for improvement. The norms in this lab are based on healthy young adults, so a score above the mean may or may not be realistic for you. Instead, you may want to set a specific goal based on time rather than rating; for example, set a goal of improving your time by 10%. Imbalances in muscular endurance have been linked with back problems, so if your rating is significantly lower for one of the three tests, you should focus particular attention on that area of the body.

Goal: _____

What should you do next? Enter the results of this lab in the Preprogram Assessment column in Appendix D. If you've set a goal for improvement, begin a program of low-back exercises such as that suggested in this chapter. After several weeks of your program, complete this lab again and enter the results in the Postprogram Assessment column of Appendix D. How do the results compare?

LABORATORY ACTIVITIES

LAB 5.4 *Posture Evaluation*

For each row, have a partner record the point total that corresponds to the illustration that most closely matches your posture.

5 points	3 points	1 point	Your Score
 Head erect (gravity line passes directly through center)	 Head twisted or turned to one side slightly	 Head twisted or turned to one side markedly	_____
 Shoulders level (horizontally)	 One shoulder slightly higher than other	 One shoulder markedly higher than other	_____
 Spine straight	 Spine slightly curved laterally	 Spine markedly curved laterally	_____
 Hips level (horizontally)	 One hip slightly higher	 One hip markedly higher	_____
 Feet pointed straight ahead	 Feet pointed out		_____
 Arches high	 Arches lower, feet slightly flat	 Arches low; feet markedly flat	_____

Feet pointed out markedly; ankles sag in (pronation)

	5 points	3 points	1 point	Your Score

 Neck erect, chin in, head in balance directly above shoulders

 Neck slightly forward, chin slightly out

 Neck markedly forward, chin markedly out

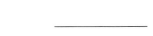

 Chest elevated (breast-bone farthest forward part of body)

 Chest slightly depressed

 Chest markedly depressed (flat)

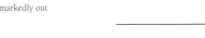

 Shoulders centered

 Shoulders slightly forward

 Shoulders markedly forward (shoulder blades protruding in rear)

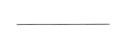

 Upper back normally rounded

 Upper back slightly more rounded

 Upper back markedly rounded

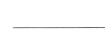

 Trunk erect

 Trunk inclined to rear slightly

Trunk inclined to rear markedly

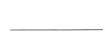

 Abdomen flat

 Abdomen protruding

 Abdomen protruding and sagging

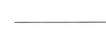

 Lower back normally curved

 Lower back slightly hollow

 Lower back markedly hollow

TOTAL SCORE (from both pages) (Scores should be between 13 and 65.) _____

If your posture needs improvement, review the information in the box on good posture and low-back health on p. 147. If you scored "1 point" for any item in the evaluation, you may want to consider seeing a physician; professional advice, physical therapy, orthotic devices, or other therapies may help you improve your posture.

SOURCE: Reproduced with the permission of The University of the State of New York, author, and publisher.

6

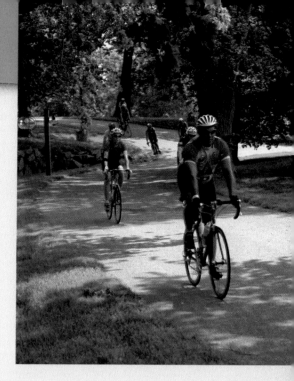

Body Composition

LOOKING AHEAD

After reading this chapter, you should be able to

• Define fat-free mass, essential fat, and nonessential fat and describe their functions in the body

• Explain how body composition affects overall health and wellness

• Describe how body mass index, body composition, and body fat distribution are measured and assessed

• Explain how to determine recommended body weight and body fat distribution

TEST YOUR KNOWLEDGE

1. Exercise helps reduce the risks associated with over-weight and obesity even if it doesn't result in improvements in body composition.
   True or false?

2. Which of the following is the most significant risk factor for the most common type of diabetes (type 2 diabetes)?
   a. smoking
   b. low-fiber diet
   c. overweight or obesity
   d. inactivity

3. In women, excessive exercise and low energy (calorie) intake can cause which of the following?
   a. unhealthy reduction in body fat levels
   b. amenorrhea (absent menstruation)
   c. bone density loss and osteoporosis
   d. muscle wasting and fatigue

ANSWERS

1. TRUE. Regular physical activity provides protection against the health risks of overweight and obesity. People who are fit and obese live longer, healthier lives than normal weight people who are sedentary. However, it is best to both be active and maintain a healthy weight.

2. C. All four are risk factors for diabetes, but overweight/obesity is the most significant. It's estimated that 90% of cases of type 2 diabetes could be prevented if people adopted healthy lifestyle behaviors.

3. ALL FOUR. Very low levels of body fat, and the behaviors used to achieve them, have serious health consequences for both men and women.

ViW Fit and Well Online Learning Center   www.mhhe.com/fahey

Visit the *Fit and Well* Online Learning Center for study aids, online labs, additional information about body composition, links, Internet activities that explore how body composition can influence wellness, and much more.

ody composition, the body's relative amount of fat and fat-free mass, is an important component of fitness for health and wellness. People whose body composition is optimal tend to be healthier, to move more efficiently, and to feel better about themselves. They also have a lower risk of many chronic diseases. To reach wellness, you must determine what body composition is right for you and then work to achieve and maintain it.

Although people pay lip service to the idea of exercising for health, a more immediate goal for many is to look fit and healthy. Unfortunately, many people don't succeed in their efforts to obtain a fit and healthy body because they set unrealistic goals and emphasize short-term weight loss rather than the permanent changes in lifestyle that lead to fat loss and a healthy body composition. Successful management of body composition requires the long-term, consistent coordination of many aspects of a wellness program. However, even in the absence of changes in body composition, an active lifestyle can improve wellness (see the box "Can You Be Fit and Fat?"). This chapter focuses on defining and measuring body composition. The aspects of lifestyle that affect body composition are discussed in detail in other chapters: physical activity and exercise in Chapters 2–5 and 7, sound nutritional habits in Chapter 8, specific strategies for weight management in Chapter 9, and healthy techniques for managing stress in Chapter 10.

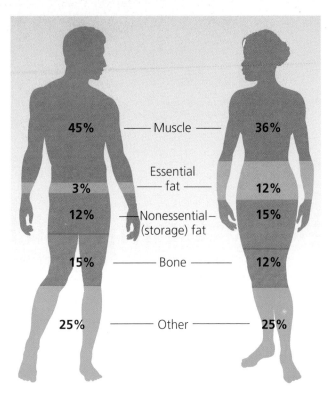

Figure 6.1   Body composition of a typical man and woman, 20–24 years old.   SOURCE: Adapted from Brooks, G. A., et al. 2005. *Exercise Physiology: Human Bioenergetics and Its Applications,* 4th ed. New York: McGraw-Hill.

WHAT IS BODY COMPOSITION, AND WHY IS IT IMPORTANT?

The human body can be divided into fat-free mass and body fat. Fat-free mass is composed of all the body's nonfat tissues: bone, water, muscle, connective tissue, organ tissues, and teeth. Body fat includes both essential and nonessential (storage) body fats (Figure 6.1). **Essential fat** includes lipids incorporated into the nerves, brain, heart, lungs, liver, and mammary glands. These fat deposits, crucial for normal body functioning,

make up approximately 3–5% of total body weight in men and 8–12% in women. (The larger percentage in women is due to fat deposits in the breasts, uterus, and other sites specific to females.) **Nonessential (storage) fat** exists primarily within fat cells, or **adipose tissue,** often located just below the skin and around major organs. The amount of storage fat varies from individual to individual based on many factors, including gender, age, heredity, metabolism, diet, and activity level. Excess storage fat is usually the result of consuming more energy (as food) than is expended (in metabolism and physical activity).

Overweight and Obesity Defined

How much body fat is too much for health and wellness? In the past, many people relied on height-weight tables based on insurance company mortality statistics to answer this question. Unfortunately, these tables can be highly inaccurate for some people; at best, they provide only an indirect measure of fatness. Because, as explained in Chapter 4, muscle tissue is denser and heavier than fat, a fit person can easily weigh more and an unfit person weigh less than recommended weights on a height-weight table.

The most important consideration when a person is looking at body composition is the proportion of the

Terms

essential fat The fat in the body necessary for normal body functioning.

nonessential (storage) fat Extra fat or fat reserves stored in the body.

adipose tissue Connective tissue in which fat is stored.

percent body fat The percentage of total body weight that is composed of fat.

overweight Characterized by a body weight above a recommended range for good health; ranges are set through large-scale population surveys.

obese Severely overweight, characterized by an excessive accumulation of body fat; overfat. Obesity may also be defined in terms of some measure of total body weight.

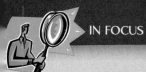
If a larger percentage of the population became physically active, the public health burden associated with obesity would be greatly reduced. This conclusion should not be interpreted to dismiss the health risks associated with obesity, but rather to emphasize the moderating influence of physical activity and physical fitness on these risks.

This quote from a recent article in the *President's Council on Physical Fitness and Sports Research Digest*—based on years of scientific studies—indicates that for adults, it may be possible to be both fit and fat.

Obesity is linked to many serious diseases and physical problems, including cardiovascular disease, diabetes, certain cancers, gallbladder disease, arthritis, and premature death. Regular physical activity can help prevent obesity, but activity is also extremely important for health even if it results in no changes in body composition. Exercise blocks many of the destructive health effects of obesity even in individuals who remain overweight. It improves blood pressure, blood fat and blood glucose levels, and body fat distribution; it lowers the risk of diabetes, heart disease, and early death. Researchers have found that active obese people have fewer health problems and live longer than normal weight people who are inactive.

Is physical activity or physical fitness more important for fighting the adverse health effects of obesity? The results of a large number of published studies suggest that physical activity and fitness are both important—the more fit and active you are, the lower your risk of dying prematurely or having health problems. Of the two, however, daily physical activity appears to be more important for health than physical fitness. Studies have further shown that people who are active and not overweight have a lower risk of death than inactive or overweight people; however, people who are overweight but active have a lower risk of death than those who are not overweight but inactive

(see figure below). So, while reducing body fat and building fitness are important for wellness, many health benefits can be obtained by simply being more physically active each day.

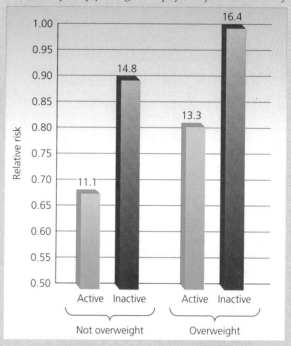

Risk of death relative to physical activity and overweight status. The numbers on the bars indicate mortality rates per 1000.

SOURCES: Katzmarzyk, P. T., et al. 2003. Physical inactivity, excess adiposity, and premature mortality. *Obesity Reviews* 4(4): 257–290. Blair, S. N., Y. Cheng, and J. S. Holder. 2001. Is physical activity or physical fitness more important in defining health benefits? *Medicine and Science in Sports and Exercise* 33(Suppl): S379–S399. Welk, G. J., and S. N. Blair. 2000. Physical activity protects against the health risks of obesity. *President's Council on Physical Fitness and Sports Research Digest* 3(12).

body's total weight that is fat—the **percent body fat.** For example, two women may both be 5 feet, 5 inches tall and weigh 130 pounds. But one women, a runner, may have only 20% of her body weight as fat, whereas the second, sedentary woman could have 40% body fat. Although neither woman is overweight by most standards, the second woman is overfat. Too much body fat (not total weight) has a negative effect on health and well-being.

Some of the most commonly used methods to assess and classify body composition are described later in the chapter. Although less accurate than standards based on body fat, some methods are based on total body weight because it is easier to measure. **Overweight** is usually defined as total body weight above the recommended range for good health (as determined by large-scale population surveys). **Obesity** is defined as a more serious degree of overweight; the cutoff point for obesity may be

set in terms of percent body fat or in terms of some measure of total body weight.

Prevalence of Overweight and Obesity Among Americans

By any measure, Americans are getting fatter. The prevalence of obesity has increased from about 13% in 1960 to about 31% today, and more than 60% of American adults are now overweight (Figure 6.2, p. 170). Possible explanations for this increase include more time spent in sedentary work and leisure activities, fewer short trips on foot and more by automobile, fewer daily gym classes for students, more meals eaten outside the home, greater consumption of fast food, increased portion sizes, and increased consumption of soft drinks and convenience foods. Fewer than half of Americans meet the minimum recommendation of 30 minutes per day of moderate physical activity,

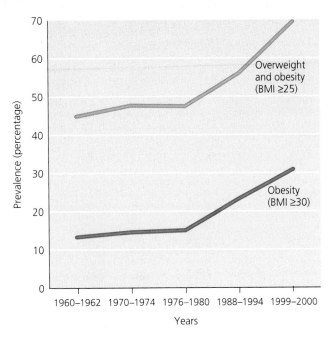

Figure 6.2 **Prevalence of overweight and obesity among Americans.** SOURCE: National Center for Health Statistics. 2003. *Health, United States, 2003.* Hyattsville, Md.: National Center for Health Statistics.

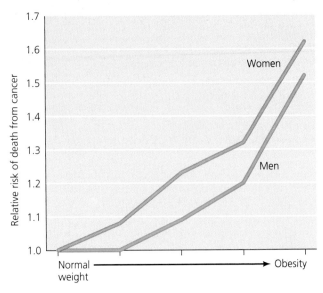

Figure 6.3 **Body weight and cancer mortality.** For both men and women, overweight and obesity are associated with significantly higher rates of death from cancer. SOURCE: Calle, E. E., et al. 2003. Overweight, obesity, and mortality from cancer in a prospectively studied cohort of U.S. adults. *New England Journal of Medicine* 348(17): 1625–1638.

and the Centers for Disease Control and Prevention has estimated that caloric intake has increased by 100–300 calories a day during the past decade. (For more on the causes of obesity, see Chapter 9.)

MOTIVATION FOR CHANGE! Do a check of your home living space to eliminate cues that trigger behaviors you are trying to reduce or eliminate and to add cues that trigger behaviors you want to develop or increase. For example, do you have unhealthy snacks stuffed into your desk drawers or in easy reach in the kitchen? If so, remove these and make healthier choices just as available. Where are your exercise clothes located? Placing them in an easily accessible and obvious location can help them serve as a reminder and motivate you to be active by making it more convenient. Place motivational notes and reminders in appropriate locations—on the bathroom mirror, on the refrigerator, by the front door. Once you've shaped your home environment to support your behavior change program, repeat the process in other locations—your office or study space, your car, and so on.

Excess Body Fat and Wellness

As rates of overweight and obesity increase, so do the problems associated with them. Obesity causes more than 400,000 premature deaths each year and costs the United States more than $100 billion annually. If current trends continue, obesity will soon surpass cigarette smoking as the leading cause of disability and death among Americans.

Excess body fat can impact overall wellness through its effects on chronic disease risk, ability to perform physical activities, and body image.

Risk of Chronic Disease and Premature Death
Obese people have an overall mortality rate almost twice that of nonobese people, and even mild to moderate overweight is associated with a substantial increase in the risk of premature death. Obesity is associated with unhealthy blood fat levels, impaired heart function, and death from cardiovascular disease. It is estimated that if all Americans had a healthy body composition, the incidence of coronary heart disease would drop by more than 24%. Obesity is also associated with increased risk of death from many types of cancer (Figure 6.3). Other health problems associated with obesity include hypertension, impaired immune function, gallbladder and kidney diseases, skin problems, sleep and breathing disorders, impotence, pregnancy complications, impaired immune function, back pain, arthritis, and other bone and joint disorders. Of particular note is the strong association between excess body fat and diabetes mellitus: Obese people are more than three times as likely as nonobese people to develop diabetes, and the incidence of diabetes among Americans has increased dramatically as the rate of obesity has climbed (see the box "Diabetes").

The distribution of fat is also an important indicator of future health. Studies suggest that people who tend to gain weight in the abdominal area ("apples") have a risk of coronary heart disease, high blood pressure, diabetes, and stroke twice as high as that of people who tend to

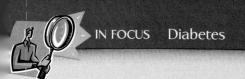

Diabetes mellitus is a disease that causes a disruption of normal metabolism. The pancreas, a long, thin organ located behind the stomach, normally secretes the hormone insulin, which stimulates cells to take up glucose to produce energy. In a person with diabetes, this process is disrupted, causing a buildup of glucose in the bloodstream. Over the long term, diabetes is associated with kidney failure; nerve damage; circulation problems; retinal damage and blindness; and increased rates of heart attack, stroke, and hypertension. The rate of diabetes has increased steadily over the past 40 years, jumping a dramatic 33% in the 1990s; it is currently the sixth leading cause of death in the United States.

Types of Diabetes

Approximately 18 million (1 in 14) Americans have one of two major forms of diabetes. About 5–10% of people with diabetes have the more serious form, known as type 1 diabetes. In this type of diabetes, the pancreas produces little or no insulin, so daily doses of insulin are required. (Without insulin, a person with type 1 can lapse into a coma.) Type 1 diabetes usually strikes before age 30.

The remaining 90% of Americans with diabetes have type 2 diabetes. This condition can develop slowly, and about half of affected individuals are unaware of their condition. In type 2 diabetes, the pancreas doesn't produce enough insulin, cells are resistant to insulin, or both. This condition is usually diagnosed in people over age 40, but the recent rise in rates of obesity has led to a significant increase in the number of children and young adults with type 2 diabetes. About one-third of people with type 2 diabetes must inject insulin; others may take medications that increase insulin production or stimulate cells to take up glucose.

A third type of diabetes occurs in about 2–5% of women during pregnancy. So-called gestational diabetes usually disappears after pregnancy but more than half of women who experience it eventually develop type 2 diabetes.

In 2002, the U.S. Department of Health and Human Services and the American Diabetes Association adopted the term *pre-diabetes* to describe blood glucose levels that are higher than normal but not high enough for a diagnosis of full-blown diabetes. About 41 million Americans have pre-diabetes, and most people with the condition will develop type 2 diabetes within 10 years unless they adopt preventive lifestyle measures.

The major factors involved in the development of diabetes are age, obesity, physical inactivity, a family history of diabetes, and lifestyle. Excess body fat reduces cell sensitivity to insulin, and it is a major risk factor for type 2 diabetes. Ethnic background also plays a role. African Americans and people of Hispanic background are 55% more likely than non-Hispanic whites to develop type 2 diabetes; more than 20% of Hispanics over age 65 have diabetes. Native Americans also have a higher-than-average incidence of diabetes.

Treatment

There is no cure for diabetes, but it can be successfully managed by keeping blood sugar levels within safe limits through diet, exercise, and, if necessary, medication. Blood sugar levels can be monitored using a home test, and close control of glucose levels can significantly reduce the rate of serious complications. Nearly 90% of people with type 2 diabetes are overweight when diagnosed, and an important step in treatment is to lose weight. Even a small amount of exercise and weight loss can be beneficial. People with diabetes should obtain carbohydrate from whole grains, fruits, vegetables, and low-fat dairy products; carbohydrate and monounsaturated fat together should provide 60–70% of total daily calories. Regular exercise and a healthy diet are often sufficient to control type 2 diabetes.

Prevention

It is estimated that 90% of cases of type 2 diabetes could be prevented if people adopted healthy lifestyle behaviors, including regular physical activity, a moderate diet, and modest weight loss. For people with pre-diabetes, lifestyle measures are more effective than medication for delaying or preventing the development of diabetes. Exercise (endurance and/or strength training) makes cells more sensitive to insulin and helps stabilize blood glucose levels; it also helps keep body fat at healthy levels.

Eating a moderate diet to help control body fat is perhaps the most important dietary recommendation for the prevention of diabetes. However, there is some evidence that the composition of the diet may also be important. Studies have linked diets low in fiber and high in sugar, refined carbohydrates, saturated fat, red meat, and high-fat dairy products to increased risk of diabetes; diets rich in whole grains, fruits, vegetables, legumes, fish, and poultry may be protective. Specific foods linked to higher diabetes risk include regular (nondiet) cola beverages, white bread, white rice, french fries, processed meats (bacon, sausage, hot dogs), and sugary desserts. (See Chapter 8 for more information on different types of carbohydrates.)

Warning Signs and Testing

A wellness lifestyle that includes a healthy diet and regular exercise is the best strategy for preventing diabetes. If you do develop diabetes, the best way to avoid complications is to recognize the symptoms and get early diagnosis and treatment. Be alert for the following warning signs:

- Frequent urination
- Extreme hunger or thirst
- Unexplained weight loss
- Extreme fatigue
- Blurred vision
- Frequent infections
- Cuts and bruises that are slow to heal
- Tingling or numbness in the hands and feet
- Generalized itching, with no rash

Type 2 diabetes is often asymptomatic in the early stages, and major health organizations now recommend routine screening for people over age 45 and anyone younger who is at high risk, including anyone who is obese. (The Web site for the American Diabetes Association, listed in the For Further Exploration section at the end of the chapter, includes an interactive diabetes risk assessment). Screening involves a blood test to check glucose levels after either a period of fasting or the administration of a set dose of glucose. A fasting glucose level of 126 mg/dl or higher indicates diabetes; a level of 110–125 mg/dl indicates pre-diabetes. If you are concerned about your risk for diabetes, talk with your physician about being tested.

If you gaze into the mirror and wish you could change the way your body looks, consider getting some exercise—not to reshape your contours but to firm up your body image and enhance your self-esteem. In a recent study, 82 adults completed a 12-week aerobic exercise program (using cycle ergometry) and had 12 months of follow-up. Compared with the control group, the participants improved their fitness and also benefited psychologically in tests of mood, anxiety, and self-concept. These same physical and psychological benefits were still significant at the 1-year follow-up.

One reason for the findings may be that people who exercise regularly often gain a sense of mastery and competence that enhances their self-esteem and body image. In addition, exercise contributes to a more toned look, which many adults prefer. Research suggests that physically active people are more comfortable with their bodies and their image than sedentary people are. In one workplace study, 60 employees were asked to complete a 36-session stretching program whose main purpose was to prevent muscle strains at work. At the end of the program, besides the significant increase by all participants in measurements of flexibility, their perceptions of their bodies improved and so did their overall sense of self-worth.

Similar results were obtained in a Norwegian study, in which 219 middle-aged people at risk for heart disease were randomly assigned to one of four groups: diet, diet plus exercise, exercise, and no intervention. The greater the participation of individuals in the exercise component of the program, the higher were their scores in perceived competence/self-esteem and coping.

SOURCES: DiLorenzo, T. M., et al. 1999. Long-term effects of aerobic exercise on psychological outcomes. *Preventive Medicine* 28(1): 75–85. Sorensen, M., et al. 1999. The effect of exercise and diet on mental health and quality of life in middle-aged individuals with elevated risk factors for cardiovascular disease. *Journal of Sports Science* 17(5): 369–377. Moore, T. M. 1998. A workplace stretching program. *AAOHN Journal* 46(12): 563–568.

gain weight in the hip area ("pears"). The reason for this increased risk is not entirely clear, but it appears that fat in the abdomen is more easily mobilized and sent into the bloodstream, increasing disease-related blood fat levels. In general, men tend to gain weight in the abdominal area and women in the hip area, but women who exhibit the male pattern of fat distribution face the increased health risks associated with it. Researchers have also found ethnic differences in the relative significance of increased abdominal fat, but more studies are needed to clarify the relationships among fat distribution, ethnicity, and disease.

Performance of Physical Activities   Too much body fat makes all types of physical activity more difficult because just moving the body through everyday activities means working harder and using more energy. In general, overfat people are less fit than others and don't have the muscular strength, endurance, and flexibility that make normal activity easy. Because exercise is more difficult, they do less of it, depriving themselves of an effective way to improve body composition.

Self-Image   The "fashionable" body image has changed dramatically during the past 50 years, varying from slightly plump to an almost unhealthy thinness. Today, a fit and healthy-looking body, developed through a healthy lifestyle, is the goal for most people (see the box "Exercise, Body Image and Self-Esteem"). The key to this "look" is a balance of proper nutrition and exercise—in short, a lifestyle that emphasizes wellness.

Goals for body composition should be realistic, however; a person's ability to change body composition through diet and exercise depends not only on a wellness program, but also on heredity. The "ideal" body presented in the media—from dolls and action figures to fashion models—is an unrealistic goal for the vast majority of Americans. Unrealistic expectations about body composition can have a negative impact on self-image and can lead to the development of eating disorders. (For more information on body image and eating disorders, see Chapter 9.)

For most people, body fat percentage falls somewhere between ideal and a level that is significantly unhealthy. If they consistently maintain a wellness lifestyle that includes a healthy diet and regular exercise, the right body composition will naturally develop.

Wellness for Life   A healthy body composition is vital for wellness throughout life. Strong scientific evidence suggests that controlling your weight will increase your life span; reduce the risk of heart disease, cancer, diabetes, insulin resistance, and back pain; increase your energy level; and improve your self-esteem.

Problems Associated with Very Low Levels of Body Fat

Though not as prevalent a problem as overweight or obesity, having too little body fat is also dangerous. Essential fat is necessary for the functioning of the body, and health experts generally view too little body fat—less than about 8–12% for women and 3–5% for men—as a threat to health and well-being. Extreme leanness is linked with reproductive, circulatory, and immune system disorders. Extremely lean people may experience muscle wasting and fatigue. They are also more likely to suffer from dangerous eating disorders, which are described in more detail in Chapter 9. For women, an extremely low percentage of body fat is associated with **amenorrhea** and loss of bone mass (see the box "The Female Athlete Triad").

While obesity is at epidemic levels in the United States, many girls and women strive for unrealistic thinness in response to pressure from peers and a society obsessed with appearance. This quest for thinness has led to an increasingly common, underreported condition called the **female athlete triad.**

The triad consists of three interrelated disorders: abnormal eating patterns (and excessive exercising), followed by lack of menstrual periods (amenorrhea), followed by decreased bone density (premature osteoporosis). Left untreated, the triad can lead to decreased physical performance, increased incidence of bone fractures, disturbances of heart rhythm and metabolism, and even death.

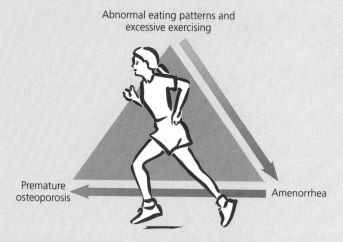

Abnormal eating patterns and excessive exercising

Premature osteoporosis

Amenorrhea

Abnormal eating is the event from which the other two components of the triad flow. Abnormal eating ranges from moderately restricting food intake, to binge eating and purging (bulimia), to severely restricting food intake (anorexia nervosa). Whether serious or relatively mild, eating disorders prevent women from consuming enough calories to meet their bodies' needs.

Disordered eating, combined with intense exercise and emotional stress, can suppress the hormones that control the menstrual cycle. If the menstrual cycle stops for three consecutive months, the condition is called amenorrhea. Prolonged amenorrhea can lead to osteoporosis; bone density may erode to the point that a woman in her 20s will have the bone density of a woman in her 60s. Women with osteoporosis have fragile, easily fractured bones. Some researchers have found that even a few missed menstrual periods can decrease bone density.

All physically active women and girls have the potential to develop one or more components of the female athlete triad; for example, it is estimated that 5–20% of women who exercise regularly and vigorously may develop amenorrhea. But the triad is most prevalent among athletes who participate in certain sports: those in which appearance is highly important, those that emphasize a prepubertal body shape, those that require contour-revealing clothing for competition, those that require endurance, and those that use weight categories for participation. Such sports include gymnastics, figure skating, swimming, distance running, cycling, cross-country skiing, track, volleyball, rowing, horse racing, and cheerleading.

The female athlete triad can be life-threatening, and health professionals are taking it seriously. Typical signs of the eating disorders that trigger the condition are extreme weight loss, dry skin, loss of hair, brittle fingernails, cold hands and feet, low blood pressure and heart rate, swelling around the ankles and hands, and weakening of the bones. Female athletes who have repeated stress fractures may be suffering from the condition. Early intervention is the key to stopping this series of interrelated conditions. Unfortunately, once the condition has progressed, long-term consequences, especially bone loss, are unavoidable. Teenagers may need only to learn about good eating habits; college-age women with a long-standing problem may require intense psychological counseling.

SOURCES: Otis, C. 1998. Too slim, amenorrheic, fracture-prone: The female athlete triad. *ACSM's Health and Fitness Journal* 2(1): 20–25. Smith, A. 1996. The female athlete triad: Causes, diagnosis, and treatment. *Physician and Sportsmedicine* 24(7). Art: Adapted from Yeager, K. K., et al. 1993. The female athlete triad: Disordered eating, amenorrhea, osteoporosis. *Medicine and Science in Sports and Exercise* 25:775–777. Reprinted by permission of Lippincott, Williams and Wilkins.

ASSESSING BODY MASS INDEX, BODY COMPOSITION, AND BODY FAT DISTRIBUTION

The morning weighing ritual on the bathroom scale can't reveal whether a fluctuation in weight is due to a change in muscle, body water, or fat and can't differentiate between overweight and overfat. A 260-pound football player may be overweight according to population height-weight standards yet may actually have much less body fat than average. Likewise, a 40-year-old woman may weigh the same as she did 20 years earlier yet have a considerably different body composition.

There are a number of simple, inexpensive ways to estimate healthy body weight and healthy body composition that are more accurate than the bathroom scale. These assessments can provide you with information about the health risks associated with your current body weight and body composition. They can also help you

amenorrhea Absent or infrequent menstruation, sometimes related to low levels of body fat and excessive quantity or intensity of exercise.

female athlete triad A condition consisting of three interrelated disorders: abnormal eating patterns (and excessive exercising) followed by lack of menstrual periods (amenorrhea) and decreased bone density (premature osteoporosis).

Terms

Table 6.1 Body Mass Index (BMI) Classification and Disease Risk

Classification	BMI (kg/m²)	Obesity Class	DISEASE RISK RELATIVE TO NORMAL WEIGHT AND WAIST CIRCUMFERENCEᵃ	
			Men ≤ 40 in. (102 cm) Women ≤ 35 in. (88 cm)	> 40 in. (102 cm) > 35 in. (88 cm)
Underweightᵇ	<18.5		—	—
Normalᶜ	18.5–24.9		—	—
Overweight	25.0–29.9		Increased	High
Obesity	30.0–34.9	I	High	Very high
	35.0–39.9	II	Very high	Very high
Extreme obesity	≥ 40.0	III	Extremely high	Extremely high

ᵃDisease risk for type 2 diabetes, hypertension, and cardiovascular disease. The waist circumference cutoff points for increased risk are 40 inches (102 cm) for men and 35 inches (88 cm) for women.

ᵇResearch suggests that a low BMI can be healthy in some cases, as long as it is not the result of smoking, an eating disorder, or an underlying disease process. A BMI of 17.5 or less is sometimes used as a diagnostic criterion for the eating disorder anorexia nervosa.

ᶜIncreased waist circumference can also be a marker for increased risk, even in persons of normal weight.

SOURCE: Adapted from National Heart, Lung, and Blood Institute. 1998. *Clinical Guidelines on the Identification, Evaluation, and Treatment of Overweight and Obesity in Adults: The Evidence Report.* Bethesda, Md.: National Institutes of Health.

establish reasonable goals and set a starting point for current and future decisions about weight loss and weight gain.

Calculating Body Mass Index

Body mass index (BMI) is a measure of body weight that is useful for classifying the health risks of body weight if you don't have access to more sophisticated methods. Though more accurate than height-weight tables, body mass index is also based on the concept that a person's weight should be proportional to their height. BMI is a fairly accurate measure of the health risks of body weight for average people, and it is easy to calculate and rate. Researchers frequently use BMI in studies that examine the health risks associated with body weight. However, because BMI doesn't distinguish between fat weight and fat-free weight, it can be very inaccurate for some groups, including people of short stature, muscular athletes, and people who train frequently with weights. If you are in one of these groups, do not use BMI as your primary means of assessing whether your current weight is healthy; instead, try one of the methods described in the next section for estimating percent body fat.

BMI is calculated by dividing your body weight (expressed in kilograms) by the square of your height (expressed in meters). The formula appears below. Space for your own calculations can be found in Lab 6.1, and a complete BMI chart appears in Lab 6.2.

1. Divide body weight in pounds by 2.2 to convert weight to kilograms.
2. Multiple height in inches by 0.0254 to convert height to meters.
3. Multiply the result in step 2 by itself to obtain the square of the height measurement.
4. Divide the result of step 1 by the result of step 3 to obtain BMI.

For example, a person who weighs 130 pounds (130 ÷ 2.2 = 59.1 kg) and is 5 feet, 3 inches tall (63 inches × 0.0254 = 1.6 meters) has a BMI of 59.1 kg ÷ (1.6 m)², or 23 kg/m².

Under new federal guidelines from the National Institutes of Health (NIH), a person is classified as overweight if he or she has a BMI of 25 or above and obese if he or she has a BMI of 30 or above (Table 6.1). More than 60% of American adults have a BMI of 25 or above. At high values of BMI (over 25), the risk of arthritis, diabetes, hypertension, endometrial cancer, and other disorders increases substantially. The increased risk of type 2 diabetes at even fairly low values of BMI, especially among women, is of particular concern (Figure 6.4).

In classifying the health risks associated with overweight and obesity, the NIH guidelines consider body fat distribution and other disease risk factors in addition to BMI. As described earlier, excess fat in the abdomen is of greater concern than excess fat in other areas. Methods of assessing body fat distribution are discussed later in the chapter; the NIH guidelines use

Terms

body mass index (BMI) A measure of relative body weight correlating highly with more direct measures of body fat, calculated by dividing total body weight (in kilograms) by the square of body height (in meters).

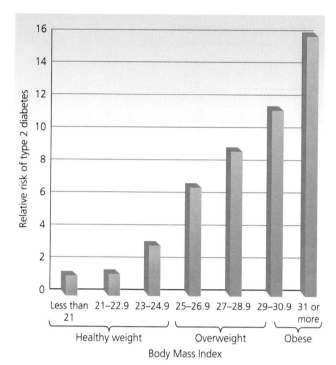

Figure 6.4   Body mass index (BMI) and risk of type 2 diabetes in women.   The risk of diabetes goes up even for women at the high end of the healthy BMI range, but it is extremely high in overweight and obese women.   SOURCE: Hankinson, S. E., et al. 2001. *Healthy Women, Healthy Lives: A Guide to Preventing Disease from the Landmark Nurses' Health Study.* New York: Simon and Schuster.

Table 6.2   **Percent Body Fat Classification**

PERCENT BODY FAT (%)

	20–39 years	40–59 years	60–79 years
Women			
Essential[a]	8–12	8–12	8–12
Low/athletic[b]	13–20	13–22	13–23
Recommended	21–32	23–33	24–35
Overfat[c]	33–38	34–39	36–41
Obese[c]	≥39	≥40	≥42
Men			
Essential[a]	3–5	3–5	3–5
Low/athletic[b]	6–7	6–10	6–12
Recommended	8–19	11–21	13–24
Overfat[c]	20–24	22–27	25–29
Obese[c]	≥25	≥28	≥30

The cutoffs for recommended, overfat, and obese ranges in this table are based on a study that linked body mass index classifications from the National Institutes of Health with predicted percent body fat (measured using dual energy X-ray absorptiometry).

[a]Essential body fat is necessary for the basic functioning of the body.

[b]Percent body fat in the low/athletic range may be appropriate for some people as long as it is not the result of illness or disordered eating habits; see pp. 172–173 for more on low levels of percent body fat.

[c]Health risks increase as percent body fat exceeds the recommended range.

SOURCES: Gallagher, D., et al. 2000. Healthy percentage body fat ranges: An approach for developing guidelines based on body mass index. *American Journal of Clinical Nutrition* 72: 694–701. American College of Sports Medicine. 2001. *ACSM's Resource Manual for Guidelines for Exercise Testing and Prescription.* 4th ed. Philadelphia: Lippincott, Williams and Wilkins.

measurement of waist circumference (see Table 6.1). At a given level of overweight, people with a large waist circumference and/or additional disease risk factors are at greater risk for health problems. For example, a man with a BMI of 27, a waist circumference of more than 40 inches, and high blood pressure is at greater risk for health problems than another man who has a BMI of 27 but has a smaller waist circumference and no other risk factors.

Thus, optimal BMI for good health depends on many factors; if your BMI is 25 or above, consult a physician for help in determining a healthy BMI for you. (Weight loss recommendations based on the NIH guidelines are discussed further in Chapter 9.) Despite its widespread use, BMI does have limitations. Although it is good for large population studies, it is less useful for measuring changes in body composition in individuals.

Estimating Percent Body Fat

Assessing body composition involves estimating percent body fat. The only method for directly measuring the percentage body weight that is fat is autopsy—the dissection and chemical analysis of the body. However, there are other indirect techniques that can provide an estimate of percent body fat. One of the most accurate is underwater weighing. Other techniques include skinfold measurements, the Bod Pod, and bioelectrical impedance analysis.

All of these methods have a margin of error, so it is important not to focus too much on precise values. For example, underwater weighing has an error of about ±3%, meaning that if a person's percent body fat is actually 17%, the test result may be between 14% and 20%; skinfold measurements have an error rate of about ±6%. The results of different methods may also vary, so if you plan to track changes in body composition over time, be sure to use the same method each time to perform the assessment. Table 6.2 provides estimated ranges for healthy percent body fat.

Underwater Weighing   Hydrostatic (underwater) weighing is the standard used for other techniques, including skinfold measurements. For this method, an individual is submerged and weighed under water. The percentages of fat and fat-free weight are calculated from body density. Muscle has a higher density and fat a lower density than water (1.1 grams per cubic centimeter for fat-free mass,

0.91 gram per cubic centimeter for fat, and 1 gram per cubic centimeter for water). Therefore, fat people tend to float and weigh less under water, and lean people tend to sink and weigh more under water. Most university exercise physiology departments or sports medicine laboratories have an underwater weighing facility. If you want an accurate assessment of your body composition, find a place that does underwater weighing.

Skinfold Measurements   Skinfold measurement is a simple, inexpensive, and practical way to assess body composition. Skinfold measurements can be used to assess body composition because equations can link the thickness of skinfolds at various sites to percent body fat calculations from more precise laboratory techniques.

Skinfold assessment typically involves measuring the thickness of skinfolds at several different sites on the body. You can use these measurements in different ways. You can sum up the skinfold values as an indirect measure of body fatness. For example, if you plan to create a fitness (and dietary change) program to improve body composition, you can compare the sum of skinfold values over time as an indicator of your program's progress and of improvements in body composition. You can also plug your skinfold values into equations like those in Lab 6.1 that predict percent body fat. When using these equations, however, it is important to remember that they have a fairly substantial margin of error—don't focus too much on specific values. The sum represents only a relative measure of body fatness.

Skinfolds are measured with a device called a **caliper,** which consists of a pair of spring-loaded, calibrated jaws. High-quality calipers are made of metal and have parallel jaw surfaces and constant spring tension. Inexpensive plastic calipers are also available; to ensure accuracy, plastic calipers should be spring-loaded and have metal jaws. Refer to Lab 6.1 for instructions on how to take skinfold measurements. Taking accurate measurements with calipers requires patience, experience, and considerable practice. It's best to take several measurements at each site (or have several different people take each measurement) to help ensure accuracy. Be sure to take the measurements in the exact location called for in the procedure. Because the amount of water in your body changes during the day, skinfold measurements taken in the morning and evening often differ. If you repeat the measurements in the future to track changes in your body composition, measure skinfolds at approximately the same time of day.

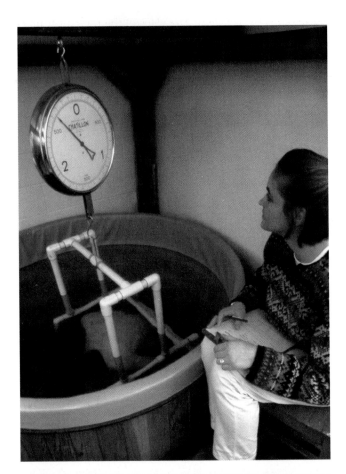

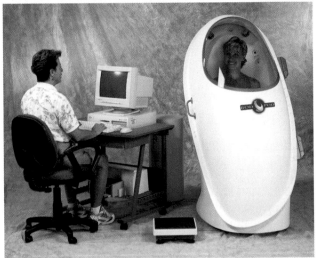

In underwater weighing (top) percent body fat is calculated from body density; muscle has a higher density than water, so people with more muscle weigh relatively more under water. The Bod Pod (bottom) measures air displacement, which can be used to calculate percent body fat.

The Bod Pod   The Bod Pod, a small chamber containing computerized sensors, measures body composition by air displacement rather than water displacement. It determines the percentage of fat by calculating how much air is displaced by the person sitting inside the chamber. Many people prefer this short, 5-minute test over underwater

---

Terms

caliper A pressure-sensitive measuring instrument with two jaws that can be adjusted to determine thickness.

weighing because it takes the place of the difficult "dunking" process and is about as accurate.

Bioelectrical Impedance Analysis (BIA) The BIA technique works by sending a small electrical current through the body and measuring the body's resistance to it. Fat-free tissues, where most body water is located, are good conductors of electrical current, whereas fat is not. Thus, the amount of resistance to electrical current is related to the amount of fat-free tissue in the body (the lower the resistance, the greater the fat-free mass) and can be used to estimate percent body fat. Bioelectrical impedance analysis is fairly accurate for most people (about the same as skinfold measurements). To avoid error, it is important to follow the manufacturer's instructions carefully and to avoid overhydration or underhydration (more or less body water than normal). Because measurement varies with the type of BIA analyzer, use the same instrument to compare measurements over time.

There are other methods of estimating percent body fat, but many require sophisticated and expensive equipment. For example, the DXA (dual energy X-ray absorptiometry) technique measures body fat by splitting an X-ray beam into two levels. The TOBEC (total body electrical conductivity) technique estimates lean body mass by passing a body through a magnetic field. You may find these and additional body composition assessment methods in some fitness centers and sports medicine research facilities.

Assessing Body Fat Distribution

Researchers have studied many different methods for determining the risk associated with body fat distribution. Two of the simplest to perform are waist circumference measurement and waist-to-hip ratio calculation. In the first method, you measure your waist circumference; in the second, you divide your waist circumference by your hip circumference. Waist circumference has been found to be a better indicator of abdominal fat than waist-to-hip ratio. More research is needed to determine the precise degree of risk associated with specific values for these two assessments of body fat distribution. However, a total waist measurement of more than 40 inches (102 cm) for men and 35 inches (88 cm) for women and a waist-to-hip ratio above 0.94 for young men and 0.82 for young women are associated with a significantly increased risk of disease. Follow the instructions in Lab 6.1 to measure and rate your body fat distribution.

SETTING BODY COMPOSITION GOALS

If assessment tests indicate that fat loss would be beneficial for your health, your first step is to establish a goal.

You can use the ratings in Table 6.1 or Table 6.2 to choose a target value for BMI or percent body fat (depending on which assessment you completed).

Make sure your goal is realistic and will ensure good health. Genetics limits your capacity to change your body composition, and few people can expect to develop the body of a fashion model or competitive bodybuilder. However, you can improve your body composition through a program of regular exercise and a healthy diet. If your body composition is in or close to the recommended range, you may want to set a lifestyle goal rather than a specific percent body fat or BMI goal. For example, you might set a goal of increasing your daily physical activity from 20 to 60 minutes or beginning a program of weight training, and then let any improvements in body composition occur as a secondary result of your primary target (physical activity).

If you are significantly overfat or if you have known risk factors for disease (such as high blood pressure or high cholesterol), consult your physician to determine a body composition goal for your individual risk profile. For people who are obese, small losses of body weight (5–15%) over a 6–12 month period can result in significant health improvements. And as described earlier, a lifestyle that includes regular exercise may be more important for health than trying to reach any "ideal" weight.

Once you've established a body composition goal, you can then set a target range for body weight. Although body weight is not an accurate method of assessing body composition, it's a useful method for tracking progress in a program to change body composition. If you're losing a small or moderate amount of weight and exercising, you're probably losing fat while building muscle mass. Lab 6.2 will help you determine a range for recommended body weight.

Using percent body fat or BMI will generate a fairly accurate target body weight for most people. However, it's best not to stick rigidly to a recommended body weight calculated from any formula; individual genetic, cultural, and lifestyle factors are also important. Decide whether the body weight that the formulas generate for you is realistic, meets all your goals, is healthy, *and* is reasonable for you to maintain.

MAKING CHANGES IN BODY COMPOSITION

Chapter 9 includes specific strategies for losing or gaining weight and improving body composition. In general, lifestyle should be your focus—regular physical activity, endurance exercise, strength training, and a moderate energy intake. Making significant cuts in food intake in order to lose weight and body fat is a difficult strategy to maintain; focusing on increased physical activity is a better approach for many people. In studies of people who have lost weight and maintained the loss, physical activity was the key to long-term success.

You can track your progress toward your target body composition by checking your body weight periodically. However, it is best not to focus too much on body weight, especially if your goal is modest. Look instead at other factors, such as how much energy you have and how your clothes fit.

To get a more accurate idea of your progress, you should directly reassess your body composition occasionally during your program: Body composition changes as weight changes. Losing a lot of weight usually includes losing some muscle mass no matter how hard a person exercises, partly because carrying less weight requires the muscular system to bear a smaller burden. (Conversely, a large gain in weight without exercise still causes some gain in muscle mass because muscles are working harder to carry the extra weight.)

> **MOTIVATION FOR CHANGE!** If modifying your body composition is one of your fitness goals, choose a method of monitoring your progress that works for you. For some people, too close attention to body weight or percent body fat can lead to unhealthy behaviors and actually reduce motivation; for others, frequent weighing or body fat checks help keep a program on track. If you fall into the first group, consider scheduling regular but infrequent checks of your weight or body composition; in the interim periods, track such factors as your level of physical activity or your daily energy level. Changes in body composition require long-term effort, so working toward short-term goals that focus on factors other than specific amounts of fat-loss can provide more opportunities for rewards and positive feedback.

SUMMARY

- The human body is composed of fat-free mass (which includes bone, muscle, organ tissues, and connective tissues) and body fat (essential and nonessential).

- Having too much body fat has negative health consequences, especially in terms of cardiovascular disease and diabetes. Distribution of fat is also a significant factor in health.

- A fit and healthy-looking body, with the right body composition for a particular person, develops from habits of proper nutrition and exercise.

- Measuring body weight is not an accurate way to assess body composition because it does not differentiate between muscle weight and fat weight.

> ### Tips for Today
>
> Your current body composition is the result of many factors, including gender, heredity, and your activity and eating habits. A healthy body composition reduces your risk of premature death and many diseases, and it improves the quality of your life. Adopting a wellness lifestyle can lead naturally to a body composition that is healthy and appropriate for you.
>
> *Right now you can*
>
> - Find out what types of body composition assessment techniques are available at facilities on your campus or in your community.
>
> - Do 15 minutes of physical activity—walk, jog, bike, swim, or climb stairs.
>
> - Drink a glass of water instead of a regular (nondiet) soda, and include a high-fiber food such as whole-grain bread or cereal, popcorn, apples, berries, or beans in your next snack or meal. (These types of dietary changes are associated with reduced risk for type 2 diabetes.)
>
> - Think about your image of the ideal body type for your sex. Consider where your idea comes from, whether you use this image to judge your own body shape and body composition, and whether it is a realistic goal for you. Write down five positive things about your body.

- Body mass index (calculated from weight and height measurements) can help classify the health risks associated with overweight.

- Techniques for estimating percent body fat include underwater weighing, skinfold measurements, the Bod Pod, and bioelectrical impedance analysis.

- Body fat distribution can be assessed through the total waist measurement or the waist-to-hip ratio.

- Recommended body composition and weight can be determined by choosing a target BMI or target body fat percentage. Keep heredity in mind when setting a goal, and focus on positive changes in lifestyle.

FOR FURTHER EXPLORATION

W *Fit and Well* Online Learning Center
(www.mhhe.com/fahey)

Use the learning objectives, study guide questions, and glossary flashcards to review key terms and concepts and prepare for exams. You can extend your knowledge of body composition and gain experience in using the Internet as a resource by completing the activities and checking out the Web links for the topics in Chapter 6 marked with the World Wide Web icon. For this chapter, Internet activities explore the health risks of too much

COMMON QUESTIONS ANSWERED

Is spot reducing effective?   No. Spot reducing refers to attempts to lose body fat in specific parts of the body by doing exercises for those parts. For example, a person might try to spot reduce in the legs by doing leg lifts. Spot-reducing exercises contribute to fat loss only to the extent that they burn calories. The only way you can reduce fat in any specific area is to create an overall negative energy balance: Take in less energy (food) than you use up through exercise and metabolism.

How does exercise affect body composition?   Cardiorespiratory endurance exercise burns calories, thereby helping create a negative energy balance. Weight training does not use many calories and therefore is of little use in creating a negative energy balance. However, weight training increases muscle mass, which maintains a high metabolic rate (the body's energy level) and helps improve body composition. To minimize body fat and increase muscle mass, thereby improving body composition, combine cardiorespiratory endurance exercise and weight training (Figure 6.5).

How do I develop a toned, healthy-looking body?   The development of a healthy-looking body requires regular exercise, proper diet, and other good health habits. However, it helps to have heredity on your side. Some people put on or take off fat more easily than others just as some people are taller than others. Be realistic in your goals, and be satisfied with the improvements in body composition you can make by observing the principles of a wellness lifestyle.

Are people who have a desirable body composition physically fit?   Having a healthy body composition is not necessarily associated with overall fitness. For example, many bodybuilders have very little body fat but have poor cardiorespiratory capacity and flexibility. To be fit, you must rate high on all the components of fitness.

What is liposuction, and will it help me lose body fat? Suction lipectomy, popularly known as liposuction, has become the most popular type of elective surgery in the United States. The procedure involves removing limited amounts of fat from specific areas. Typically, no more than 2.5 kg (5.5 lb) of adipose tissue is removed at a time. The procedure is usually successful if the amount of excess fat is limited and skin elasticity is good. The procedure is most effective if integrated into a program of dietary restriction and exercise. Side effects include infection, dimpling, and wavy skin contours. Liposuction has a death rate of 1 in 5000 patients, primarily from pulmonary thromboembolism (a blood clot in the lungs) or fat embolism (circulatory blockage caused by a dislodged piece of fat). Other serious complications include shock, bleeding, and impaired blood flow to vital organs.

What is cellulite, and how do I get rid of it?   Cellulite is the name commonly given to ripply, wavy fat deposits that collect just under the skin. However, these rippling fat deposits are really the same as fat deposited anywhere else in the body. The only way to control them is to create a negative energy balance—burn up more calories than are taken in. There are no creams or lotions that will rub away surface (subcutaneous) fat deposits, and spot reducing is also ineffective. The solution is sensible eating habits and exercise.

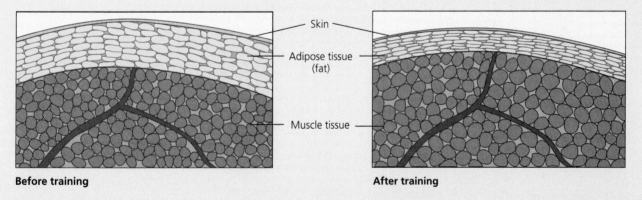

Before training   **After training**

Figure 6.5   Effects of exercise on body composition. Endurance exercise and strength training reduce body fat and increase muscle mass.

or too little body fat, body mass index, and diabetes; there are also Web links for major chapter topics.

Daily Fitness and Nutrition Journal

Fill in the body composition portion of the fitness program plan. If you plan to make changes in your body composition, you may also want to begin reviewing the steps in the weight management section of the journal.

HealthQuest

As a shortcut, use the body mass index calculator included on the HealthQuest CD-ROM (look in the Wellness Activities for the Fitness module or the Nutrition and Weight Control module).

Books

American Diabetes Association. 2002. *American Diabetes Association Complete Guide to Diabetes*, 3d ed. New York: McGraw-Hill. *Explains the causes, symptoms, diagnosis, treatment, and self-care of diabetes.*

Bray, G. A., and C. A. Bray. 2002. *An Atlas of Obesity and Weight Control.* London: CRC Press. *Provides detailed information about assessment, classification, and treatment of obesity.*

Gaesser, G. A. 2002. *Big Fat Lies: The Truth About Your Weight and Your Health.* Updated Edition. Carlsbad, Calif.: Gurze Books. *Emphasizes the importance of diet and exercise in maintaining metabolic health.*

Heyward, V. H., and D. R. Wagner. 2004. *Applied Body Composition Assessment.* 2nd ed. Champaign, Ill.: Human Kinetics. *Describes different methods of measuring and assessing body composition.*

Otis, C. L., and R. Goldingay. 2000. *The Athletic Woman's Survival Guide.* Champaign, Ill.: Human Kinetics. *Information on the female athlete triad and suggestions for changing attitudes toward weight, self-esteem, and body image.*

⩗⩗ Organizations and Web Sites

American Diabetes Association. Provides information, a free newsletter, and referrals to local support groups; the Web site includes an online diabetes risk assessment.

800-342-2383
http://www.diabetes.org

National Heart, Lung, and Blood Institute. Provides information on the latest federal obesity standards and a BMI calculator.

http://www.nhlbi.nih.gov/guidelines/obesity/ob_home.htm

National Institute of Diabetes and Digestive and Kidney Diseases Health Information/Nutrition and Obesity. Provides information about adult obesity: how it is defined and assessed, the risk factors associated with it, and its causes.

877-946-4627
http://www.niddk.nih.gov/health/nutrit/nutrit.htm

Shape Up America. A site devoted to promoting healthy weight management; calculates and rates BMI and looks at why BMI is an important measure of health.

http://shapeup.org

USDA Food and Nutrition Information Center: Reports and Studies on Obesity. Provides links to recent reports and studies on the issue of obesity among Americans.

http://www.nal.usda.gov/fnic/reports/obesity.html

See also the listings for Chapters 2, 8, and 9.

SELECTED BIBLIOGRAPHY

American College of Sports Medicine. 2001. *ACSM's Resource Manual for Guidelines for Exercise Testing and Prescription,* 4th ed. Philadelphia: Lippincott Williams and Wilkins.

American Diabetes Association. 2003. *Pre-Diabetes* (http://www.diabetes.org:80/main/info/pre-diabetes.jsp: retrieved December 28, 2003).

American Diabetes Association. 2002. Evidence-based nutrition principles and recommendations for the treatment and prevention of diabetes and related complications. *Diabetes Care* 25:148–198.

Calle, E. E., et al. 2003. Overweight, obesity, and mortality from cancer in a prospectively studied cohort of U.S. adults. *New England Journal of Medicine* 348(17): 1625–1638.

Centers for Disease Control and Prevention. 2004. National Diabetes Fact Sheet (http://www.cdc.gov/diabetes/pubs/general.htm; retrieved April 30, 2004).

Deurenberg, P. 2003. Validation of body composition methods and assumptions. *British Journal of Nutrition* 90(3): 485–486.

Fang, J., et al. 2003. Exercise, body mass index, caloric intake, and cardiovascular mortality. *American Journal of Preventive Medicine* 25(4): 283–289.

Fenicchia, L. M., et al. 2004. Influence of resistance exercise training on glucose control in women with type 2 diabetes. *Metabolism* 53(3): 284–289.

Fontaine, K. R., et al. 2003. Years of life lost due to obesity. *Journal of the American Medical Association* 289(2): 187–193.

Frankenfield, D. C., et al. 2001. Limits of body mass index to detect obesity and predict body composition. *Nutrition* 17(1): 26–30.

Guagnano, M. T., et al. 2001. Large waist circumference and risk of hypertension. *International Journal of Obesity Related Metabolic Disorders* 25(9): 1360–1364.

Hoffman, C. J., and L. A. Hildebrandt. 2001. Use of the air displacement plethysmograph to monitor body composition: A beneficial tool for dietitians. *Journal of the American Dietetic Association* 101(9): 986, 988.

Holten, M. K., et al. 2004. Strength training increases insulin-mediated glucose uptake, GLUT4 content, and insulin signaling in skeletal muscle in patients with type 2 diabetes. *Diabetes* 53(2): 294–305.

Jiang, R., et al. 2004. Body iron stores in relation to risk of type 2 diabetes in apparently healthy women. *Journal of the American Medical Association* 291(6): 711–717.

Katzmarzyk, P. T., et al. 2003. Physical inactivity, excess adiposity, and premature mortality. *Obesity Reviews* 4(4): 257–290.

Knowler, W. C., et al. 2002. Reduction in the incidence of type 2 diabetes with lifestyle intervention or metformin. *New England Journal of Medicine* 346(6): 393–403.

Mokdad, A. H., et al. 2004. Actual causes of death in the United States, 2000. *Journal of the American Medical Association* 291(10): 1238–1245.

Mokdad, A. H., et al. 2003. Prevalence of obesity, diabetes, and obesity-related health risk factors, 2001. *Journal of the American Medical Association* 289(1): 76–79.

National Heart, Lung, and Blood Institute. 1998. *Clinical Guidelines on the Identification, Evaluation, and Treatment of Overweight and Obesity in Adults: The Evidence Report.* Bethesda, Md.: National Institutes of Health.

Nielsen, S. J., and B. M. Popkin. 2003. Patterns and trends in food portion sizes, 1977–1996. *Journal of the American Medical Association* 289(4): 450–453.

Saris, W. H., et al. 2003. How much physical activity is enough to prevent unhealthy weight gain? Outcome of the IASO 1st Stock Conference and consensus statement. *Obesity Reviews* 4(2): 101–114.

Siani, A., et al. 2002. The relationship of waist circumference to blood pressure. *American Journal of Hypertension* 15(9): 780–786.

Suk, S-H., et al. 2003. Abdominal obesity and risk of ischemic stroke. *Stroke* 34:1586–1592.

Tuomilehto, J., et al. 2001. Prevention of type 2 diabetes mellitus by changes in lifestyle among subjects with impaired glucose tolerance. *New England Journal of Medicine* 344(18): 1343–1350.

Van Dam, R. M., et al. 2002. Dietary patterns and risk for type 2 diabetes mellitus in U.S. men. *Annals of Internal Medicine* 136(3): 201–209.

Wong, S. L., et al. 2004. Cardiorespiratory fitness is associated with lower abdominal fat independent of body mass index. *Medicine and Science in Sports and Exercise* 36(2): 286–291.

LAB 6.1 *Assessing Body Mass Index and Body Composition*

Body Mass Index

Equipment

1. Weight scale
2. Tape measure or other means of measuring height

Instructions

Measure your height and weight, and record the results. Be sure to record the unit of measurement.

Height: _____   Weight: _____

Calculating BMI (see also the shortcut chart of BMI values in Lab 6.2)

1. Convert your body weight to kilograms by dividing your weight in pounds by 2.2.

   Body weight _____ lb ÷ 2.2 lb/kg = body weight _____ kg

2. Convert your height measurement to meters by multiplying your height in inches by 0.0254.

   Height _____ in. × 0.0254 m/in. = height _____ m

3. Square your height measurement.

   Height _____ m × height _____ m = height _____ m²

4. BMI equals body weight in kilograms divided by height in meters squared (kg/m²).

   Body weight _____ kg ÷ height _____ m² = BMI _____ kg/m²
                    (from step 1)   (from step 3)

Rating Your BMI

Refer to the table for a rating of your BMI. Record the results below and on the final page of this lab.

Classification	BMI (kg/m²)
Underweight	<18.5
Normal	18.5–24.9
Overweight	25.0–29.9
Obesity (I)	30.0–34.9
Obesity (II)	35.0–39.9
Extreme obesity (III)	≥40.0

(See complete version of table on p. 174 for additional information.)

BMI _____ kg/m²

Classification (from table) _____

Skinfold Measurements

Equipment

1. Skinfold calipers
2. Partner to take measurements
3. Marking pen (optional)

Instructions

1. *Select and locate the correct sites for measurement.* All measurements should be taken on the right side of the body with the subject standing. Skinfolds are normally measured on the natural fold line of the skin, either vertically or at a slight angle. The skinfold measurement sites for males are chest, abdomen, and thigh; for females, triceps, suprailium, and thigh. If the person taking skinfold measurements is inexperienced, it may be helpful to mark the correct sites with a marking pen.

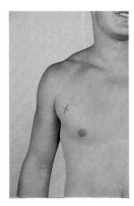 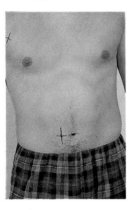 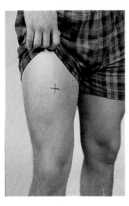 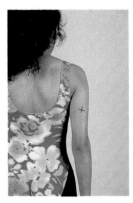 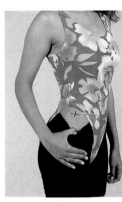

(a) Chest   (b) Abdomen   (c) Thigh   (d) Triceps   (e) Suprailium

(a) Chest. Pinch a diagonal fold halfway between the nipple and the shoulder crease. *(b) Abdomen.* Pinch a vertical fold about 1 inch to the right of the umbilicus (navel). *(c) Thigh.* Pinch a vertical fold midway between the top of the hipbone and the kneecap. *(d) Triceps.* Pinch a vertical skinfold on the back of the right arm midway between the shoulder and elbow. The arm should be straight and should hang naturally. *(e) Suprailium.* Pinch a fold at the top front of the right hipbone. The skinfold here is taken slightly diagonally according to the natural fold tendency of the skin.

2. *Measure the appropriate skinfolds.* Pinch a fold of skin between your thumb and forefinger. Pull the fold up so that no muscular tissue is included; don't pinch the skinfold too hard. Hold the calipers perpendicular to the fold and measure the skinfold about 0.25 inch away from your fingers. Allow the tips of the calipers to close on the skinfold and let the reading settle before marking it down. Take readings to the nearest half-millimeter. Continue to repeat the measurements until two consecutive measurements match, releasing and repinching the skinfold between each measurement. Make a note of the final measurement for each site.

Time of day of measurements: _____

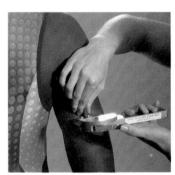

Men	*Women*
Chest: _____ mm	Triceps: _____ mm
Abdomen: _____ mm	Suprailium: _____ mm
Thigh: _____ mm	Thigh: _____ mm

Determining Percent Body Fat

Add the measurements of your three skinfolds. Use this sum as a point of comparison for future assessments and/or find the percent body fat that corresponds to your total in the appropriate table. For example, a 19-year-old female with measurements of 16 mm, 19 mm, and 22 mm would have a skinfold sum of 57 mm; according to the table on page 183, her percent body fat is 22.7.

Sum of three skinfolds: _____ mm   Percent body fat: _____ %

Percent Body Fat Estimate for Women: Sum of Triceps, Suprailium, and Thigh Skinfolds

Sum of Skinfolds (mm)	Age								
	Under 22	23–27	28–32	33–37	38–42	43–47	48–52	53–57	Over 57
23–25	9.7	9.9	10.2	10.4	10.7	10.9	11.2	11.4	11.7
26–28	11.0	11.2	11.5	11.7	12.0	12.3	12.5	12.7	13.0
29–31	12.3	12.5	12.8	13.0	13.3	13.5	13.8	14.0	14.3
32–34	13.6	13.8	14.0	14.3	14.5	14.8	15.0	15.3	15.5
35–37	14.8	15.0	15.3	15.5	15.8	16.0	16.3	16.5	16.8
38–40	16.0	16.3	16.5	16.7	17.0	17.2	17.5	17.7	18.0
41–43	17.2	17.4	17.7	17.9	18.2	18.4	18.7	18.9	19.2
44–46	18.3	18.6	18.8	19.1	19.3	19.6	19.8	20.1	20.3
47–49	19.5	19.7	20.0	20.2	20.5	20.7	21.0	21.2	21.5
50–52	20.6	20.8	21.1	21.3	21.6	21.8	22.1	22.3	22.6
53–55	21.7	21.9	22.1	22.4	22.6	22.9	23.1	23.4	23.6
56–58	22.7	23.0	23.2	23.4	23.7	23.9	24.2	24.4	24.7
59–61	23.7	24.0	24.2	24.5	24.7	25.0	25.2	25.5	25.7
62–64	24.7	25.0	25.2	25.5	25.7	26.0	26.7	26.4	26.7
65–67	25.7	25.9	26.2	26.4	26.7	26.9	27.2	27.4	27.7
68–70	26.6	26.9	27.1	27.4	27.6	27.9	28.1	28.4	28.6
71–73	27.5	27.8	28.0	28.3	28.5	28.8	29.0	29.3	29.5
74–76	28.4	28.7	28.9	29.2	29.4	29.7	29.9	30.2	30.4
77–79	29.3	29.5	29.8	30.0	30.3	30.5	30.8	31.0	31.3
80–82	30.1	30.4	30.6	30.9	31.1	31.4	31.6	31.9	32.1
83–85	30.9	31.2	31.4	31.7	31.9	32.2	32.4	32.7	32.9
86–88	31.7	32.0	32.2	32.5	32.7	32.9	33.2	33.4	33.7
89–91	32.5	32.7	33.0	33.2	33.5	33.7	33.9	34.2	34.4
92–94	33.2	33.4	33.7	33.9	34.2	34.4	34.7	34.9	35.2
95–97	33.9	34.1	34.4	34.6	34.9	35.1	35.4	35.6	35.9
98–100	34.6	34.8	35.1	35.3	35.5	35.8	36.0	36.3	36.5
101–103	35.3	35.4	35.7	35.9	36.2	36.4	36.7	36.9	37.2
104–106	35.8	36.1	36.3	36.6	36.8	37.1	37.3	37.5	37.8
107–109	36.4	36.7	36.9	37.1	37.4	37.6	37.9	38.1	38.4
110–112	37.0	37.2	37.5	37.7	38.0	38.2	38.5	38.7	38.9
113–115	37.5	37.8	38.0	38.2	38.5	38.7	39.0	39.2	39.5
116–118	38.0	38.3	38.5	38.8	39.0	39.3	39.5	39.7	40.0
119–121	38.5	38.7	39.0	39.2	39.5	39.7	40.0	40.2	40.5
122–124	39.0	39.2	39.4	39.7	39.9	40.2	40.4	40.7	40.9
125–127	39.4	39.6	39.9	40.1	40.4	40.6	40.9	41.1	41.4
128–130	39.8	40.0	40.3	40.5	40.8	41.0	41.3	41.5	41.8

SOURCE: Jackson, A. S., and M. L. Pollock. 1985. Practical assessment of body composition. *Physician and Sportsmedicine* 13(5): 76–90. Reproduced by permission of The McGraw-Hill Companies.

LABORATORY ACTIVITIES

Percent Body Fat Estimate for Men: Sum of Chest, Abdomen, and Thigh Skinfolds

Sum of Skinfolds (mm)	Age								
	Under 22	23–27	28–32	33–37	38–42	43–47	48–52	53–57	Over 57
8–10	1.3	1.8	2.3	2.9	3.4	3.9	4.5	5.0	5.5
11–13	2.2	2.8	3.3	3.9	4.4	4.9	5.5	6.0	6.5
14–16	3.2	3.8	4.3	4.8	5.4	5.9	6.4	7.0	7.5
17–19	4.2	4.7	5.3	5.8	6.3	6.9	7.4	8.0	8.5
20–22	5.1	5.7	6.2	6.8	7.3	7.9	8.4	8.9	9.5
23–25	6.1	6.6	7.2	7.7	8.3	8.8	9.4	9.9	10.5
26–28	7.0	7.6	8.1	8.7	9.2	9.8	10.3	10.9	11.4
29–31	8.0	8.5	9.1	9.6	10.2	10.7	11.3	11.8	12.4
32–34	8.9	9.4	10.0	10.5	11.1	11.6	12.2	12.8	13.3
35–37	9.8	10.4	10.9	11.5	12.0	12.6	13.1	13.7	14.3
38–40	10.7	11.3	11.8	12.4	12.9	13.5	14.1	14.6	15.2
41–43	11.6	12.2	12.7	13.3	13.8	14.4	15.0	15.5	16.1
44–46	12.5	13.1	13.6	14.2	14.7	15.3	15.9	16.4	17.0
47–49	13.4	13.9	14.5	15.1	15.6	16.2	16.8	17.3	17.9
50–52	14.3	14.8	15.4	15.9	16.5	17.1	17.6	18.2	18.8
53–55	15.1	15.7	16.2	16.8	17.4	17.9	18.5	19.1	19.7
56–58	16.0	16.5	17.1	17.7	18.2	18.8	19.4	20.0	20.5
59–61	16.9	17.4	17.9	18.5	19.1	19.7	20.2	20.8	21.4
62–64	17.6	18.2	18.8	19.4	19.9	20.5	21.1	21.7	22.2
65–67	18.5	19.0	19.6	20.2	20.8	21.3	21.9	22.5	23.1
68–70	19.3	19.9	20.4	21.0	21.6	22.2	22.7	23.3	23.9
71–73	20.1	20.7	21.2	21.8	22.4	23.0	23.6	24.1	24.7
74–76	20.9	21.5	22.0	22.6	23.2	23.8	24.4	25.0	25.5
77–79	21.7	22.2	22.8	23.4	24.0	24.6	25.2	25.8	26.3
80–82	22.4	23.0	23.6	24.2	24.8	25.4	25.9	26.5	27.1
83–85	23.2	23.8	24.4	25.0	25.5	26.1	26.7	27.3	27.9
86–88	24.0	24.5	25.1	25.7	26.3	26.9	27.5	28.1	28.7
89–91	24.7	25.3	25.9	26.5	27.1	27.6	28.2	28.8	29.4
92–94	25.4	26.0	26.6	27.2	27.8	28.4	29.0	29.6	30.2
95–97	26.1	26.7	27.3	27.9	28.5	29.1	29.7	30.3	30.9
98–100	26.9	27.4	28.0	28.6	29.2	29.8	30.4	31.0	31.6
101–103	27.5	28.1	28.7	29.3	29.9	30.5	31.1	31.7	32.3
104–106	28.2	28.8	29.4	30.0	30.6	31.2	31.8	32.4	33.0
107–109	28.9	29.5	30.1	30.7	31.3	31.9	32.5	33.1	33.7
110–112	29.6	30.2	30.8	31.4	32.0	32.6	33.2	33.8	34.4
113–115	30.2	30.8	31.4	32.0	32.6	33.2	33.8	34.5	35.1
116–118	30.9	31.5	32.1	32.7	33.3	33.9	34.5	35.1	35.7
119–121	31.5	32.1	32.7	33.3	33.9	34.5	35.1	35.7	36.4
122–124	32.1	32.7	33.3	33.9	34.5	35.1	35.8	36.4	37.0
125–127	32.7	33.3	33.9	34.5	35.1	35.8	36.4	37.0	37.6

SOURCE: Jackson, A. S., and M. L. Pollock. 1985. Practical assessment of body composition. *Physician and Sportsmedicine* 13(5): 76–90. Reproduced by permission of The McGraw-Hill Companies.

LABORATORY ACTIVITIES

Rating Your Body Composition

Refer to the figure to rate your percent body fat. Record it below and in the chart at the end of this lab.

Rating: _____

Percent Body Fat Classification

	Percent Body Fat (%)				Percent Body Fat (%)		
	20–39 years	40–59 years	60–79 years		20–39 years	40–59 years	60–79 years
Women				**Men**			
Essential[a]	8–12	8–12	8–12	Essential[a]	3–5	3–5	3–5
Low/athletic[b]	13–20	13–22	13–23	Low/athletic[b]	6–7	6–10	6–12
Recommended	21–32	23–33	24–35	Recommended	8–19	11–21	13–24
Overfat[c]	33–38	34–39	36–41	Overfat[c]	20–24	22–27	25–29
Obese[c]	≥39	≥40	≥42	Obese[c]	≥25	≥28	≥30

The cutoffs for recommended, overfat, and obese ranges in this table are based on a study that linked body mass index classifications from the National Institutes of Health with predicted percent body fat (measured using dual energy X-ray absorptiometry).

[a]Essential body fat is necessary for the basic functioning of the body

[b]Percent body fat in the low/athletic range may be appropriate for some people as long as it is not the result of illness or disordered eating habits; see pp. 172–173 for more on low levels of percent body fat.

[c]Health risks increase as percent body fat exceeds the recommended range.

SOURCES: Gallagher, D., et al. 2000. Healthy percentage body fat ranges: An approach for developing guidelines based on body mass index. *American Journal of Clinical Nutrition* 72: 694–701. American College of Sports Medicine. 2001. *ACSM's Resource Manual for Guidelines for Exercise Testing and Prescription.* 4th ed. Philadelphia: Lippincott, Williams and Wilkins.

Other Methods of Assessing Percent Body Fat

If you use a different method, record the name of the method and the result below and in the chart at the end of this lab. Find your body composition rating on the chart above.

Method used: _____ Percent body fat: _____ % Rating (from chart above): _____

Waist Circumference and Waist-to-Hip Ratio

Equipment

1. Tape measure
2. Partner to take measurements

Preparation

Wear clothes that will not add significantly to your measurements.

Instructions

Stand with your feet together and your arms at your sides. Raise your arms only high enough to allow for taking the measurements. Your partner should make sure the tape is horizontal around the entire circumference and pulled snugly against your skin. The tape shouldn't be pulled so tight that it causes indentations in your skin. Record measurements to the nearest millimeter or one-sixteenth of an inch.

Waist. Measure at the smallest waist circumference. If you don't have a natural waist, measure at the level of your navel. Waist measurement: _____

Hip. Measure at the largest hip circumference. Hip measurement: _____

Waist-to-Hip Ratio: You can use any unit of measurement (for example, inches or centimeters), as long as you're consistent. Waist-to-hip ratio equals waist measurement divided by hip measurement.

Waist-to-hip ratio: _____ ÷ _____ = _____
     (waist measurement)   (hip measurement)

Determining Your Risk

The table below indicates values for waist circumference and waist-to-hip ratio above which the risk of health problems increases significantly. If your measurement or ratio is above either cutoff point, put a check on the appropriate line below and in the chart at the end of this lab.

Waist circumference: _____ (✔ high risk)   Waist-to-hip ratio: _____ (✔ high risk)

Body Fat Distribution

Cutoff Points for High Risk

	Waist Circumference	Waist-to-Hip Ratio
Men	more than 40 in. (102 cm)	more than 0.94
Women	more than 35 in. (88 cm)	more than 0.82

SOURCES: National Heart, Lung, and Blood Institute. 1998. *Clinical Guidelines on the Identification, Evaluation, and Treatment of Overweight and Obesity in Adults: The Evidence Report.* Bethesda, Md.: National Institutes of Health. American College of Sports Medicine. 2001. *ACSM's Resource Manual for Guidelines for Exercise Testing and Prescription,* 4th ed. Philadelphia: Lippincott, Williams and Wilkins.

Rating Your Body Composition

Assessment	Value	Classification
BMI	_____ kg/m^2	_____
Skinfold measurements or alternative method of determining percent body fat Specify method: _____	_____ % body fat	_____
Waist circumference Waist-to-hip ratio	_____ in. or cm _____ (ratio)	_____ (✔ high risk) _____ (✔ high risk)

Using Your Results

How did you score? Are you at all surprised by your ratings for body composition and body fat distribution? Are your current ratings in the range for good health? Are you satisfied with your current body composition? Why or why not?

If you're not satisfied, set a realistic goal for improvement: _____

What should you do next? Enter the results of this lab in the Preprogram Assessment column in Appendix D. If you've determined that you need to improve your body composition, set a specific goal by completing Lab 6.2, and then plan your program using the labs in Chapters 8 and 9 and the weight management section of the Daily Fitness and Nutrition Journal. After several weeks or months of an exercise and/or dietary change program, complete this lab again and enter the results in the Postprogram Assessment column of Appendix D. How do the results compare?

Name _____ Section _____ Date _____

LAB 6.2 *Determining a Target Body Weight*

Complete this lab if the results of Lab 6.1 indicate that a change in body composition would be beneficial for your health and well-being. This lab will help you set a target body weight based on a goal for BMI or percent body fat. Remember, though, that a wellness lifestyle that includes a sensible diet and regular exercise is more important for most people than achieving any specific target weight. In addition, you may have other health risk factors that could affect your body composition goals. You may decide to choose a lifestyle goal for your body composition target instead of a specific BMI, percent body fat, or target body weight. For example, you may set goals of increasing physical activity and improving your diet, and then let your body composition change as a result. Choose an approach that best fits your goals and preferences.

Equipment

Calculator (or pencil and paper for calculations)

Preparation

Determine percent body fat and/or calculate BMI as described in Lab 6.1. Keep track of height and weight as measured for these calculations.

Height: _____ Weight: _____

Instructions: Target Body Weight from Target BMI

Use the chart below to find the target body weight that corresponds to your target BMI. Find your height in the left column and then move across the appropriate row until you find the weight that corresponds to your target BMI. Remember, BMI is only an indirect measurement of body composition. It is possible to improve body composition without any significant change in weight. For example, a weight training program may result in increased muscle mass and decreased fat mass without any change in overall weight. For this reason, you may want to set alternative or additional goals, such as improving the fit of your clothes or decreasing your waist measurement.

	<18.5 Underweight		18.5–24.9 Normal						25–29.9 Overweight					30–34.9 Obesity (Class I)					35–39.9 Obesity (Class II)					≥40 Extreme Obesity
BMI	17	18	19	20	21	22	23	24	25	26	27	28	29	30	31	32	33	34	35	36	37	38	39	40
Height											Body Weight (pounds)													
4' 10"	81	86	91	96	101	105	110	115	120	124	129	134	139	144	148	153	158	163	168	172	177	182	187	192
4' 11"	84	89	94	99	104	109	114	119	124	129	134	139	144	149	154	159	163	168	173	178	183	188	193	198
5'	87	92	97	102	108	113	118	123	128	133	138	143	149	154	159	164	169	174	179	184	190	195	200	205
5' 1"	90	95	101	106	111	117	122	127	132	138	143	148	154	159	164	169	175	180	185	191	196	201	207	212
5' 2"	93	98	104	109	115	120	126	131	137	142	148	153	159	164	170	175	181	186	191	197	202	208	213	219
5' 3"	96	102	107	113	119	124	130	136	141	147	153	158	164	169	175	181	186	192	198	203	209	215	220	226
5' 4"	99	105	111	117	122	128	134	140	146	152	157	163	169	175	181	187	192	198	204	210	216	222	227	233
5' 5"	102	108	114	120	126	132	138	144	150	156	162	168	174	180	186	192	198	204	210	216	222	229	235	241
5' 6"	105	112	118	124	130	136	143	149	155	161	167	174	180	186	192	198	205	211	217	223	229	236	242	248
5' 7"	109	115	121	128	134	141	147	153	160	166	173	179	185	192	198	204	211	217	224	230	236	243	249	256
5' 8"	112	118	125	132	138	145	151	158	165	171	178	184	191	197	204	211	217	224	230	237	244	250	257	263
5' 9"	115	122	129	136	142	149	156	163	169	176	183	190	197	203	210	217	224	230	237	244	251	258	264	271
5' 10"	119	126	133	139	146	153	160	167	174	181	188	195	202	209	216	223	230	237	244	251	258	265	272	279
5' 11"	122	129	136	143	151	158	165	172	179	187	194	201	208	215	222	230	237	244	251	258	265	273	280	287
6'	125	133	140	148	155	162	170	177	184	192	199	207	214	221	229	236	243	251	258	266	273	280	288	295
6' 1"	129	137	144	152	159	167	174	182	190	197	205	212	220	228	235	243	250	258	265	273	281	288	296	303
6' 2"	132	140	148	156	164	171	179	187	195	203	210	218	226	234	242	249	257	265	273	281	288	296	304	312
6' 3"	136	144	152	160	168	176	184	192	200	208	216	224	232	240	248	256	264	272	280	288	296	304	312	320
6' 4"	140	148	156	164	173	181	189	197	206	214	222	230	238	247	255	263	271	280	288	296	304	312	321	329

SOURCE: Ratings from the National Heart, Lung, and Blood Institute. 1998. *Clinical Guidelines on the Identification, Evaluation, and Treatment of Overweight and Obesity in Adults.* Bethesda, Md.: National Institutes of Health.

Current BMI _____ Target BMI _____ Target body weight (from chart) _____

Alternative/additional goals _____

_____

Note: You can calculate target body weight from target BMI more precisely by using the following formula: (1) convert your height measurement to meters, (2) square your height measurement, (3) multiply this number by your target BMI to get your target weight in kilograms, and (4) convert your target weight from kilograms to pounds:

1. Height _____ in. $\times$ 0.0254 m/in. = height _____ m

2. Height _____ m $\times$ height _____ m = _____ m^2

3. Target BMI _____ $\times$ height _____ m^2 = target weight _____ kg

4. Target weight _____ kg $\times$ 2.2 lb/kg = target weight _____ lb

Instructions: Target Body Weight from Target Body Fat Percentages

Use the formula below to determine the target body weight that corresponds to your target percent body fat.

Current percent body fat _____ Target percent body fat _____

Formula

*Example: 180-lb male,
current percent body fat of 24%, goal of 21%*

1. To determine the fat weight in your body, multiply your current weight by percent body fat (determined through skinfold measurements and expressed as a decimal).

180 lb $\times$ 0.24 = 43.2 lb

2. Subtract the fat weight from your current weight to get your current fat-free weight.

180 lb $-$ 43.2 lb = 136.8 lb

3. Subtract your target percent body fat from 1 to get target percent fat-free weight.

1 $-$ 0.21 = 0.79

4. To get your target body weight, divide your fat-free weight by your target percent fat-free weight.

136.8 lb $\div$ 0.79 = 173 lb

Note: Weight can be expressed in either pounds or kilograms, as long as the unit of measurement is used consistently.

1. Current body weight _____ $\times$ percent body fat _____ = fat weight _____

2. Current body weight _____ $-$ fat weight _____ = fat-free weight _____

3. 1 $-$ target percent body fat _____ = target percent fat-free weight _____

4. Fat-free weight _____ $\div$ target percent fat-free weight _____ = target body weight _____

Setting a Goal

Based on these calculations and other factors (including heredity, individual preference, and current health status), select a target weight or range of weights for yourself.

Target body weight: _____

7

Putting Together a Complete Fitness Program

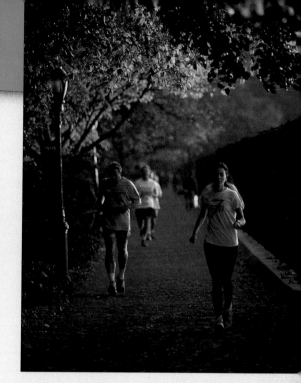

LOOKING AHEAD

After reading this chapter, you should be able to

- Explain the steps for putting together a successful personal fitness program
- Describe strategies that can help you maintain a fitness program over the long term
- Tailor a fitness program to accommodate special health concerns and different life stages

TEST YOUR KNOWLEDGE

1. In surveys, how many Americans report that they've engaged in no physical activity in the past month?
   a. 7%
   b. 17%
   c. 27%

2. Falling asleep in a boring class means a person needs more sleep.
   True or false?

3. Exercise is not recommended for people with asthma or diabetes.
   True or false?

ANSWERS

1. **C.** More than a quarter of Americans are completely sedentary, putting them at risk for early death and a wide variety of diseases and disabling conditions.

2. **TRUE.** A fully rested person may become bored during an uninteresting or monotonous event but will not fall asleep. Daytime sleepiness is a sign of inadequate sleep, which negatively affects health and athletic performance.

3. **FALSE.** Although special precautions may be needed, people with many types of chronic conditions can exercise safely and obtain significant health benefits. Regular exercise reduces the risks of acute asthma attacks and improves insulin sensitivity.

Understanding the physiological basis and wellness benefits of health-related physical fitness, as explained in Chapters 1–6, is the first step toward creating a well-rounded exercise program. The next challenge is to combine activities into a program that develops all the fitness components and maintains motivation.

This chapter presents a step-by-step procedure for creating and maintaining a well-rounded program. Following the chapter, you'll find sample programs based on popular activities. The structure these programs provide can be helpful if you're beginning an exercise program for the first time.

DEVELOPING A PERSONAL FITNESS PLAN

If you're ready to create a complete fitness program based around the activities you enjoy most, begin by preparing the program plan and contract in Lab 7.1. By carefully developing your plan and signing a contract, you'll increase your chances of success. The step-by-step procedure outlined here (adapted from *Your Guide to Getting Fit*, by Ivan Kusinitz and Morton Fine) will guide you through the steps of Lab 7.1 to the creation of an exercise program that's right for you. Refer to Figure 7.1 for a sample personal fitness program plan and contract.

If you'd like additional help in setting up your program, choose one of the sample programs at the end of this chapter. Sample programs are provided for walking/jogging/running, cycling, swimming, and inline skating; they include detailed instructions for starting a program and developing and maintaining fitness.

1. Set Goals

Setting goals to reach through exercise is a crucial first step. Ask yourself, "What do I want from my fitness program?" Develop different types of goals—general and specific, long term and short term. General or long-term goals might include things like lowering your risk for chronic disease, improving posture, having more energy, and improving the fit of your clothes. It's a good idea to also develop some specific, short-term goals based on measurable factors. Specific goals might be raising $\dot{V}O_{2max}$ by 10%, reducing the time it takes you to jog 2 miles from 22 minutes to 19 minutes, increasing the number of push-ups you can do from 15 to 25, and lowering BMI from 26 to 24.5. Having specific goals will allow you to track your progress and enjoy the measurable changes brought about by your fitness program.

Physical fitness assessment tests are essential to determining your goals. They help you decide which types of exercise you should emphasize, and they help you understand the relative difficulty of attaining specific goals. If you have health problems, such as high blood pressure, heart disease, obesity, or serious joint or muscle disabilities,

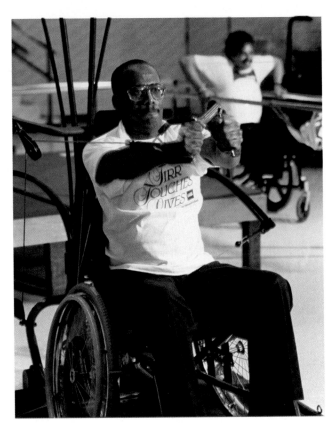

Weight training does little to develop cardiorespiratory endurance but is excellent for developing muscular strength and endurance. An overall fitness program includes exercises to develop all the components of physical fitness.

see your physician before taking assessment tests. Measure your progress by taking these tests about every 3 months.

You'll find it easier to stick with your program if you choose goals that are both important to you and realistic. Remember that heredity, your current fitness level, and other individual factors influence the amount of improvement and the ultimate level of fitness you can expect to obtain through physical training. Fitness improves most quickly during the first 6 months of an exercise program. After that, gains come more slowly and usually require a higher-intensity program. So don't expect to improve indefinitely. Improve your fitness to a reasonable target level, and then train consistently to maintain it. Sometimes you may lose fitness—due to illness, injury, missed workouts, or a vacation—so you must begin again at a lower level. Developing fitness is a dynamic process that involves gains and losses. Even if you lose ground occasionally, stay with your program, and you'll be able to achieve your goals.

Think carefully about your reasons for exercising, and then fill in the goals portion of your plan in Lab 7.1.

2. Select Activities

If you have already chosen activities and created separate program plans for different fitness components in Chapters 3, 4, and 5, you can put those plans together

A. I   Tracie Kaufman   am contracting with myself to follow a physical
   (name)
fitness program to work toward the following goals:

Specific or short-term goals

1. Improving cardiorespiratory fitness by raising my $\dot{V}O_{2max}$ from 34 to 37 ml/kg/min
2. Improving upper body muscular strength and endurance rating from fair to good
3. Improving body composition (from 28% to 25% body fat)
4. Improving my tennis game (hitting 20 playable shots in a row against the ball machine)

General or long-term goals

1. Developing a more positive attitude about myself
2. Improving the fit of my clothes
3. Building and maintaining bone mass to reduce my risk of osteoporosis
4. Increasing my life expectancy and reducing my risk for diabetes and heart disease

B. My program plan is as follows:

| Activities | Components (Check ✓) | | | | | Frequency (Check ✓) | | | | | | | Intensity* | Time |
	CRE	MS	ME	F	BC	M	Tu	W	Th	F	Sa	Su		
Swimming	✓	✓	✓	✓	✓	✓		✓		✓			140–170 bpm	35min
Tennis	✓	✓	✓	✓	✓						✓		RPE i 13–16	90min
Weight training		✓	✓	✓	✓		✓		✓		✓		see Lab 4-3	30min
Stretching				✓		✓		✓		✓	✓		—	25min

*List your target heart rate range or an RPE value if appropriate.

C. My program will begin on   Sept. 21.   My program includes the following schedule
   of mini-goals. For each step in my program, I will give myself the reward listed.

Completing 2 full weeks of program	Oct 5	movie with friends
(mini-goal 1)	(date)	(reward)
$\dot{V}O_{2max}$ of 35 ml/kg/min	Nov 2	new CD
(mini-goal 2)	(date)	(reward)
Completing 10 full weeks of program	Nov 30	new sweater
(mini-goal 3)	(date)	(reward)
Percent body fat of 27%	Dec 22	weekend away
(mini-goal 4)	(date)	(reward)
$\dot{V}O_{2max}$ of 36 ml/kg/min	Jan 18	new CD
(mini-goal 5)	(date)	(reward)

D. My program will include the addition of physical activity to my daily routine (such
   as climbing stairs or walking to class):

1. Walking to and from campus job
2. Taking the stairs to dorm room instead of elevator
3. Bicycling to the library instead of driving
4. Doing one active chore a day
5.

E. I will use the following tools to monitor my program and my progress toward
   my goals: I'll use a chart that lists the number of laps and minutes I swim and the
   charts for strength and flexibility from Labs 4-3 & 5-2.

I sign this contract as an indication of my personal commitment to reach my goal.

Tracie Kaufman   Sept 10
(your signature)   (date)

I have recruited a helper who will witness my contract and
swim with me three days per week
(list any way your helper will participate in your program)

Russell Walter   Sept 10
(witness's signature)   (date)

Figure 7.1   A sample personal fitness program plan and contract.

Table 7.1   A Summary of Sports and Fitness Activities

This table classifies sports and activities as high (H), moderate (M), or low (L) in terms of their ability to develop each of the five components of physical fitness: cardiorespiratory endurance (CRE), muscular strength (MS), muscular endurance (ME), flexibility (F), and body composition (BC). The skill level needed to obtain fitness benefits is noted: Low (L) means little or no skill is required to obtain fitness benefits; moderate (M) means average skill is needed to obtain fitness benefits; and high (H) means much skill is required to obtain fitness benefits. The fitness prerequisite, or conditioning needs of a beginner, is also noted: Low (L) means no fitness prerequisite is required, moderate (M) means some preconditioning is required, and high (H) means substantial fitness is required. The last two columns list the calorie cost of each activity when performed moderately and vigorously. To determine how many calories you burn, multiply the value in the appropriate column by your body weight and then by the number of minutes you exercise. Work up to using 300 or more calories per workout.

| Sports and Activities | COMPONENTS | | | | | Skill Level | Fitness Prerequisite | APPROXIMATE CALORIE COST (CAL/LB/MIN) | |
	CRE	MS*	ME*	F*	BC			Moderate	Vigorous
Aerobic dance	H	M	H	H	H	L	L	.046	.062
Backpacking	H	M	H	M	H	L	M	.032	.078
Badminton, skilled, singles	H	M	M	M	H	M	M	—	.071
Ballet (floor combinations)	M	M	H	H	M	M	L	—	.058
Ballroom dancing	M	L	M	L	M	M	L	.034	.049
Baseball (pitcher and catcher)	M	M	H	M	M	H	M	.039	—
Basketball, half court	H	M	H	M	H	M	M	.045	.071
Bicycling	H	M	H	M	H	M	L	.049	.071
Bowling	L	L	L	L	L	L	L	—	—
Calisthenic circuit training	H	M	H	M	H	L	L	—	.060
Canoeing and kayaking (flat water)	M	M	H	M	M	M	M	.045	—
Cheerleading	M	M	M	M	M	M	L	.033	.049
Fencing	M	M	H	H	M	M	L	.032	.078
Field hockey	H	M	H	M	H	M	M	.052	.078
Folk and square dancing	M	L	M	L	M	L	L	.039	.049
Football, touch	M	M	M	M	M	M	M	.049	.078
Frisbee, ultimate	H	M	H	M	H	M	M	.049	.078
Golf (riding cart)	L	L	L	M	L	L	L	—	—
Handball, skilled, singles	H	M	H	M	H	M	M	—	.078
Hiking	H	M	H	L	H	L	M	.051	.073
Hockey, ice and roller	H	M	H	M	H	M	M	.052	.078
Horseback riding	M	M	M	L	M	M	M	.052	.065
Interval circuit training	H	H	H	M	H	L	L	—	.062
Jogging and running	H	M	H	L	H	L	L	.060	.104

*Ratings are for the muscle groups involved.

into a single program. It's usually best to include exercises to develop each of the health-related components of fitness.

- Cardiorespiratory endurance is developed by activities such as walking, cycling, and aerobic dance that involve continuous rhythmic movements of large-muscle groups like those in the legs (see Chapter 3).
- Muscular strength and endurance are developed by training against resistance (see Chapter 4).
- Flexibility is developed by stretching the major muscle groups (see Chapter 5).
- Healthy body composition can be developed by combining a sensible diet and a program of regular exercise, including cardiorespiratory endurance

exercise to burn calories and resistance training to build muscle mass (see Chapter 6).

Table 7.1 rates many popular activities for their ability to develop each of the health-related components of fitness. Check the ratings of the activities you're considering to make sure the program you put together will develop all fitness components and help you achieve your goals. One strategy is to select one activity for each component of fitness—bicycling, weight training, and stretching, for example. Another strategy applies the principle of **cross-training**, using several different activities to develop a particular fitness component—aerobics classes, swimming, and volleyball for cardiorespiratory endurance, for example. Cross-training is discussed in the next section.

If you select activities that support your commitment rather than activities that turn exercise into a chore, the

Table 7.1   *A Summary of Sports and Fitness Activities (continued)*

Sports and Activities	COMPONENTS					Skill Level	Fitness Prerequisite	APPROXIMATE CALORIE COST (CAL/LB/MIN)	
	CRE	MS*	ME*	F*	BC			Moderate	Vigorous
Judo	M	H	H	M	M	M	L	.049	.090
Karate	H	M	H	H	H	L	M	.049	.090
Lacrosse	H	M	H	M	H	H	M	.052	.078
Modern dance (moving combinations)	M	M	H	H	M	L	L	—	.058
Orienteering	H	M	H	L	H	L	M	.049	.078
Outdoor fitness trails	H	M	H	M	H	L	L	—	.060
Popular dancing	M	L	M	M	M	M	L	—	.049
Racquetball, skilled, singles	H	M	M	M	H	M	M	.049	.078
Rock climbing	M	H	H	H	M	H	M	.033	.033
Rope skipping	H	M	H	L	H	M	M	.071	.095
Rowing	H	H	H	H	H	L	L	.032	.097
Rugby	H	M	H	M	H	M	M	.052	.097
Sailing	L	L	M	L	L	M	L	—	—
Skating, ice, roller, and in-line	M	M	H	M	M	H	M	.049	.095
Skiing, alpine	M	H	H	M	M	H	M	.039	.078
Skiing, cross-country	H	M	H	M	H	M	M	.049	.104
Soccer	H	M	H	M	H	M	M	.052	.097
Squash, skilled, singles	H	M	M	M	H	M	M	.049	.078
Stretching	L	L	L	H	L	L	L	—	—
Surfing (including swimming)	M	M	M	M	M	H	M	—	.078
Swimming	H	M	H	M	H	M	L	.032	.088
Synchronized swimming	M	M	H	H	H	H	M	.032	.052
Table tennis	M	L	M	M	M	M	L	—	.045
Tennis, skilled, singles	H	M	M	M	H	M	M	—	.071
Volleyball	M	L	M	M	M	M	M	—	.065
Walking	H	L	M	L	H	L	L	.029	.048
Water polo	H	M	H	M	H	H	M	—	.078
Water skiing	M	M	H	M	M	H	M	.039	.055
Weight training	L	H	H	H	M	L	L	—	—
Wrestling	H	H	H	H	H	H	H	.065	.094
Yoga	L	L	M	H	L	H	L	—	—

*Ratings are for the muscle groups involved.

SOURCE: Kusinitz, I., and M. Fine. 1983. From *Physical Fitness for Practically Everybody*, Consumer Reports, 1983. Copyright © 1996 by the Consumers Union of the United States, Inc., Yonkers, NY 10703-1057, a nonprofit organization. Reprinted with permission for educational purposes only. No commercial use or photo-copying permitted. To subscribe, call 1-800-234-1645 or visit us at www.ConsumerReports.org.

right program will be its own incentive for continuing. Consider the following factors in making your choices.

• *Fun and interest.* Your fitness program is much more likely to be successful if you choose activities that you enjoy doing. Start by considering any activities you currently engage in and enjoy. Often you can modify your current activities to fit your fitness program. As you consider new activities, ask yourself, "Is this activity fun?" "Will it hold my interest over time?" For new activities, it is a good idea to undertake a trial period before making a final choice. Table 7.2 shows a number of popular fitness activities you may enjoy.

• *Your current skill and fitness level.* Although many activities are appropriate for beginners, some sports and activities require participants to have a moderate level of

skill to obtain fitness benefits. For example, a beginning tennis player will probably not be able to sustain rallies long enough to develop cardiorespiratory endurance. Refer to the skill level column in Table 7.1 to determine the level of skill needed for full participation in the activities you're considering. If your current skill level doesn't meet the requirement, you may want to begin your program with a different activity. For example, a beginning tennis player may be better off with a walking program while improving his or her tennis game—or

cross-training Alternating two or more activities to improve a single component of fitness.

Terms

Activity	Number of Participants (millions)
Table 7.2	Popular Fitness Activities of Americans
Exercise walking[a]	82.2
Swimming[a]	54.7
Exercising with equipment[a]	50.2
Cycling/mountain biking[b]	41.4
Aerobic exercising[a]	29.0
Weight lifting[a]	28.1
Running/jogging[a]	24.7
In-line skating[b]	18.8

[a]Participants are those age 7 and over who participated in the activity more than five times per year.

[b]Participants are those age 7 and over who participated in the activity more than once per year.

SOURCE: National Sporting Goods Association, Mt. Prospect, IL 60056. Reprinted with permission.

practicing with a ball machine to guarantee steady activity. To build skill for a particular activity, consider taking a class or getting some instruction from a coach or fellow participant.

Your current fitness level may also limit the activities that are appropriate for your program. For example, if you have been inactive, a walking program would be more appropriate than a jogging program. Activities in which participants control the intensity of effort—walking, cycling, and swimming, for example—are more appropriate for a beginning fitness program than sports and activities that are primarily "other paced"—soccer, basketball, and tennis, for example. Refer to the fitness prerequisite column of Table 7.1 to determine the minimum level of fitness required for participation in the activities you're considering. However, staying active is the most important thing. If you like to play tennis but don't like to take walks or jog, then play tennis.

• *Time and convenience.* Unless exercise fits easily into your daily schedule, you are unlikely to maintain your program over the long term. As you consider activities, think about whether a special location or facility is required. Can you participate in the activity close to your residence, school, or job? Are the necessary facilities open and available at times convenient to you (see Lab 7.2)? Do you need a partner or a team to play? Can you participate in the activity year-round, or will you need to find an alternative during the summer or winter? Would a home treadmill make you more likely to exercise regularly?

• *Cost.* Some sports and activities require equipment, fees, or some type of membership investment. If you are on a tight budget, limit your choices to activities that are inexpensive or free. Investigate the facilities on your campus, which you may be able to use at little or no cost. Many activities require no equipment beyond an appropriate pair of shoes (see the box "Choosing Exercise Footwear" for more information). Refer back to Chapters 2 and 3 for consumer guidelines for evaluating exercise equipment and facilities.

• *Special health needs.* If you have special exercise needs due to a particular health problem, choose activities that will conform to your needs and enhance your ability to cope. If necessary, consult your physician about how best to tailor an exercise program to your particular needs and goals. Guidelines and safety tips for exercisers with common chronic conditions are provided later in the chapter.

MOTIVATION FOR CHANGE! To add variety and enjoyment to your workouts and to boost your motivation, try exercising to music. Researchers have found that working out to music can boost mood and even keep people working out longer and harder without feeling like they are expending extra effort. Just make sure that music provides a safe distraction and doesn't increase your risk of injury; for example, don't wear headphones while walking or jogging on the street.

3. Set a Target Frequency, Intensity, and Time (Duration) for Each Activity

The next step is to apply the FITT principle and set a starting frequency, intensity, and time (duration) for each type of activity you've chosen (see the sample in Figure 7.1). Refer to the calculations and plans you completed in Chapters 3, 4, and 5.

Cardiorespiratory Endurance Exercise An appropriate frequency for cardiorespiratory endurance exercise is 3–5 times per week. For intensity, note your target heart rate zone or RPE value. Your target total workout time (duration) should be about 20–60 minutes, depending on the intensity of the activity (shorter durations are appropriate for high-intensity activities, longer durations for activities of more moderate intensity). You can exercise in a single session or in multiple sessions of 10 or more minutes. One way to check whether the total duration you've set is appropriate is to use the **calorie costs** (calories per minute per pound of body weight) given in Table 7.1. Your goal should be to work up to burning about 300 calories per workout; beginners should start with a calorie cost of about 100–150 calories per workout. You can calculate the calorie cost of your activities by multiplying the appropriate factor from Table 7.1 by your body weight and the duration of your workout. For example, walking at a moderate pace burns about 0.029 calorie per minute per pound of body weight. A person weighing 150 pounds could begin her

Terms

calorie cost The amount of energy used to perform a particular activity, usually expressed in calories per minute per pound of body weight.

Footwear is perhaps the most important item of equipment for almost any activity. Shoes protect and support your feet and improve your traction. When you jump or run, you place as much as six times more force on your feet than when you stand still. Shoes can help cushion against the stress that this additional force places on your lower legs, thereby preventing injuries. Some athletic shoes are also designed to help prevent ankle rollover, another common source of injury.

General Guidelines

When choosing athletic shoes, first consider the activity you've chosen for your exercise program. Shoes appropriate for different activities have very different characteristics. For example, running shoes typically have highly cushioned midsoles, rubber outsoles with elevated heels, and a great deal of flexibility in the forefoot. The heels of walking shoes tend to be lower, less padded, and more beveled than those designed for running. For aerobic dance, shoes must be flexible in the forefoot and have straight, nonflared heels to allow for safe and easy lateral movements. Court shoes also provide substantial support for lateral movements; they typically have outsoles made from white rubber that will not damage court surfaces.

Also consider the location and intensity of your workouts. If you plan to walk or run on trails, you should choose shoes with water-resistant, highly durable uppers and more outsole traction. If you work out intensely or have a relatively high body weight, you'll need thick, firm midsoles to avoid bottoming-out the cushioning system of your shoes.

Foot type is another important consideration. If your feet tend to roll inward excessively, you may need shoes with additional stability features on the inner side of the shoe to counteract this movement. If your feet tend to roll outward excessively, you may need highly flexible and cushioned shoes that promote foot motion. For aerobic dancers with feet that tend to roll inward or outward, mid-cut to high-cut shoes may be more appropriate than low-cut aerobic shoes or cross-trainers (shoes designed to be worn for several different activities). Compared with men, women have narrower feet overall and narrower heels relative to the forefoot. Most women will get a better fit if they choose shoes that are specifically designed for women's feet rather than those that are downsized versions of men's shoes.

Successful Shopping

For successful shoe shopping, keep the following strategies in mind:

- Shop at an athletic shoe or specialty store that has personnel trained to fit athletic shoes and a large selection of styles and sizes.

- Shop late in the day or, ideally, following a workout. Your foot size increases over the course of the day and as a result of exercise.

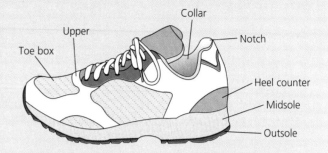

- Wear socks like those you plan to wear during exercise. If you have an old pair of athletic shoes, bring them with you. The wear pattern on your old shoes can help you select a pair with extra support or cushioning in the places you need it the most.

- Ask for help. Trained salespeople know which shoes are designed for your foot type and your level of activity. They can also help fit your shoes properly.

- Don't insist on buying shoes in what you consider to be your typical shoe size. Sizes vary from shoe to shoe. In addition, foot sizes change over time, and many people have one foot that is larger or wider than the other. Try several sizes in several widths, if necessary. Don't buy shoes that are too small.

- Try on both shoes and wear them around for 10 or more minutes. Try walking on a noncarpeted surface. Approximate the movements of your activity: walk, jog, run, jump, and so on.

- Check the fit and style carefully:

  Is the toe box roomy enough? Your toes will spread out when your foot hits the ground or you push off. There should be at least one thumb's width of space from the longest toe to the end of the toe box.

  Do the shoes have enough cushioning? Do your feet feel supported when you bounce up and down? Try bouncing on your toes and on your heels.

  Do your heels fit snugly into the shoe? Do they stay put when you walk, or do they rise up?

  Are the arches of your feet right on top of the shoes' arch supports?

  Do the shoes feel stable when you twist and turn on the balls of your feet? Try twisting from side to side while standing on one foot.

  Do you feel any pressure points?

- If the shoes are not comfortable in the store, don't buy them. Don't expect athletic shoes to stretch over time in order to fit your feet properly.

- Replace athletic shoes about every 3 months or 500 miles of jogging or walking.

Name Tracie Kaufman

Enter time, distance, or another factor to track your progress.

Activity/Date	M	Tu	W	Th	F	S	S	Weekly Total	M	Tu	W	Th	F	S	S	Weekly Total
1 Swimming	800 yd		725 yd		800 yd			2325 yd	800 yd		800 yd		850 yd			2450 yd
2 Tennis				90 min				90 min						95 min		95 min
3 Weight Training		✓		✓		✓				✓		✓		✓	✓	
4 Stretching	✓		✓		✓	✓				✓		✓	✓	✓	✓	

Figure 7.2   A sample program log.

exercise program by walking for 30 minutes, burning about 130 calories. Once her fitness improves, she might choose to start cycling for her cardiorespiratory endurance workouts. Cycling at a moderate pace has a higher calorie cost than walking (0.049 calorie per minute per pound), and if she cycled for 40 minutes, she would burn the target 300 calories during her workout.

Muscular Strength and Endurance Training   A frequency of 2–3 days per week for strength training is recommended. As described in Chapter 4, a general fitness strength training program includes 1 or more sets of 8–12 repetitions of 8–10 exercises that work all major muscle groups. For intensity, choose a weight that is heavy enough to fatigue your muscles but not so heavy that you cannot complete the full number of repetitions with proper form.

Flexibility Training   Stretches should be performed when muscles are warm at least 2–3 days per week. Stretches should be performed for all major muscle groups. For each exercise, stretch to the point of slight tension or mild discomfort and hold the stretch for 10–30 seconds; do at least 4 repetitions of each exercise.

4. Set Up a System of Mini-Goals and Rewards

To keep your program on track, it is important to set up a system of goals and rewards. Break your specific goals into several steps, and set a target date for each step. For example, if one of the goals of an 18-year-old male student's program is to improve upper-body strength and endurance, he could use the push-up test in Lab 4.2 to set intermediate goals. If he can currently perform 15 push-ups (for a rating of "very poor"), he might set intermediate goals of 17, 20, 25, and 30 push-ups (for a final rating of "fair"). By allowing several weeks between mini-goals and specifying rewards, he'll be able to track his progress and reward himself as he moves toward his final goal. Reaching a series of small goals is more satisfying than working toward a single, more challenging goal that may take months to achieve. Realistic goals, broken into achievable mini-goals, can boost your chances of success.

For more on choosing appropriate rewards, refer to page 17 in Chapter 1 and Activity 4 in the Behavior Change Workbook at the end of the text.

5. Include Lifestyle Physical Activity in Your Program

As described in Chapter 2, daily physical activity is an important part of a fit and well lifestyle. As part of your fitness program plan, specify ways to be more active during your daily routine. You may find it helpful to first use your health journal to track your activities for several days. Review the records in your journal, identify routine opportunities to be more active, and add these to your program plan in Lab 7.1.

6. Develop Tools for Monitoring Your Progress

A record that tracks your daily progress will help remind you of your ongoing commitment to your program and give you a sense of accomplishment. Figure 7.2 shows you how to create a general program log and record the activity type, frequency, and times (durations). Or if you wish, complete specific activity logs like those in Labs 3.2, 4.3, and 5.2 in addition to, or instead of, a general log. Post your log in a place where you'll see it often as a reminder and as an incentive for improvement. If you have specific, measurable goals, you can also graph your weekly or monthly progress toward your goal (Figure 7.3). To monitor the overall progress of your fitness program, you may choose to reassess your cardiorespiratory endurance, muscular strength and endurance, flexibility, and body composition every 3 months or so during the improvement phase of your program. Because the results of different fitness tests vary, be sure to compare results for the same assessments over time.

7. Make a Commitment

Your final step in planning your program is to make a commitment by signing a contract. Find a witness for your contract—preferably one who will be actively

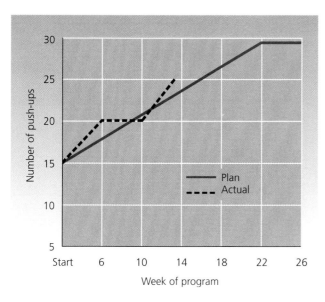

Figure 7.3   A sample program progress chart.

involved in your program. Keep your contract in a visible spot to remind you of your commitment.

PUTTING YOUR PLAN INTO ACTION

Once you've developed a detailed plan and signed your contract, you are ready to begin your fitness program. Refer to the specific training suggestions provided in Chapters 2–5 for advice on beginning and maintaining your program. Many people find it easier to plan a program than to put their plan into action and stick with it over time. For that reason, adherence to healthy lifestyle programs has become an important area of study for psychologists and health researchers. The guidelines below and in the next section reflect research into strategies that help people succeed in sticking with an exercise program:

• *Start slowly and increase fitness gradually.* Overzealous exercising can result in discouraging discomforts and injuries. Your program is meant to last a lifetime. The important first step is to break your established pattern of inactivity. Be patient and realistic. Once your body has adjusted to your starting level of exercise, slowly increase the amount of overload. Small increases are the key— achieving a large number of small improvements will eventually result in substantial gains in fitness. It's usually best to increase duration and frequency before increasing intensity.

• *Find an exercise buddy.* The social side of exercise is an important factor for many regular exercisers. Working out with a friend will make exercise more enjoyable and increase your chances of sticking with your program. Find an exercise partner who shares your goals and general fitness level.

• *Vary your activities.* You can make your program more fun over the long term if you participate in a variety of different activities that you enjoy. You can also add interest by strategies such as varying the routes you take when walking, running, biking, or in-line skating; finding a new tennis or racquetball partner; changing your music for aerobic dance; or switching to a new volleyball or basketball court.

Varying your activities, a strategy known as cross-training, has other benefits. It can help you develop balanced, total body fitness. For example, by alternating running with swimming, you build both upper- and lower-body strength. Cross-training can thus prepare you for a wider range of activities and physical challenges. It can also reduce the risk of injury and overtraining because the same muscles, bones, and joints are not continuously subjected to the stresses of the same activity. Cross-training can be done either by choosing different activities on different days or by alternating activities within a single workout.

• *Cycle the volume and intensity of your workouts.* Olympic athletes use a training technique called periodization of training, meaning that they vary the volume and intensity of their workouts. Sometimes they exercise very intensely; at other times they train lightly or rest. You can use the same technique to improve fitness faster and make your training program more varied and enjoyable. For example, if your program consists of walking, weight training, and stretching, pick one day a week for each activity to train a little harder or longer than you normally do. If you usually walk 2 miles in 16 minutes per mile, increase the pace to 15 minutes per mile once a week. If you lift weights twice a week, train more intensely during one of the workouts by using more resistance or performing multiple sets.

• *Adapt to changing environments and schedules.* Most people are creatures of habit and have trouble adjusting to change. Don't use wet weather or a new job as excuses to give up your exercise program. If you walk in the summer, put on a warm coat and walk in the winter. If you can't go out because of darkness, join a gym and walk on a treadmill. Changes in your job or family situation can also affect your exercise program. Taking a job with a longer commute or having a new baby can rob you of the time you used to spend exercising. Remember that physical activity is important for your energy level, self-esteem, and well-being. You owe it to yourself to include physical activity in your day. Try to exercise before going to work or do some physical activity during your lunch hour—even if it's only a short walk or a few trips up and down the stairs.

• *Expect fluctuations and lapses.* On some days, your progress will be excellent, but on others, you'll barely be able to drag yourself through your scheduled activities. Don't let off-days or lapses discourage you or make you feel guilty. Instead, feel a renewed commitment for your fitness program (see the box "Getting Your Fitness Program Back on Track" on p. 198).

Lapses are a normal part of any behavior change program. The important point is to move on and avoid becoming discouraged. Try again, and keep trying. Know that continued effort will lead to success.

- Don't judge yourself harshly. Focus on the improvements you've already obtained from your program and how good you feel after exercise—both physically and mentally.

- Visualize what it will be like to reach your goals. Keep these pictures in your mind as an incentive to stick with your program.

- Use your exercise journal to identify thoughts and behaviors that are causing noncompliance. Devise strategies to combat these problematic patterns. If needed, make additional changes in your environment or obtain more social support. Call a friend to walk with you. Put your exercise clothes in your car or backpack.

- Make changes in your plan and reward system to help renew your enthusiasm and commitment to your program. Try changing fitness activities or your exercise schedule. Build in more opportunities to reward yourself.

- Plan ahead for difficult situations. Think about what circumstances might make it tough to keep up your fitness routine. Develop strategies to increase your chances of sticking with your program. For example, devise strategies for your program during vacation, travel, bad weather, and so on.

- If you're in a bad mood or just don't feel like exercising, remind yourself that physical activity is probably the one thing you can do that will make you feel better. Even if you can only do half your scheduled workout, you'll boost your energy, improve your mood, and help keep your program on track.

MOTIVATION FOR CHANGE!   In addition to tracking the basic progress of your fitness program, you may find that directly monitoring some of your program's benefits can help keep you motivated and on track. For example, try tracking your energy level. Develop a point scale (1–10 or 1–20), record a value for your energy level each day, and graph the results. Most people find that increasing physical activity quickly boosts their energy level.

MAINTAINING YOUR PROGRAM: FIT FOR LIFE

Exercise should not be something you do just during January and February to satisfy a New Year's resolution—or during a class to satisfy a course requirement. You must make it a permanent part of your life. Choose activities you enjoy and make them part of your daily routine, just like sleeping, eating, brushing your teeth, and going to school and work. Scientists gather more evidence every year that regular exercise is the most important activity you can do to contribute to wellness. It is not a frill or a treat—it is a necessity. You will be a healthier, more vital person if you make physical activity a habit. The following strategies can help keep you active for life:

- *Be safe.* Minimize the risk of injury or problems from activity by following safety guidelines, using proper technique and equipment, respecting signals from your body that something may be wrong, and treating any injuries that occur. Warm up, cool down, and drink plenty of fluids before and after exercise.

- *Have several exercise options.* Don't depend on a single location, activity, or person to be active. Cultivate many enjoyable activities that can be done in all seasons and circumstances. Take up a new sport or activity to keep your program fresh and enjoyable. And don't forget to include lifestyle physical activity in your daily routine.

- *Keep an exercise journal.* A journal can help keep your program on track, identify sources of problems, and give you a continuing sense of accomplishment.

- *Reward yourself.* Don't stop rewarding yourself once you reach your fitness goals. Continue to give yourself regular rewards for sticking with your program.

- *Choose other healthy lifestyle behaviors.* Exercise provides huge benefits for your health, but other behaviors are also important. Choose a nutritious diet and avoid harmful habits like smoking and overconsumption of alcohol. Don't skimp on sleep, which has a mutually beneficial relationship with exercise. Physical activity improves sleep, and adequate sleep can improve physical performance (see the box "Sleep").

EXERCISE GUIDELINES FOR PEOPLE WITH SPECIAL HEALTH CONCERNS

Regular, appropriate exercise is safe and beneficial for many people with chronic conditions or other special health concerns. For example, people with heart disease or hypertension who exercise may lower their blood pressure and improve their cholesterol levels. For people with diabetes, exercise can improve insulin sensitivity and body composition. For people with asthma, regular exercise may reduce the risk of acute attacks during exertion. For many people with special health concerns, the risks associated with *not* exercising are far greater than those associated with a moderate program of regular exercise.

The fitness recommendations for the general population presented in this text can serve as a general guideline for any exercise program. However, for people with special health concerns, certain precautions and monitoring

If you could do something simple, safe, and free to dramatically improve your mental, physical, and psychological health, would you do it? The opportunity is yours starting tonight—all you have to do is go to bed earlier! The majority of Americans suffer from chronic sleep deprivation. Most of us get between one-half and two fewer hours of sleep each night than we need in order to be fully alert during the day. One hundred years ago, Americans slept on average one and a half more hours each night than we do now. With the advent of electric lights, sleep times decreased dramatically.

Many people view sleep as a luxury or a waste of time, but sleep is absolutely essential for life and health. Humans and other animals who are deprived of sleep for many days will become ill and even die. Less extreme sleep deprivation over a long period of time makes us vulnerable to a wide variety of illnesses including CVD, diabetes, high blood pressure, and psychological disorders such as anxiety and depression. Inadequate sleep also depresses the immune system, making people more likely to become ill with infectious diseases. Inadequate sleep affects learning, memory, and attention span, all critical to academic performance. Athletes who fail to get sufficient sleep cannot perform at their peak because fatigue slows reaction time and lessens endurance. Every aspect of life is easier and more pleasurable when you are well rested.

Sleep deprivation also takes a huge toll on society. The National Sleep Foundation estimates that sleepy employees cost U.S. businesses $18 billion every year in lost productivity alone. The costs are much higher if you factor in mistakes, accidents, and health problems caused by lack of sleep. Drowsiness is a factor in at least one-third of all auto crashes; it impairs driving ability as much as alcohol use. Many of us think that no matter how tired we may be, we can force ourselves to be alert. Researchers have found that people who are sleep deprived may think they are wide awake but often fall asleep at the wheel for brief periods without even realizing it.

College students are particularly vulnerable to sleep deprivation and poor quality of sleep. Most students lead hectic lives as they juggle studies, work, socializing, and family obligations. Students who live in dormitories are often awakened by nighttime noise. Partying, especially if alcohol and other drugs are used, further disrupts sleep. To make matters worse, teens and young adults actually need more sleep than older individuals—more than 9 hours of sleep a night—to be well rested.

Financial necessity dictates that many students work part time or even full time. Realistically, there are only so many hours in the day, and many working students find it nearly impossible to get enough sleep to function well in school or at work. What can you do if you are faced with this dilemma? Cut back on work hours if at all possible. Obtaining financial aid or a loan or taking an extra year to get your degree may be worth it to preserve your health and happiness.

How do you know if you're getting enough sleep? If you need an alarm to get yourself up every morning, rather than awakening naturally at the appropriate time, chances are you are significantly sleep deprived. Another clue is if you fall asleep within just a few minutes of getting into bed, or if you fall asleep during the day when you don't intend to, such as during lectures or while reading or watching TV. Sleep you need but don't get is referred to as "sleep debt." Whenever you get less sleep than your body requires, you add to your sleep debt. Week after week, sleep debt can build, leaving you chronically groggy. If you have a large sleep debt, sleeping in a few extra hours on the weekends won't solve the problem, although it can help a bit. The real solution is to make sleep a priority in your daily life. Remember that the time you spend sleeping will pay for itself in increased productivity. For example, if you go to bed one hour earlier instead of trying to study when you're half awake, you are likely to get the work done in a fraction of the time when you're more alert the next day. Knowing that the quality of your life depends on getting adequate sleep, make sleep a priority part of your wellness lifestyle.

may be required. Anyone with special health concerns should consult a physician before beginning an exercise program. Guidelines and cautions for some common conditions are described below.

Arthritis

- Begin an exercise program as early as possible in the course of the disease.
- Warm up thoroughly before each workout to loosen stiff muscles and lower the risk of injury.
- For cardiorespiratory endurance exercise, avoid high-impact activities that may damage arthritic joints; consider swimming, water walking, or another type of exercise in a warm pool.
- Strength train the whole body; pay special attention to muscles that support and protect affected joints (for example, build quadriceps, hamstring, and calf strength for the knee). Start with small loads and build intensity gradually.

- Perform flexibility exercises regularly to maintain joint mobility.

Asthma

- Exercise regularly. Acute attacks are more likely if you exercise only occasionally.
- Carry medication during workouts and avoid exercising alone. Use your inhaler before exercise, if recommended by your physician.
- Warm up and cool down slowly to reduce the risk of acute attacks.
- When starting an exercise program, choose self-paced endurance activities, especially those involving **interval training** (short bouts of exercise

interval training A training technique that alternates exercise intervals with rest intervals or intense exercise intervals with low to moderate intervals. Terms

followed by a rest period). Increase the intensity of cardiorespiratory endurance exercise gradually.

- Educate yourself about circumstances that may trigger an asthma attack, and act accordingly. For example, cold, dry air can trigger or worsen an attack. Pollen, dust, and polluted air can also trigger an attack. To avoid attacks in dry air, drink water before, during, and after a workout to moisten your airways. In cold weather, cover your mouth with a mask or scarf to warm and humidify the air you breathe. Also, avoid outdoor activities during pollen season or when the air is polluted or dusty.

Diabetes

- Don't begin an exercise program unless your diabetes is under control and you have checked about exercise safety with your physician. Because people with diabetes have an increased risk for heart disease, an exercise stress test may be recommended.
- Don't exercise alone. Wear a bracelet identifying yourself as having diabetes.
- If you are taking insulin or another medication, you may need to adjust the timing and amount of each dose. Work with your physician and check your blood sugar levels regularly so you can learn to balance your energy intake and output and your medication dosage.
- To prevent abnormally rapid absorption of injected insulin, inject it over a muscle that won't be exercised and wait at least an hour before exercising.
- Check blood sugar levels before, during, and after exercise and adjust your diet or insulin dosage if needed. Carry high-carbohydrate foods during a workout. Avoid exercises if your blood sugar level is above 250 mg/dl and ingest carbohydrates prior to exercise if your blood sugar level is below 100 mg/dl.
- Don't lift heavy weights. Straining can damage blood vessels.
- If you have poor circulation or numbness in your extremities, check your skin regularly for blisters and abrasions, especially on your feet. Avoid high-impact activities and wear comfortable shoes.
- For maximum benefit and minimum risk, choose low-to-moderate-intensity activities.

Heart Disease and Hypertension

- Check with your physician about exercise safety before increasing your activity level.
- Exercise at a moderate rather than a high intensity. Keep your heart rate below the level at which abnormalities appear on an exercise stress test.
- Warm-up and cool-down sessions should be gradual and last at least 10 minutes.
- Monitor your heart rate during exercise and stop if you experience dizziness or chest pain.

- If your physician has prescribed it, carry nitroglycerin with you during exercise. If you are taking beta-blockers for hypertension, use RPE rather than heart rate to monitor exercise intensity (beta-blockers reduce heart rate). Exercise at an RPE level of "somewhat hard"; your breathing should be unlabored, and you should be able to talk.
- Don't hold your breath when exercising. Doing so can cause sudden, steep increases in blood pressure. Take special care during weight training; don't lift extremely heavy loads.
- Increase exercise frequency, intensity, and time very gradually.

Obesity

- For maximum benefit and minimum risk, begin by choosing low-to-moderate-intensity activities. Increase intensity slowly as your fitness improves. Studies of overweight people show that exercising at moderate to high intensities causes more fat loss than training at low intensities.
- The National Academies and the World Health Organization recommend that people who want to lose weight or maintain lost weight exercise moderately 60 minutes or more every day. To get the benefit of 60 minutes of exercise, you can exercise all at once or divide your total activity time into sessions of 10, 20, or 30 minutes.
- Choose non- or low-weight-bearing activities such as swimming, water exercises, cycling, or walking. Low-impact activities are less likely to lead to joint problems or injuries.

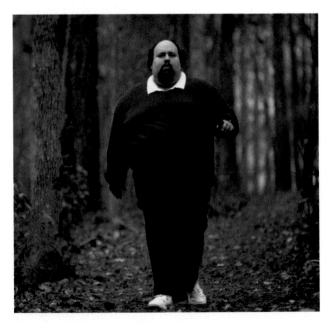

Low-impact activities like walking are a good choice for people who are overweight because they can provide a good workout and are less likely than high-impact activities to cause joint problems or injuries. This man lost 100 pounds in the year after this photo was taken.

- Stay alert for symptoms of heat-related problems during exercise (see Chapter 3). People who are obese are particularly vulnerable to problems with heat intolerance.
- Ease into an exercise program and increase overload gradually. Increase time and frequency of exercise before increasing intensity.
- Include strength training in your fitness program to build or maintain muscle mass.
- Try to include as much lifestyle physical activity in your daily routine as possible.

Osteoporosis

- For cardiorespiratory endurance activities, exercise at the maximum intensity that causes no significant discomfort. If possible, choose low-impact weight-bearing activities to help safely maintain bone density (see Chapter 8 for more strategies for building and maintaining bone density).
- To prevent fractures, avoid any activity or movement that stresses the back or carries a risk of falling.
- Include weight training in your exercise program to improve strength and balance and reduce the risk of falls and fractures. Avoid lifting heavy loads.

Exercise guidelines for people with disabilities are discussed in Chapter 2 and for people with low-back pain, in Chapter 5.

> **MOTIVATION FOR CHANGE!** If you have a special health concern and have hesitated becoming more active, one helpful strategy is to take a class or join an exercise group specifically designed for your condition. Many health centers and support groups sponsor specially tailored activity programs. Such a class can provide you with both expert advice and exercise partners who share your concerns and goals.

EXERCISE GUIDELINES FOR LIFE STAGES

A fitness program may also need to be adjusted to accommodate the requirements of different life stages.

Children and Adolescents

Only about half of all young people age 12–21 in the United States participate regularly in vigorous activity, and 25% report no vigorous activity at all. This lack of physical activity has led to alarming increases in overweight and obesity in children and adolescents. If you have children or are in a position to influence children, keep these guidelines in mind:

- Provide opportunities for children and adolescents to exercise every day. Minimize sedentary activities, such as watching television and playing video games.

Children and adolescents should aim for 60 minutes of moderate activity most, but preferably all, days.

- During family outings, choose dynamic activities. For example, go for a walk, park away from a mall and then walk to the stores, and take the stairs instead of the escalator.
- For children younger than 12 years, emphasize skill development and fitness rather than excellence in competitive sports. For adolescents, combine participation and training in lifetime sports with traditional, competitive sports.
- Make sure children are developmentally capable of participating in an activity. For example, catching skills are difficult for young children because their nervous system is not developed enough to fully master the skill. When teaching a child to catch a ball, start with a large ball and throw it from a short range. Gradually increase the complexity of the skill once the child has mastered the simpler skill.
- Make sure children get plenty of water when exercising in the heat. Make sure they are dressed properly when doing sports in the cold.

Pregnant Women

Exercise is important during pregnancy, but women should be cautious because some types of exercise can pose increased risk to the mother and the unborn child. The following guidelines are consistent with the recommendations of the American College of Obstetrics and Gynecology.

- See your physician about possible modifications needed for your particular pregnancy.
- Continue mild-to-moderate exercise routines at least three times a week. Avoid exercising vigorously or to exhaustion, especially in the third trimester. Monitor exercise intensity by assessing how you feel rather than by monitoring your heart rate.
- Favor non- or low-weight-bearing exercises such as swimming or cycling over weight-bearing exercises, which can carry increased risk of injury.
- Avoid exercise in a supine position—lying on your back—after the first trimester. Research indicates that this position restricts blood flow to the uterus. Also avoid prolonged periods of motionless standing.
- Avoid exercise that could cause loss of balance, especially in the third trimester, and exercise that might injure the abdomen, stress the joints, or carry a risk of falling (such as contact sports, vigorous racquet sports, skiing, and in-line skating).
- Avoid activities involving extremes in altitude—for example, scuba diving and mountain climbing.
- Especially during the first trimester, drink plenty of fluids and exercise in well-ventilated areas to avoid heat stress.
- Do 3–5 sets of 10 Kegel exercises daily. These exercises involve tightening the muscles of the pelvic

floor for 5–15 seconds. Kegel exercises are thought to help prevent incontinence (involuntary loss of urine) and speed recovery after giving birth.

- After giving birth, resume prepregnancy exercise routines gradually, based on how you feel.

Older Adults

Older people readily adapt to endurance exercise and strength training. Exercise principles are the same as for younger people, but some specific guidelines apply:

- Include the three basic types of exercise—resistance, endurance, and flexibility.
- For strength training, the ACSM recommends that older adults use a lighter weight and perform more (10–15) repetitions than that recommended for young adults.
- Drink plenty of water and avoid exercising in excessively hot or cold environments. (Older people sometimes have a decreased ability to regulate body temperature during exercise.) Wear clothes that speed heat loss in warm environments and that prevent heat loss in cold environments.
- Warm up slowly and carefully. Increase intensity and duration of exercise gradually.
- Cool down slowly, continuing very light exercise until the heart rate is below 100.
- To help prevent soft tissue pain, do static stretching after a normal workout.

Sample fitness programs begin on p. 204.

Tips for Today

A complete fitness program includes activities to build and maintain cardiorespiratory endurance, muscular strength and endurance, and flexibility. It takes time, energy, and commitment to begin and maintain a fitness program, but the many benefits are well worth the effort. Begin today, and you'll be on your way to enjoying fitness and wellness for the rest of your life.

Right now you can

- Obtain a journal to track your daily physical activity and exercise routine.
- Put away your remote control devices—every bit of physical activity can benefit your health.
- Put the clothes and equipment for your next workout in a convenient and obvious location.
- Set a firm time for your next workout with your training partner (buddy).
- Plan to go to bed 15 minutes earlier than usual.
- Make a list of situations such as bad weather that may challenge your ability to stick with your fitness program. develop a strategy for dealing with each one.

SUMMARY

- Steps for putting together a complete fitness program include (1) setting realistic goals; (2) selecting activities to develop all the health-related components of fitness; (3) setting a target frequency, intensity, and time (duration) for each activity; (4) setting up a system of mini-goals and rewards; (5) making lifestyle physical activity a part of the daily routine; (6) developing tools for monitoring progress; and (7) making a commitment.
- In selecting activities, consider fun and interest, your current skill and fitness levels, time and convenience, cost, and any special health concerns.
- Keys to beginning and maintaining a successful program include starting slowly, increasing intensity and duration gradually, finding a buddy, varying the activities and intensity of the program, and expecting fluctuations and lapses.
- Regular exercise is appropriate and highly beneficial for people with special health concerns or in particular stages of life; program modifications may be necessary to maximize safety.

FOR FURTHER EXPLORATION

W *Fit and Well* **Online Learning Center (www.mhhe.com/fahey)**

Use the learning objectives, study guide questions, and glossary flashcards to review key terms and concepts and prepare for exams. You can extend your knowledge of personal fitness and gain experience in using the Internet as a resource by completing the activities and checking out the Web links for the topics in Chapter 7 marked with the World Wide Web icon. For this chapter, Internet activities explore fitness activities and strategies for creating a complete fitness program; there are also helpful Web links for chapter topics.

Daily Fitness and Nutrition Journal

Complete the program plan and fitness contract, and begin your program. Use the journal to record your activities and track your progress.

HealthQuest

Use the Fitness Wizard on the HealthQuest CD-ROM to create a schedule for your complete fitness program; select the Fitness Wizard option from the Fitness Planner portion of the Wellness Activities in the Fitness module. Once in the Fitness Wizard, choose the Physical Fitness Program option to build a program that includes activities to build all the health-related fitness components.

W Books, Organizations, and Web Sites

See the listings for Chapters 2–7.

COMMON QUESTIONS ANSWERED

Should I exercise every day? Some daily exercise is beneficial, and health experts recommend that you engage in at least
30 minutes of moderate physical activity over the course of
every day. Back experts suggest that you also do back pain
prevention exercises daily. However, if you train intensely every
day without giving yourself a rest, you will likely get injured or
become overtrained. When strength training, for example, rest
at least 48 hours between workouts before exercising the same
muscle group. For cardiorespiratory endurance exercise, rest or
exercise lightly the day after an intense or long-duration workout. Balancing the proper amount of rest and exercise will help
you feel better and improve your fitness faster.

***I'm just starting an exercise program. How much activity
should I do at first?*** Be conservative. Walking is a good way
to begin almost any fitness program. At first, walk for approximately 10 minutes, and then increase the distance and pace.
After several weeks, you can progress to something more vigorous. Let your body be your guide. If the intensity and duration of a workout seem easy, increase them a little the next
time. The key is to be progressive; don't try to achieve physical
fitness in one or two workouts. Build your fitness gradually.

***What are kickboxing and Tae Bo? Are they effective forms of
exercise?*** Kickboxing and Tae Bo are group fitness workouts
that combine martial arts maneuvers, boxing moves, and
traditional group exercise activities. Participants in martial arts
workouts repetitively execute a variety of punches and kicks,
building movement combinations that involve the entire body.

Workouts are often choreographed to moderately paced popular music and are continuous. Although more research is
needed to clarify the actual training effects, the workouts
certainly develop cardiovascular endurance, muscular endurance, and flexibility. Because of the potential for injury,
classes should be led either by a certified fitness professional
who has had ancillary training in teaching martial arts skills or
a martial artist with qualifications as a fitness instructor. Other
key safety elements include precise skill modeling and verbal
instruction, moderate pacing, and an emphasis on health-
related fitness development.

***I'm concerned about my safety when I go for a jog or walk.
What can I do to make sure that my training sessions are safe
and enjoyable?*** A person exercising alone in the park can be
a tempting target for criminals. Don't exercise alone. You are
much safer training in a group or with a partner. Another
alternative is to take an exercise class. Classes are fun and
much safer than exercising by yourself. If you must train
alone, try to exercise where there are plenty of people. A good
bet is the local high school or college track.

Make sure you're wearing proper safety equipment. If
you're riding a bike, wear a helmet. If you're playing racquetball or handball, wear eye protectors. Don't go in-line skating
unless you're wearing the proper pads and protective equipment. If you are jogging at night, wear reflective clothing that
can be seen easily.

Refer to Appendix A for more on personal safety.

SELECTED BIBLIOGRAPHY

American College of Obstetrics and Gynecology Committee on Obstetric
Practice. 2002. Exercise during pregnancy and the postpartum period.
Committee Opinion No. 267. *International Journal of Gynaecology and
Obstetrics* 77:79–81.

American College of Sports Medicine. 2001. *ACSM's Resource Manual for
Guidelines for Exercise Testing and Prescription,* 4th ed. Philadelphia:
Lippincott Williams and Wilkins.

American College of Sports Medicine. 2000. *ACSM's Guidelines for Exercise
Testing and Prescription,* 6th ed. Baltimore, Md.: Lippincott Williams and
Wilkins.

American College of Sports Medicine. 1998. ACSM position stand: Exercise
and physical activity for older adults. *Medicine and Science in Sports and
Exercise* 30(6): 992–1008.

American Diabetes Association. 2003. Physical activity/exercise and diabetes mellitus. *Diabetes Care* 26:S73–S77.

American Heart Association. 2003. Exercise and physical activity in the
prevention and treatment of atherosclerotic cardiovascular disease.
Circulation 107:3109–3116.

Bernstein, M. S., M. C. Costanza, and A. Morabia. 2004. Association of physical activity intensity levels with overweight and obesity in a population-
based sample of adults. *Preventive Medicine* 38(1): 94–104.

Fenicchia, L. M., et al. 2004. Influence of resistance exercise training on
glucose control in women with type 2 diabetes. *Metabolism* 53(3):
284–289.

Heesch, K. C., et al. 2003. Does adherence to a lifestyle physical activity intervention predict changes in physical activity? *Journal of Behavioral
Medicine* 26(4): 333–348.

Mazzeo, R. S., and H. Tanaka. 2001. Exercise prescription for the elderly:
Current recommendations. *Sports Medicine* 31(11): 809–818.

National Sleep Foundation. 2002. *2002 Sleep in America Poll* (http://www.
sleepfoundation.org/2002poll.html; retrieved May 14, 2002).

Nieman, D. C. 2002. How do I adapt current ACSM exercise prescription
guidelines for my obese clients? *ACSM Health and Fitness Journal,*
January/February.

Olson, M. D., and H. N. Williford. 1999. Martial arts exercise. *ACSM's
Health and Fitness Journal* 3(6): 6–14.

Pescatello, L. S., et al. 2004. American College of Sports Medicine Position
Stand: Exercise and hypertension. *Medicine and Science in Sports and
Exercise* 36(3): 533–553.

Satta, A. 2000. Exercise training in asthma. *Journal of Sports Medicine and
Physical Fitness* 40(4): 277–283.

Seguin, R., and M. E. Nelson. 2003. The benefits of strength training for
older adults. *American Journal of Preventive Medicine* 25(3 Suppl 2):
141–149.

Simonen, R. L., et al. 2003. Factors associated with exercise lifestyle—a
study of monozygotic twins. *International Journal of Sports Medicine*
24(7): 499–505.

Trost, S. G., et al. 2002. Correlates of adults' participation in physical
activity: Review and update. *Medicine and Science in Sports and Exercise*
34(12): 1996–2001.

Walters, P. H. 2000. Sleep facts. *ACSM's Health and Fitness Journal* 4(6):
17–19, 28.

World Health Organization/FAO Expert Consultation. 2003. *Diet, Nutrition
and the Prevention of Chronic Diseases.* WHO Technical Report Series 916.
Geneva: World Health Organization.

Sample programs based on four different types of cardiorespiratory activities—walking/jogging/running, bicycling, swimming, and in-line skating—are presented below. Each sample program includes regular cardiorespiratory endurance exercise, resistance training, and stretching. To choose a sample program, first compare your fitness goals with the benefits of the different types of endurance exercise featured in the sample programs (see Table 7.1). Identify the programs that meet your fitness needs. Next, read through the descriptions of the programs you're considering, and decide which will work best for you based on your present routine, the potential for enjoyment, and adaptability to your lifestyle. If you choose one of these programs, complete the personal fitness program plan in Lab 7.1, just as if you had created a program from scratch.

No program will produce enormous changes in your fitness level in the first few weeks. Give your program a good chance. Follow the specifics of the program for 3–4 weeks. Then if the exercise program doesn't seem suitable, make adjustments to adapt it to your particular needs. But retain the basic elements of the program that make it effective for developing fitness.

GENERAL GUIDELINES

The following guidelines can help make the activity programs more effective for you.

- *Frequency and time.* To experience training effects, you should exercise for 20–60 minutes at least three times a week.

- *Intensity.* To work effectively for cardiorespiratory endurance training or to improve body composition, you must raise your heart rate into its target zone. Monitor your pulse or use rates of perceived exertion to monitor your intensity.

  If you've been sedentary, begin very slowly. Give your muscles a chance to adjust to their increased workload. It's probably best to keep your heart rate below target until your body has had time to adjust to new demands. At first you may not need to work very hard to keep your heart rate in its target zone, but as your cardiorespiratory endurance improves, you will probably need to increase intensity.

- *Interval training.* Some of the sample programs involve continuous activity. Others rely on interval training, which calls for alternating a relief interval with exercise (walking after jogging, for example, or coasting after biking uphill). Interval training is an effective way to achieve progressive overload: When your heart rate gets too high, slow down to lower your pulse rate until you're at the low end of your target zone. Interval training can also prolong the total time you spend in exercise and delay the onset of fatigue.

- *Warm-up and cool-down.* Begin each exercise session with a 10-minute warm-up. Begin your activity at a slow pace and work up gradually to your target heart rate. Always slow down gradually at the end of your exercise session to bring your system back to its normal state. It's a good idea to do stretching exercises to increase your flexibility after cardiorespiratory exercise or strength training because your muscles will be warm and ready to stretch.

- *Record keeping.* After each exercise session, record your daily distance or time on a progress chart.

WALKING/JOGGING/RUNNING SAMPLE PROGRAM

Walking, jogging, and running are the most popular forms of training for people who want to improve cardiorespiratory endurance; they also improve body composition and muscular endurance of the legs. It's not always easy to distinguish among these three endurance activities. For clarity and consistency, we'll consider walking to be any on-foot exercise of less than 5 miles per hour, jogging any pace between 5 and 7.5 miles per hour, and running any pace faster than that. Table 1 divides walking, jogging, and running into nine categories, with rates of speed (in both miles per hour and minutes per mile) and calorie costs for each. The faster your pace or the longer you exercise, the more calories you burn. The greater the number of calories burned, the higher the potential training effects of these activities. Tables 2 and 3 contain sample walking/jogging programs by time and distance.

Equipment and Technique

These activities require no special skills, expensive equipment, or unusual facilities. Comfortable clothing, well-fitted walking or running shoes, and a stopwatch or ordinary watch with a second hand are all you need.

Developing Cardiorespiratory Endurance

The four variations of the basic walking/jogging/running sample program that follow are designed to help you regulate the intensity, duration, and frequency of your program. Use the following guidelines to choose the variation that is right for you.

- *Variation 1: Walking (Starting).* Choose this program if you have medical restrictions, are recovering from illness or surgery, tire easily after short walks, are obese, or have a sedentary lifestyle, and if you want to prepare for the advanced walking program to improve cardiorespiratory endurance, body composition, and muscular endurance.

- *Variation 2: Advanced Walking.* Choose this program if you already can walk comfortably for 30 minutes and if you want to develop and maintain cardiorespiratory fitness, a lean body, and muscular endurance.

- *Variation 3: Preparing for a Jogging Program.* Choose this program if you already can walk comfortably for 30 minutes and if you want to prepare for the jogging/running program to improve cardiorespiratory endurance, body composition, and muscular endurance.

SAMPLE PROGRAM TABLE 1   *Calorie Costs for Walking/Jogging/Running*

This table gives the calorie costs of walking, jogging, and running for slow, moderate, and fast paces. Calculations for calorie costs are approximate and assume a level terrain. A hilly terrain would result in higher calorie costs. To get an estimate of the number of calories you burn, multiply your weight by the calories per minute per pound for the speed at which you're doing the activity, and then multiply that by the number of minutes you exercise.

| | SPEED | | Calories per Minute per Pound |
Activity	Miles per Hour	Minutes: Seconds per Mile	
Walking			
Slow	2.0	30:00	.020
	2.5	24:00	.023
Moderate	3.0	20:00	.026
	3.5	17:08	.029
Fast	4.0	15:00	.037
	4.5	13:20	.048
Jogging			
Slow	5.0	12:00	.060
	5.5	11:00	.074
Moderate	6.0	10:00	.081
	6.5	9:00	.088
Fast	7.0	8:35	.092
	7.5	8:00	.099
Running			
Slow	8.5	7:00	.111
Moderate	9.0	6:40	.116
Fast	10.0	6:00	.129
	11.0	5:30	.141

SOURCE: Kusinitz, I., and M. Fine. 1983. From *Physical Fitness for Practically Everybody,* Consumer Reports, 1983. Copyright © 1996 by the Consumers Union of the United States, Inc., Yonkers, NY 10703-1057, a nonprofit organization. Reprinted with permission for educational purposes only. No commercial use or photo-copying permitted. To subscribe, call 1-800-234-1645 or visit us at www.ConsumerReports.org.

• *Variation 4: Jogging/Running.* Choose this program if you already can jog comfortably without muscular discomfort, if you already can jog for 15 minutes without stopping or 30 minutes with brief walking intervals within your target heart rate range, and if you want to develop and maintain a high level of cardiorespiratory fitness, a lean body, and muscular endurance.

Variation 1: Walking (Starting)

FIT—frequency, intensity, and time: Walk at first for 15 minutes at a pace that keeps your heart rate below your target zone. Gradually increase to 30-minute sessions. The distance you travel will probably be 1–2 miles. At the beginning, walk every

other day. You can gradually increase to daily walking if you want to burn more calories (helpful if you want to change body composition).

Calorie cost: Work up to using 90–135 calories in each session (see Table 1). To increase calorie costs to the target level, walk for a longer time or for a longer distance rather than sharply increasing speed.

At the beginning: Start at whatever level is most comfortable. Maintain a normal, easy pace, and stop to rest as often as you need to. Never prolong a walk past the point of comfort. When walking with a friend (a good motivation), let a comfortable conversation be your guide to pace.

As you progress: Once your muscles have become adjusted to the exercise program, increase the duration of your sessions—but by no more than 10% each week. Increase your intensity only enough to keep your heart rate just below your target. When you're able to walk 1.5 miles in 30 minutes, using 90–135 calories per session, you should consider moving on to variation 2 or 3. Don't be discouraged by lack of immediate progress and don't try to speed things up by overdoing. Remember that pace and heart rate can vary with the terrain, the weather, and other factors.

Variation 2: Advanced Walking

FIT—frequency, intensity, and time: Start at a pace at the lower end of your target heart rate zone and begin soon afterward to increase your pace. This might boost your heart rate into the upper levels of your target zone, which is fine for brief periods. But don't overdo the intervals of fast walking. Slow down after a short time to drop your pulse rate. Vary your pattern to allow for intervals of slow, medium, and fast walking. Walk at first for 30 minutes and gradually increase your walking time until eventually you reach 60 minutes, all the while maintaining your target heart rate. The distance you walk will probably be 2–4 miles. Walk at least every other day.

Calorie cost: Work up to using about 200–350 calories in each session (see Table 1).

At the beginning: Begin by walking somewhat faster than you did in Variation 1. Check your pulse to make sure you keep your heart rate within your target zone. Slow down when necessary to lower your heart rate when going up hills or when extending the duration of your walks.

As you progress: As your heart rate adjusts to the increased workload, gradually increase your pace and your total walking time. Gradually lengthen the periods of fast walking and shorten the relief intervals of slow walking, always maintaining target heart rate. Eventually, you will reach the fitness level you would like to maintain. And to maintain that level of fitness, continue to burn the same amount of calories in each session.

Vary your program by changing the pace and distance walked, or by walking routes with different terrains and views. Gauge your progress toward whatever calorie goal you've set by using Table 1.

Variation 3: Preparing for a Jogging Program

FIT—frequency, intensity, and time: Start by walking at a moderate pace (3–4 miles per hour or 15–20 minutes per mile).

SAMPLE PROGRAM TABLE 2 *Walking/Jogging Progression by Time*

This table is based on a walking interval of 3.75 miles per hour, measured in seconds, and a jogging interval of 5.5 miles per hour, measured in minutes:seconds. The combination of the two intervals equals a single set. In the Number of Sets column, the higher figure represents the maximum number of sets to be completed.

	Walk Interval (sec)	Jog Interval (min:sec)	Number of Sets	Total Distance (mi)	Total Time (min:sec)
Stage 1	:60	:30	10–15	1.0–1.7	15:00–22:30
Stage 2	:60	:60	8–13	1.2–2.0	16:00–26:00
Stage 3	:60	2:00	5–19	1.3–2.3	15:00–27:00
Stage 4	:60	3:00	5–7	1.6–2.4	16:00–28:00
Stage 5	:60	4:00	3–6	1.5–2.7	15:00–30:00

SOURCE: Kusinitz, I., and M. Fine. 1983. From *Physical Fitness for Practically Everybody*, Consumer Reports, 1983. Copyright © 1996 by the Consumers Union of the United States, Inc., Yonkers, NY 10703-1057, a nonprofit organization. Reprinted with permission for educational purposes only. No commercial use or photo-copying permitted. To subscribe, call 1-800-234-1645 or visit us at www.ConsumerReports.org.

SAMPLE PROGRAM TABLE 3 *Walking/Jogging Progression by Distance*

This table is based on a walking interval of 3.75 miles per hour, measured in yards, and a jogging interval of 5.5 miles per hour, also measured in yards. The combination of the two intervals equals a single set. (One lap around a typical track is 440 yards.)

	Walk Interval (yd)	Jog Interval (yd)	Number of Sets	Total Distance (mi)	Total Time (min:sec)
Stage 1	110	55	11–21	1.0–2.0	15:00–28:12
Stage 2	110	110	16	2.0	26:56
Stage 3	110	220	11	2.0	26:02
Stage 4	110	330	8	2.0	24:24
Stage 5	110	440	7	2.2	26:05
Stage 6	110	440	8	2.5	29:49

SOURCE: Kusinitz, I., and M. Fine. 1983. From *Physical Fitness for Practically Everybody*, Consumer Reports, 1983. Copyright © 1996 by the Consumers Union of the United States, Inc., Yonkers, NY 10703-1057, a nonprofit organization. Reprinted with permission for educational purposes only. No commercial use or photo-copying permitted. To subscribe, call 1-800-234-1645 or visit us at www.ConsumerReports.org.

Staying within your target heart rate zone, begin to add brief intervals of slow jogging (5–6 miles per hour or 10–12 minutes per mile). Keep the walking intervals constant at 60 seconds or at 110 yards, but gradually increase the jogging intervals until eventually you jog 4 minutes for each minute of walking. You'll probably cover between 1.5 and 2.5 miles. Each exercise session should last 15–30 minutes. Exercise every other day. If your goals include changing body composition and you want to exercise more frequently, walk on days you're not jogging.

Calorie cost: Work up to using 200–350 calories in each session (see Table 1).

At the beginning: Start slowly. Until your muscles adjust to jogging, you may need to exercise at less than your target heart rate. At the outset, expect to do two to four times as much walking as jogging, even more if you're relatively inexperienced. Be guided by how comfortable you feel—and by your heart rate—in setting the pace for your progress. Follow the guidelines presented in Chapter 3 for exercising in hot or cold weather. Drink enough liquids to stay adequately hydrated, particularly in hot weather. In addition, use the proper running technique, described below.

- Run with your back straight and your head up. Look straight ahead, not at your feet. Shift your pelvis forward and tuck your buttocks in.

- Hold your arms slightly away from your body. Your elbows should be bent so that your forearms are parallel to the ground. You may cup your hands, but do not clench your fists. Allow your arms to swing loosely and rhythmically with each stride.

- Your heel should hit the ground first in each stride. Then roll forward onto the ball of your foot and push off for the next stride. If you find this difficult, you can try a more flat-footed style, but don't land on the balls of your feet.

- Keep your steps short by allowing your foot to strike the ground in line with your knee. Keep your knees bent at all times.

- Breathe deeply through your mouth. Try to use your abdominal muscles rather than just your chest muscles to take deep breaths.
- Stay relaxed.

As you progress: Adjust your ratio of walking to jogging to keep within your target heart rate zone as much as possible. When you have progressed to the point where most of your 30-minute session is spent jogging, consider moving on to Variation 4. To find a walking/jogging progression that suits you, refer to Tables 2 and 3 (one uses time, the other distance). Which one you choose will depend, to some extent, on where you work out. If you have access to a track or can use a measured distance with easily visible landmarks to indicate yardage covered, you may find it convenient to use distance as your organizing principle. If you'll be using parks, streets, or woods, time intervals (measured with a watch) would probably work better. The progressions in Tables 2 and 3 are not meant to be rigid; they are guidelines to help you develop your own rate of progress. Let your progress be guided by your heart rate and increase your intensity and duration only to achieve your target zone.

Variation 4: Jogging/Running

FIT—frequency, intensity, and time: The key is to exercise within your target heart rate zone. Most people who sustain a continuous jog/run program will find that they can stay within their target heart rate zone with a speed of 5.5–7.5 miles per hour (8–11 minutes per mile). Start by jogging steadily for 15 minutes. Gradually increase your jog/run session to a regular 30–60 minutes (or about 2.5–7 miles). Exercise at least every other day. Increasing frequency by doing other activities on alternate days will place less stress on the weight-bearing parts of your lower body than will a daily program of jogging/running.

Calorie cost: Use about 300–750 calories in each session (see Table 1).

At the beginning: The greater number of calories you burn per minute makes this program less time-consuming for altering body composition than the three other variations in the walking/jogging/running program.

As you progress: If you choose this variation, you probably already have a moderate-to-high level of cardiorespiratory fitness. To stay within your target heart rate zone, increase your distance or both pace and distance as needed. Add variety to your workouts by varying your route, intensity, and duration. Alternate short runs with long ones. If you run for 60 minutes one day, try running for 30 minutes the next session. Or try doing sets that alternate hard and easy intervals—even walking, if you

feel like it. You can also try a road race now and then, but be careful not to do too much too soon.

Developing Muscular Strength and Endurance

Walking, jogging, and running provide muscular endurance workouts for your lower body; they also develop muscular strength of the lower body to a lesser degree. To develop muscular strength and endurance of the upper body, and to make greater and more rapid gains in lower-body strength, you need to include resistance training in your fitness program. Use the general wellness weight training program from Chapter 4, or tailor one to fit your personal fitness goals. If you'd like to increase your running speed and performance, you might want to focus your program on lower-body exercises. (Don't neglect upper-body strength, however; it is important for overall wellness.) Regardless of the strength training exercises you choose, follow the guidelines for successful training:

- Train 2–3 days per week.
- Perform 1 or more sets of 8–12 repetitions of 8–10 exercises.
- Include exercises that work all the major muscle groups: neck, shoulders, chest, arms, upper and lower back, abdomen, thighs, and calves.

Depending on the amount of time you are able to set aside for exercise, you may find it more convenient to alternate between your cardiorespiratory endurance workouts and your muscular strength and endurance workouts. In other words, walk or jog one day and strength train the next day.

Developing Flexibility

To round out your fitness program, you also need to include exercises that develop flexibility. The best time for a flexibility workout is when your muscles are warm, as they are immediately following cardiorespiratory endurance exercise or strength training. Perform the stretching routine presented in Chapter 5 or one that you have created to meet your own goals and preferences. Be sure to pay special attention to the hamstrings and quadriceps, which are not worked through their complete range of motion during walking or jogging. As you put your program together, remember the basic structure of a successful flexibility program:

- Stretch at least 2–3 days per week, preferably when muscles are warm.
- Stretch all the major muscle groups.
- Stretch to the point of mild discomfort and hold for 10–30 seconds.
- Repeat each stretch at least 4 times.

BICYCLING SAMPLE PROGRAM

Bicycling can also lead to large gains in physical fitness. For many people, cycling is a pleasant and economical alternative to driving and a convenient way to build fitness.

Equipment and Technique

Cycling has its own special array of equipment, including headgear, lighting, safety pennants, and special shoes. The bike is the most expensive item, ranging from about $100 to well over $1000. Avoid making a large investment until you're sure you'll

use your bike regularly. While investigating what the marketplace has to offer, rent or borrow a bike. Consider your intended use of the bike. Most cyclists who are interested primarily in fitness are best served by a sturdy 10-speed rather than a mountain bike or sport bike. Stationary cycles are good for rainy days and areas that have harsh winters.

Clothing for bike riding shouldn't be restrictive or binding, nor should it be so loose-fitting or so long that it might get caught in the chain. Clothing worn on the upper body should be comfortable but not so loose that it catches the wind and slows you down. Always wear a helmet to help prevent injury in case of a fall or crash. Wearing glasses or goggles can protect the eyes from dirt, small objects, and irritation from wind.

To avoid saddle soreness and injury, choose a soft or padded saddle and adjust it to a height that allows your legs to almost reach full extension while pedaling. Make certain the saddle doesn't put too much pressure on sensitive areas. Wear a pair of well-padded gloves if your hands tend to become numb while riding or if you begin to develop blisters or calluses. To prevent backache and neck strain, warm up thoroughly and periodically shift the position of your hands on the handlebars and your body in the saddle. Keep your arms relaxed and don't lock your elbows. To protect your knees from strain, pedal with your feet pointed straight ahead or very slightly inward and don't pedal in high gear for long periods.

Bike riding requires a number of precise skills that practice makes automatic. If you've never ridden before, consider taking a course. In fact, many courses are not just for beginners. They'll help you develop skills in braking, shifting, and handling emergencies, as well as teach you ways of caring for and repairing your bike. For safe cycling, follow these rules:

- Always wear a helmet.
- Keep on the correct side of the road. Bicycling against traffic is usually illegal and always dangerous.
- Obey all traffic signs and signals.
- On public roads, ride in single file, except in low-traffic areas (if the law permits). Ride in a straight line; don't swerve or weave in traffic.
- Be alert; anticipate the movements of other traffic and pedestrians. Listen for approaching traffic that is out of your line of vision.
- Slow down at street crossings. Check both ways before crossing.
- Use hand signals—the same as for automobile drivers—if you intend to stop or turn. Use audible signals to warn those in your path.
- Maintain full control. Avoid anything that interferes with your vision. Don't jeopardize your ability to steer by carrying anything (including people) on the handlebars.
- Keep your bicycle in good shape. Brakes, gears, saddle, wheels, and tires should always be in good condition.
- See and be seen. Use a headlight at night and equip your bike with rear reflectors. Use side reflectors on pedals, front and rear. Wear light-colored clothing or use reflective tape at night; wear bright colors or use fluorescent tape by day.
- Be courteous to other road users. Anticipate the worst and practice preventive cycling.
- Use a rear-view mirror.

Developing Cardiorespiratory Endurance

Cycling is an excellent way to develop and maintain cardiorespiratory endurance and a healthy body composition.

FIT—frequency, intensity, and time: If you've been inactive for a long time, begin your cycling program at a heart rate that is 10–20% below your target zone. Beginning cyclists should pedal at about 80–100 revolutions per minute; adjust the gear so that you can pedal at that rate easily. Your bicycle may display different types of useful information, including speed, distance traveled, heart rate, altitude, and revolutions per minute, and it may provide a cadence signal to help you maintain your pace. Once you feel at home on your bike, try 1 mile at a comfortable speed, and then stop and check your heart rate. Increase your speed gradually until you can cycle at 12–15 miles per hour (4–5 minutes per mile), a speed fast enough to bring most new cyclists' heart rate into their target zone. Allow your pulse rate to be your guide: More highly fit individuals may need to ride faster to achieve their target heart rate. Cycling for at least 20 minutes three times a week will improve your fitness.

Calorie cost: Use Table 4 to determine the number of calories you burn during each outing. You can increase the number of calories burned by cycling faster or for a longer time (it's usually better to increase distance rather than to add speed).

At the beginning: It may require several outings to get the muscles and joints of your legs and hips adjusted to this new activity. Begin each outing with a 10-minute warm-up that includes stretches for your hamstrings and your back and neck muscles. Until you become a skilled cyclist, select routes with the fewest hazards and avoid heavy automobile traffic.

As you progress: Interval training is also effective with bicycling. Simply increase your speed for periods of 4–8 minutes or for specific distances, such as 1–2 miles. Then coast for 2–3 minutes. Alternate the speed intervals and slow intervals for a total of 20–60 minutes, depending on your level of fitness. Hilly terrain is also a form of interval training.

Developing Muscular Strength and Endurance

Bicycling develops a high level of endurance and a moderate level of strength in the muscles of the lower body. To develop muscular strength and endurance of the upper body—and to make greater and more rapid gains in lower-body strength—you need to include resistance training as part of your fitness program. Use the general wellness weight training program from Chapter 4, or tailor one to fit your personal fitness goals. If one of your goals is to increase your cycling speed and performance, be sure to include exercises for the quadriceps, hamstrings, and buttocks muscles in your strength training program. No matter which exercises you include in your program, follow the general guidelines for successful and safe training:

- Train 2–3 days per week.
- Perform 1 or more sets of 8–12 repetitions of 8–10 exercises.
- Include exercises that work all the major muscle groups: neck, shoulders, chest, arms, upper and lower back, abdomen, things, and calves.

Depending on your schedule, you may find it more convenient to alternate between your cardiorespiratory endurance workouts and your muscular strength and endurance workouts. In other words, cycle one day and strength train the next day.

Developing Flexibility

A complete fitness program also includes exercises that develop flexibility. The best time for a flexibility workout is when your muscles are warm, as they are immediately following a session of cardiorespiratory endurance exercise or strength training. Perform the stretching routine presented in Chapter 5, or

This table gives the approximate calorie costs per pound of body weight for cycling from 5 to 60 minutes for distances of .50 mile up to 15 miles on a level terrain. To use the table, find on the horizontal line the time most closely approximating the number of minutes you cycle. Next, locate on the vertical column the approximate distance in miles you cover. The figure at the intersection represents an estimate of the calories used per minute per pound of body weight. Multiply this figure by your own body weight. Then multiply the product of these two figures by the number of minutes you cycle to get the total number of calories burned. For example, assuming you weigh 154 pounds and cycle 6 miles in 40 minutes, you would burn 260 calories: $154 \times .042$ (calories per pound, from table) $= 6.5 \times 40$ (minutes) $= 260$ calories burned.

Distance (mi)	TIME (MIN)											
	5	10	15	20	25	30	35	40	45	50	55	60
.50	.032											
1.00	.062	.032										
1.50		.042	.032									
2.00		.062	.039	.032								
3.00			.062	.042	.036	.032						
4.00				.062	.044	.039	.035	.032				
5.00				.097	.062	.045	.041	.037	.035	.032		
6.00					.088	.062	.047	.042	.039	.036	.034	.032
7.00						.081	.062	.049	.043	.040	.038	.036
8.00							.078	.062	.050	.044	.041	.039
9.00								.076	.062	.051	.045	.042
10.00								.097	.074	.062	.051	.045
11.00									.093	.073	.062	.052
12.00										.088	.072	.062
13.00											.084	.071
14.00												.081
15.00												.097

SOURCE: Kusinitz, I., and M. Fine. 1983. From *Physical Fitness for Practically Everybody,* Consumer Reports, 1983. Copyright © 1996 by the Consumers Union of the United States, Inc., Yonkers, NY 10703-1057, a nonprofit organization. Reprinted with permission for educational purposes only. No commercial use or photo-copying permitted. To subscribe, call 1-800-234-1645 or visit us at www.ConsumerReports.org.

develop one that meets your own goals and preferences. Pay special attention to the hamstrings and quadriceps, which are not worked through their complete range of motion during bike riding, and to the muscles in your lower back, shoulders, and neck. As you put your stretching program together, remember these basic guidelines:

• Stretch at least 2–3 days per week, preferably when muscles are warm.

• Stretch all the major muscle groups.

• Stretch to the point of mild discomfort and hold for 10–30 seconds.

• Repeat each stretch at least 4 times.

SWIMMING SAMPLE PROGRAM

Swimming is excellent for developing all-around fitness. Because water supports the body weight of the swimmer, swimming places less stress than weight-bearing activities on joints, ligaments, and tendons and tends to cause fewer injuries.

Equipment and Safety Guidelines

Aside from having access to a swimming pool, the only equipment required for a swimming program is a swimsuit and a pair of swimming goggles (that fit and do not leak) to protect the eyes from irritation in chlorinated pools. Following these few

simple rules can help keep you safe and healthy during your swimming sessions:

• Swim only in a pool with a qualified lifeguard on duty.

• Always walk carefully on wet surfaces.

• Dry your ears well after swimming. If you experience the symptoms of swimmer's ear (itching, discharge, or even a partial hearing loss), consult your physician. If you swim while recovering from swimmer's ear, protect your ears with a few drops of lanolin on a wad of lamb's wool.

- To avoid back pain, try not to arch your back excessively when you swim.
- Be courteous to others in the pool.

If you swim in a setting other than a pool with a lifeguard, remember the following important rules:

- Don't swim beyond your skill and endurance limits.
- Avoid being chilled: don't swim in water colder than 70°F.
- Never drink alcohol before going swimming.
- Never swim alone.

Developing Cardiorespiratory Endurance

Any one or any combination of common swimming strokes—front crawl stroke, breaststroke, backstroke, butterfly stroke, sidestroke, or elementary backstroke—can help develop and maintain cardiorespiratory fitness. (Swimming may not be as helpful as walking, jogging, or cycling for body fat loss.)

FIT—frequency, intensity, and time: Because swimming is not a weight-bearing activity and is not done in an upright position, it elicits a lower heart rate per minute. Therefore, you need to adjust your target heart rate zone. To calculate your target heart rate for swimming, use this formula:

Maximum swimming heart rate (MSHR) = 205 − age

Target heart rate zone = 65 − 90% of MSHR

For example, a 19-year-old would calculate her target heart rate zone for swimming as follows:

MSHR = 205 − 19 = 186 bpm

65% intensity: 0.65 × 186 = 121 bpm

90% intensity: 0.90 × 186 = 167 bpm

Base your duration of swimming on your intensity and target calorie costs. Swim at least three times a week.

Calorie cost: Calories burned while swimming are the result of the pace: how far you swim and how fast (see Table 5). Work up to using at least 300 calories per session.

At the beginning: If you are an inexperienced swimmer, invest the time and money for instruction. You'll make more rapid gains in fitness if you learn correct swimming technique. If you've been sedentary and haven't done any swimming for a long time, begin your program with 2–3 weeks, three times a week, of leisurely swimming at a pace that keeps your heart rate 10–20% below your target zone. Start swimming laps of the width of the pool if you can't swim the length. To keep your heart rate below target, take rest intervals as needed. Swim one lap, then rest 15–90 seconds as needed. Start with 10 minutes of swim/rest intervals and work up to 20 minutes. How long it takes will depend on your swimming skills and muscular fitness.

As you progress: Gradually increase the duration, or the intensity, or both duration and intensity of your swimming to raise your heart rate to a comfortable level within your target zone. Gradually increase your swimming intervals and decrease your rest intervals as you progress. Once you can swim the length of the pool at a pace that keeps your heart rate on target, continue swim/rest intervals for 20 minutes. Your rest intervals should be 30–45 seconds. You may find it helpful to get out of the pool during your rest intervals and walk until you've lowered your heart rate. Next, swim two laps of the pool length per swim

SAMPLE PROGRAM TABLE 5 *Calorie Costs for Swimming*

To use this table, find on the top horizontal row the distance in yards that most closely approximates the distance you swim. Next, locate on the appropriate vertical column (below the distance in yards) the time it takes you to swim the distance. Then locate in the first column on the left the approximate number of calories burned per minute per pound for the time and distance. To find the total number of calories burned, multiply your weight by the calories per minute per pound. Then multiply the product of these two numbers by the time it takes you to swim the distance (minutes: seconds). For example, assuming you weigh 130 pounds and swim 500 yards in 20 minutes, you would burn 106 calories: 130 × .041 (calories per pound, from table) = 5.33 × 20 (minutes) = 106 calories burned.

Calories per Minute per Pound	DISTANCE (YD)					
	25	100	150	250	500	750
.033	1:15	5:00	7:30	12:30	25:00	30:30
.041	1:00	4:00	6:00	10:00	20:00	30:00
.049	0:50	3:20	5:00	8:20	18:40	25:00
.057	0:43	2:52	4:18	7:10	17:20	21:30
.065	0:37.5	2:30	3:45	6:15	10:00	
.073	0:33	2:13	3:20	5:30	8:50	
.081	0:30	2:00	3:00	5:00	8:00	
.090	0:27	1:48	2:42	4:30	7:12	
.097	0:25	1:40	2:30	4:10	6:30	

SOURCE: Kusinitz, I., and M. Fine. 1983. From *Physical Fitness for Practically Everybody,* Consumer Reports, 1983. Copyright © 1996 by the Consumers Union of the United States, Inc., Yonkers, NY 10703-1057, a nonprofit organization. Reprinted with permission for educational purposes only. No commercial use or photo-copying permitted. To subscribe, call 1-800-234-1645 or visit us at www.ConsumerReports.org.

interval and continue swim/rest intervals for 30 minutes. For the 30-second rest interval, walk (or rest) until you've lowered your heart rate. Gradually increase the number of laps you swim consecutively and the total duration of your session until you reach your target calorie expenditure and fitness level. But take care not to swim at too fast a pace: It can raise your heart rate too high and limit your ability to sustain your swimming. Alternating strokes can rest your muscles and help prolong your swimming time. A variety of strokes will also let you work more muscle groups. You can also vary your program by incorporating kick boards, pull-buoys, hand paddles, or fins into some of your workouts.

Developing Muscular Strength and Endurance

The swimming program outlined in this section will result in moderate gains in strength and large gains in endurance in the muscles used during the strokes you've chosen. To develop strength and endurance in all the muscles of the body, you need to include resistance training as part of your fitness program. Use the general wellness weight training program from Chapter 4, or tailor one to fit your personal fitness goals. To improve your swimming performance, include exercises that work key muscles. For example, if you swim primarily front crawl, include exercises to increase strength in your shoulders, arms, and upper back. (Training the muscles you use during swimming can also help prevent injuries.) Regardless of which strength training exercise you include in your program, follow the general guidelines for successful training:

- Train 2–3 days per week.
- Perform 1 or more sets of 8–12 repetitions of 8–10 exercises.
- Include exercises that work all the major muscle groups: neck, shoulders, chest, arms, upper and lower back, abdomen, thighs, and calves.

Depending on the amount of time you have for exercise, you might want to schedule your cardiorespiratory endurance workouts and your muscular strength and endurance workouts on alternate days. In other words, swim one day and strength train the next day.

Developing Flexibility

For a complete fitness program, you also need to include exercises that develop flexibility. The best time for a flexibility workout is when your muscles are warm, as they are immediately following cardiorespiratory endurance exercise or strength training. Perform the stretching routine presented in Chapter 5 or one you have created to meet your own goals and preferences. Be sure to pay special attention to the muscles you use during swimming, particularly the shoulders and back. As you put your program together, remember the basic structure of a successful flexibility program:

- Stretch at least 2–3 days per week, preferably when muscles are warm.
- Stretch all the major muscle groups.
- Stretch to the point of mild discomfort and hold for 10–30 seconds.
- Repeat each stretch at least 4 times.

IN-LINE SKATING SAMPLE PROGRAM

In-line skating is convenient and inexpensive (after the initial outlay for equipment); it can be done on city streets, on paved bike paths and trails, and in parks. If done intensively enough, skating can provide a cardiorespiratory endurance workout comparable to the workouts provided by jogging and cycling. Studies indicate that skating consumes about as many calories as jogging. An advantage of skating over jogging is that skating is low impact, so it is less harmful to the knees and ankles. An advantage of skating over bicycling is that it works the hamstring muscle in the back of the thigh. Skating develops lower-body strength and endurance, working all the muscles of the leg and hip and strengthening the muscles and connective tissues surrounding the ankles, knees, and hips.

Equipment

To skate safely and enjoyably, you will need a pair of comfortable, sturdy, quality skates and adequate safety equipment. The skate consists of a hard polyurethane shell or outer boot; a padded foam liner; and a frame or chassis that holds the wheels, bearings, spacers, and brake. If you want to try out the sport before making a commitment, rent your skates and equipment from a skate shop. If you are buying, plan to spend about $110–$200 for skates that meet the basic needs of most recreational skaters. Shop for the best combination of price, quality, comfort, and service.

Essential safety equipment includes a helmet, elbow pads, knee pads, and wrist guards. (Wrist injuries are the most common in-line skating injury.) You may want to put reflective tape on your skates for those occasions when you don't get home before dark. Carry moleskin or adhesive bandages with you in case you start to develop a blister while skating. (For more on safety, see Appendix A.)

Technique

In-line skating uses many of the skills and techniques of ice skating, roller skating, and skiing, so if you have ever participated in any of those activities, you will probably take to in-line skating fairly readily. Many people begin without instruction, but instruction will allow you to progress more quickly.

To begin, center your weight equally over both skates, bend your knees slightly so your nose, knees, and toes are all in the same line, and look straight ahead. Keep your weight forward over the balls of your feet; don't lean back.

To skate, use a stroke, glide, stroke, glide rhythm (rather than a series of quick, short strokes). Push with one leg while gliding with the other. Shift your body weight back and forth so it is always centered over the gliding skate.

To stop, use your brake, located on the back of the right skate in most skates. With knees bent and arms extended in front of your body, move the right foot forward, shift your weight to your left leg, and lift your right toe until the brake pad touches the ground and stops you. An alternative stop is the T-stop, in which you drag one skate behind the other at a 90-degree angle to the direction of your forward motion.

If you lose your balance and are about to fall, lower your center of gravity by bending at the waist and putting your hands on your knees. If you can't regain your balance, try to fall forward, directing the impact to your wrist guards and knee pads. Try not to fall backward.

Again, instruction can help you learn many moves and techniques that will make the sport safer and more enjoyable.

Developing Cardiorespiratory Endurance

Studies have shown that in-line skaters raise their heart rates and oxygen consumption comparably to joggers, bicyclers, and walkers. Skaters reached 60–75% of $\dot{V}O_{2max}$ by skating continuously (not pushing off and gliding for several seconds) at 10.6–12.5 mph for 20–30 minutes. It may be difficult for recreational skaters to safely skate this fast for this long, however, given the typical constraints of city and suburban streets. Experts suggest skating uphill as much as possible to reach the level of intensity that builds cardiorespiratory endurance. If you can reach and maintain higher speeds in parks or on paved paths, do so, but always skate safely.

FIT—frequency, intensity, and time: Start your early skating sessions at a pace that keeps your heart rate about 10–20% below your target zone. Skate for 5–10 minutes, and then check your heart rate. Increase your speed gradually until you can skate at about 10 miles per hour (6 minutes per mile). Use your pulse as a guide to speed, aiming for 65% of your target heart rate zone. To achieve cardiorespiratory benefits, you will have to skate at a continuous and relatively intense pace for at least 20 minutes three times a week. The more fit you are, the more intensively you will need to skate to reach your target heart rate.

Calorie cost: Use Table 6 to determine the approximate number of calories you burn during each outing. You can increase the number of calories burned by skating faster, for a longer time, or uphill.

At the beginning: If you are a beginner, practice skating in an empty schoolyard or a parking lot. As you become confident with the basic techniques, you can move on to streets, parks, and paved bike trails. Maintain an easy pace, alternating stroking and gliding.

Begin each outing with a 5- to 10-minute warm-up of walking, jogging, or even slow skating. Once your muscles are warm, you can do some stretches to help loosen and warm up the primary muscles used during skating. These muscles include the quadriceps, hamstrings, buttocks, hips, groin, ankles, calves, and lower back. You can also save the stretches for the end of the workout.

To launch an in-line skating fitness program, aim for slow, long-distance workouts at first. Start by skating for 15 minutes and gradually increase your sessions to 20–30 minutes of continuous skating (about 3.5–5 miles). Try to skate about 20 miles a week, or 5 miles a day (about 30 minutes) 4 days a week.

As you progress: After the first week or two, add about a mile a day, up to 40 miles per week (60 minutes a day). To increase intensity, add some hills, sprints (bursts of short, rapid striding), and interval training (periods of intensive exercise at your target heart rate alternating with timed rest periods when your heart rate drops below your target zone). Try to skate 30–60 minutes a day four or more times a week.

The harder and faster you skate, the more intensive your workout will be and the more your cardiorespiratory endurance and muscular strength will improve. The longer and more often you skate, the more your endurance will increase.

Developing Muscular Strength and Endurance

In-line skating develops the muscles in the entire upper leg, buttocks, and hip; lower back; and upper arms and shoulders when arms are swung vigorously. To make greater gains in lower-body strength and to develop the entire upper body, include resistance training in your overall fitness program. Use the general wellness weight training program from Chapter 4, or tailor one to fit your personal fitness goals. No matter which exercises you include in your program, follow the general guidelines for successful and safe training:

- Train 2–3 days per week.
- Perform 1 or more sets of 8–12 repetitions of 8–10 exercises.
- Include exercises that work all the major muscle groups: neck, shoulders, chest, arms, upper and lower back, thighs, and calves.

Depending on your schedule, you may find it more convenient to skate and strength train on alternate days.

Developing Flexibility

The best times for a flexibility workout are when your muscles are warm, so stretch after a short warm-up at the beginning of your skating session, or after your skating session, or after a weight training session. Use the stretching routine presented in Chapter 5, or develop one that meets your own goals and preferences. Pay particular attention to your quadriceps, hamstrings, buttocks, hips, groin, ankles, calves, and lower back. Remember these basic guidelines:

- Stretch at least 2–3 days per week, preferably when muscles are warm.
- Stretch all the major muscle groups.
- Stretch to the point of mild discomfort and hold for 10–30 seconds.
- Repeat each stretch at least 4 times.

Name _____ **Section** _____ **Date** _____

LAB 7.1 *A Personal Fitness Program Plan and Contract*

A. I, _____ , am contracting with myself to follow a physical fitness pro-
　　　　　　(name)

gram to work toward the following goals:

Specific or short-term goals (include current status for each)

1. _____

2. _____

3. _____

4. _____

General or long-term goals

1. _____

2. _____

3. _____

4. _____

B. My program plan is as follows:

Activities	Components (Check ✓)					Frequency (Check ✓)							Intensity*	Time (duration)
	CRE	MS	ME	F	BC	M	Tu	W	Th	F	Sa	Su		

*Conduct activities for achieving CRE goals in your target range for heart rate or RPE.

C. My program will begin on _____ . My program includes the following schedule of mini-goals. For each step
　　　　　　　　　　　　(date)

in my program, I will give myself the reward listed.

_____ _____ _____
(mini-goal 1)　　　　　　　　　(date)　　　　　　(reward)

_____ _____ _____
(mini-goal 2)　　　　　　　　　(date)　　　　　　(reward)

_____ _____ _____
(mini-goal 3)　　　　　　　　　(date)　　　　　　(reward)

_____ _____ _____
(mini-goal 4)　　　　　　　　　(date)　　　　　　(reward)

_____ _____ _____
(mini-goal 5)　　　　　　　　　(date)　　　　　　(reward)

D. My program will include the addition of physical activity to my daily routine (such as climbing stairs or walking to class):

1. _____

2. _____

3. _____

4. _____

5. _____

E. I will use the following tools to monitor my program and my progress toward my goals:

_____

(list any charts, graphs, or journals you plan to use)

_____

_____

I sign this contract as an indication of my personal commitment to reach my goal.

_____   _____

(your signature)   (date)

I have recruited a helper who will witness my contract and _____

_____

(list any way your helper will participate in your program)

_____

_____   _____

(witness's signature)   (date)

Name _____ **Section** _____ **Date** _____

LAB 7.2 *Getting to Know Your Fitness Facility*   **WW**

To help create a successful training program, take time out to learn more about the fitness facility you plan to use.

Basic Information

Name and location of facility: _____

Hours of operation: _____

Times available for general use: _____

Times most convenient for your schedule: _____

Can you obtain an initial session or consultation with a trainer to help you create a program? _____ yes _____ no

If so, what does the initial planning session involve? _____
_____

Are any of the staff certified? Do any have special training? If yes, list/describe: _____
_____

What types of equipment are available for the development of cardiorespiratory endurance? Briefly list/describe:
_____
_____
_____

Are any group activities or classes available? If so, briefly describe: _____
_____
_____

What types of weight training equipment are available for use? _____
_____

Yes   No

___ ___ Is there a fee for using the facility? If so, how much? $ _____

___ ___ Is a student ID required for access to the facility?

___ ___ Do you need to sign up in advance to use the facility or any of the equipment?

___ ___ Is there typically a line or wait to use the equipment during the times you use the facility?

___ ___ Is there a separate area with mats for stretching and/or cool-down?

___ ___ Do you need to bring your own towel?

___ ___ Are lockers available? If so, do you need to bring your own lock? _____ yes _____ no

___ ___ Are showers available? If so, do you need to bring your own soap and shampoo? _____ yes _____ no

___ ___ Is drinking water available? (If not, be sure to bring your own bottle of water.)

Describe any other amenities, such as vending machines or saunas, that are available at the facility.
_____
_____

Information About Equipment

Fill in the specific equipment and exercise(s) that you can use to develop cardiorespiratory endurance and each of the major muscle groups. For cardiorespiratory endurance, list the type(s) of equipment and a sample starting workout: frequency, intensity, time, and other pertinent information (such as a setting for resistance or speed). For muscular strength and endurance, list the equipment, exercises, and finally indicate the order in which you'll complete them during a workout session (see p. 96 for suggestions on order of weight training exercises).

Cardiorespiratory Endurance Equipment

Equipment	Sample Starting Workout

Muscular Strength and Endurance Equipment

Order	Muscle Groups	Equipment	Exercises(s)
	Neck		
	Chest		
	Shoulders		
	Upper back		
	Front of arms		
	Back of arms		
	Buttocks		
	Abdomen		
	Lower back		
	Front of thighs		
	Back of thighs		
	Calves		
	Other:		
	Other:		

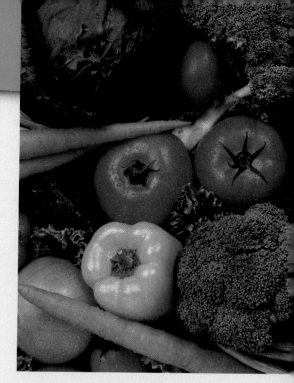

8

Nutrition

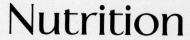

LOOKING AHEAD

After reading this chapter, you should be able to

- List the essential nutrients and describe the functions they perform in the body
- Describe the guidelines that have been developed to help people choose a healthy diet, avoid nutritional deficiencies, and protect themselves from diet-related chronic diseases
- Discuss nutritional guidelines for vegetarians and for special population groups
- Explain how to use food labels and other consumer tools to make informed choices about foods
- Put together a personal nutrition plan based on affordable foods that you enjoy and that will promote wellness, today and in the future

TEST YOUR KNOWLEDGE

1. Three ounces of chicken or meat, the amount considered to be one serving, is approximately the size of which of the following?
   a. a domino
   b. a deck of cards
   c. a small paperback book

2. Candy is the leading source of added sugars in the American diet.
   True or false?

3. Which of the following is NOT a whole grain?
   a. brown rice
   b. wheat flour
   c. popcorn

ANSWERS

1. **B.** Many people underestimate the size of the servings they eat, leading to overconsumption of calories and fat.

2. **FALSE.** Regular (nondiet) sodas are the leading source, with an average of 54 gallons consumed per person per year. Each 12-ounce soda supplies about 10 teaspoons of sugar, the total recommended daily limit for a 2000-calorie diet.

3. **B.** Unless labeled "whole wheat," wheat flour is processed to remove the bran and germ and is not a whole grain.

Fit and Well Online Learning Center   www.mhhe.com/fahey

Visit the *Fit and Well* Online Learning Center for study aids, online labs, additional information about nutrition, links, Internet activities that explore the role of nutrition in wellness, and much more.

In your lifetime, you'll spend about 6 years eating—about 70,000 meals and 60 tons of food. What you eat affects your energy level, well-being, and overall health (see the box "Eating Habits and Total Wellness"). Of particular concern is the connection between lifetime nutritional habits and risk of the major chronic diseases, including heart disease, cancer, stroke, and diabetes. Choosing foods that provide adequate amounts of the nutrients you need while limiting the substances linked to disease should be an important part of your daily life. The food choices you make will significantly influence your health—both now and in the future.

Creating a diet plan to support maximum fitness and protect against disease is a two-part project. First, you have to know which nutrients are necessary and in what amounts. Second, you have to translate those requirements into a diet consisting of foods you like to eat that are both available and affordable. Once you have an idea of what constitutes a healthy diet for you, you may also have to make adjustments in your current diet to bring it into line with your goals.

This chapter provides the basic principles of **nutrition**. It introduces the six classes of essential nutrients, explaining their role in the functioning of the body. It also provides different sets of guidelines that you can use to design a healthy diet plan. Finally, it offers practical tools and advice to help you apply the guidelines to your own life. Diet is an area of your life in which you have almost total control. Using your knowledge and understanding of nutrition to create a healthy diet plan is a significant step toward wellness.

NUTRITIONAL REQUIREMENTS: COMPONENTS OF A HEALTHY DIET

When you think about your diet, you probably do so in terms of the foods you like to eat—a turkey sandwich and a glass of milk, or a steak and a baked potato. What's important for your health, though, are the nutrients contained in those foods. Your body requires proteins, fats, carbohydrates, vitamins, minerals, and water—about 45

Terms

ViW

nutrition The science of food and how the body uses it in health and disease.

essential nutrients Substances the body must get from food because it cannot manufacture them at all or fast enough to meet its needs. These nutrients include proteins, fats, carbohydrates, vitamins, minerals, and water.

digestion The process of breaking down foods in the gastrointestinal tract into compounds the body can absorb.

macronutrients Essential nutrients required by the body in relatively large amounts.

micronutrients Essential nutrients required by the body in minute amounts.

kilocalorie A measure of energy content in food; 1 kilocalorie represents the amount of heat needed to raise the temperature of 1 liter of water 1°C; commonly referred to as *calorie*.

MOTIVATION FOR CHANGE! A nutrition journal can be a very useful tool for evaluating and improving your diet. The very act of recording everything you eat may improve your dietary habits—you'll find yourself thinking before you eat and avoiding some unhealthy choices so that you don't have to record them in your journal. A nutrition journal can significantly boost your awareness of both your food choices and your portion sizes. Keeping a journal also demonstrates and reinforces your commitment, and it can help you maintain your motivation to change your behavior during a dietary improvement program.

essential nutrients. The word *essential* in this context means that you must get these substances from food because your body is unable to manufacture them at all, or at least not fast enough to meet your physiological needs. The six classes of nutrients, along with their functions and major sources, are listed in Table 8.1.

Nutrients are released into the body by the process of **digestion,** which breaks them down into compounds that the gastrointestinal tract can absorb and the body can use (Figure 8.1, p. 220). A diet containing adequate amounts of all essential nutrients is vital because various nutrients provide energy, build and maintain body tissues, and regulate body functions. Some essential nutrients are needed by the body in relatively large amounts. These **macronutrients** include protein, fat, and carbohydrate. **Micronutrients,** such as vitamins and minerals, are required in much smaller amounts.

The energy in foods is expressed as **kilocalories.** One kilocalorie represents the amount of heat it takes to raise the temperature of 1 liter of water 1°C. A person needs about 2000 kilocalories a day to meet energy needs. In common usage, people usually refer to kilocalories as *calories,* which is a much smaller energy unit: 1 kilocalorie contains 1000 calories. We'll use the familiar word *calorie* in this chapter to stand for the larger energy unit; you'll also find the word *calorie* used on food labels.

Of the six classes of essential nutrients, three supply energy:

- Fat = 9 calories per gram
- Protein = 4 calories per gram
- Carbohydrate = 4 calories per gram

(Alcohol, although it is not an essential nutrient, also supplies energy, providing 7 calories per gram.) The high caloric content of fat is one reason experts often advise against high fat consumption; most of us do not need the extra calories to meet energy needs. Calories consumed in excess of energy needs are converted to fat and stored in the body.

But just meeting energy needs is not enough; our bodies need adequate amounts of all the essential nutrients to grow and function properly. Practically all foods contain mixtures of nutrients, although foods are commonly

Healthy eating does more than nourish your body—it enhances your ability to enjoy life to the fullest by improving overall wellness, both physical and mental. A recent study examined a group of adults who followed a healthy eating plan for four years. At the end of this period, the study subjects were more confident with their food choices and more satisfied with their lives in general than their peers who did not make any dietary changes. The reverse is also true—when people overeat they often have feelings of guilt, anger, discouragement, and even self-loathing. Out-of-control eating can erode self-confidence and lead to depression. How we eat is a reflection of how we feel about ourselves. Enjoying food and eating well is a major part of a healthy and happy life.

Can individual foods affect the way we feel? Limited scientific evidence points to some correlation between certain foods and one's mood. Many people, especially women, seem to crave chocolate when they are "blue." Studies show that chocolate, in small quantities, may indeed give you a lift. Sugary foods tend to temporarily raise serotonin levels in the brain, which can improve mood (serotonin is a neurotransmitter associated with a calm, relaxed state). The fat found in chocolate acts to increase endorphins, brain chemicals that reduce pain and increase feelings of well-being. Chocolate also contains caffeine, theobromine, phenylethylamine, and a variety of other less studied chemicals that may have a positive impact on mood.

A commonly held belief about the connection between food and the mind is that eating sugary foods makes people (especially children) hyperactive. Parents often comment on the wild behavior observed at parties and festive events where lots of sweets are consumed. However, several carefully controlled studies showed no correlation between behavior and the consumption of sugary foods. Researchers speculate that high-sugar foods tend to be eaten at birthday parties and other exciting occasions when children tend to be highly stimulated regardless of what they eat.

Some recent research shows that eating certain carbohydrate-rich foods, such as a plain baked potato or a bagel with jelly, can have a temporary calming effect. Scientists postulate that this occurs because carbohydrates stimulate insulin release, which improves the transport of the amino acid tryptophan (the major building block for serotonin) into the brain. This effect is most pronounced when rapidly digestible carbohydrates are consumed alone, with no fats or protein in the meal. The practical implications of this research are uncertain.

If you are looking for a mental boost, some scientists think that eating a meal consisting primarily of protein-rich foods may be helpful. The theory is that proteins contain the amino acid tyrosine, which is used by the body to manufacture the neurotransmitters dopamine and norepinephrine. Some researchers postulate that eating protein-containing foods could increase the synthesis of these neurotransmitters, which can speed reaction time and increase alertness. Whether this really works, especially in well-nourished individuals who have not been lacking these nutrients to begin with, remains to be seen. In the meantime, it wouldn't hurt, and might even help, to include some protein in the meal you eat prior to your next big exam.

What we know about how food affects mood remains limited. But evidence points to the commonsense conclusion that enjoying reasonable portions of a variety of healthy and tasty foods is a great way to optimize your physical and mental health.

Table 8.1	The Six Classes of Essential Nutrients	
Nutrient	**Function**	**Major Sources**
Proteins (4 calories/gram)	Form important parts of muscles, bone, blood, enzymes, some hormones, and cell membranes; repair tissue; regulate water and acid-base balance; help in growth; supply energy	Meat, fish, poultry, eggs, milk products, legumes, nuts
Carbohydrates (4 calories/gram)	Supply energy to cells in brain, nervous system, and blood; supply energy to muscles during exercise	Grains (breads and cereals), fruits, vegetables, milk
Fats (9 calories/gram)	Supply energy; insulate, support, and cushion organs; provide medium for absorption of fat-soluble vitamins	Animal foods, grains, nuts, seeds, fish, vegetables
Vitamins	Promote (initiate or speed up) specific chemical reactions within cells	Abundant in fruits, vegetables, and grains; also found in meat and dairy products
Minerals	Help regulate body functions; aid in the growth and maintenance of body tissues; act as catalysts for the release of energy	Found in most food groups
Water	Makes up 50–70% of body weight; provides a medium for chemical reactions; transports chemicals; regulates temperature; removes waste products	Fruits, vegetables, and liquids

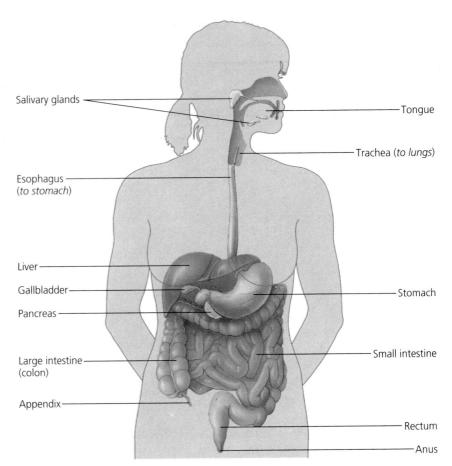

Figure 8.1 The digestive system. Food is partially broken down by being chewed and mixed with saliva in the mouth. As food moves through the digestive tract, it is mixed by muscular contractions and broken down by chemicals. After traveling to the stomach via the esophagus, food is broken down further by stomach acids. Most absorption of nutrients occurs in the small intestine, aided by secretions from the pancreas, gallbladder, and intestinal lining. The large intestine reabsorbs excess water; the remaining solid wastes are collected in the rectum and excreted through the anus.

classified according to their predominant nutrients. For example, spaghetti is considered a carbohydrate food although it contains small amounts of other nutrients. Let's take a closer look at the functions and sources of the six classes of nutrients.

Proteins—The Basis of Body Structure

Proteins form important parts of the body's main structural components: muscles and bones. Proteins also form important parts of blood, enzymes, cell membranes, and some hormones. As mentioned above, protein can also provide energy at 4 calories per gram of protein weight.

Amino Acids   The building blocks of proteins are called **amino acids.** Twenty common amino acids are found in food; nine of these are essential: histidine, isoleucine, leucine, lysine, methionine, phenylalanine, threonine, tryptophan, and valine. The other eleven amino acids can be produced by the body as long as the necessary components are supplied by foods.

Complete and Incomplete Proteins   Individual protein sources are considered "complete" if they supply all the essential amino acids in adequate amounts and "incomplete" if they do not. Meat, fish, poultry, eggs, milk, cheese, and soy provide complete proteins. Incomplete proteins, which come from plant sources such as **legumes** and

nuts, are good sources of most essential amino acids, but are usually low in one or two.

Combining two vegetable proteins, such as wheat and peanuts in a peanut butter sandwich, allows each vegetable protein to make up for the amino acids missing in the other protein. The combination yields a complete protein. Your concern with amino acids and complete protein in your diet should focus on what you consume throughout the day, rather than at each meal. It was once believed that vegetarians had to "complement" their proteins at each meal in order to receive the benefit of a complete protein. It is now known, however, that proteins consumed throughout the course of the day can complement each other to form a pool of amino acids from which the body can draw to produce the necessary proteins. (Healthy vegetarian diets are discussed later in the chapter.)

Recommended Protein Intake   In the most recent set of research-based recommendations, the Food and Nutrition Board of the Institute of Medicine defined adequate daily intake of protein for adults as 0.8 gram per kilogram (0.36 gram per pound) of body weight, or about 56 grams of protein per day for men and 46 grams of protein per day for women. This amount of protein is easily obtained from popular foods: 3 ounces of lean meat, poultry, or fish or ½ cup of tofu contains about 20–25 grams of protein; 1 cup of legumes such as pinto and kidney beans, 15–20 grams; 1 cup of milk or yogurt or

1½ ounces of cheese, 8–12 grams; and cereals, grains, nuts, and vegetables, about 2–4 grams of protein per serving.

Most Americans meet or exceed the protein intake needed for adequate nutrition. Protein consumed beyond what the body needs is synthesized into fat for energy storage or burned for energy requirements. Consuming somewhat above our needs is not harmful, but it does contribute fat to the diet because protein-rich foods are often fat-rich as well. A very high protein intake can strain the kidneys and lead to dehydration. A fairly broad range of protein intake is associated with good health, and the Food and Nutrition Board recommends that the amount adults eat should fall within the range of 10–35% of the total daily calorie intake. The average American diet includes about 15–16% of total daily calories as protein. (See Chapter 9 for more information about high-protein diets advocated for weight loss.)

Fats—Essential in Small Amounts

Fats, also known as lipids, are the most concentrated source of energy, at 9 calories per gram. The fats stored in your body represent usable energy, help insulate your body, and support and cushion your organs. Fats in the diet help your body absorb fat-soluble vitamins and add important flavor and texture to foods. Fats are the major fuel for the body during periods of rest and light activity. Two fats—linoleic acid and alpha-linolenic acid—are essential to the diet; they are key regulators of such body functions as the maintenance of blood pressure and the progress of a healthy pregnancy.

Types and Sources of Fats   Most of the fats in food are in the form of triglycerides, which are composed of a glycerine molecule (an alcohol) plus three fatty acids. A fatty acid is made up of a chain of carbon atoms with oxygen attached at the end and hydrogen atoms attached along the length of the chain. Fatty acids differ in the length of their carbon atom chains and in their degree of saturation (the number of hydrogens attached to the chain). If every available bond from each carbon atom in a fatty acid chain is attached to a hydrogen atom, the fatty acid is said to be **saturated** (Figure 8.2). If not all the available bonds are taken up by hydrogens, the carbon atoms in the chain will form double bonds with each other. Such fatty acids are called unsaturated fats. If there is only one double bond, the fatty acid is called **monounsaturated.** If there are two or more double bonds, the fatty acid is called **polyunsaturated.** The essential fatty acids, linoleic and alpha-linolenic acids, are both polyunsaturated. The different types of fatty acids have different characteristics and different effects on your health.

Food fats are often composed of both saturated and unsaturated fatty acids; the dominant type of fatty acid determines the fat's characteristics. Food fats containing large amounts of saturated fatty acids are usually solid at room temperature; they are generally found naturally in animal products. The leading sources of saturated fat in

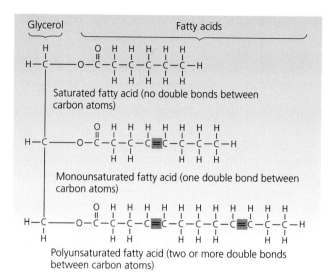

Figure 8.2   Chemical structures of saturated and unsaturated fatty acids.   This example of a triglyceride consists of a molecule of glycerol with three fatty acids attached. Fatty acids can differ in the length of their carbon chains and their degree of saturation.

the American diet are red meats (hamburger, steak, roasts), whole milk, cheese, and hot dogs and lunch meats. Food fats containing large amounts of monounsaturated and polyunsaturated fatty acids are usually from plant sources and are liquid at room temperature. Olive, canola, safflower, and peanut oils contain mostly monounsaturated fatty acids. Corn, soybean, and cottonseed oils contain mostly polyunsaturated fatty acids.

There are notable exceptions to these generalizations. When unsaturated vegetable oils undergo the process of **hydrogenation,** a mixture of saturated and unsaturated fatty acids is produced. Hydrogenation turns many of the double bonds in unsaturated fatty acids into single bonds, increasing the degree of saturation and producing a more solid fat from a liquid oil. Hydrogenation also changes

protein An essential nutrient; a compound made of amino acids that contains carbon, hydrogen, oxygen, and nitrogen.

amino acids The building blocks of proteins.

legumes Vegetables such as peas and beans that are high in fiber and are also important sources of protein.

saturated fat A fat with no carbon-carbon double bonds; usually solid at room temperature.

monounsaturated fat A fat with one carbon-carbon double bond; liquid at room temperature.

polyunsaturated fat A fat containing two or more carbon-carbon double bonds; liquid at room temperature.

hydrogenation A process by which hydrogens are added to unsaturated fats, increasing the degree of saturation and turning liquid oils into solid fats. Hydrogenation produces a mixture of saturated fatty acids and standard and trans forms of unsaturated fatty acids.

Terms

some unsaturated fatty acids into **trans fatty acids,** unsaturated fatty acids with an atypical shape that affects their behavior in the body. Food manufacturers use hydrogenation to increase the stability of an oil so it can be reused for deep frying; to improve the texture of certain foods (to make pastries and pie crusts flakier, for example); and to extend the shelf life of foods made with oil. Hydrogenation is also used to transform liquid vegetable oils into margarine or shortening.

Many baked and fried foods are prepared with hydrogenated vegetable oils, so they can be relatively high in saturated and trans fatty acids. Leading sources of trans fats in the American diet are deep-fried fast foods such as french fries and fried chicken (typically fried in vegetable shortening rather than oil); baked and snack foods such as pot pies, cakes, cookies, pastries, doughnuts, and chips; and stick margarine. In general, the more solid a hydrogenated oil is, the more saturated and trans fats it contains; for example, stick margarines typically contain more saturated and trans fats than do tub or squeeze margarines. Small amounts of trans fatty acids are also found naturally in meat and milk.

Hydrogenated vegetable oils are not the only plant fats that contain saturated fats. Palm and coconut oils, although derived from plants, are also highly saturated. Yet fish oils, derived from an animal source, are rich in polyunsaturated fats.

Fats and Health   Different types of fats have very different effects on health. Many studies have examined the effects of dietary fat intake on blood **cholesterol** levels and the risk of heart disease. Saturated and trans fatty acids raise blood levels of **low-density lipoprotein (LDL),** or "bad" cholesterol, thereby increasing a person's risk of heart disease. Unsaturated fatty acids, on the other hand, lower LDL. Monounsaturated fatty acids, such as those found in olive and canola oils, may also increase levels of **high-density lipoproteins (HDL),** or "good" cholesterol, providing even greater benefits for heart health. In large amounts, trans fatty acids may lower HDL. Thus, to reduce the risk of heart disease, it is important to choose unsaturated fats instead of saturated and trans fats. (See Chapter 11 for more on cholesterol and a heart-healthy diet.)

Most Americans consume more saturated fat than trans fat (12% versus 2–4% of total daily calories). However, health experts are particularly concerned about trans fats because of their double negative effect on heart health—they both raise LDL and lower HDL—and because there is less public awareness of trans fats. The saturated fat content of prepared foods has been listed on nutrition labels since 1994. In 2003, the FDA mandated that the trans fat content must also be listed on food labels, allowing consumers to determine the total amount of unhealthy fats that a food contains; however, food manufacturers have until 2006 to comply with the new regulation. Until trans fat content appears on food labels, consumers can check for the presence of trans fats by examining the ingredient list of a food: If a food contains "partially hydrogenated oil" or "vegetable shortening," it contains trans fat.

For heart health, it's important to limit your consumption of both saturated and trans fats. The best way to reduce saturated fat in your diet is to lower your intake of meat and full-fat dairy products (whole milk, cream, butter, cheese, ice cream). To lower trans fats, decrease your intake of deep-fried foods and baked goods made with hydrogenated vegetable oils; use liquid oils rather than margarine or shortening for cooking; and favor tub or squeeze margarines or those labeled low-trans or transfree over standard stick margarines. Remember, the softer or more liquid a fat is, the less saturated and trans fat it is likely to contain.

Although saturated and trans fats pose health hazards, other fats are beneficial. Monounsaturated fatty acids, as found in avocados, most nuts, and olive, canola, peanut, and safflower oils, improve cholesterol levels and may help protect against some cancers. **Omega-3 fatty acids,** a form of polyunsaturated fat found primarily in fish, may be even more healthful. Omega-3s are produced when the endmost double bond of a polyunsaturated fat occurs three carbons from the end of the fatty acid chain. (The polyunsaturated fatty acid shown in Figure 8.2 is an omega-3 form.) Omega-3s have a number of heart-healthy effects: They reduce the tendency of blood to clot, inhibit inflammation and abnormal heart rhythms, and reduce blood pressure and risk of heart attack and stroke in some people. Because of these benefits, nutritionists recommend that Americans increase the proportion of omega-3s in their diet by eating fish two or more times a week. Salmon, tuna, trout, mackerel, herring, sardines, and anchovies are all good sources of omega-3s; lesser amounts are found in plant sources, including dark-green leafy vegetables; walnuts; flaxseeds; and canola, walnut, and flaxseed oils.

Another form of polyunsaturated fat, omega-6 fatty acid, is produced if the endmost double bond occurs at the sixth carbon atom. Most of the polyunsaturated fats currently consumed by Americans are omega-6s, primarily from corn oil and soybean oil. Foods rich in omega-6s are important because they contain the essential nutrient linoleic acid. However, some nutritionists recommend that people reduce the proportion of omega-6s they consume in favor of omega-3s. To make this adjustment, use canola oil rather than corn oil in cooking, and check for corn, soybean, or cottonseed oil in products such as mayonnaise, margarine, and salad dressing.

In addition to its effects on heart disease risk, dietary fat can affect health in other ways. Diets high in fatty red meat are associated with an increased risk of certain forms of cancer, especially colon cancer. A high-fat diet can also make weight management more difficult. Because fat is a concentrated source of calories (9 calories per gram versus 4 calories per gram for protein and carbohydrate), a high-fat diet is often a high-calorie diet that can lead to

Type of Fatty Acid	Found In[a]	Possible Effects on Health
Keep Intake Low		
SATURATED	Animal fats (especially fatty meats and poultry fat and skin) Butter, cheese, and other high-fat dairy products Palm and coconut oils	Raises total cholesterol and "bad" (LDL) cholesterol levels Increases risk of heart disease May increase risk of colon and prostate cancers
TRANS	French fries and other deep-fried fast foods Stick margarines, shortening Packaged cookies and crackers Processed snacks and sweets	Raises total cholesterol and "bad" (LDL) cholesterol levels Lowers "good" (HDL) cholesterol levels May increase risk of heart disease and breast cancer
Choose Moderate Amounts		
MONOUNSATURATED	Olive, canola, and safflower oils Avocados, olives Peanut butter (without added fat) Many nuts, including almonds, cashews, pecans, pistachios	Lowers total cholesterol and "bad" (LDL) cholesterol levels May reduce blood pressure and lower triglyceride levels (a risk factor for CVD) May reduce risk of heart disease, stroke, and some cancers
POLYUNSATURATED (two groups)[b]		
Omega-3 fatty acids	Fatty fish, including salmon, white albacore tuna, mackerel, anchovies, and sardines Lesser amounts in walnut, flaxseed, canola, and soybean oils; tofu; walnuts; flaxseeds; and dark-green, leafy vegetables	Reduces blood clotting and inflammation and inhibits abnormal heart rhythms Lowers triglyceride levels (a risk factor for CVD) May lower blood pressure in some people May reduce risk of fatal heart attack, stroke, and some cancer
Omega-6 fatty acids	Corn, soybean, and cottonseed oils (often used in margarine, mayonnaise, and salad dressing)	Lowers total cholesterol and "bad" (LDL) cholesterol levels May lower "good" (HDL) cholesterol levels May reduce risk of heart disease May slightly increase risk of cancer if omega-6 intake is high and omega-3 intake is low

[a] Food fats contain a combination of types of fatty acids in various proportions; for example, canola oil is composed mainly of monounsaturated fatty acids (62%) but also contains polyunsaturated (32%) and saturated (6%) fatty acids. Food fats are categorized here according to their predominant fatty acid.

[b] The essential fatty acids are polyunsaturated: Linoleic acid is an omega-6 fatty acid and alpha-linolenic acid is an omega-3 fatty acid.

Figure 8.3 Types of fatty acids and their possible effects on health.   The health effects of dietary fats are still being investigated. In general, nutritionists recommend that we consume a diet moderate in fat overall and that we substitute unsaturated fats for saturated and trans fats. Monounsaturated fats and omega-3 polyunsaturated fats may be particularly good choices for promoting health. Eating lots of fat of any type can provide excess calories because all types of fats are rich sources of energy (9 calories per gram).

weight gain. In addition, there is some evidence that calories from fat are more easily converted to body fat than calories from protein or carbohydrate.

Although more research is needed on the precise effects of different types and amounts of fat on overall health, a great deal of evidence points to the fact that most people benefit from lowering their overall fat intake to recommended levels and choosing unsaturated fats instead of saturated and trans fats. The types of fatty acids and their effects on health are summarized in Figure 8.3.

Recommended Fat Intake   To meet the body's need for essential fats, adult men need about 17 grams per day of linoleic acid and 1.6 grams per day of alpha-linolenic acid; for women, the daily need is 12 grams of linoleic acid and 1.1 grams of alpha-linolenic acid. About 3–4 teaspoons (15–20 grams) of vegetable oil per day incorporated into your diet will supply the essential fats. Most Americans consume sufficient amounts of the essential

fats, and limiting unhealthy fats is a much greater health concern.

trans fatty acid A type of unsaturated fatty acid produced during the process of hydrogenation; trans fats have an atypical shape that affects their chemical activity.

cholesterol A waxy substance found in the blood and cells and needed for cell membranes, vitamin D, and hormone synthesis.

low-density lipoprotein (LDL) Blood fat that transports cholesterol to organs and tissues; excess amounts result in the accumulation of fatty deposits on artery walls.

high-density lipoprotein (HDL) Blood fat that helps transport cholesterol out of the arteries, thereby protecting against heart disease.

omega-3 fatty acids Polyunsaturated fatty acids commonly found in fish oils that are beneficial to cardiovascular health; the endmost double bond occurs three carbons from the end of the fatty acid chain.

Terms

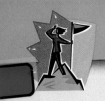

Goals have been established by the Food and Nutrition Board to help ensure adequate intake of the essential amino acids, fatty acids, and carbohydrate. The daily goals for adequate intake for adults are as follows:

	Men	Women
Protein	56 grams	46 grams
Fat: Linoleic acid	17 grams	12 grams
Alpha-linolenic acid	1.6 grams	1.1 grams
Carbohydrate	130 grams	130 grams

Protein intake goals can be calculated more specifically by multiplying your body weight in kilograms by 0.8 or your body weight in pounds by 0.36. (Refer to the Nutrition Resources section at the end of the chapter for information for specific age groups and life stages.)

To meet your daily energy needs, you need to consume more than the minimally adequate amounts of the energy-providing nutrients listed above, which alone supply only about 800–900 calories. The Food and Nutrition Board provides additional guidance in the form of Acceptable Macronutrient Distribution Ranges (AMDRs). The ranges can help you balance your intake of the energy-providing nutrients in ways that ensure adequate intake while reducing the risk of chronic disease. The AMDRs for protein, total fat, and carbohydrate are as follows:

Protein	10–35% of total daily calories
Total fat	20–35% of total daily calories
Carbohydrate	45–65% of total daily calories

To set individual goals, begin by estimating your total daily energy (calorie) needs; if your weight is stable, your current energy intake is the number of calories you need to maintain your weight at your current activity level. Next, select percentage goals for protein, fat, and carbohydrate. You can allocate your total daily calories among the three classes of macronutrients to suit your preferences; just make sure that the three percentage values you select total 100% and that you meet the minimum intake goals listed. Two samples reflecting different total energy intake and nutrient intake goals are shown in the table below.

To translate your own percentage goals into daily intake goals expressed in calories and grams, multiply the appropriate percentages by total calorie intake and then divide the results by the corresponding calories per gram. For example, a fat limit of 35% applied to a 2200-calorie diet would be calculated as follows: $0.35 \times 2200 = 770$ calories of total fat; $770 \div 9$ calories per gram = 86 grams of total fat. (Remember that fat has 9 calories per gram and that protein and carbohydrate have 4 calories per gram.)

Two Sample Macronutrient Distributions

Nutrient	AMDR	Sample 1 Individual Goals	Sample 1 Amounts for a 1600-calorie diet	Sample 2 Individual Goals	Sample 2 Amounts for a 2800-calorie diet
Protein	10–35%	15%	240 calories = 60 grams	20%	560 calories = 140 grams
Fat	20–35%	30%	480 calories = 53 grams	20%	560 calories = 62 grams
Carbohydrate	45–65%	55%	880 calories = 220 grams	60%	1680 calories = 420 grams

SOURCE: Food and Nutrition Board, Institute of Medicine, National Academies. 2002. *Dietary Reference Intakes: Energy, Carbohydrate, Fiber, Fat, Fatty Acids, Cholesterol, Protein, and Amino Acids.* Washington, D.C.: National Academy Press. Reprinted with permission from *Dietary Reference Intakes: Applications in Dietary Planning.* Copyright © 2003 by the National Academy of Sciences. Courtesy of the National Academies Press, Washington, D.C.

Limits for total, saturated, and trans fat intake have been set by a number of government and research organizations. In 2002, the Food and Nutrition Board released recommendations for the balance of energy sources in a healthful diet. These new recommendations, called Acceptable Macronutrient Distribution Ranges (AMDRs), are based on ensuring adequate intake of essential nutrients while also reducing the risk of chronic diseases like heart disease and cancer. As with protein, a range of levels of fat intake is associated with good health; the AMDR for total fat is 20–35% of total calories. Although more difficult for consumers to monitor, AMDRs have also been set for omega-6 fatty acids (5–10%) and omega-3 fatty acids (0.6–1.2%) as part of total fat intake. Because any amount of saturated and trans fat increases the risk of heart disease, the Food and Nutrition Board recommends that saturated and trans fat intake be kept as low as possible and that most fat in a healthy diet should be unsaturated. American adults currently consume about 33% of total calories as fat, including 11–12% of calories as saturated fat and 2–4% as trans fat.

For advice on setting individual intake goals, see the box, "Setting Intake Goals for Protein, Fat, and Carbohydrate." To determine how close you are to meeting these intake goals for fat, keep a running total over the course of the day. For prepared foods, food labels list the number of grams of fat, protein, and carbohydrate; the breakdown for many foods and popular fast-food items can be found in Appendixes B and C. Nutrition information is also available in many grocery stores, in published nutrition guides, and online (see For Further Exploration at the end of the chapter). By checking these resources, you can keep track of the total grams of fat, protein, and carbohydrate you eat and assess how close your current diet is to the recommended intake goals.

In reducing fat intake to recommended levels, the emphasis should be on lowering saturated and trans fats (see Figure 8.3). You can still eat high-fat foods, but it makes good sense to limit the size of your portions and to balance your intake with low-fat foods. For example, peanut butter is high in fat, with 8 grams (72 calories) of fat in each 90-calorie tablespoon. Two tablespoons of peanut butter eaten on whole-wheat bread and served with a banana, carrot sticks, and a glass of nonfat milk makes a nutritious lunch—high in protein and carbohydrate, relatively low in total and saturated fat (500 calories, 18 grams of total fat, 4 grams of saturated fat). Four tablespoons of peanut butter on high-fat crackers with potato chips, cookies, and whole milk is a less healthy combination (1000 calories, 62 grams of total fat, 15 grams of saturated fat). So although it's important to evaluate individual food items for their fat content, it is more important to look at them in the context of your overall diet.

Carbohydrates—An Ideal Source of Energy

Carbohydrates are needed in the diet primarily to supply energy to body cells. Some cells, such as those in the brain and other parts of the nervous system and in the blood, use only carbohydrates for fuel. During high-intensity exercise, muscles also get most of their energy from carbohydrates.

Simple and Complex Carbohydrates Carbohydrates are classified into two groups: simple and complex. Simple carbohydrates contain only one or two sugar units in each molecule; they include sucrose (table sugar), fructose (fruit sugar, honey), maltose (malt sugar), and lactose (milk sugar). Providing much of the sweetness in foods, they are found naturally in fruits and milk and are added to soft drinks, fruit drinks, candy, and sweet desserts. There is no evidence that any type of simple sugar is more nutritious than any other.

Complex carbohydrates consist of chains of many sugar molecules; they include starches and most types of dietary fiber. Starches are found in a variety of plants, especially grains (wheat, rye, rice, oats, barley, millet), legumes, and tubers (potatoes and yams). Most other vegetables contain a mix of starches and simple carbohydrates. Fiber, discussed in the next section, is found in fruits, vegetables, and grains.

During digestion in the mouth and small intestine, your body breaks down starches and double sugars into single sugar molecules, such as **glucose,** for absorption.

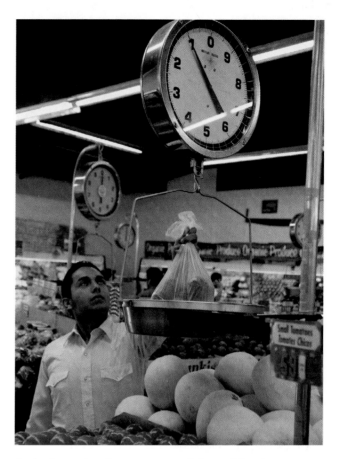

Our bodies require adequate amounts of all essential nutrients—water, proteins, carbohydrates, fats, vitamins, and minerals—to grow and function properly. Choosing foods to satisfy these nutritional requirements is an important part of a healthy lifestyle.

Once the glucose is in the bloodstream, the pancreas releases insulin, which allows cells to take up glucose and use it for energy. The liver and muscles also take up glucose and store it in the form of a starch called **glycogen.** The muscles use glucose from glycogen as fuel during endurance events or long workouts. Carbohydrates consumed in excess of the body's energy needs are changed into fat and stored. Whenever calorie intake exceeds calorie expenditure, fat storage can lead to weight gain. This is true whether the excess calories come from carbohydrates, proteins, fat, or alcohol.

Refined Carbohydrates Versus Whole Grains Complex carbohydrates can be further divided between refined, or processed, carbohydrates and unrefined carbohydrates, or whole grains. Before they are processed, all

carbohydrate An essential nutrient; sugars, starches, and dietary fiber are all carbohydrates.	Terms
glucose A simple sugar that is the body's basic fuel.	
glycogen An animal starch stored in the liver and muscles.	

What Are Whole Grains?

The first step in increasing your intake of whole grains is to correctly identify them. The following are whole grains:

whole wheat	whole-grain corn
whole rye	popcorn
whole oats	brown rice
oatmeal	barley

Other choices include bulgur (cracked wheat), millet, kasha (roasted buckwheat kernels), quinoa, teff, wheat and rye berries, amaranth, graham flour, whole-grain kamut, whole-grain spelt, and whole-grain triticale.

Wheat flour, unbleached flour, enriched flour, and degerminated corn meal are not whole grains. Wheat germ and wheat bran are also not whole grains, but they are the constituents of wheat typically left out when wheat is processed and so are healthier choices than regular wheat flour, which typically contains just the endosperm.

Reading Food Packages to Find Whole Grains

To find packaged foods rich in whole grains, read the list of ingredients and check for special health claims related to whole grains. *The first item on the list of ingredients should be one of the whole grains listed above.* In addition, the FDA allows manufacturers to include special health claims for foods that contain 51% or more whole-grain ingredients. Such products may contain a statement such as the following on their packaging: "Rich in whole grain," "Made with 100% whole grain," or "Diets rich in whole-grain foods may help reduce the risk of heart disease and certain cancers." However, many whole-grain products will not carry such claims.

Incorporating Whole Grains into Your Daily Diet

- *Bread:* Look for sandwich breads, bagels, English muffins, buns, and pita breads with a whole grain listed as the first ingredient. Color and name can be misleading; always check the list of ingredients.

- *Breakfast cereals:* Whole-grain choices include oatmeal, muesli, shredded wheat, and some types of raisin bran, bran flakes, wheat flakes, toasted oats, and granola. Check the ingredient list for whole grains.

- *Rice:* Choose brown rice or rice blends that include brown rice.

- *Pasta:* Look for whole-wheat, whole-grain kamut, or whole-grain spelt pasta.

- *Tortillas:* Choose whole-wheat or whole-corn tortillas.

- *Crackers and snacks:* Some varieties of crackers are made from whole grains, including some flatbreads or crispbreads, woven wheat crackers, and rye crackers. Other whole-grain snack possibilities include popcorn, popcorn cakes, brown rice cakes, whole-corn tortilla chips, and whole-wheat fig cookies. Be sure to check food labels for fat content, as many popular snacks are also high in fat.

- *Mixed-grain dishes:* Combine whole grains with other foods to create healthy mixed dishes such as tabouli; soups made with hulled barley or wheat berries; and pilafs, casseroles, and salads made with brown rice, whole-wheat couscous, kasha, millet, wheat bulgur, and quinoa.

If your grocery store doesn't carry these items, try your local health food store.

---

grains are **whole grains**, consisting of an inner layer of germ, a middle layer called the endosperm, and an outer layer of bran. During processing, the germ and bran are often removed, leaving just the starchy endosperm. The refinement of whole grains transforms whole-wheat flour to white flour, brown rice to white rice, and so on.

Refined carbohydrates usually retain all the calories of their unrefined counterparts, but they tend to be much lower in fiber, vitamins, minerals, and other beneficial compounds. Unrefined carbohydrates tend to take longer to chew and digest than refined ones; they also enter the bloodstream more slowly. This slower digestive pace tends to make people feel full sooner and for a longer period, lessening the chance that they will overeat. Also, a slower rise in blood glucose levels following consumption of complex carbohydrates may help in the prevention and management of diabetes. Whole grains are also high in dietary fiber and so have all the benefits of fiber. Consumption of whole grains has been linked to reduced risk for heart disease, diabetes, high blood pressure, stroke, and certain forms of cancer. For all these reasons, whole

grains are recommended over those that have been refined. This does not mean that you should never eat refined carbohydrates such as white bread or white rice, simply that whole-wheat bread, brown rice, and other whole grains are healthier choices. See the box "Choosing More Whole-Grain Foods" for tips on increasing your intake of whole grains.

Glycemic Index   Insulin and glucose levels rise and fall following a meal or snack containing any type of carbohydrate. Some foods cause a quick and dramatic rise in glucose and insulin levels; others have a slower, more moderate effect. A food that has a strong effect on blood glucose levels is said to have a high **glycemic index.** A meal containing high glycemic index foods may increase appetite in some people; over the long term, diets rich in high glycemic index foods are linked to increased risk of diabetes and heart disease.

Attempting to base food choices on glycemic index is a difficult task, however. Although one can say generally that unrefined complex carbohydrates and high-fiber foods tend to have a low glycemic index, patterns are less clear for other types of foods and do not follow a simple distinction such as that of simple versus complex carbohydrates. For example, some fruits with fairly high levels of simple carbohydrates have only a moderate effect on blood glucose levels, while white rice, potatoes, and white bread, which are rich in complex carbohydrates, have a high glycemic index. Watermelon has a glycemic index more than twice that of strawberries, and the glycemic index of a banana changes dramatically as it ripens. Spaghetti has a glycemic index half that of white bread, even when the two items are made from the same ingredients. The acid and fat content of a food also affect glycemic index—the more acidic and higher in fat a food is, the lower its effect on glucose levels.

This complexity is one reason why major health organizations have not issued specific guidelines for glycemic index. For people with particular health concerns, glycemic index may be an important consideration; however, it should not be the sole criterion for food choices. For example, ice cream and chocolate have much lower glycemic index values than brown rice and carrots—but that doesn't make them healthier choices overall. Glycemic index and its effects on appetite and heart health are discussed further in Chapters 9 and 11. For now, remember that most unrefined grains, fruits, vegetables, and legumes are rich in nutrients and have a low-to-moderate glycemic index. Choose a variety of vegetables daily, and avoid heavy consumption of white potatoes.

Recommended Carbohydrate Intake On average, Americans consume 200–300 grams of carbohydrate per day, well above the 130 grams needed to meet the body's requirement for essential carbohydrate. A range of intakes is associated with good health, and experts recommend that adults consume 45–65% of total daily calories as carbohydrate, about 225–325 grams of carbohydrate for someone consuming 2000 calories per day. The focus should be on consuming a variety of foods rich in complex carbohydrates, especially whole grains.

Health experts offer separate guidelines for intake of added sugars as part of total carbohydrate consumption. The Food and Nutrition Board set an AMDR for added sugars of 25% or less of total daily calories, but many health experts recommend a substantially lower intake. Guidelines released by the World Health Organization in 2003 suggested a limit of 10% of total daily calories from added sugars. Foods high in added sugar are generally high in calories and low in nutrients and fiber, thus providing "empty" calories. To reduce your intake of added sugars, limit soft drinks, candy, sweet desserts, and sweetened fruit drinks. The simple carbohydrates in your diet should come from food sources in which they are found naturally—including fruits, which are excellent sources of vitamins and minerals, and from milk, which is high in protein and calcium.

Athletes in training can especially benefit from high-carbohydrate diets (60–70% of total daily calories), which enhance the amount of carbohydrates stored in their muscles (as glycogen) and therefore provide more carbohydrate fuel for use during endurance events or long workouts. In addition, carbohydrates consumed during prolonged athletic events can help fuel muscles and extend the availability of the glycogen stored in muscles. Caution is in order, however, because overconsumption of carbohydrates can lead to feelings of fatigue and underconsumption of other nutrients. (For more on the special nutritional needs of athletes, see pp. 242–244.)

Dietary Fiber—A Closer Look

Fiber is the term given to nondigestible carbohydrates provided mainly by plants. Instead of being digested, like starch, fiber passes through the intestinal tract and provides bulk for feces in the large intestine, which in turn facilitates elimination. In the large intestine, some types of fiber are broken down by bacteria into acids and gases, which explains why consuming too much fiber can lead to intestinal gas. Because humans cannot digest fiber, it is not a source of carbohydrate in the diet; however, the consumption of fiber is necessary for good health.

Types of Dietary Fiber The Food and Nutrition Board has defined two types of fiber: dietary fiber and functional fiber. **Dietary fiber** refers to nondigestible carbohydrates and lignin that are present naturally in plants such as grains, legumes, and vegetables. **Functional fiber** refers to nondigestible carbohydrates that have been either isolated from natural sources or synthesized in a lab and then added to a food product or supplement. **Total fiber** is the sum of dietary and functional fiber.

Fibers have different properties that lead to different physiological effects in the body. **Soluble (viscous) fiber** slows the body's absorption of glucose and binds cholesterol-containing compounds in the intestine, lowering blood cholesterol levels and reducing the risk of

---

whole grain The entire edible portion of a grain such as wheat, rice, or oats, including the germ, endosperm, and bran. During milling or processing, parts of the grain are removed, often leaving just the endosperm.

glycemic index A measure of how the ingestion of a particular food affects blood glucose levels.

dietary fiber Nondigestible carbohydrates and lignin that are intact in plants.

functional fiber Nondigestible carbohydrates either isolated from natural sources or synthesized; these may be added to foods and dietary supplements.

total fiber The total amount of dietary fiber and functional fiber in the diet.

soluble (viscous) fiber Fiber that dissolves in water or is broken down by bacteria in the large intestine.

Terms
VW

cardiovascular disease. **Insoluble fiber** binds water, making the feces bulkier and softer so they pass more quickly and easily through the intestines.

Both kinds of fiber contribute to disease prevention. A diet high in soluble fiber can help people manage diabetes and high blood cholesterol levels. A diet high in insoluble fiber can help prevent a variety of health problems, including constipation, hemorrhoids, and **diverticulitis.** Some studies have linked diets high in fiber-rich fruits, vegetables, and grains with a lower risk of some kinds of cancer; however, it is unclear whether fiber or other food components are responsible for this reduction in risk.

Sources of Dietary Fiber All plant foods contain some dietary fiber, but fruits, legumes, oats (especially oat bran), barley, and psyllium (found in some cereals and laxatives) are particularly rich in it. Wheat (especially wheat bran), cereals, grains, and vegetables are all good sources of insoluble fiber. However, the processing of packaged foods can remove fiber, so it's important to depend on fresh fruits and vegetables and foods made from whole grains as sources of dietary fiber.

Recommended Intake of Dietary Fiber To reduce the risk of chronic disease and maintain intestinal health, the Food and Nutrition Board recommends a daily fiber intake of 38 grams for adult men and 25 grams for adult women. Americans currently consume about half this amount. Fiber should come from foods, not supplements, which should be used only under medical supervision.

To increase the amount of fiber in your diet, try the following:

- Look for breads, crackers, and cereals that list whole grain first in the ingredient list: Whole-wheat flour, whole-grain oats, and whole-grain rice are whole grains; wheat flour is not. Choose a breakfast cereal with 5 or more grams of fiber per serving.
- Eat whole, unpeeled fruits rather than drinking fruit juice. Top cereals, yogurt, and desserts with berries, apple slices, or other fruit.
- Include beans in soups and salads. Combine raw vegetables with pasta, rice, or beans in salads.

Terms

insoluble fiber Fiber that does not dissolve in water and is not broken down by bacteria in the large intestine.

diverticulitis A digestive disorder in which abnormal pouches form in the walls of the intestine and become inflamed.

vitamins Organic substances needed in small amounts to help promote and regulate chemical reactions and processes in the body.

antioxidant A substance that protects against the breakdown of body constituents by free radicals; actions include binding oxygen, donating electrons to free radicals, and repairing damage to molecules.

- Substitute bean dip for cheese-based or sour cream–based dips or spreads. Use raw vegetables rather than chips for dipping.

Vitamins—Organic Micronutrients

Vitamins are organic (carbon-containing) substances required in very small amounts to regulate various processes within living cells (Table 8.2). Humans need 13 vitamins. Four are fat-soluble (A, D, E, and K), and nine are water-soluble (C and the eight B-complex vitamins: thiamin, riboflavin, niacin, vitamin B-6, folate, vitamin B-12, biotin, and pantothenic acid). Solubility affects how a vitamin is absorbed, transported, and stored in the body. The water-soluble vitamins are absorbed directly into the bloodstream, where they travel freely; excess water-soluble vitamins are detected and removed by the kidneys and excreted in urine. Fat-soluble vitamins require a more complex absorptive process; they are usually carried in the blood by special proteins and are stored in the body in fat tissues rather than excreted.

Functions of Vitamins Many vitamins help chemical reactions take place. They provide no energy to the body directly but help unleash the energy stored in carbohydrates, proteins, and fats. Vitamins are critical in the production of red blood cells and the maintenance of the nervous, skeletal, and immune systems. Some vitamins also form substances that act as **antioxidants,** which help preserve healthy cells in the body. Key vitamin antioxidants include vitamin E, vitamin C, and the vitamin A precursor beta-carotene. (The actions of antioxidants are described later in the chapter.)

Sources of Vitamins The human body does not manufacture most of the vitamins it requires and must obtain them from foods. Vitamins are abundant in fruits, vegetables, and grains. In addition, many processed foods, such as flour and breakfast cereals, contain added vitamins. A few vitamins are made in certain parts of the body: The skin makes vitamin D when it is exposed to sunlight, and intestinal bacteria make vitamin K. Nonetheless, you still need to obtain vitamin D and vitamin K from foods.

Vitamin Deficiencies and Excesses If your diet lacks sufficient amounts of a particular vitamin, characteristic symptoms of deficiency develop (see Table 8.2). For example, vitamin A deficiency can cause blindness, and vitamin B-6 deficiency can cause seizures. Vitamin deficiency diseases are most often seen in developing countries; they are relatively rare in the United States because vitamins are readily available from our food supply. However, intakes below recommended levels can have adverse effects on health even if they are not low enough to cause a deficiency disease. For example, low intake of folate increases a woman's chance of giving birth to a baby with a neural tube defect (a congenital malformation of the central nervous system). Low

Table 8.2   *Facts About Vitamins*

Vitamin	Important Dietary Sources	Major Functions	Signs of Prolonged Deficiency	Toxic Effects of Megadoses
Fat-Soluble				
Vitamin A	Liver, milk, butter, cheese, and fortified margarine; carrots, spinach, and other orange and deep-green vegetables and fruits	Maintenance of vision, skin, linings of the nose, mouth, digestive and urinary tracts, immune function	Night blindness; dry, scaling skin; increased susceptibility to infection; loss of appetite; anemia; kidney stones	Liver damage, miscarriage and birth defects, headache, vomiting and diarrhea, vertigo, double vision, bone abnormalities
Vitamin D	Fortified milk and margarine, fish oils, butter, egg yolks (sunlight on skin also produces vitamin D)	Development and maintenance of bones and teeth, promotion of calcium absorption	Rickets (bone deformities) in children; bone softening, loss, and fractures in adults	Kidney damage, calcium deposits in soft tissues, depression, death
Vitamin E	Vegetable oils, whole grains, nuts and seeds, green leafy vegetables, asparagus, peaches	Protection and maintenance of cellular membranes	Red blood cell breakage and anemia, weakness, neurological problems, muscle cramps	Relatively nontoxic, but may cause excess bleeding or formation of blood clots
Vitamin K	Green leafy vegetables; smaller amounts widespread in other foods	Production of proteins essential for blood clotting and bone metabolism	Hemorrhaging	None reported
Water-Soluble				
Biotin	Cereals, yeast, egg yolks, soy flour, liver; widespread in foods	Synthesis of fat, glycogen, and amino acids	Rash, nausea, vomiting, weight loss, depression, fatigue, hair loss	None reported
Folate	Green leafy vegetables, yeast, oranges, whole grains, legumes, liver	Amino acid metabolism, synthesis of RNA and DNA, new cell synthesis	Anemia, weakness, fatigue, irritability, shortness of breath, swollen tongue	Masking of vitamin B-12 deficiency
Niacin	Eggs, poultry, fish, milk, whole grains, nuts, enriched breads and cereals, meats, legumes	Conversion of carbohydrates, fats, and protein into usable forms of energy	Pellagra (symptoms include diarrhea, dermatitis, inflammation of mucous membranes, dementia)	Flushing of the skin, nausea, vomiting, diarrhea, liver dysfunction, glucose intolerance
Pantothenic acid	Animal foods, whole grains, broccoli, potatoes; widespread in foods	Metabolism of fats, carbohydrates, and proteins	Fatigue, numbness and tingling of hands and feet, gastrointestinal disturbances	None reported
Riboflavin	Dairy products, enriched breads and cereals, lean meats, poultry, fish, green vegetables	Energy metabolism; maintenance of skin, mucous membranes, and nervous system structures	Cracks at corners of mouth, sore throat, skin rash, hypersensitivity to light, purple tongue	None reported
Thiamin	Whole-grain and enriched breads and cereals, organ meats, lean pork, nuts, legumes	Conversion of carbohydrates into usable forms of energy, maintenance of appetite and nervous system function	Beriberi (symptoms include muscle wasting, mental confusion, anorexia, enlarged heart, nerve changes)	None reported
Vitamin B-6	Eggs, poultry, fish, whole grains, nuts, soybeans, liver, kidney, pork	Metabolism of amino acids and glycogen	Anemia, convulsions, cracks at corners of mouth, dermatitis, nausea, confusion	Neurological abnormalities and damage
Vitamin B-12	Meat, fish, poultry, fortified cereals	Synthesis of blood cells; other metabolic reactions	Anemia, fatigue, nervous system damage, sore tongue	None reported
Vitamin C	Peppers, cruciferous vegetables, spinach, citrus fruits, strawberries, tomatoes, potatoes, other fruits and vegetables	Maintenance and repair of connective tissue, bones, teeth, and cartilage; promotion of healing; aid in iron absorption	Scurvy, anemia, reduced resistance to infection, loosened teeth, joint pain, poor wound healing, hair loss, poor iron absorption	Urinary stones in some people, acid stomach from ingesting supplements in pill form, nausea, diarrhea, headache, fatigue

SOURCES: Food and Nutrition Board, Institute of Medicine, National Academies. 2001. *Dietary Reference Intakes Tables* (http://www.iom.edu/board. asp?id=3788; retrieved November 15, 2003). The complete Dietary Reference Intake reports are available from the National Academy Press (http:// www.nap.edu). National Research Council. 1989. *Recommended Dietary Allowances*, 10th ed. Washington, D.C.: National Academy Press. Shils, M. E., et al., eds. 1998. *Modern Nutrition in Health and Disease*, 9th ed. Baltimore: Williams and Wilkins.

intake of folate and vitamins B-6 and B-12 has been linked to increased heart disease risk. Many Americans consume less-than-recommended amounts of vitamins A, C, B-6, and E.

Extra vitamins in the diet can be harmful, especially when taken as supplements. High doses of vitamin A are toxic and increase the risk of birth defects, for example. Vitamin B-6 can cause irreversible nerve damage when taken in large doses. Megadoses of fat-soluble vitamins are particularly dangerous because the excess will be stored in the body rather than excreted, increasing the risk of toxicity. Even when supplements are not taken in excess, relying on them for an adequate intake of vitamins can be a problem: There are many substances in foods other than vitamins and minerals, and some of these compounds may have important health effects. Later in the chapter we discuss specific recommendations for vitamin intake and when a supplement is advisable. For now, keep in mind that it's best to obtain most of your vitamins from foods rather than supplements.

When preparing foods, remember that vitamins and minerals in vegetables can be easily lost or destroyed during storage or cooking. To retain their value, eat or process vegetables immediately after buying them. If you can't do this, then store them in a cool place, covered to retain moisture—either in the refrigerator (for a few days) or in the freezer (for a longer term). To reduce nutrient losses during food preparation, minimize the amount of water used and the total cooking time. Develop a taste for a crunchier texture in cooked vegetables. Baking, steaming, broiling, and microwaving are all good methods of preparing vegetables.

Minerals—Inorganic Micronutrients

Minerals are inorganic (non-carbon-containing) elements you need in small amounts to help regulate body functions, aid in the growth and maintenance of body tissues, and help release energy (Table 8.3). There are about 17 essential minerals. The major minerals, those that the body needs in amounts exceeding 100 milligrams, include calcium, phosphorus, magnesium, sodium, potassium, and chloride. The essential trace minerals, those that you

need in minute amounts, include copper, fluoride, iodine, iron, selenium, and zinc.

Characteristic symptoms develop if an essential mineral is consumed in a quantity too small or too large for good health. The minerals most commonly lacking in the American diet are iron, calcium, magnesium, and potassium. Focus on good food choices for these nutrients (see Table 8.3). Lean meats are rich in iron; low-fat or fat-free dairy products are excellent choices for calcium. Plant foods such as whole grains and leafy vegetables are good sources of magnesium. Potassium-rich foods include spinach and other leafy greens, cantaloupe, bananas, mushrooms, and potatoes. Iron-deficiency **anemia** is a problem in some age groups, and researchers fear poor calcium intakes are sowing the seeds for future **osteoporosis,** especially in women. See the box "Eating for Healthy Bones" on p. 232 to learn more.

Water—A Vital Component

Water is the major component in both foods and the human body: You are composed of about 60% water. Your need for other nutrients, in terms of weight, is much less than your need for water. You can live up to 50 days without food but only a few days without water.

Water is distributed all over the body, among lean and other tissues and in urine and other body fluids. Water is used in the digestion and absorption of food and is the medium in which most of the chemical reactions take place within the body. Some water-based fluids like blood transport substances around the body; other fluids serve as lubricants or cushions. Water also helps regulate body temperature.

Water is contained in almost all foods, particularly in liquids, fruits, and vegetables. The foods and fluids you consume provide 80–90% of your daily water intake; the remainder is generated through metabolism. You lose water each day in urine, feces, and sweat and through evaporation in your lungs.

As described in Chapter 3, severe dehydration causes weakness and can lead to death. However, most people maintain a healthy water balance by consuming beverages at meals and drinking fluids in response to thirst. In 2004, the Food and Nutrition Board set levels of adequate water intake to maintain hydration (Table 8.4, p. 232); all fluids, including those containing caffeine, can count toward your total daily fluid intake. Water and other beverages typically make up about 80% of your fluid intake; the remainder comes from foods. So, for example, in consuming 2.7 liters of total water per day, an adult woman would consume about 2.2 liters (9 cups) of water and other beverages, while the remaining 0.5 liter would come from foods, especially fruits and vegetables. If you exercise vigorously or live in a hot climate, you need to consume additional fluids to maintain a balance between water consumed and water lost. See p. 244 for more on the fluid needs of athletes and active people.

Terms
Vi̵w

minerals Inorganic compounds needed in small amounts for regulation, growth, and maintenance of body tissues and functions.

anemia A deficiency in the oxygen-carrying material in the red blood cells.

osteoporosis A condition in which the bones become thin and brittle and break easily.

free radical An electron-seeking compound that can react with fats, proteins, and DNA, damaging cell membranes and mutating genes in its search for electrons; produced through chemical reactions in the body and by exposure to environmental factors such as sunlight and tobacco smoke.

Table 8.3   Facts About Selected Minerals

Mineral	Important Dietary Sources	Major Functions	Signs of Prolonged Deficiency	Toxic Effects of Megadoses
Calcium	Milk and milk products, tofu, fortified orange juice and bread, green leafy vegetables, bones in fish	Formation of bones and teeth; control of nerve impulses, muscle contraction, blood clotting	Stunted growth in children, bone mineral loss in adults; urinary stones	Kidney stones, calcium deposits in soft tissues, inhibition of mineral absorption, constipation
Fluoride	Fluoridated water, tea, marine fish eaten with bones	Maintenance of tooth and bone structure	Higher frequency of tooth decay	Increased bone density, mottling of teeth, impaired kidney function
Iodine	Iodized salt, seafood, processed foods	Essential part of thyroid hormones, regulation of body metabolism	Goiter (enlarged thyroid), cretinism (birth defect)	Depression of thyroid activity, hyperthyroidism in susceptible people
Iron	Meat and poultry, fortified grain products, dark-green vegetables, dried fruit	Component of hemoglobin, myoglobin, and enzymes	Iron-deficiency anemia, weakness, impaired immune function, gastrointestinal distress	Nausea, diarrhea, liver and kidney damage, joint pains, sterility, disruption of cardiac function, death
Magnesium	Widespread in foods and water (except soft water); especially found in grains, legumes, nuts, seeds, green vegetables, milk	Transmission of nerve impulses, energy transfer, activation of many enzymes	Neurological disturbances, cardiovascular problems, kidney disorders, nausea, growth failure in children	Nausea, vomiting, diarrhea, central nervous system depression, coma; death in people with impaired kidney function
Phosphorus	Present in nearly all foods, especially milk, cereal, peas, eggs, meat	Bone growth and maintenance, energy transfer in cells	Impaired growth, weakness, kidney disorders, cardiorespiratory and nervous system dysfunction	Drop in blood calcium levels, calcium deposits in soft tissues, bone loss
Potassium	Fruits and vegetables, especially leafy greens, cantaloupe, bananas, mushrooms, potatoes	Basic functioning of cells, water balance, acid-base balance	Elevated blood pressure, bone mineral loss, kidney stones, increased salt sensitivity, cardiac arrhythmia, muscle weakness	Cardiac arrhythmia and arrest, gastrointestinal discomfort
Selenium	Seafood, meat, eggs, whole grains	Defense against oxidative stress and regulation of thyroid hormone action	Muscle pain and weakness, heart disorders	Hair and nail brittleness and loss, nausea and vomiting, weakness, irritability
Sodium	Salt, soy sauce, fast food, and processed foods, especially lunch meats, canned soups and vegetables, salty snacks, and processed cheese	Body water balance, acid-base balance, nerve function	Muscle weakness, loss of appetite, nausea, vomiting; deficiency is rarely seen	Increased blood pressure (even at fairly low levels of intake), renal stones, edema
Zinc	Whole grains, meat, eggs, liver, seafood (especially oysters)	Synthesis of proteins, RNA, and DNA; wound healing; immune response; ability to taste	Growth failure, loss of appetite, impaired taste acuity, skin rash, impaired immune function, poor wound healing	Vomiting, impaired immune function, decline in blood HDL levels, impaired copper absorption

SOURCES: Food and Nutrition Board, Institute of Medicine, National Academies. 2004. *Dietary Reference Intakes for Water, Potassium, Sodium, Chloride, and Sulfate*. Washington, D.C.: National Academies Press. Food and Nutrition Board, Institute of Medicine, National Academies. 2001. *Dietary Reference Intakes Tables* (http://www.iom.edu/board.asp?id=3788; retrieved November 15, 2003). The complete Dietary Reference Intake reports are available from the National Academy Press (http://www.nap.edu). Shils, M. E., et al., eds. 1998. *Modern Nutrition in Health and Disease*, 9th ed. Baltimore: Williams and Wilkins.

Other Substances in Food

There are many substances in food that are not essential nutrients but that may influence health.

Antioxidants   When the body uses oxygen or breaks down certain fats or proteins as a normal part of metabolism, it gives rise to substances called **free radicals.**

Environmental factors such as cigarette smoke, exhaust fumes, radiation, excessive sunlight, certain drugs, and stress can increase free radical production. A free radical is a chemically unstable molecule that is missing an electron; it will react with any molecule it encounters from which it can take an electron. In their search for electrons, free radicals react with fats, proteins, and DNA, damaging cell membranes and mutating genes. Because

Osteoporosis is a condition in which the bones become danger-ously thin and fragile over time. It currently afflicts over 28 mil-lion Americans, 80% of them women, and results in over 1.5 million bone fractures each year. Most bone mass is built by age 18. After bone density peaks between the ages of 25 and 35, bone mass is slowly lost over time. To prevent osteoporosis, the best strategy is to build as much bone as possible during your young years and then do everything you can to maintain it as you age. Up to 50% of bone loss is determined by controllable lifestyle factors. Key nutrients include the following:

Calcium   Consuming an adequate amount of calcium is important throughout life to build and maintain bone mass. Milk, yogurt, and calcium-fortified orange juice, bread, and cereals are all good sources.

Vitamin D   Vitamin D is necessary for bones to absorb calcium, a daily intake of 5 mg is recommended for adults age 19–50 years. Vitamin D can be obtained from foods and is man-ufactured by the skin when exposed to sunlight. Candidates for vitamin D supplements include people who don't eat many foods rich in vitamin D; those who don't expose their face, arms, and hands to the sun (without sunscreen) for 5–15 minutes a few times each week; and people who live north of an imaginary line roughly between Boston and the Oregon–California border (the sun is weaker in northern latitudes).

Vitamin K   Vitamin K promotes the synthesis of proteins that help keep bones strong. Broccoli and leafy-green vegeta-bles are rich in vitamin K.

Other Nutrients   Other nutrients that may play an important role in bone health include vitamin C, magnesium, potassium, manganese, zinc, copper, and boron. On the flip side, there are several dietary substances that may have a *negative* effect on bone health, especially if consumed in excess: alcohol, sodium, caffeine, and retinol (a form of vitamin A). Drinking lots of soda, which often replaces milk in the diet and which is high in phosphorus (a mineral that may interfere with calcium absorption), has been shown to increase the risk of bone fracture in teenage girls. For healthy bones, it is important to be moderate in your consumption of alcohol, sodium, caffeine, retinol, and sodas.

The effect of protein intake on bone mass depends on other nutrients: Protein helps build bone as long as calcium and vitamin D intake are adequate; but if intake of calcium and vitamin D is low, high protein intake can lead to bone loss.

Finally, it is important to combine a healthy diet with other wellness behaviors. Weight-bearing aerobic activities, if per-formed regularly, help build and maintain bone mass through-out life. Strength training improves bone density, muscle mass, strength, and balance, protecting against both bone loss and falls, a major cause of fractures. Drinking alcohol only in mod-eration, refraining from smoking, and managing depression and stress are also important for maintaining strong bones. For peo-ple who do develop osteoporosis, a variety of medications is available to treat the condition.

Table 8.4	Adequate Daily Water Intake	
Life stage	Total water intake from fluids and food	Fluid intake (water and beverages) as part of total water intake
Children 1–3 years	1.3 liters	0.9 liters (about 4 cups)
4–8 years	1.7 liters	1.2 liters (about 5 cups)
Males 9–13 years	2.4 liters	1.8 liters (about 8 cups)
14–18 years	3.3 liters	2.6 liters (about 11 cups)
19 years and older	3.7 liters	3.0 liters (about 13 cups)
Females 9–13 years	2.1 liters	1.6 liters (about 7 cups)
14–18 years	2.3 liters	1.8 liters (about 8 cups)
19 years and older	2.7 liters	2.2 liters (about 9 cups)

Infant fluid intake (0.7–0.8 liters/day) is assumed to be from human milk and, for infants 7–12 months, from complementary foods and beverages.

SOURCE: Food and Nutrition Board, Institute of Medicine, National Academies. 2004. *Dietary Reference Intakes: Water, Potassium, Sodium, Chloride, and Sulfate.* Washington, D.C.: National Academies Press.

of this, free radicals have been implicated in aging, can-cer, cardiovascular disease, and other degenerative dis-eases like arthritis.

Antioxidants found in foods can help protect the body by blocking the formation and action of free radicals and repairing the damage they cause. Some antioxidants, such as vitamin C, vitamin E, and selenium, are also essential nutrients; others, such as carotenoids, found in yellow, orange, and dark-green leafy vegetables, are not. Many fruits and vegetables are rich in antioxidants.

Phytochemicals   Antioxidants are a particular type of **phytochemical**, a substance found in plant foods that may help prevent chronic disease. Researchers have just begun to identify and study all the different compounds found in foods, and many preliminary findings are promising. For example, certain proteins found in soy foods may help lower cholesterol levels. Sulforaphane, a compound isolated from broccoli and other **cruciferous vegetables**, may render some carcinogenic compounds harmless. Allyl sulfides, a group of chemicals found in garlic and onions, appear to boost the activity of cancer-fighting immune cells. Further research on phytochemicals may extend the role of nutrition to the prevention and treatment of many chronic diseases.

To increase your intake of phytochemicals, it is best to obtain them by eating a variety of fruits and vegetables rather than relying on supplements. Like many vitamins and minerals, isolated phytochemicals may be harmful if taken in high doses. In addition, it is likely that their health benefits are the result of chemical substances working in combination. The role of phytochemicals in disease prevention is discussed further in Chapters 11 and 12.

NUTRITIONAL GUIDELINES: PLANNING YOUR DIET

The second part of putting together a healthy food plan—after you've learned about necessary nutrients—is choosing foods that satisfy nutritional requirements and meet your personal criteria. Various tools have been created by scientific and government groups to help people design healthy diets. The **Dietary Reference Intakes (DRIs)** are standards for nutrient intake designed to prevent nutritional deficiencies and reduce the risk of chronic disease. The **Food Guide Pyramid** translates these nutrient recommendations into a balanced food-group plan that includes all essential nutrients. To provide further guidance, **Dietary Guidelines for Americans** have been established to address the prevention of diet-related chronic diseases. Together, these tools make up a complete set of resources for dietary planning.

Dietary Reference Intakes (DRIs)

How much vitamin C, iron, calcium, and other nutrients do you need to stay healthy? The Food and Nutrition Board of the National Academy of Sciences establishes dietary standards, or recommended intake levels, for Americans of all ages. The current set of standards, called Dietary Reference Intakes (DRIs), is relatively new, having been introduced in 1997. An earlier set of standards, called the **Recommended Dietary Allowances (RDAs)**, focused on preventing nutritional deficiency diseases such as anemia; the RDAs were established in 1941 and updated periodically, most recently in 1989. The newer DRIs have a broader focus because recent research has looked not just at the prevention of nutrient deficiencies but also at the role of nutrients in promoting optimal health and preventing chronic diseases such as cancer, osteoporosis, and heart disease.

The DRIs include standards for both recommended intakes and maximum safe intakes. The recommended intake of each nutrient is expressed as either a *Recommended Dietary Allowance (RDA)* or *Adequate Intake (AI)*. An AI is set when there is not enough information available to set an RDA value; regardless of the type of standard used, however, the DRI represents the best available estimate of intake for optimal health. The *Tolerable Upper Intake Level (UL)* sets the maximum daily intake by a healthy person that is unlikely to cause health problems. For example, the RDA for calcium for an 18-year-old female is 1300 mg per day; the UL is 2500 mg per day. Because of lack of data, ULs have not been set for all nutrients. This does not mean that people can tolerate chronic intakes of these vitamins and minerals above recommended levels. Like all chemical agents, nutrients can produce adverse effects if intakes are excessive. There is no established benefit from consuming nutrients at levels above the RDA or AI. The DRIs can be found in the Nutrition Resources section at the end of the chapter. For more information, visit the Web site of the National Academies' Food and Nutrition Board (see For Further Exploration at the end of the chapter.)

Should You Take Supplements?   The aim of the DRIs is to guide you in meeting your nutritional needs primarily with food, rather than with vitamin and mineral supplements. This goal is important because recommendations have not yet been set for some essential nutrients. Many supplements contain only nutrients with established

Terms

phytochemical A naturally occurring substance found in plant foods that may help prevent and treat chronic diseases such as heart disease and cancer; *phyto* means plant.

cruciferous vegetables Vegetables of the cabbage family, including cabbage, broccoli, brussels sprouts, kale, and cauliflower; the flower petals of these plants form the shape of a cross, hence the name.

Dietary Reference Intakes (DRIs) An umbrella term for four types of nutrient standards: Adequate Intake (AI), Estimated Average Requirement (EAR), and Recommended Dietary Allowance (RDA) set levels of intake considered adequate to prevent nutrient deficiencies and reduce the risk of chronic disease; Tolerable Upper Intake Level (UL) sets the maximum daily intake that is unlikely to cause health problems.

Food Guide Pyramid A food-group plan that provides practical advice to ensure a balanced intake of the essential nutrients.

Dietary Guidelines for Americans General principles of good nutrition intended to help prevent certain diet-related diseases.

Recommended Dietary Allowances (RDAs) Amounts of certain nutrients considered adequate to prevent deficiencies in most healthy people; will eventually be replaced by the Dietary Reference Intakes (DRIs).

recommendations, so using them to meet nutrient needs can leave you deficient in other nutrients. Supplements also lack potentially beneficial phytochemicals that are found only in whole foods. Nutrition scientists generally agree that most Americans can obtain most of the vitamins and minerals they need by consuming a varied, nutritionally balanced diet.

The question of whether to take supplements is a serious one. Some vitamins and minerals are dangerous when ingested in excess, as described in Tables 8.2 and 8.3. Large doses of particular nutrients can also cause health problems by affecting the absorption of other vitamins and minerals. For all these reasons, you should think carefully about whether to take supplements; consider consulting a physician or registered dietitian.

In setting the DRIs, the Food and Nutrition Board recommended supplements of particular nutrients for the following groups:

• Women who are capable of becoming pregnant should take 400 μg per day of folic acid (the synthetic form of the vitamin folate) from fortified foods and/or supplements in addition to folate from a varied diet. Research indicates that this level of folate intake will reduce the risk of neural tube defects. (This defect occurs early in pregnancy, before most women know they are pregnant; therefore, the recommendation for the folate intake applies to all women of reproductive age rather than only to pregnant women.) Since 1998, enriched breads, flours, corn meals, rice, noodles, and other grain products have been fortified with small amounts of folic acid. Folate is found naturally in leafy green vegetables, legumes, oranges and orange juice, and strawberries.

• People over age 50 should consume foods fortified with vitamin B-12, B-12 supplements, or a combination of the two in order to meet the majority of the DRI of 2.4 mg of B-12 daily. Up to 30% of people over 50 may have problems absorbing protein-bound B-12 in foods. Vitamin B-12 in supplements and fortified foods is more readily absorbed and can help prevent a deficiency.

Because of the oxidative stress caused by smoking, the Food and Nutrition Board also recommends that smokers consume 35 mg *more* vitamin C per day than the DRI intake level set for their age and sex (for adults, recommended daily vitamin C intakes for nonsmokers are 90 mg for men and 75 mg for women). However, supplements are not usually needed because this extra vitamin C can easily be obtained from foods. For example, one cup of orange juice has about 100 mg of vitamin C.

Supplements may also be recommended in other cases. Women with heavy menstrual flows may need extra iron to compensate for the monthly loss. Some vegetari-

ans may need supplemental calcium, iron, zinc, and vitamin B-12, depending on their food choices. Newborns need a single dose of vitamin K, which must be administered under the direction of a physician. People who consume few calories, who have certain diseases, or who take certain medications may need specific vitamin and mineral supplements; such supplement decisions must be made by a physician because some vitamins and minerals counteract the actions of certain medications.

In deciding whether to take a vitamin and mineral supplement, consider whether you already regularly consume a fortified breakfast cereal. Many breakfast cereals contain almost as many nutrients as a vitamin pill! If you do decide to take a supplement, choose a balanced formulation that contains 50–100% of the Daily Value for vitamins and minerals. Avoid supplements containing large doses of particular nutrients. See pp. 246–247 for more on choosing and using supplements.

Daily Values Because the DRIs are far too cumbersome to use as a basis for food labels, the U.S. Food and Drug Administration developed another set of dietary standards, the **Daily Values.** The Daily Values are based on several different sets of guidelines and include standards for fat, cholesterol, carbohydrate, dietary fiber, and selected vitamins and minerals. The Daily Values represent appropriate intake levels for a 2000-calorie diet. The percent Daily Value shown on a food label shows how well that food contributes to your recommended daily intake. Food labels are described in detail later in the chapter.

The Food Guide Pyramid

The Food Guide Pyramid is a food-group plan developed by the U.S. Department of Agriculture that gives a recommended number of servings for five different major food groups (Figure 8.4). A range of servings is given for each group: The smaller number is for people who consume about 1600 calories a day, such as many sedentary women; the larger number is for those who consume about 2800 calories a day, such as active men. Serving sizes and examples of foods are described below for each group. The fundamental principles of the Food Guide Pyramid are moderation, variety, and balance—a theme echoed throughout this chapter.

It is important to choose a variety of foods within each group because different foods have different combinations of nutrients: for example, within the vegetable group, potatoes are high in vitamin C, and spinach is a rich source of vitamin A. Foods also vary in their amount of calories and nutrients. People who do not need many calories should focus on nutrient-dense foods within each group (foods that are high in nutrients relative to the number of calories they contain). For example, whole-grain bread is more nutrient-dense than white bread, and 100% orange juice is more nutrient-dense than an orange-flavored drink. Many foods you eat contain servings from more than one food group.

Terms
V̇i̇w

Daily Values A simplified version of the RDAs used on food labels; also included are values for nutrients with no established RDA.

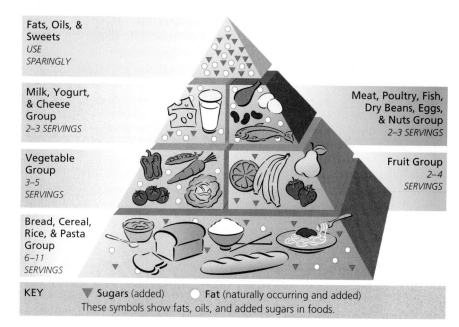

Fats, Oils, &
Sweets
*USE
SPARINGLY*

Milk, Yogurt,
& Cheese
Group
2–3 SERVINGS

Meat, Poultry, Fish,
Dry Beans, Eggs,
& Nuts Group
2–3 SERVINGS

Vegetable
Group
*3–5
SERVINGS*

Fruit Group
*2–4
SERVINGS*

Bread, Cereal,
Rice, & Pasta
Group
*6–11
SERVINGS*

KEY   ▼ Sugars (added)   ○ Fat (naturally occurring and added)
These symbols show fats, oils, and added sugars in foods.

Figure 8.4   The Food Guide Pyramid: A guide to daily food choices. The Pyramid is an outline of what to eat each day—not a rigid prescription, but a general guide that lets you choose a healthful diet that's right for you. It calls for eating a variety of foods to get the nutrients you need and at the same time the right amount of calories to maintain a healthy weight. The Pyramid also focuses on fat because many Americans eat too much fat, especially saturated fat.   SOURCE: USDA. Center for Nutrition Policy and Information. 1996. *Food Guide Pyramid.* USDA Home and Garden Bulletin no. 252.

The USDA Pyramid is not universally accepted. Critics say that its advice is too general and that it doesn't differentiate enough between sources of fat, protein, and carbohydrate. (The Dietary Guidelines, described in the next section, address some of these issues, but they are not reflected in the Pyramid graphic.) In addition, many other countries have their own dietary guidelines. Alternatives to the basic USDA Pyramid and food-group plan have been proposed by a variety of organizations and experts—to address its perceived shortcomings and to adapt its advice to special populations. Three alternative food plans appear in the Nutrition Resources section at the end of the chapter: a food pyramid for vegetarians, the Harvard Healthy Eating Pyramid, and Canada's Food Guide to Healthy Eating.

The USDA began the process of revising its own basic pyramid in 2003; the new version is scheduled for release in 2005. Information on some of the key proposed changes to the basic USDA pyramid appears in the discussion of the basic food groups. For more on the current pyramid, the 2005 version of the pyramid, and alternative pyramids for special populations such as young children and people choosing particular ethnic diets, visit the *Fit and Well* Online Learning Center and/or contact the USDA's Center for Nutrition Policy and Promotion (see For Further Exploration at the end of the chapter).

Food Guide Pyramid Serving Sizes   The number of servings recommended for each group in the Food Guide Pyramid is based on specific serving sizes that may be more or less than your own typical portion sizes and the serving sizes listed on food labels. For example, one Food Guide Pyramid serving of pasta is ½ cup; if your portion at a meal is 1½ cups of pasta, it would count as 3 servings toward your daily total from the breads, cereal, rice, and pasta food group. One Food Guide Pyramid serving of

french fries is about 10 small fries; most restaurant portions are considerably larger. When evaluating your current diet or planning dietary changes, it is very important to consider the serving sizes given in the pyramid. If you are one of the many people who have trouble identifying an ounce of cereal or a half-cup of rice, see the strategies in the box "Judging Serving Sizes" on p. 236. Additional tools and assessments relating to servings sizes can be found on the Online Learning Center.

Bread, Cereals, Rice, and Pasta (6–11 Servings)
Foods from this group are usually low in fat and rich in complex carbohydrates, dietary fiber (if grains are unrefined), and many vitamins and minerals, including thiamin, riboflavin, iron, niacin, folate, and zinc. Although 6–11 servings may seem like a large amount of food, many people eat several servings at a time. A single serving is the equivalent of the following:

- 1 slice of bread or half a hamburger bun, English muffin, or bagel
- 1 small roll, biscuit, or muffin
- 1 ounce of ready-to-eat cereal
- ½ cup cooked cereal, rice, or pasta
- 5–6 small or 2–3 large crackers
- 1 7-inch corn or flour tortilla

Choose foods that are typically made with little fat or sugars (bread, rice, pasta) over those that are high in fat and sugars (croissants, chips, cookies, doughnuts). For maximum nutrition, choose 3–5 servings per day from whole grains, such as whole-wheat bread, high-fiber cereal, whole-wheat pasta, and brown rice.

Vegetables (3–5 Servings)   Vegetables are rich in carbohydrates, dietary fiber, vitamin A, vitamin C, folate, magnesium, and other nutrients. They are also naturally

Studies have shown that most people underestimate the size of their food portions, in many cases by as much as 50%. If you need to retrain your eye, try using measuring cups and spoons and an inexpensive kitchen scale when you eat at home. With a little practice, you'll learn the difference between 3 and 8 ounces of chicken or meat and what a half-cup of rice really looks like. For quick estimates, use these equivalents:

- 1 teaspoon of margarine = the tip of your thumb

- 1 ounce of cheese = your thumb, four dice stacked together, or an ice cube

- 3 ounces of chicken or meat = a deck of cards or an audio-cassette tape

- ½ cup of rice or cooked vegetables = an ice cream scoop or one-third of a soda can

- 2 tablespoons of peanut butter = a Ping-Pong ball or large marshmallow

- 1 cup of pasta = a small fist or a tennis ball

- 1 medium potato = a computer mouse

- 1 2-ounce bagel = a hockey puck or yo-yo

- 1 2-ounce muffin or roll = a plum or a large egg

- 1 medium fruit (apple or orange) = a baseball

- ¼ cup nuts = a golf ball

- small cookie or cracker = a poker chip

low in fat. A serving of vegetables is equivalent to the following:

- 1 cup raw leafy vegetables
- ½ cup raw or cooked vegetables
- ½ cup tomato sauce
- ¾ cup vegetable juice
- ½ cup cooked dry beans (legumes)
- 1 cup bean or vegetable soup

Because vegetables vary in the nutrients they provide, it is important to consume a variety of types of vegetables to obtain maximum nutrition. Many Americans consume only a few different types of vegetables, with white potatoes (baked or served as french fries) being the most popular. To help boost variety, initial proposals for the 2005 version of the Food Guide Pyramid broke the vegetables group into five subgroups, with suggested weekly intakes for each subgroup. Try to consume at least one serving from each of the following vegetable groups on most days of the week:

- Dark-green vegetables like spinach, chard, collards, broccoli, romaine, and turnip and mustard greens

- Deep-yellow and orange vegetables like carrots, winter squash, sweet potatoes, and pumpkin

- Legumes like pinto beans, kidney beans, black beans, lentils, chickpeas, and tofu; legumes can be counted as servings of vegetables *or* as alternatives to meat

- Starchy vegetables like corn, green peas, and white potatoes

- Other vegetables; tomatoes, bell peppers (red, orange, yellow, or green), green beans, and cruciferous vegetables like cauliflower are good choices

Fruits (2–4 Servings) Like vegetables, fruits are rich in carbohydrates, dietary fiber, and many vitamins, especially vitamin C. They are low in fat and sodium. The serving sizes used in the Pyramid are as follows:

- 1 medium (apple, banana, peach, orange, pear) or 2 small (apricot, plum) whole fruit(s)

- 1 melon wedge
- ½ cup berries, cherries, or grapes
- ½ grapefruit
- ½ cup chopped, cooked, canned, or frozen fruit
- ¾ cup fruit juice (100% juice)
- ¼ cup dried fruit

Good choices from this group are citrus fruits and juices, melons, pears, apples, bananas, and berries. Choose whole fruits often—they are higher in fiber and often lower in calories than fruit juices. Fruit *juices* typically contain more nutrients than fruit *drinks*. For canned fruits, choose those packed in their own juice rather than in syrup.

Milk, Yogurt, and Cheese (2–3 Servings) Foods from this group are high in protein, carbohydrate, calcium, riboflavin, and vitamin D. To limit the fat in your diet, choose servings of low-fat or nonfat items from this group:

- 1 cup milk or yogurt
- 1½ ounces cheese
- 2 ounces processed cheese

Cottage cheese is lower in calcium than most other cheeses, and 1 cup of cottage cheese counts as only half a serving for this food group. Ice cream is also lower in calcium than many other dairy products (½ cup is equivalent to ⅓ serving); in addition, it is high in sugar and fat.

Meat, Poultry, Fish, Dry Beans, Eggs, and Nuts (2–3 Servings) This food group provides protein, niacin, iron, vitamin B-6, zinc, and thiamin; the animal foods in the group also provide vitamin B-12. The Pyramid recommends 2–3 servings each day of foods from this group. The total amount of these servings should be the equivalent of 5–7 ounces of cooked lean meat, poultry, or fish a day. Many people misjudge what makes up a single serving for this food group:

- 2–3 ounces cooked lean meat, poultry, or fish (an average hamburger or a medium chicken breast half is about 3 ounces; 4 slices of bologna, 6 slices of hard salami, or ½ cup of drained canned tuna counts as about 2 ounces)

- The following portions of nonmeat foods are equivalent to 1 ounce of lean meat: ½ cup cooked dry beans (if not counted as a vegetable), 1 egg, 2 tablespoons peanut butter, ⅓ cup nuts, ¼ cup seeds, and ½ cup tofu

One egg at breakfast, a cup of pinto beans at lunch, and a hamburger at dinner would add up to the equivalent of 6 ounces of lean meat for the day. To limit your intake of fat and saturated fat, choose lean cuts of meat and skinless poultry, eat nuts and seeds in moderation, and watch your serving sizes carefully. Choose at least one serving of such plant proteins as black beans, lentils, or tofu every day.

Fats, Oils, and Sweets The tip of the Pyramid includes fats, oils, and sweets—foods such as salad dressings, oils, butter, margarine, gravy, mayonnaise, soft drinks, sugar, candy, jellies and jams, syrups, and sweet desserts. Foods from the Pyramid tip provide calories but few nutrients; they should not replace foods from the other groups. The total amount of fats, oils, and sweets you consume should be determined by your overall energy needs.

The colored triangles and circles in the Pyramid appear in all the other food groups to remind you that food choices in those groups can also be high in fats and added sugars. ("Added sugars" are sugars added in processing, not those found naturally in fruits and milk.) Foods that come from animals (the meat and milk groups) are naturally higher in fats than foods that come from plants, which is why it's important to choose lean meats and low-fat dairy products. Fruits, vegetables, and grains are naturally lower in fat, but they are often prepared in ways that make them higher-fat choices, such as french fries, baked potatoes with sour cream and cheese, fettuccine Alfredo, and baked goods like cookies and pies. Added sugars are common in the milk group (ice cream, sweetened yogurt), the fruit group (canned fruit in syrup), and the grain group (bakery goods). Reduced-fat versions of prepared foods are often *very* high in added sugars and consequently just as high in calories as their full-fat versions.

The Food Guide Pyramid suggests fairly strict limits on added sugars: 6 teaspoons in a diet with 1600 calories per day, 18 teaspoons in a diet with 2800 calories per day. Many Americans exceed the recommended limit for added sugar intake. Initial proposals for the 2005 version of the Pyramid also include suggested limits for "additional fats," defined as fats that are added in cooking, at the table, or when higher fat items are selected from the food groups (for example, whole milk instead of fat-free milk). Stressing the importance of favoring unsaturated fats over those that are saturated, the proposed limits for additional fats are divided into two groups—solid fats and oils and soft margarines—and lower limits are suggested for solid fats. For example, in a 2000-calorie diet,

a limit of 40 g of additional fats is suggested, with 60% coming in the form of oils and soft margarines.

The Current U.S. Diet Versus the Pyramid The average American diet currently includes more fat and added sugars than recommended. You can moderate your fat intake by making low-fat choices from each group and minimizing the use of fat in cooking or as toppings such as sour cream and heavy sauces. Consumption of large amounts of sugars adds empty calories to the diet and can make weight management more difficult.

Analysis of the average diet of Americans has revealed that the number of servings from the fruit, dairy, and meat groups is below the recommended ranges, and servings from the grain and vegetable groups are near the bottom of the recommended ranges (Table 8.5, p. 238). Overconsumption of fat and added sugars leaves fewer calories available for healthier food choices from the five major food groups. For example, the average daily diet among American women includes about 9 teaspoons (36 grams) of added sugars and 5 grams of fat above recommended limits. The 200 calories in these extra sugars and fats could be better used to increase the number of servings from the food groups for which women typically fall short of Pyramid recommendations.

General strategies for controlling intake of fat and added sugars include choosing lower-fat foods within each food group, eating fewer foods that are high in sugar and fat and low in other nutrients, and limiting the amount of fats and sugars added to foods during cooking or at the table. Consider the nutrient density of your food choices, and favor foods that are rich in nutrients relative to the number of calories they contain.

The Food Guide Pyramid is a general guide to what you should eat every day. By eating a balanced variety of foods from each of the six food groups and including some plant proteins, you can ensure that your daily diet is adequate in all nutrients. A diet using low-fat food choices contains only about 1600 calories but meets all known nutritional needs, except possibly for iron in some women who have heavy menstrual periods. For these women, foods fortified in iron, such as breakfast cereals, can make up the deficit.

Dietary Guidelines for Americans

To provide further guidance for choosing a healthy diet, the U.S. Department of Agriculture (USDA) and the U.S. Department of Health and Human Services (DHHS) have issued Dietary Guidelines for Americans, most recently in 2000. (The Dietary Guidelines are being revised along with the Food Guide Pyramid, and an updated version is expected to be released in 2005; for more information, visit the Web site for the USDA's Center for Nutrition Policy and Promotion.) Following these guidelines promotes health and reduces risk for chronic diseases, including heart disease, cancer, diabetes, stroke, osteoporosis, and

Table 8.5   *Food Guide Pyramid Recommendations Compared with the Average American Diet*

	RECOMMENDED DIETS AT THREE CALORIE LEVELS[a]			AVERAGE AMERICAN DIET	
				Women (1600 calories)	Men (2400 calories)
	1600	2200	2800		
Grain group (servings)	6	9	11	5.7	7.9
Vegetable group (servings)	3	4	5	2.9	3.9
Fruit group (servings)	2	3	4	1.5	1.5
Dairy group (servings)[b]	2–3	2–3	2–3	1.1	1.5
Meat group (ounces)[c]	5	6	7	4.0	6.7
Total fat (grams)[d]	53	73	93	58.1	90.1
Total added sugars (teaspoons)[d,e]	6	12	18	15.4	22.2

[a]The bottom of the recommended range of servings (1600 calories) is about right for many sedentary women and older adults. The middle range (2200 calories) is about right for most children, teenage girls, active women, and many sedentary men. The top of the range (2800 calories) is about right for teenage boys, many active men, and some very active women.

[b]Women who are pregnant or lactating, teenagers, and young adults to age 24 need 3 servings.

[c]The Pyramid recommends 2–3 servings a day, the equivalent of 5–7 ounces of cooked lean meat, poultry, or fish.

[d]Values for total fat and added sugars include fat and added sugars that are in food choices from the five major food groups as well as fat and added sugars from foods in the Fats, Oils, and Sweets group. The total for added sugars does not include sugars that occur naturally in foods such as fruit and milk. The recommended fat totals are based on a limit of 30% of total calories as fat.

[e]A teaspoon of sugar is equivalent to 4 grams (16 calories).

SOURCES: USDA Agricultural Research Service. 2000. *Pyramid Servings Intakes: CNRG Table Set No. 1.* Beltsville, Md.: Community Nutrition Research Group. Shaw, A., et al. 1997. *Using the Food Guide Pyramid: A Resource for Nutrition Educators.* Washington, D.C.: USDA Center for Nutrition Policy and Promotion.

obesity. Ten guidelines are provided, organized under three messages, the "ABCs for Health":

Aim for fitness.

Build a healthy base.

Choose sensibly.

Here is a brief summary of the guidelines.

Aim for Fitness   The two guidelines in this category emphasize that a lifestyle combining sensible eating with regular physical activity promotes long-term health and fitness and enables people to enjoy life and feel their best.

AIM FOR A HEALTHY WEIGHT   Evaluate your body weight in terms of body mass index (BMI); see Chapter 6 for instructions on how to determine your BMI. If your current weight is healthy, aim to avoid weight gain. Do so by eating vegetables, fruits, and whole grains with little added fat or sugar; also focus on selecting sensible portion sizes. If you are overweight, first aim to prevent further weight gain, and then lose weight to improve your health. Plan to lose weight gradually—about 10% of your weight over about 6 months—through a combination of sensible eating, physical activity, and behavior change. Loss of ½ to 2 pounds a week is usually safe. Your health is more likely to improve over the long term if you achieve and maintain a healthy weight than if you lose and regain weight several times. But even if

you have regained weight in the past, it's worthwhile to try again.

BE PHYSICALLY ACTIVE EVERY DAY   Become active if you are inactive, and maintain or increase physical activity if you are already active. Aim to accumulate at least 30 minutes (adults) or 60 minutes (children) of moderate physical activity on most days, preferably every day. You can do the activity all at once or spread it out over two to three periods during the day. If you already get 30 minutes of physical activity daily, you can gain even more health benefits by increasing the intensity or duration of your activity. Aerobic activities and activities for strength and flexibility are especially beneficial.

Physical activity and nutrition work together for better health. For example, physical activity increases the amount of calories you use, which in turn makes it easier to get the nutrients you need. For those who have intentionally lost weight, being active makes it easier to maintain the weight loss. However, to maintain a healthy weight after weight loss, adults will likely need more than 30 minutes of activity daily.

Build a Healthy Base   The four guidelines in this category provide a foundation for healthy eating.

LET THE PYRAMID GUIDE YOUR FOOD CHOICES   To ensure that you get all the nutrients and other substances you need, choose the recommended number of daily servings from each of the five major food groups shown in the Food Guide Pyramid (see Figure 8.4). Healthy eating patterns start with plant foods, represented in the three food groups at the base of the Pyramid: grains, vegetables, and fruits. Plan your meals around a variety of foods from these groups, keeping a close eye on serving sizes. Be flexible and adventurous—try new choices in place of some of the less nutritious foods you usually eat. Everyone, especially adolescent girls and women, should take special care to meet their recommended intakes for calcium, iron, and folic acid.

People's food choices are affected by culture, family background, religion, moral beliefs, the cost and availability of food, life experience, food intolerances, and allergies. The Pyramid provides a good guide to healthy eating no matter how the foods are prepared or combined. However, if you avoid all foods from any of the five major groups, be sure to get enough nutrients from other groups. For example, if you eat few dairy products, choose other foods that are good sources of calcium and make sure you get enough vitamin D. If you avoid animal products, be sure you get enough iron, vitamin B-12, calcium, and zinc. Some people may need to consume fortified foods or take a vitamin or mineral supplement to meet a specific nutrient need; however, you should not depend on supplements to meet your usual nutritional needs.

EAT A VARIETY OF GRAINS DAILY, ESPECIALLY WHOLE GRAINS Grains such as wheat, oats, corn, and rice are rich in complex carbohydrates and tend to be low in fat; whole grains provide more fiber and nutrients than refined grains. Make grains the foundation of your diet—eat six or more servings daily. If your calorie needs are low, eat only six servings of a sensible size. Include several servings of whole grains daily, choosing a variety of grains, such as whole wheat, brown rice, oats, and whole corn. Prepare or choose grain products with little added saturated fat and sugar.

EAT A VARIETY OF FRUITS AND VEGETABLES DAILY Different fruits and vegetables are rich in different nutrients, so it's important to choose a variety. For example, carrots, dark-green leafy vegetables, and cantaloupe are excellent sources of carotenoids; citrus fruits, potatoes, and broccoli are rich in vitamin C; spinach, legumes, and orange juice are high in folate; and bananas, winter squash, and dried fruits are good sources of potassium. Fresh fruits and vegetables, especially when eaten with the peel, are also good sources of dietary fiber.

Eat at least two servings of fruit and three servings of vegetables daily. Choose fresh, frozen, dried, or canned forms and a variety of colors and kinds. Favor dark-green leafy vegetables, bright orange fruits and vegetables, and cooked dried peas and beans.

KEEP FOOD SAFE TO EAT Safe foods are those that pose little risk from harmful bacteria, viruses, parasites, or chemical contaminants. It is especially important to be careful with perishable foods such as eggs, meats, poultry, fish, shellfish, milk products, and fresh fruits and vegetables. If food has been left out for too long or refrigerated for too long, it may not be safe to eat even if it looks and smells fine. Refer to the section "Preventing and Treating Foodborne Illness" on p. 248 for specific food safety tips.

Choose Sensibly The four guidelines in this category help you make food choices that promote health and reduce the risk of certain chronic diseases.

CHOOSE A DIET LOW IN SATURATED FAT AND CHOLESTEROL AND MODERATE IN TOTAL FAT A diet low in saturated fat (less than 10% of daily calories) and cholesterol (less than 300 milligrams per day) helps keep blood cholesterol levels low and reduces the risk of cardiovascular disease. Moderate total fat intake also helps with weight control. The Dietary Guidelines suggest a limit of 30% of total calories as fat, while the Food and Nutrition Board allows up to 35%. The Food and Nutrition Board also recommends keeping intake of saturated and trans fats and cholesterol as low as possible. Refer to the box "Reducing the Fat in Your Diet" on p. 240 for specific strategies for meeting these guidelines.

Cholesterol is found only in animal foods. To limit your cholesterol intake, follow the Pyramid recommendations for consumption of animal foods and pay particular attention to serving sizes. In addition, limit your intake of foods that are particularly high in cholesterol, including egg yolks, dairy fats, and liver and other organ meats. Food labels provide the fat, saturated fat, and cholesterol content of foods.

CHOOSE BEVERAGES AND FOODS TO MODERATE YOUR INTAKE OF SUGARS Sugar doesn't cause hyperactivity, but it does promote tooth decay and it may lower HDL cholesterol levels. In addition, many foods high in sugar are relatively

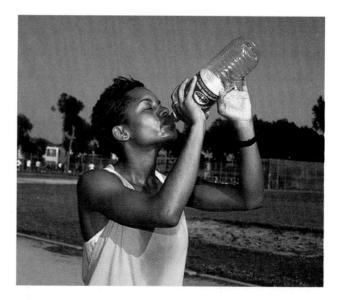

No matter what your dietary choices or challenges, you need to include water and other beverages in your daily diet. Drink about 9–13 cups of fluid a day—more if you live in a hot climate or if you exercise vigorously.

Your overall goal is to limit total fat intake to no more than 35% of total calories. Within that limit, favor unsaturated fats from vegetable oils, nuts, and fish over saturated and trans fats from animal products and foods made with hydrogenated vegetable oils or shortening. Saturated and trans fat intake should be kept as low as possible within a nutritionally adequate diet.

- Be moderate in your consumption of foods high in fat, including fast food, commercially prepared baked goods and desserts, deep-fried foods, meat, poultry, nuts and seeds, and regular dairy products.

- When you do eat high-fat foods, limit your portion sizes, and balance your intake with foods low in fat.

- Choose lean cuts of meat, and trim any visible fat from meat before and after cooking. Remove skin from poultry before or after cooking.

- Drink fat-free or low-fat milk instead of whole milk, and use lower-fat varieties in puddings, soups, and baked products. Substitute plain low-fat yogurt, blender-whipped low-fat cottage cheese, or buttermilk for sour cream.

- To reduce saturated and trans fat, use vegetable oil instead of butter or margarine. Use tub or squeeze margarine instead of stick margarine. Look for margarines that are free of trans fats.

- Season vegetables, seafood, and meats with herbs and spices rather than with creamy sauces, butter, or margarine.

- Try lemon juice on salad, or use a yogurt-based salad dressing instead of mayonnaise or sour cream dressings.

- Steam, boil, bake, or microwave vegetables, or stir-fry them in a small amount of vegetable oil.

- Roast, bake, or broil meat, poultry, or fish so that fat drains away as the food cooks.

- Use a nonstick pan for cooking so that added fat will be unnecessary; use a vegetable spray for frying.

- Chill broths from meat or poultry until the fat becomes solid. Spoon off the fat before using the broth.

- Substitute egg whites for whole eggs when baking; limit the number of egg yolks when scrambling eggs.

- Choose fruits as desserts most often.

- Eat a low-fat vegetarian main dish at least once a week.

---

high in calories but low in other nutrients; consuming excess calories from added sugars may contribute to weight gain or lower consumption of more nutritious foods. The Pyramid recommends no more than about 6 teaspoons (24 g) of added sugars a day if you eat 1600 calories, 12 teaspoons (48 g) at 2200 calories, or 18 teaspoons (72 g) at 2800 calories. Most Americans consume much more than this—one can of regular soda, the leading source of added sugars in the American diet, supplies about 10 teaspoons of sugar. On average, Americans consume more than 50 gallons of soda and 25 pounds of candy per year.

To reduce sugar consumption, cut back on soft drinks, candies, sweet desserts (cakes, cookies, pies), fruit drinks, and other foods high in added sugars. A food is likely high in sugar if one of the following ingredients appears first or second in the list of ingredients or if several are listed: sugar (any type, including beet, brown, raw, and cane), corn syrup or sweetener, fruit juice concentrate, honey, malt syrup, molasses, syrup, cane juice, or dextrose, fructose, glucose, lactose, maltose, mannitol, or sucrose. Try drinking water rather than sweetened drinks and don't let sodas and other sweets crowd out more nutritious foods, such as low-fat milk and fruit.

CHOOSE AND PREPARE FOODS WITH LESS SALT   Many people can reduce their chance of developing high blood pressure by consuming less salt. Salt is made up of the minerals sodium and chloride, both of which are essential for normal body functioning. However, we need only a small amount of salt to meet our body's daily requirement, and consuming excess salt raises blood pressure. The Dietary Guidelines suggest that adults reduce their sodium intake to no more than 2400 mg per day, the equivalent of about one teaspoon of salt; most Americans currently consume more than this amount. In 2004, the Food and Nutrition Board recommended an even lower intake; their report stated that adults 18–50 years of age need only 1500 mg of sodium per day, an amount equivalent to about two-thirds of a teaspoon of salt. The Food and Nutrition Board also set a UL (upper limit) of 2300 mg per day. It is estimated that more than 95% of American men and 75% of American women consume sodium in excess of this upper limit.

Most sodium in the American diet comes from processed and prepared foods; some may also be added during cooking or at the table. To lower your intake of salt, choose fresh or plain frozen meat, poultry, seafood, and vegetables most often; they are lower in salt than more processed forms. Check and compare the sodium content in processed foods, including luncheon meats, frozen dinners, cheeses, soups, salad dressings, sauces, and canned vegetables and mixed dishes. Limit intake of heavily salted snack foods like chips. Add less salt during cooking and at the table, and limit your use of high-sodium condiments like soy sauce, ketchup, mustard, pickles, and olives. Use lemon juice, herbs, and spices instead of salt to enhance the flavor of foods. (See Appendixes B and C for the sodium content of many foods.)

IF YOU DRINK ALCOHOLIC BEVERAGES, DO SO IN MODERATION   Alcoholic beverages supply calories but few nutrients; excess alcohol alters judgment and can lead to dependency and other serious health problems (see

Chapter 13). Drinking in moderation is defined as no more than one drink a day for women and no more than two drinks a day for men. People who should not drink at all include individuals who cannot restrict their drinking to moderate levels, women who are or may become pregnant, individuals who plan to drive or operate machinery, and individuals taking medications that can interact with alcohol. If you choose to drink alcoholic beverages, do so sensibly, moderately, and with meals; never drink in situations where it may put you or others at risk.

> **MOTIVATION FOR CHANGE!**   Maintaining a healthy diet can be a challenge in an environment filled with convenient but less-than-ideal food choices. To help increase your commitment and motivation, complete an analysis of the short-term and long-term advantages and disadvantages of your current diet and your goal diet (see Chapter 1 for tips on completing this type of analysis). Keep your list of the advantages of change handy to help overcome challenging situations.

The Vegetarian Alternative

Some people choose a diet with one essential difference from the diets we've already described: Foods of animal origin (meat, poultry, fish, eggs, milk) are eliminated or restricted. Many do so for health reasons; vegetarian diets tend to be lower in saturated fat, cholesterol, and animal protein and higher in complex carbohydrates, dietary fiber, folate, vitamins C and E, carotenoids, and phytochemicals. Some people adopt a vegetarian diet out of concern for the environment, for financial considerations, or for reasons related to ethics or religion.

Types of Vegetarian Diets   There are various vegetarian styles; the wider the variety of the diet eaten, the easier it is to meet nutritional needs. **Vegans** eat only plant foods. **Lacto-vegetarians** eat plant foods and dairy products. **Lacto-ovo-vegetarians** eat plant foods, dairy products, and eggs. According to recent polls, about 5 million American adults never eat meat, poultry, or fish and fall into one of these three groups. Others can be categorized as **partial vegetarians, semivegetarians,** or **pescovegetarians;** these individuals eat plant foods, dairy products, eggs, and usually a small selection of poultry, fish, and other seafood. Many other people choose vegetarian meals frequently but are not strictly vegetarian. Including some animal protein (such as dairy products) in a vegetarian diet makes planning easier, but it is not necessary.

A Food Pyramid for Vegetarians   The basic USDA pyramid can be adapted for use by vegetarians with only a few key modifications (see Figure 1 in the Nutrition Resources section at the end of the chapter):

- Bread, cereal, rice, and pasta group (6–11 servings per day)

- Vegetable group (3–5 servings per day)
- Fruit group (2–4 servings per day)
- Milk, yogurt, and cheese group (0–3 servings per day); vegans and other vegetarians who do not consume any dairy products must find other rich sources of calcium (see below)
- Dry beans, nuts, seeds, eggs, and meat substitutes group (2–3 servings per day); this group includes such foods as soy milk, legumes, eggs or egg whites, nuts, seeds, tofu (soybean curd), tempeh (a cultured soy product), and peanut butter

A healthy vegetarian diet emphasizes a wide variety of plant foods. Although plant proteins are generally incomplete, choosing a variety of plant foods will supply all of the essential amino acids. Choosing minimally processed and unrefined foods will maximize nutrient value and provide ample dietary fiber. Daily consumption of a variety of plant foods in amounts that meet total energy needs can provide all needed nutrients, except vitamin B-12 and possibly vitamin D. Strategies for obtaining these and other nutrients of concern include the following:

- *Vitamin B-12* is found naturally only in animal foods; if dairy products and eggs are limited or avoided, B-12 can be obtained from fortified foods such as ready-to-eat cereals, soy beverages, meat substitutes, and special yeast products or from supplements.
- *Vitamin D* can be obtained by spending 5–15 minutes a day out in the sun, by consuming vitamin D-fortified products like ready-to-eat cereals and soy or rice milk, or by taking a supplement.
- *Calcium* is found in legumes, tofu processed with calcium, dark-green leafy vegetables, nuts, tortillas made from lime-processed corn, and fortified orange juice, soy milk, bread, and other foods.
- *Iron* is found in whole grains, fortified bread and breakfast cereals, dried fruits, green leafy vegetables, nuts and seeds, legumes, and soy foods. The iron in plant foods is more difficult for the body to absorb than the iron from animal sources; consuming a good source of vitamin C with most meals is helpful because vitamin C improves iron absorption.
- *Zinc* is found in whole grains, nuts, legumes, and soy foods.

It takes a little planning and common sense to put together a good vegetarian diet. If you are a vegetarian

> **vegan** A vegetarian who eats no animal products at all.
>
> **lacto-vegetarian** A vegetarian who includes milk and cheese products in the diet.
>
> **lacto-ovo-vegetarian** A vegetarian who eats no meat, poultry, or fish, but does eat eggs and milk products.
>
> **partial vegetarian, semivegetarian,** or **pescovegetarian** A vegetarian who includes eggs, dairy products, and small amounts of poultry and seafood in the diet.
>
> Terms
>
> **W̶w̶**

or are considering becoming one, devote some extra time and thought to your diet. It's especially important that you eat as wide a variety of foods as possible to ensure that all your nutritional needs are satisfied. Consulting with a registered dietitian will make your planning even easier. Vegetarian diets for children, teens, and pregnant and lactating women warrant professional guidance.

Dietary Challenges for Special Population Groups

The Food Guide Pyramid and Dietary Guidelines for Americans provide a basis that everyone can use to create a healthy diet. However, some population groups face special dietary challenges.

Women   Women tend to be smaller and to weigh less than men, meaning they have lower energy needs and therefore consume fewer calories. Because of this, women have more difficulty getting adequate amounts of all the essential nutrients and need to focus on nutrient-dense foods. Two nutrients of special concern are calcium and iron, minerals for which many women fail to meet the RDAs. Low calcium intake may be linked to the development of osteoporosis in later life. The *Healthy People 2010* report sets a goal of increasing from 40% to 75% the proportion of women age 20–49 who meet the dietary recommendation for calcium. Nonfat and low-fat dairy products and fortified cereal, bread, and orange juice are good choices. Iron is also a concern: Menstruating women have higher iron requirements than other groups, and a lack of iron in the diet can lead to iron-deficiency anemia. Lean red meat, green leafy vegetables, and fortified breakfast cereals are good sources of iron. As discussed earlier, all women capable of becoming pregnant should consume adequate folic acid from fortified foods and/or supplements.

Men   Men are seldom thought of as having nutritional deficiencies because they generally have high-calorie diets. However, many men have a diet that does not follow the Food Guide Pyramid but that includes more red meat and fewer fruits, vegetables, and grains than recommended. This dietary pattern is linked to heart disease and some types of cancer. A high intake of calories can lead to weight gain in the long term if a man's activity level decreases as he ages. Men should use the Food Guide Pyramid as a basis for their overall diet and focus on increasing their consumption of fruits, vegetables, and grains to obtain vitamins, minerals, dietary fiber, and phytochemicals. The "5 A Day for Better Health" program created by the National Cancer Institute and Department of Health and Human Services to promote increased intake of fruits and vegetables has been adapted to create the "Shoot for 9 for Better Health" message for men; for strategies and guidelines for consuming more fruits and vegetables, visit http://5aday.gov/9aday.

College Students   Foods that are convenient for college students are not always the healthiest choices. It is easy for students who eat in buffet-style dining halls to overeat, and the foods offered are not necessarily high in essential nutrients and low in fat. The same is true of meals at fast-food restaurants, another convenient source of quick and inexpensive meals for busy students. Although no food is entirely "bad," consuming a wide variety of foods is critical for a healthy diet. See the box "Eating Strategies for College Students" for tips on making healthy eating convenient and affordable.

Older Adults   As people age, they tend to become less active, so they require fewer calories to maintain their weight. At the same time, the absorption of nutrients tends to be lower in older adults because of age-related changes in the digestive tract. Thus, they must consume nutrient-dense foods to meet their nutritional requirements. As discussed earlier, foods fortified with vitamin B-12 and/or B-12 supplements are recommended for people over age 50. Because constipation is a common problem, consuming foods high in dietary fiber and obtaining adequate fluids are important goals.

Athletes   Key dietary concerns for athletes are meeting increased energy and fluid requirements for training and making healthy food choices throughout the day.

ENERGY INTAKE   Individuals engaged in vigorous training programs expend more energy (calories) than sedentary and moderately active individuals and may have energy needs ranging from 2000 to more than 6000 calories per day. For athletes, the American Dietetic Association recommends a diet with 60–65% of calories coming from carbohydrate, 10–15% from protein, and no more than 30% from fat. Athletes for whom maintaining low body weight and body fat is important—such as gymnasts, skaters, and wrestlers—should consume adequate calories and nutrients and avoid falling into unhealthy patterns of eating. The combination of low levels of body fat, high physical activity, disordered eating habits, and, in women, amenorrhea, is associated with stress fractures and other injuries and with osteoporosis. The female athlete triad was discussed in Chapter 6; see Chapter 9 for more on eating disorders.

CARBOHYDRATE   Endurance athletes involved in competitive events lasting longer than 90 minutes may benefit from increasing carbohydrate intake to 65–70% of total calories; this increase should come in the form of complex, rather than simple, carbohydrates. High carbohydrate intake builds and maintains muscle glycogen stores, resulting in greater endurance and delayed fatigue during competitive events. Some endurance athletes engage in "carbohydrate loading"—a practice that involves increasing carbohydrate intake in the days before a competition. Before exercise, the ACSM recommends that an active adult or athlete consume a meal or snack that is relatively

General Guidelines

- Eat slowly and enjoy your food. Set aside a separate time to eat. Don't eat while you study.

- Eat a colorful, varied diet. The more colorful your diet is, the more varied and rich in fruits and vegetables it will be. Many Americans eat few fruits and vegetables, despite the fact that these foods are typically inexpensive, delicious, rich in nutrients, and low in fat and calories. Don't limit your vegetable choices to french fries, which are typically high in saturated and trans fats.

- Consider nutrient density in your food choices, and avoid large servings of foods that provide calories but few essential nutrients. "Spend" your daily calorie budget wisely on healthy, nutrient-rich foods.

- Check out the labels and ingredient lists of foods you commonly eat so that you are aware of their general nutrient profile.

- Eat breakfast. You'll have more energy in the morning and be less likely to grab an unhealthy snack later on. Whole-grain cereals or whole-grain toast are excellent breakfast choices.

- Choose healthy snacks—fruits, vegetables, grains, and cereals—as often as you can.

- Drink water more often than soft drinks or other sweetened beverages. Rent a mini-refrigerator for your dorm room and stock up on healthy beverages.

- Pay attention to portion sizes. Read food labels carefully, and take special note of serving sizes and the total number of servings in the package. You may find that your favorite bottled drinks and packaged snack foods—which you treat as a single serving—actually provide multiple servings and that you are consuming more calories, fat, and added sugars than you realize.

- Combine physical activity with healthy eating. You'll look and feel better and have a much lower risk of many chronic diseases. Even a little exercise is better than none.

Eating in the Dining Hall

- Choose a meal plan that includes breakfast—and don't skip it.

- Accept that dining hall food is not going to be as good as home cooking. Find dishes that you like that are nutritious.

- If menus are posted or distributed, decide what you want to eat before getting in line and stick to your choices. Consider what you plan to do and eat for the rest of the day before making your choices.

- Ask for large servings of vegetables and small servings of meat and other high-fat main dishes. Build your meals around grains and vegetables.

- Try whole grains like brown rice, whole-wheat bread, and whole-grain cereals.

- Choose leaner poultry, fish, or bean dishes rather than high-fat meats and fried entrees.

- Ask that gravies and sauces be served on the side; limit your intake.

- Choose broth-based or vegetable soups rather than cream soups.

- At the salad bar, load up on leafy greens, beans, and fresh vegetables. Avoid mayonnaise-coated salads, bacon, croutons, and high-fat dressings. Put dressing on the side; dip your fork into it rather than pouring it over the salad.

- Drink nonfat milk, water, mineral water, or 100% fruit juice rather than heavily sweetened fruit drinks, whole milk, soft drinks, or beer.

- Choose fruit for dessert rather than pastries, cookies, or cakes.

- Do some research about the foods and preparation methods used in your dining hall or cafeteria. Discuss any suggestions you have with your food service manager.

Eating in Fast-Food Restaurants

- Most fast-food chains can provide a brochure with a nutritional breakdown of the foods on the menu. Ask for it and identify the healthiest options. (See also the information in Appendix C.)

- Order small single burgers with no cheese instead of double burgers with many toppings. If possible, ask for them broiled instead of fried.

- Ask for items to be prepared without mayonnaise, tartar sauce, sour cream, or other high-fat sauces. Ketchup, mustard, and fat-free mayonnaise or sour cream are better choices and are available at many fast-food restaurants.

- Choose whole-grain buns or bread for burgers, hot dogs, and sandwiches.

- Choose chicken items made from chicken breast, not processed chicken.

- Order vegetable pizzas without extra cheese.

- If you order french fries or onion rings, get the smallest size and/or share them with a friend.

Fast-food meals are a health concern not just because of what they typically provide—significant amounts of calories, fat, added sugars, and sodium—but also because of what they often lack—fiber and many vitamins and minerals. A large cheeseburger, large order of fries, and large (32 oz) nondiet soda may provide about 1600 calories, 75 grams of fat, and 30 teaspoons of added sugars. It is important to balance any fast-food meals you consume by choosing healthy, nutrient-rich foods during the rest of the day.

Eating on the Run

Are you chronically short of time? The following healthy and filling items can be packed for a quick snack or meal: fresh or dried fruit, fruit juices, raw fresh vegetables, plain bagels, bread sticks, whole-wheat fig bars, low-fat cheese sticks or cubes, low-fat crackers or granola bars, nonfat or low-fat yogurt, snack-size cereal boxes, pretzels, rice or corn cakes, plain popcorn, soup (if you have access to a microwave), or water.

high in carbohydrate, moderate in protein, and low in fat. Soon after exercise, particularly following a strenuous competition or training session, a mixed meal containing carbohydrates, protein, and fat should be consumed to replace muscle glycogen and provide amino acids for building and repairing muscle tissue. Consuming some simple carbohydrate immediately after exercise can help replenish glycogen stores in the liver and muscle.

PROTEIN   For endurance athletes, the ACSM recommends a protein intake of 1.2–1.4 grams of protein per kilogram (0.55–0.64 gram per pound) of body weight per day, up from the standard DRI of 0.8 gram per kilogram (0.36 gram per pound); for athletes engaged in heavy strength training, protein needs may be as high as 1.6–1.7 grams per kilogram (0.73–0.77 gram per pound) of body weight. This level of protein intake is easily obtainable from foods, however. A 160-pound athlete consuming 3500 calories per day needs to obtain only 12% of total calories to achieve the upper end of the protein range for endurance athletes. The average American diet includes about 16% of total calories as protein, and a balanced high-carbohydrate, moderate protein, moderate-fat diet can provide the nutrients athletes need.

There is no evidence that consuming supplements containing vitamins, minerals, protein, or specific amino acids will build muscle or improve sports performance. Strength and muscle are built with exercise, not extra protein, and carbohydrates provide the fuel needed for muscle-building exercise. Strenuous physical activity does increase the need for protein and some vitamins and minerals; however, the increased energy intake of athletes more than compensates for this increased need.

FLUIDS   Moderately active people should consume adequate fluids according to the guidelines in Table 8.4. People who exercise heavily and/or live in a hot climate need to consume additional fluids to maximize performance and prevent heat illness. For a strenuous endurance event, prepare yourself the day before by drinking plenty of fluid. On the day of the event, the ACSM recommends that you consume 14–22 oz (400–600 ml) of fluid about 2 hours before exercise, and then 6–12 oz (150–350 ml) of fluid every 15–20 minutes during exercise—or as much of this amount as you can tolerate. Afterwards, drink enough to replace lost fluids—16–24 oz for every pound of weight lost. (Weight loss during a workout or athletic event comes primarily from fluid loss through sweat; as described in Chapter 3, checking your weight can help you monitor your fluid balance.)

Water is a good choice for fluid replacement for workouts and events lasting less than 60–90 minutes, especially if you are trying to avoid the additional calories in many other beverages. However, for workouts or events lasting longer, a sports drink can be a good choice. These contain water, electrolytes, and carbohydrates. The advantage of sports drinks is that they can provide you with some extra energy (in the form of rapidly digestible carbohydrates that help maintain blood glucose levels) and replace electrolytes like sodium that are lost in sweat.

There have been rare instances of athletes consuming too much water and developing *hyponatremia* ("water intoxication"), a condition characterized by lung congestion, muscle weakness, and nervous system problems. Hyponatremia may result from consumption of too much water, too few electrolytes, or both; it is usually associated with water consumption during or after more than 4–6 hours of prolonged stressful exercise. Following the ACSM fluid guidelines above, including consumption of sports drinks containing electrolytes during long exercise sessions, can prevent hyponatremia.

People with Special Health Concerns   Many Americans have special health concerns that affect their dietary needs. For example, women who are pregnant or breastfeeding require extra calories, vitamins, and minerals. People with diabetes benefit from a well-balanced diet that is low in simple sugars, high in complex carbohydrates, and relatively rich in monounsaturated fats. And people with high blood pressure need to limit their sodium consumption and control their weight. If you have a health problem or concern that may require a special diet, discuss your situation with a physician or registered dietitian.

NUTRITIONAL PLANNING: MAKING INFORMED CHOICES ABOUT FOOD

Now that you know the nutrients you need and the amounts required for maximum wellness, you are almost ready to create a diet that works for you. Depending on your needs and dietary habits, you may have some specific areas of concern you want to address first, such as interpreting food labels, understanding food additives, or avoiding foodborne illnesses. We turn to these and other topics next.

Food Labels—A Closer Look

Consumers can get help in applying the principles of the Food Guide Pyramid and the Dietary Guidelines for Americans from food labels. Since 1994, all processed foods regulated by either the FDA or the USDA have included standardized nutrition information on their labels. Every food label shows serving sizes and the amount of fat, saturated fat, cholesterol, protein, dietary fiber, and sodium in each serving. To make intelligent choices about food, learn to read and understand food labels (see the box "Using Food Labels"). Research has shown that people who read food labels eat less fat.

Because most meat, poultry, fish, fruits, and vegetables are not processed, they were not covered by the 1994 law. You can obtain information on the nutrient content of these items from basic nutrition books, registered dietitians, nutrient analysis computer software, the World Wide Web, and the companies that produce or distribute

Food labels are designed to help consumers make food choices based on the nutrients that are most important to good health. In addition to listing nutrient content by weight, the label puts the information in the context of a daily diet of 2000 calories that includes no more than 65 grams of fat (approximately 30% of total calories). For example, if a serving of a particular product has 13 grams of fat, the label will show that the serving represents 20% of the daily fat allowance. If your daily diet contains fewer or more than 2000 calories, you need to adjust these calculations accordingly.

Food labels contain uniform serving sizes. This means that if you look at different brands of salad dressing, for example, you can compare calories and fat content based on the serving amount. (Food label serving sizes may be larger or smaller than Food Guide Pyramid serving sizes, however.) Regulations also require that foods meet strict definitions if their packaging includes the terms *light, low-fat,* or *high-fiber* (see below). Health claims such as "good source of dietary fiber" or "low in saturated fat" on packages are signals that those products can wisely be included in your diet. Overall, the food label is an important tool to help you choose a diet that conforms to the Food Guide Pyramid and the Dietary Guidelines.

Selected Nutrient Claims and What They Mean

Healthy   A food that is low in fat, is low in saturated fat, has no more than 360–480 mg of sodium and 60 mg of cholesterol, *and* provides 10% or more of the Daily Value for vitamin A, vitamin C, protein, calcium, iron, or dietary fiber.

Light or lite   One-third fewer calories or 50% less fat than a similar product.

Reduced or fewer   At least 25% less of a nutrient than a similar product; can be applied to fat ("reduced fat"), saturated fat, cholesterol, sodium, and calories.

Extra or added   10% or more of the Daily Value per serving when compared to what a similar product has.

Good source   10–19% of the Daily Value for a particular nutrient.

High, rich in, or excellent source of   20% or more of the Daily Value for a particular nutrient.

Low calorie   40 calories or less per serving.

High fiber   5 g or more of fiber per serving.

Good source of fiber   2.5–4.9 g of fiber per serving.

Fat-free   Less than 0.5 g of fat per serving.

Low-fat   3 g of fat or less per serving.

Saturated fat-free   Less than 0.5 g of saturated fat and 0.5 g of trans fatty acids per serving.

Low saturated fat   1 g or less of saturated fat per serving and no more than 15% of total calories.

Cholesterol-free   Less than 2 mg of cholesterol and 2 g or less of saturated fat per serving.

Low cholesterol   20 mg or less of cholesterol and 2 g or less of saturated fat per serving.

Low sodium   140 mg or less of sodium per serving.

Very low sodium   35 mg or less of sodium per serving.

Lean   Cooked seafood, meat, or poultry with less than 10 g of fat, 4.5 g or less of saturated fat, and less than 95 mg of cholesterol per serving.

Extra lean   Cooked seafood, meat, or poultry with less than 5 g of fat, 2 g of saturated fat, and 95 mg of cholesterol per serving.

Note: As of May 2004, the FDA had not yet defined nutrient claims relating to carbohydrate, so foods labeled low- or reduced-carbohydrate do not conform to any approved standard.

1. Serving size: Determine how many servings there are in the food package and compare it to how much you actually eat. You may need to adjust the rest of the nutrient values based on your typical serving size.

2. Calories and calories from fat: Note whether a serving is high in calories and fat. The sample food shown here is low in fat, with only 30 of its 235 calories from fat.

3. Daily Values: Based on a 2000-calorie diet, Daily Value percentages tell you whether the nutrients in a serving of food contribute a lot or a little to your total daily diet.

    5% or less is low
    20% or more is high

4. Limit these nutrients: Look for foods low in fat, saturated fat, trans fat, cholesterol, and sodium. *(Trans fat content must be included on the label by January 2006 for any food with more than 0.5g trans fat per serving.)*

5. Get enough of these nutrients: Look for foods high in dietary fiber, vitamin A, vitamin C, calcium, and iron.

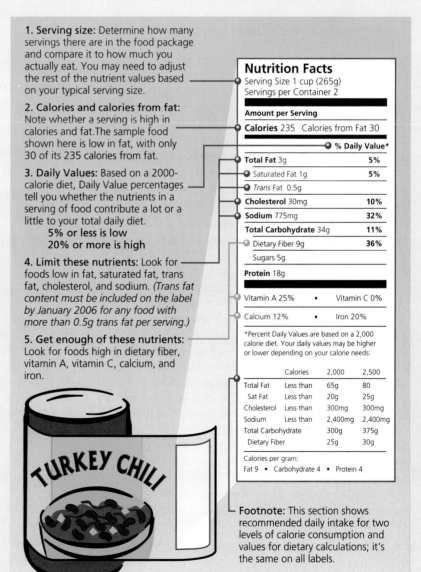

Nutrition Facts
Serving Size 1 cup (265g)
Servings per Container 2

Amount per Serving

Calories 235   Calories from Fat 30

	% Daily Value*
Total Fat 3g	5%
Saturated Fat 1g	5%
Trans Fat 0.5g	
Cholesterol 30mg	10%
Sodium 775mg	32%
Total Carbohydrate 34g	11%
Dietary Fiber 9g	36%
Sugars 5g	
Protein 18g	

Vitamin A 25%	•	Vitamin C 0%
Calcium 12%	•	Iron 20%

*Percent Daily Values are based on a 2,000 calorie diet. Your daily values may be higher or lower depending on your calorie needs:

		Calories	2,000	2,500
Total Fat	Less than		65g	80
Sat Fat	Less than		20g	25g
Cholesterol	Less than		300mg	300mg
Sodium	Less than		2,400mg	2,400mg
Total Carbohydrate			300g	375g
Dietary Fiber			25g	30g

Calories per gram:
Fat 9 • Carbohydrate 4 • Protein 4

Footnote: This section shows recommended daily intake for two levels of calorie consumption and values for dietary calculations; it's the same on all labels.

these foods. Also, supermarkets often have large posters or pamphlets listing the nutrient contents of these foods. Lab 8.3 gives you the opportunity to compare foods using the information provided on their labels.

Dietary Supplement Labels— New Requirements

Dietary supplements include vitamins, minerals, amino acids, herbs, enzymes, and other compounds. Although dietary supplements are often thought to be safe and "natural," they do contain powerful, bioactive chemicals that have the potential for harm. About one-quarter of all pharmaceutical drugs are derived from botanical sources, and even essential vitamins and minerals can have toxic effects if consumed in excess.

In the United States, supplements are not legally considered drugs and are not regulated the way drugs are. Before they are approved by the FDA and put on the market, drugs undergo clinical studies to determine safety, effectiveness, side effects and risks; possible interactions with other substances; and appropriate dosages. The FDA does not authorize or test dietary supplements, and supplements are not required to demonstrate either safety or effectiveness before they are marketed. Although dosage guidelines exist for some of the compounds in dietary supplements, dosages for many are not well established.

Many ingredients in dietary supplements are classified by the FDA as "generally recognized as safe," but some have been found to be dangerous on their own or to interact with prescription or over-the-counter drugs in dangerous ways. Garlic supplements, for example, can cause bleeding if taken with anticoagulant ("blood-thinning") medications. Even products that are generally considered safe can have side effects—St. John's wort, for example, increases the skin's sensitivity to sunlight and may decrease the effectiveness of oral contraceptives, drugs used to treat HIV infection, and many other medications.

There are also key differences between drugs and supplements in their manufacture. FDA-approved medications are standardized for potency, and quality control and proof of purity are required. Dietary supplement manufacture is not so closely regulated, and there is no guarantee that a product even contains a given ingredient, let alone in the appropriate amount. The potency of herbal supplements can vary widely due to differences in growing and harvesting conditions, preparation methods, and storage. Contamination and misidentification of plant compounds are also potential problems. The FDA proposed manufacturing standards for supplements in 2003, but they aren't yet in effect.

In an effort to provide consumers with more reliable and consistent information about supplements, the FDA has developed new labeling regulations. Since March 1999, labels similar to those found on foods have been required for dietary supplements; for more information, see the box "Using Dietary Supplement Labels."

Remember that dietary supplements are no substitute for a healthy diet. Supplements do not provide all the known—or yet-to-be-discovered—benefits of whole foods. Supplements should also not be used as a replacement for medical treatment for serious illnesses.

Food Additives—Benefits and Risks

Today, some 2800 substances are intentionally added to foods for one or more of the following reasons: (1) to maintain or improve nutritional quality, (2) to maintain freshness, (3) to help in processing or preparation, or (4) to alter taste or appearance. Additives make up less than 1% of our food. The most widely used are sugar, salt, and corn syrup; these three, plus citric acid, baking soda, vegetable colors, mustard, and pepper, account for 98% by weight of all food additives used in the United States.

Food additives pose no significant health hazard to most people because the levels used are well below any that could produce toxic effects. Two additives of potential concern for some people are sulfites, used to keep vegetables from turning brown, and monosodium glutamate (MSG), used as a flavor enhancer. Sulfites can cause severe reactions in some people, and the FDA strictly limits their use and requires clear labeling on any food containing sulfites. MSG may cause some people to experience episodes of sweating and increased blood pressure. To protect yourself, eat a variety of foods in moderation. If you have any sensitivity to an additive, check food labels when you shop and ask questions when you eat out.

Foodborne Illness—An Increasing Threat

Many people worry about additives or pesticide residues in their food. However, a greater threat to the safety of the food supply comes from microorganisms that cause foodborne illnesses. Raw or undercooked animal products, such as chicken, hamburger, and oysters, pose the greatest risk for contamination. The CDC estimates that 76 million Americans become sick each year as a result of foodborne illness, 325,000 are hospitalized, and 5200 die. In most cases, foodborne illness produces acute gastroenteritis, characterized by diarrhea, vomiting, fever, and weakness. People often mistake foodborne illness for a bout of the flu. Although the effects of foodborne illness are usually not serious, some groups, such as children and older people, are at risk for severe complications, including rheumatic diseases, kidney failure, seizures, blood poisoning, and death.

Causes of Foodborne Illnesses Most cases of foodborne illness are caused by **pathogens,** disease-causing microorganisms that contaminate food, usually from improper handling. The threats are numerous and varied;

Terms   **pathogen** A microorganism that causes disease.
Vw

Since 1999, specific types of information have been required on the labels of dietary supplements. In addition to basic information about the product, labels include a "Supplement Facts" panel, modeled after the "Nutrition Facts" panel used on food labels (see the figure). Under the Dietary Supplement Health and Education Act (DSHEA) and food labeling laws, supplement labels can make three types of health-related claims.

- *Nutrient-content claims,* such as "high in calcium," "excellent source of vitamin C," or "high potency." The claims "high in" and "excellent source of" mean the same as they do on food labels. A "high potency" single-ingredient supplement must contain 100% of its Daily Value; a "high potency" multi-ingredient product must contain 100% or more of the Daily Value of at least two-thirds of the nutrients present for which Daily Values have been established.

- *Health claims,* if they have been authorized by the FDA or another authoritative scientific body. The association between adequate calcium intake and lower risk of osteoporosis is an example of an approved health claim. Since 2003, the FDA has also allowed so-called *qualified* health claims for situations in which there is emerging but as yet inconclusive evidence for a particular claim. Such claims must include qualifying language such as "scientific evidence suggests but does not prove" the claim.

- *Structure-function claims,* such as "antioxidants maintain cellular integrity" or "this product enhances energy levels." Because these claims are not reviewed by the FDA, they must carry a disclaimer (see the sample label).

Tips for Choosing and Using Dietary Supplements

- Check with your physician before taking a supplement. Many are not meant for children, elderly people, women who are pregnant or breastfeeding, people with chronic illnesses or upcoming surgery, or people taking prescription or OTC medications.

- Follow the cautions, instructions for use, and dosage given on the label.

- Look for the USP-DSVP mark on the label, indicating that the product meets minimum safety and purity standards developed under the Dietary Supplement Verification Program (DSVP) by the United States Pharmacopeia (USP). The USP-DSVP mark means that the product (1) contains the ingredients stated on the label, (2) has the declared amount and strength of ingredients, (3) will dissolve effectively, (4) has been screened for harmful contaminants, and (5) has been manufactured using safe, sanitary, and well-controlled procedures. The National Nutritional Foods Association (NNFA) has a self-regulatory testing program for its members; other, smaller associations and labs, including ConsumerLab.Com, also test and rate dietary supplements.

- Choose brands made by nationally known food and drug manufacturers or "house brands" from large retail chains. Due to their size and visibility, such sources are likely to have higher manufacturing standards.

- If you experience side effects, discontinue use of the product and contact your physician. Report any serious reactions to the FDA's MedWatch monitoring program (800-FDA-1088; http://www.fda.gov/medwatch).

For More Information About Dietary Supplements

ConsumerLab.Com: http://www.consumerlab.com

Food and Drug Administration: http://vm.cfsan.fda.gov/~dms/supplmnt.html

National Institutes of Health, Office of Dietary Supplements: http://dietary-supplements.info.nih.gov

National Nutritional Foods Association: http://www.nnfa.org

U.S. Department of Agriculture: http://www.nal.usda.gov/fnic/etext/000015.html

U.S. Pharmacopeia: http://www.usp.org/dietarysupplements

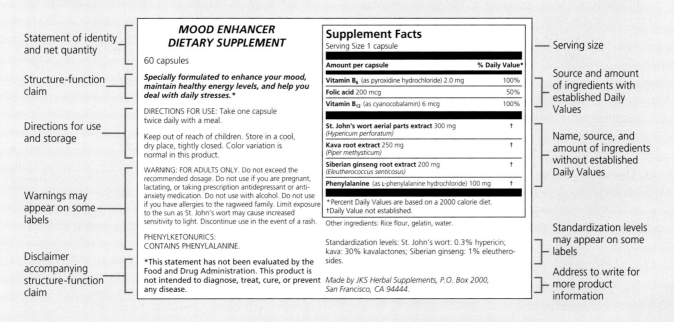

among them are the sometimes deadly *Escherichia coli* (*E. coli*) O157:H7 in meat and water; *Salmonella* in eggs, on vegetables, and on poultry; *Vibrio* in shellfish; *Cyclospora* and hepatitis A virus on fruit; *Cryptosporidium* in drinking water; *Campylobacter jejuni* in meat and poultry; and *Listeria monocytogenes* in lunch meats, sausages, and hot dogs.

You can't tell by taste, smell, or sight whether a food is contaminated. Some studies have revealed high levels of contamination. In 2003, *Consumer Reports* tested 484 chickens purchased in grocery stores and found that half were contaminated with *Campylobacter* and/or *Salmonella*. Although pathogens are usually destroyed during cooking, the U.S. government is taking steps to bring down levels of contamination by improving national testing and surveillance. Raw meat and poultry products are now sold with safe handling and cooking instructions, and all packaged, unpasteurized fresh fruit and vegetable juices carry warnings about potential contamination. It is important to note that while foodborne illness outbreaks associated with food-processing plants make headlines, most cases of illness trace back to poor food handling in the home or in food-service establishments.

A potential new threat from food is bovine spongiform encephalopathy (BSE), or "mad cow disease," a fatal degenerative neurological disease caused by an abnormal protein that forms deposits in the brain. In Britain, more than 100 cases of a related brain disease in humans have been linked to consumption of beef contaminated with central nervous system tissue from BSE-infected cows. In December 2003, the first BSE-infected cow was identified in the United States. Although the USDA states that the risk to human health from BSE is extremely low, additional steps are being taken to prevent the BSE protein from entering the food supply; visit the USDA Web site for more information (www.usda.gov/bse).

Preventing and Treating Foodborne Illness The key to protecting yourself from foodborne illness is to handle, cook, and store foods in ways that prevent bacteria from spreading and multiplying:

- Don't buy food in containers that leak, bulge, or are severely dented. Refrigerated foods should be cold, and frozen foods should be solid.
- Refrigerate perishable items as soon as possible after purchase. Use or freeze fresh meats within 3–5 days and fresh poultry, fish, and ground meat within 1–2 days.
- Thaw frozen food in the refrigerator or in the microwave oven, not on the kitchen counter.
- Thoroughly wash your hands with warm soapy water for 20 seconds before and after handling food, especially raw meat, fish, poultry, or eggs.
- Make sure counters, cutting boards, dishes, and other equipment are thoroughly cleaned before and after use. If possible, use separate cutting boards for meat and for foods that will be eaten raw, such as fruits and vegetables. Wash dishcloths and kitchen towels frequently.

- Thoroughly rinse and scrub fruits and vegetables with a brush, if possible, or peel off the skin.
- Cook foods thoroughly, especially beef, poultry, fish, pork, and eggs. Cooking kills most microorganisms, as long as an appropriately high temperature is reached. The USDA now recommends that consumers, especially high-risk individuals, use a food thermometer to verify that hamburgers are cooked to 160° F. When eating out, order red meat cooked "well done."
- Cook stuffing separately from poultry; or wash poultry thoroughly, stuff immediately before cooking, and transfer the stuffing to a clean bowl immediately after cooking.
- Refrigerate foods at or below 40°F and freeze at or below 0°F. Do not leave cooked or refrigerated foods, such as meats or salads, at room temperature for more than 2 hours. Use refrigerated leftovers within 3–4 days.
- Don't eat raw animal products, including raw eggs in Caesar salad, hollandaise sauce, or eggnog. Use only pasteurized milk and juice, and look for pasteurized eggs, which are now available in some states.
- Cook eggs until they're firm and fully cook foods containing eggs. Store eggs in the coldest part of the refrigerator, not on the door, and use them within 3–5 weeks.
- Because of possible contamination with *E. coli* O157:H7 and *Salmonella,* avoid raw sprouts, or eat them only after submerging them in boiling water for 10 seconds.
- According to the USDA, "When in doubt, throw it out."

Additional precautions are recommended for people at particularly high risk for foodborne illness—pregnant women, young children, older persons, and people with weakened immune systems or certain chronic illnesses. If you are a member of one of these groups, don't eat or drink any of the following products: unpasteurized juices; raw sprouts; raw (unpasteurized) milk and products made from unpasteurized milk; raw or undercooked meat, poultry, eggs, fish, and shellfish; and soft cheeses such as feta, Brie, Camembert, or blue-veined varieties. It's also important to avoid ready-to-eat foods such as hot dogs, luncheon meats, and cold cuts unless they are reheated until they are steaming hot.

If you think you may be having a bout of foodborne illness, drink plenty of clear fluids to prevent dehydration and rest to speed recovery. To prevent further contamination, wash your hands often and always before handling food until you recover. A fever higher than 102° F, blood in the stool, or dehydration deserves a physician's evaluation, especially if the symptoms persist for more than 2–3 days. In cases of suspected botulism—characterized by symptoms such as double vision, paralysis, dizziness, and vomiting—consult a physician immediately.

Irradiated Foods— A Technique of Biotechnology

Food irradiation is the treatment of foods with gamma rays, X rays, or high-voltage electrons to kill potentially harmful pathogens, including bacteria, parasites, insects, and fungi that cause foodborne illness. It also reduces spoilage and extends shelf life. Even though irradiation has been generally endorsed by agencies such as the World Health Organization, the Centers for Disease Control and Prevention, and the American Medical Association, few irradiated foods are currently on the market due to consumer resistance and skepticism. Studies haven't conclusively identified any harmful effects of food irradiation, and the newer methods of irradiation involving electricity and X rays do not require the use of any radioactive materials. Studies indicate that when consumers are given information about the process of irradiation and the benefits of irradiated foods, most want to purchase them.

All primary irradiated foods (meat, vegetables, and so on) are labeled with the flowerlike radura symbol and a brief information label; spices and foods that are merely ingredients do not have to be so labeled. It is important to remember that although irradiation kills most pathogens, it does not completely sterilize foods. Proper handling of irradiated foods is still critical for preventing foodborne illness.

Organic Foods—Stricter Standards for a Booming Industry

Some people who are concerned about pesticides and other environmental contaminants choose to buy foods that are **organic.** In December 2000, the USDA enacted a new national standard for organic foods to replace the older system of local, state, and private standards. To be certified as organic, foods must meet strict production, processing, handling, and labeling criteria. Organic crops must meet limits on pesticide residues; for meat, milk, eggs, and other animal products to be certified organic, animals must be given organic feed and access to the outdoors and may not be given antibiotics or growth hormones. The use of genetic engineering, ionizing radiation, and sewage sludge are prohibited. Products can be labeled "100% organic" if they contain all organic ingredients and "organic" if they contain at least 95% organic ingredients; all such products may carry the new USDA organic seal. A product with at least 70% organic ingredients can be labeled "made with organic ingredients" but cannot use the USDA seal.

Foods that are organic are not chemical-free, however. They may be contaminated with pesticides used on neighboring lands or on foods transported in the same train or truck. However, they do tend to have lower levels of pesticide residues than conventionally grown crops. There are strict pesticide limits for all foods—organic and conventional—and the debate about the potential health effects of long-term exposure to small amounts of pesticide residues is ongoing. Supporters of organic foods also note that practices associated with organic farming help maintain biodiversity of crops and are less likely to degrade soil, contaminate water, or expose farm workers to dangerous chemicals.

A PERSONAL PLAN: APPLYING NUTRITIONAL PRINCIPLES

You've learned the basics of good nutrition, know how to interpret food and supplement labels, and have some guidelines for protecting yourself from foodborne illness. With this foundation, you can now put together a diet that works for you. Based on your particular nutrition and health status, there probably is an ideal diet for you, but there is no single type of diet that provides optimal health for everyone. Many cultural dietary patterns can meet people's nutritional requirements (see the box "Ethnic Foods" on p. 250). Every individual needs to customize a food plan based on age, gender, weight, activity level, medical risk factors—and, of course, personal tastes.

Assessing and Changing Your Diet

The first step in planning a healthy diet is to examine what you currently eat. Labs 8.1 and 8.2 are designed to help you analyze your current diet and compare it with optimal dietary goals. (This analysis can be completed using Appendix B, a nutritional analysis software program, or one of several Web sites.)

Next, experiment with additions and substitutions to your current diet to bring it closer to your goals. If you are consuming too much fat, for example, try substituting fruit for a calorie-rich dessert. If you aren't getting enough iron, try adding some raisins to your cereal or garbanzo beans to your salad. If you need to plan your diet from the ground up, use the Food Guide Pyramid and the Dietary Guidelines.

To put your plan into action, use the behavioral self-management techniques and tips described in Chapter 1. If you identify several changes you want to make, focus on one at a time. You might start, for example, by substituting nonfat or low-fat milk for whole milk. When you become used to that, you can try substituting whole-wheat bread for white bread. The information on eating behavior in Lab 8.1 will help you identify and change unhealthy patterns of eating.

---

food irradiation The treatment of foods with gamma rays, X rays, or high-voltage electrons to kill potentially harmful pathogens and increase shelf life.

organic A designation applied to foods grown and produced according to strict guidelines limiting the use of pesticides, nonorganic ingredients, hormones, antibiotics, genetic engineering, irradiation, and other practices.

Terms

There is no one ethnic diet that clearly surpasses all others in providing people with healthful foods. However, every diet has its advantages and disadvantages and, within each cuisine, some foods are better choices. The dietary guidelines described in this chapter can be applied to any ethnic cuisine. For additional guidance, refer to the table below.

	Choose More Often	Choose Less Often
Chinese	Dishes that are steamed, poached (jum), boiled (chu), roasted (kow), barbecued (shu), or lightly stir-fried Hoisin sauce, oyster sauce, wine sauce, plum sauce, velvet sauce, or hot mustard Fresh fish and seafood, skinless chicken, tofu Mixed vegetables, Chinese greens Steamed rice, steamed spring rolls, soft noodles	Fried wontons or egg rolls Crab rangoon Crispy (Peking) duck or chicken Sweet-and-sour dishes made with breaded and deep-fried meat, poultry, or fish Fried rice Fried or crispy noodles
French	Dishes prepared au vapeur (steamed), en brochette (skewered and broiled), or grillé (grilled) Fresh fish, shrimp, scallops, or mussels or skinless chicken, without sauces Clear soups	Dishes prepared à la crème (in cream sauce), au gratin or gratinée (baked with cream and cheese), or en croûte (in pastry crust) Drawn butter, hollandaise sauce, and remoulade (mayonnaise-based sauce)
Greek	Dishes that are stewed, broiled, or grilled, including shish kabobs (souvlaki) Dolmas (grape leaves) stuffed with rice Tzatziki (yogurt, cucumbers, and garlic) Tabouli (bulgur-based salad) Pita bread, especially whole wheat	Moussaka, saganaki (fried cheese) Vegetable pies such as spanakopita and tyropita Baba ghanoush (eggplant and olive oil) Deep-fried falafel (chickpea patties) Gyros stuffed with ground meat Baklava
Indian	Dishes prepared masala (curry), tandoori (roasted in a clay oven), or tikke (pan roasted); kabobs Raita (yogurt and cucumber salad) and other yogurt-based dishes and sauces Dal (lentils), pullao or pilau (basmati rice) Chapati (baked bread)	Ghee (clarified butter) Korma (meat in cream sauce) Samosas, pakoras (fried dishes) Molee and other coconut milk-based dishes Poori, bhatura, or paratha (fried breads)
Italian	Pasta primavera or pasta, polenta, risotto, or gnocchi with marinara, red or white wine, white or red clam, or light mushroom sauce Dishes that are grilled or prepared cacciatore (tomato-based sauce), marsala (broth and wine sauce), or piccata (lemon sauce) Cioppino (seafood stew) Vegetable soup, minestrone or fagioli (beans)	Antipasto (cheese, smoked meats) Dishes that are prepared alfredo, frito (fried), crema (creamed), alla panna (with cream), or carbonara Veal scaloppini Chicken, veal, or eggplant parmigiana Italian sausage, salami, and prosciutto Buttered garlic bread Cannoli
Japanese	Dishes prepared nabemono (boiled), shabu-shabu (in boiling broth), mushimono (steamed), nimono (simmered), yaki (broiled), or yakimono (grilled) Sushi or domburi (mixed rice dish) Steamed rice or soba (buckwheat), udon (wheat), or rice noodles	Tempura (battered and fried) Agemono (deep fried) Katsu (fried pork cutlet) Sukiyaki Fried tofu
Mexican	Soft corn or wheat tortillas Burritos, fajitas, enchiladas, soft tacos, and tamales filled with beans, vegetables, or lean meats Refried beans, nonfat or low-fat, rice and beans Ceviche (fish marinated in lime juice) Salsa, enchilada sauce, and picante sauce Gazpacho, menudo, or black bean soup Fruit or flan for dessert	Crispy, fried tortillas Dishes that are fried, such as chile relleños, chimichangas, flautas, and tostadas Nachos and cheese, chili con queso, and other dishes made with cheese or cheese sauce Guacamole, sour cream, and extra cheese Refried beans made with lard Fried ice cream
Thai	Dishes that are barbecued, sautéed, broiled, boiled, steamed, braised, or marinated Sàté (skewered and grilled meats) Fish sauce, basil sauce, chili or hot sauces Bean thread noodles, Thai salad	Coconut milk soup Peanut sauce or dishes topped with nuts Mee-krob (crispy noodles) Red, green, and yellow curries, which typically contain coconut milk

SOURCES: National Heart, Lung, and Blood Institute. 1998. Tips for Healthy Multicultural Dining Out. In *Clinical Guidelines on the Identification, Evaluation, and Treatment of Overweight and Obesity in Adults*. Bethesda, Md.: National Institutes of Health. Duyff, R. L. 1998. *The American Dietetic Association's Complete Food and Nutrition Guide*. Minneapolis, Minn.: Chronimed. Kirby, J. 1998. *Dieting for Dummies*. Foster City, Calif.: IDG Books.

Staying Committed to a Healthy Diet

Beyond knowledge and information, you also need support in difficult situations. Keeping to your plan is easiest when you choose and prepare your own food at home. Advance planning is the key: mapping out meals and shopping appropriately, cooking in advance when possible, and preparing enough food for leftovers later in the week. A tight budget does not necessarily make it more difficult to eat healthy meals. It makes good health sense and good budget sense to use only small amounts of meat and to have a few meatless meals each week.

In restaurants, keeping to food plan goals becomes somewhat more difficult. Portion sizes in restaurants tend to be larger than serving sizes of the Food Guide Pyramid, but by remaining focused on your goals, you can eat only part of your meal and take the rest home for a meal later in the week. Don't hesitate to ask questions when you're eating in a restaurant. Most restaurant personnel are glad to explain how menu selections are prepared and to make small adjustments, such as serving salad dressings and sauces on the side so they can be avoided or used sparingly. To limit your fat intake, order meat or fish broiled or grilled rather than fried or sauteed, choose rice or a plain baked potato over french fries, and select a clear soup rather than a creamy one. Desserts that are irresistible can, at least, be shared.

Strategies like these can be helpful, but small changes cannot change a fundamentally high-fat, high-calorie meal into a moderate, healthful one. Often, the best advice is to bypass a large steak with potatoes au gratin for a flavorful but low-fat entree. Many of the selections offered in ethnic restaurants are healthy choices (refer to the box on ethnic foods for suggestions).

Fast-food restaurants offer the biggest challenge to a healthy diet. Surveys show that about 70% of 18- to 24-year-olds and 64% of 25- to 34-year-olds visit a fast-food restaurant at least once a week. Fast-food meals are often high in calories, total fat, saturated fat, trans fat, sodium, and sugar; they may be low in fiber and in some vitamins and minerals (see Appendix C). If you do eat at a fast-food restaurant, make sure the rest of your meals that day are low-fat meals rich in fruits and vegetables.

Knowledge of food and nutrition is essential to the success of your program. The information provided in this chapter should give you the tools you need to design and implement a diet that promotes long-term health and well-being. If you need additional information or have questions about nutrition, be sure the source you consult is reliable.

Tips for Today

Eating is one of life's great pleasures. There are many ways to satisfy your nutrient needs so you can create a healthy diet that takes into account your personal preferences and favorite foods. If your current eating habits are not as healthy as they could be, you can choose equally delicious foods that offer both short-term and long-term health benefits. Opportunities to improve your diet present themselves every day, and small changes add up.

Right now you can

- Substitute a healthy snack—an apple, a banana, or plain popcorn—for a bag of chips or cookies.

- Drink a glass of water and put a bottle of water in your backpack for tomorrow.

- Plan to make healthy selections when you go to dinner, such as a baked potato instead of french fries or salmon instead of steak.

- Study the box on ethnic foods in this chapter and plan to order a healthy selection the next time you eat at your favorite ethnic restaurant. Do the same with the fast-food restaurants listed in Appendix C at the end of the book.

SUMMARY

- The six classes of nutrients are carbohydrates, proteins, fats, vitamins, minerals, and water.

- The nutrients essential to humans are released into the body through digestion. Nutrients in foods provide energy, measured in kilocalories (commonly called calories); build and maintain body tissues; and regulate body functions.

- Protein, an important component of body tissue, is composed of amino acids; nine are essential to a diet. Foods from animal sources provide complete proteins; plants provide incomplete proteins.

- Fats, a major source of energy, also insulate the body and cushion the organs; 3–4 teaspoons of vegetable oil per day supplies the essential fats. For most people, dietary fat intake should be 20–35% of total calories, and unsaturated fats should be favored over saturated and trans fats.

Which should I eat—butter or margarine? Both butter and margarine are concentrated sources of fat, containing about 11 grams of fat and 100 calories per tablespoon. Butter is higher in saturated fat, which raises levels of artery-clogging LDL ("bad" cholesterol). Each tablespoon of butter has about 8 grams of saturated fat; margarine has about 2. Butter also contains cholesterol, which margarine does not.

Margarine, on the other hand, contains trans fat, which not only raises LDL but lowers HDL ("good" cholesterol). A tablespoon of stick margarine contains about 2 grams of trans fat. Butter contains a small amount of trans fat as well. Although butter has a combined total of saturated and trans fats that is twice that of stick margarine, the trans fat in stick margarine may be worse for you. Clearly, you should avoid both butter and stick margarine. To solve this dilemma, remember that softer is better. The softer or more liquid a margarine or spread is, the less hydrogenated it is and the less trans fat it contains. Tub and squeeze margarines contain less trans fat than stick margarines; some margarines are modified to be low-trans or trans-free and are labeled as such. Vegetable oils are even better choice for cooking and for table use (such as olive oil for dipping bread) because most are low in saturated fat and completely free of trans fats.

The Food Guide Pyramid seems to recommend such a large number of servings. How can I possibly follow its recommendations without gaining weight? First of all, consider how many servings from each food group are appropriate for you. The suggested number of servings is given as a range, 6–11 servings of grain products, 3–5 of vegetables, and so on. The smaller number of servings is for people who consume about 1600 calories a day, such as many sedentary women. The larger number is for those who consume about 2800 calories a day, such as active men. If the smaller number of servings is appropriate for you, concentrate on choosing nutrient-dense foods—those that are rich in nutrients but relatively low in calories, such as most grains, fruits, and vegetables.

Second, compare the serving sizes of the foods you eat with those used in the Food Guide Pyramid. Some of the Pyramid's serving sizes are smaller than what you might typically eat. For example, many people eat a cup or more of pasta or rice in a meal, which would correspond to 2 or more servings from the grain products group. You'll probably find that your current diet already includes the minimum number of servings from most of the food groups. If not, you may find that you are eating too many servings from one group and not enough from another. Make small changes in your eating habits and food choices to bring your diet into line with the recommendations in the Pyramid, paying particular attention to your consumption of fat and added sugars. The Food Guide Pyramid is designed to help you balance your food choices to ensure good health. Strategies for successful weight management are described in detail in the next chapter.

What exactly are genetically modified foods? Are they safe? How can I recognize them on the shelf, and how can I know when I'm eating them? Genetic engineering involves altering the characteristics of a plant, animal, or microorganism by adding, rearranging, or replacing genes in its DNA; the result is a genetically modified (GM) organism. New DNA may come from related species or organisms or from entirely different types of organisms. Many GM crops are already grown in the United States: About 75% of the current U.S. soybean crop has been genetically modified to be resistant to an herbicide used to kill weeds, and about a third of the U.S. corn crop carries genes for herbicide resistance or to produce a protein lethal to a destructive type of caterpillar. Products made with GM organisms include juice, soda, nuts, tuna, frozen pizza, spaghetti sauce, canola oil, chips, salad dressing, and soup.

The potential benefits of GM foods cited by supporters include improved yields overall and in difficult growing conditions, increased disease resistance, improved nutritional content, lower prices, and less use of pesticides. Critics of biotechnology argue that unexpected effects may occur: Gene manipulation could elevate levels of naturally occurring toxins or allergens, permanently change the gene pool and reduce biodiversity, and produce pesticide-resistant insects through the transfer of genes. In 2000, a form of GM corn approved for use only in animal feed was found to have comingled with other varieties of corn and to have been used in human foods; this mistake sparked fears of allergic reactions and led to

- Carbohydrates provide energy to the brain, nervous system, and blood and to muscles during high-intensity exercise. Naturally occurring simple carbohydrates and unrefined complex carbohydrates should be favored over added sugars and refined carbohydrates.

- Fiber includes plant substances that are impossible for the human body to digest. It helps reduce cholesterol levels and promotes the passage of wastes through the intestines.

- The 13 essential vitamins are organic substances that promote specific chemical and cell processes and act as antioxidants. The 17 known essential minerals are inorganic substances that regulate body functions, aid in growth and tissue maintenance, and help in

the release of energy from food. Deficiencies in vitamins and minerals can cause severe symptoms over time, but excess doses are also dangerous.

- Water aids in digestion and food absorption, allows chemical reactions to take place, serves as a lubricant or cushion, and helps regulate body temperature.

- Foods contain other substances, such as phytochemicals, that may not be essential nutrients but that may protect against chronic diseases.

- The Dietary Reference Intakes, Food Guide Pyramid, and Dietary Guidelines for Americans provide standards and recommendations for getting all essential nutrients from a varied, balanced diet and for eating in ways that protect against chronic disease.

recalls. Opposition to GM foods is particularly strong in Europe; in many developing nations that face food shortages, responses to GM crops have tended to be more positive.

In April 2000, the National Academy of Sciences released a report stating that there is no proof that GM food on the market is unsafe but that changes are needed to better coordinate regulation of GM foods and to assess potential problems. Labeling has been another major concern. Surveys indicate that the majority of Americans want to know if their foods contain GM ingredients. However, under current rules, the FDA requires special labeling only when a food's composition is changed significantly or when a known allergen is introduced. For example, soybeans that contain a gene from a peanut would have to be labeled because peanuts are a common allergen. The only foods guaranteed not to contain GM ingredients are those certified as organic.

I've heard that fish contains mercury. Is it safe to eat?

Overall, fish and shellfish are healthy sources of protein, omega-3 fats, and other nutrients; and prudent choices can minimize the risk of any possible negative health effects. Because of mercury contamination, the FDA and Environmental Protection Agency (EPA) have issued special guidelines for certain groups. To reduce exposure to the harmful effects of mercury, women who may become pregnant, pregnant women, and nursing mothers should follow these guidelines:

- Do not eat shark, swordfish, king mackerel, or tilefish.

- Eat up to 12 ounces a week of a variety of fish and shellfish that are lower in mercury; these include shrimp, canned light tuna, salmon, pollock, and catfish. Limit consumption of albacore tuna to 6 ounces per week.

- Check advisories about the safety of recreationally caught fish from local lakes, rivers, and coastal areas; if no information is available, limit consumption to 6 ounces per week.

The same FDA/EPA guidelines apply to children, although they should consume smaller servings.

Some experts have also expressed concern about the presence of toxins such as PCBs in farmed fish, especially farmed salmon. Although no federal guidelines have been set, some researchers suggest that consumers limit themselves to 8 ounces of farmed salmon per month. Beginning in October 2004, fish will be labeled with its country of origin and whether it is wild or farmed; most canned salmon is wild.

How can I tell if I'm allergic to a food?

A true food allergy is a reaction of the body's immune system to a food or food ingredient, usually a protein. This immune reaction can occur with minutes of ingesting the food, resulting in symptoms such as hives, diarrhea, difficulty breathing, or swelling of the lips or tongue. The most severe response is a systemic reaction called anaphylaxis, which involves a potentially life-threatening drop in blood pressure. Food allergies affect only about 2% of the adult population and about 4–6% of infants. Just a few foods account for more than 90% of the food allergies in the United States: cow's milk, eggs, peanuts, tree nuts (walnuts, cashews, and so on), soy, wheat, fish, and shellfish.

Many people who believe they have food allergies may actually suffer from a food intolerance, a much more common source of adverse food reactions that typically involves problems with metabolism rather than with the immune system. The body may not be able to adequately digest a food or the body may react to a particular food compound. Food intolerances have been attributed to lactose (milk sugar), gluten (a protein in some grains), tartrazine (yellow food coloring), sulfite (a food additive), MSG, and the sweetener aspartame. Although symptoms of a food intolerance may be similar to those of a food allergy, they are typically more localized and not life-threatening. Many people with food intolerance can safely and comfortably consume small amounts of the food that affects them.

If you suspect you have a food allergy or intolerance, a good first step is to keep a food diary. Note everything you eat or drink, any symptoms you develop, and how long after eating the symptoms appear. Then make an appointment with your physician to go over your diary and determine if any additional tests are needed. People at risk for severe allergic reactions must diligently avoid trigger foods and carry medications to treat anaphylaxis.

- Basic recommendations for a healthy diet include aiming for a healthy weight through diet and physical activity; building a healthy base for our diets by following the Pyramid, choosing a variety of plant foods, and handling foods safely; and making sensible choices that consider intake of fat, sugar, salt, and alcohol.

- A vegetarian diet requires special planning but can meet all human nutritional needs.

- Different population groups, such as college students and athletes, face special dietary challenges and should plan their diets to meet their particular needs.

- Consumers can get help applying nutritional principles by reading the standardized labels that appear on all packaged foods and on dietary supplements.

- Although nutritional basics are well established, no single diet provides wellness for everyone. Individuals should focus on their particular needs and adapt general dietary principles to meet them.

FOR FURTHER EXPLORATION

For reliable nutrition advice, talk to a faculty member in the nutrition department on your campus, a registered dietitian (R.D.), or your physician. Many large communities have a telephone service called Dial a Dietitian. By calling this number, you can receive free nutrition information from an R.D.

Experts on quackery suggest that you steer clear of anyone who puts forth any of the following false statements: Most diseases are caused primarily by faulty nutrition, large doses of vitamins are effective against many diseases, hair analysis can be used to determine a person's nutritional state, or a computer-scored nutritional deficiency test is a basis for prescribing vitamins. Any practitioner—licensed or not—who sells supplements in his or her office should be thoroughly scrutinized.

VW Fit and Well Online Learning Center (www.mhhe.com/fahey)

Use the learning objectives, study guide questions, and glossary flashcards to review key terms and concepts and prepare for exams. You can extend your knowledge of nutrition and gain experience in using the Internet as a resource by completing the activities and checking out the Web links for the topics in Chapter 8 marked with the World Wide Web icon. For this chapter, Internet activities explore specialized food pyramids, food composition analysis, osteoporosis prevention, and dietary supplements; there are Web links for the Vital Statistics table, the Critical Consumer boxes on food labels and dietary supplements, and the chapter as a whole.

Daily Fitness and Nutrition Journal

Review the resources and complete the activities available in the nutrition portion of the journal. Take the portion sizes quiz, complete the preprogram nutrition log, and analyze the results. Based on what you find, set healthy goals for change and complete the contract. Once you put your plan into action, complete the postprogram nutrition log to determine how successful you've been at improving your diet and moving toward the goals you've set.

HealthQuest

Learn more about your current diet by completing the dietary assessment in the Nutrition and Weight Control module of the HealthQuest CD-ROM (select How's Your Diet? from the Wellness Activities menu). Your scores will help you pinpoint dietary patterns that you could change to improve wellness. To determine if you are ready to make changes in your diet, complete the Stages of Change quiz (select Stages of Change from the Wellness Activities menu). You'll receive an assessment of your stage plus advice on moving forward toward the action and maintenance stages.

Books

Duyff, R. L. 2002. *ADA Complete Food and Nutrition Guide,* 2d ed. Chicago, Ill.: American Dietetic Association. *An excellent review of current nutrition information.*

Insel, P., R. E. Turner, and D. Ross. 2004. *Nutrition,* 2d ed. Sudbury, Mass.: Jones and Bartlett. *A comprehensive review of major concepts in nutrition.*

Jacobson, M. F., and J. Hurley. 2002. *Restaurant Confidential.* New York: Workman Publishing. *Provides information about restaurant foods, including tips for making healthier choices.*

Selkowitz, A. 2000. *The College Student's Guide to Eating Well on Campus.* Bethesda, Md.: Tulip Hill Press. *Provides practical advice for students, including how to make healthy choices when eating in a dorm or restaurant and how to stock a first pantry.*

Wardlaw, G. M. 2004. *Perspectives in Nutrition,* 6th ed. New York: McGraw-Hill. *An easy-to-understand review of major concepts in nutrition.*

Williams, M. H. 2005. *Nutrition for Health, Fitness, and Sport,* 7th ed. New York: McGraw-Hill. *An overview of the role of nutrition in enhancing health, fitness, and sport performance.*

Newsletters

Environmental Nutrition (800-829-5384); http://www.environmentalnutrition.com

Nutrition Action Health Letter (202-332-9110; http://www.cspinet.org)

Tufts University Health and Nutrition Letter (800-274-7581; http://www.healthletter.tufts.edu)

VW Organizations, Hotlines, and Web Sites

American Dietetic Association. Provides a wide variety of educational materials on nutrition.
> 800-877-1600
> http://www.eatright.org

American Heart Association: Delicious Decisions. Provides basic information about nutrition, tips for shopping and eating out, and heart-healthy recipes.
> http://www.deliciousdecisions.org

Consumer Information Center: Food. Provides government publications about fat, fiber, food safety, and other nutrition issues.
> http://www.pueblo.gsa.gov/food.htm

FDA Center for Food Safety and Applied Nutrition. Offers information about topics such as food labeling, food additives, and foodborne illness.
> http://vm.cfsan.fda.gov

Food Safety Hotlines. Provide information on the safe purchase, handling, cooking, and storage of food.
> 888-SAFEFOOD (FDA)
> 800-535-4555 (USDA Meat and Poultry Hotline)

Gateways to Government Nutrition Information. Provides access to government resources relating to food safety, including consumer advice and information on specific pathogens.
> http://www.nutrition.gov
> http://www.foodsafety.gov

Harvard School of Public Health: Nutrition Source. Provides advice on interpreting news on nutrition; an overview of the Healthy Eating Pyramid, an alternative to the basic USDA pyramid; and suggestions for building a healthy diet.
> http://www.hsph.harvard.edu/nutritionsource

Health Canada: Food and Nutrition. Provides information about Canada's Food Guide to Healthy Eating as well as advice for people with special dietary needs.
> http://www.hc-sc.gc.ca/english/lifestyles/food_nutr.html

MedlinePlus: Nutrition. Provides links to information from government agencies and major medical associations on a wide variety of nutrition topics.
> http://www.nlm.nih.gov/medlineplus/nutrition.html

National Academies' Food and Nutrition Board. Provides information about the Dietary Reference Intakes and related guidelines.
> http://www.iom.edu/board.asp?id=3788

National Cancer Institute 5 A Day Program. Promotes the consumption of fruits and vegetables per day.
> http://www.5aday.gov

National Institutes of Health: Osteoporosis and Related Bone Diseases—National Resource Center. Provides information about osteoporosis prevention and treatment; includes a special section on men and osteoporosis.
> http://www.osteo.org

National Osteoporosis Foundation. Provides information on the causes, prevention, detection, and treatment of osteoporosis.

http://www.nof.org

Tufts University Nutrition Navigator. Provides descriptions and ratings for many nutrition-related Web pages.

http://navigator.tufts.edu

USDA Center for Nutrition Policy and Promotion. Click on Interactive Healthy Eating Index for an assessment of your diet and a comparison of your diet with the Food Guide Pyramid.

http://www.usda.gov/cnpp

USDA Food and Nutrition Information Center. Provides a variety of materials relating to the Dietary Guidelines, food labels, Food Guide Pyramid, and many other topics.

http://www.nal.usda.gov/fnic

Vegetarian Resource Group. Information and links for vegetarians and people interested in learning more about vegetarian diets.

http://www.vrg.org

You can obtain nutrient breakdowns of individual food items from the following sites:

Nutrition Analysis Tools, and System

http://nat.crgq.com

USDA Food and Nutrition Information Center

http://www.nal.usda.gov/fnic/foodcomp

See also the resources listed in Chapters 9, 11, and 12.

SELECTED BIBLIOGRAPHY

American College of Sports Medicine, American Dietetic Association, and Dietitians of Canada. 2000. Joint Position Statement: Nutrition and athletic performance. *Medicine and Science in Sports and Exercise* 32(12): 2130–2145.

American Diabetes Association. 2002. Evidence-based nutrition principles and recommendations for the treatment and prevention of diabetes and related complications. *Diabetes Care* 25:148–198.

American Heart Association Nutrition Committee. 2000. AHA Dietary Guidelines: Revision 2000. *Circulation* 102:2296–2311.

Bunyard, L. B., K. E. Dennis, and B. J. Nicklas. 2002. Dietary intake and changes in lipoprotein lipids in obese, postmenopausal women placed on an American Heart Association Step 1 diet. *Journal of the American Dietetic Association* 102(1): 52–57.

Capps, O., L. Cleveland, and J. Park. 2002. Dietary behaviors associated with total fat and saturated fat intake. *Journal of the American Dietetic Association* 102(4): 490–502.

Corle, D. K., et al. 2001. Self-rated quality of life measures: Effect of change to a low-fat, high-fiber, fruit and vegetable enriched diet. *Annals of Behavioral Medicine* 23(3): 198–207.

Ervin, R. B., et al. 2004. Dietary intake of selected minerals for the United States Population: 1999–2000. *Advance Data from Vital and Health Statistics,* 341.

Food and Drug Administration. 2004. *Backgrounder for the 2004 FDA/EPA Consumer Advisory: What You Need to Know About Mercury in Fish and Shellfish* (http://www.fda.gov/oc/opacom/hottopics/mercury/backgrounder.html; retrieved April 27, 2004).

Food and Drug Administration. 2004. *Commonly Asked Questions About BSE in Product's Regulated by FDA's Center for Food Safety and Applied Nutrition.* (http://www.cfsan.fda.gov/~comm/bsefaq.html; retrieved April 28, 2004).

Food and Drug Administration. 2004. *Fact Sheet: Carbohydrates* (http://www.fda.gov/oc/initiatives/obesity/factsheet.html; retrieved April 28, 2004).

Food and Nutrition Board, Institute of Medicine. 2004. *Dietary Reference Intakes for Water, Potassium, Sodium, Chloride, and Sulfate.* Washington, D.C.: National Academies Press.

Food and Nutrition Board, Institute of Medicine. 2002. *Dietary Reference Intakes for Energy, Carbohydrate, Fiber, Fat, Fatty Acids, Cholesterol, Protein, and Amino Acids.* Washington, D.C.: National Academies Press.

Hites, R. A., et al. 2004. Global assessment of organic contaminants in farmed salmon. *Science* 303(5655): 226–229.

Jacobs, D. R., H. E. Meyer, and K. Solvoll. 2001. Reduced mortality among whole grain bread eaters in men and women in the Norwegian Country Study. *European Journal of Clinical Nutrition* 55(20): 137–143.

Joint WHO/FAO Expert Consultation. 2003. *Diet, Nutrition, and the Prevention of Chronic Diseases.* Geneva: World Health Organization.

Kant, A. K. 2000. Consumption of energy-dense, nutrient-poor foods by adult Americans: Nutritional and health implications. *American Journal of Clinical Nutrition* 72(4): 929–936.

Ludwig, D. S. 2002. The glycemic index: Physiological mechanisms relating to obesity, diabetes, and cardiovascular disease. *Journal of the American Medical Association* 287(18): 2414–2423.

Michaelsson, K., et al. 2003. Serum retinol levels and the risk of fracture. *New England Journal of Medicine* 348(4): 287–294.

Nanney, M. S., et al. 2004. Rationale for a consistent "powerhouse" approach to vegetable and fruit messages. *Journal of the American Dietetic Association* 104(3): 352–356.

National Center for Health Statistics. 2003. Dietary intake of ten key nutrients for public health, United States: 1999–2000. *Advance Data from Vital and Health Statistics* No. 334.

Of birds and bacteria. 2003. *Consumer Reports,* January.

Oomen, C. M., et al. 2001. Association between trans fatty acid intake and 10-year risk of coronary heart disease. *Lancet* 357(9258): 746–751.

Toborek, M., et al. 2002. Unsaturated fatty acids selectively induce an inflammatory environment in human endothelial cells. *American Journal of Clinical Nutrition* 75(1): 119–125.

U.S. Department of Agriculture. 2003. *Backgrounder for Revision of Food Guide Pyramid* (http://www.usda.gov/news/releases/2003/09/bg0308.htm; retrieved September 10, 2003).

U.S. Department of Agriculture and U.S. Department of Health and Human Services. 2000. *Nutrition and Your Health: Dietary Guidelines for Americans,* 5th ed. Home and Garden Bulletin No. 232.

U.S. Department of Agriculture, Center for Food Safety and Applied Nutrition. 2003. *Examples of Revised Nutrition Facts Panel Listing Trans Fat* (http://www.cfsan.fda.gov/~dms/labtr.html; retrieved January 5, 2004).

U.S. Department of Agriculture, Center for Food Safety and Applied Nutrition. 2003. *Questions and Answers About Trans Fat Nutrition Labeling* (http://www.cfsan.fda.gov/~dms/qatrans2.html; retrieved January 5, 2004).

U.S. Department of Agriculture, Center for Nutrition Policy and Promotion. 2003. *Proposed Daily Food Intake Patterns for the Food Guide Pyramid* (http://www.cnpp.usda.gov/pyramid-update-index.html; retrieved September 10, 2003).

Willett, W. C., and M. J. Stampfer. 2003. Rebuilding the food pyramid. *Scientific American,* January.

Wong, S. H. S., and S. Chung. 2003. Glycemic index: An educational tool for health and fitness professionals? *ACSM's Health and Fitness Journal,* November/December.

Wyshak, G. 2000. Teenaged girls, carbonated beverage consumption, and bone fracture. *Archives of Pediatric and Adolescent Medicine* 154:610–613.

Table 1   *Dietary Reference Intakes (DRIs): Recommended Levels for Individual Intake*

Life Stage	Group	Biotin (µg/day)	Choline (mg/day)ᵃ	Folate (µg/day)ᵇ	Niacin (mg/day)ᶜ	Pantothenic Acid (mg/day)	Riboflavin (mg/day)	Thiamin (mg/day)	Vitamin A (µg/day)ᵈ	Vitamin B-6 (mg/day)	Vitamin B-12 (µg/day)	Vitamin C (mg/day)ᵉ	Vitamin D (µg/day)ᶠ	Vitamin E (mg/day)ᵍ
Infants	0–6 months	5	125	65	2	1.7	0.3	0.2	400	0.1	0.4	40	5	4
	7–12 months	6	150	80	4	1.8	0.4	0.3	500	0.3	0.5	50	5	5
Children	1–3 years	8	200	**150**	6	2	**0.5**	0.5	300	0.5	0.9	15	5	6
	4–8 years	12	250	200	8	3	0.6	0.6	400	0.6	1.2	25	5	7
Males	9–13 years	20	375	300	12	4	0.9	0.9	600	1.0	1.8	45	5	11
	14–18 years	25	550	**400**	16	5	1.3	1.2	900	1.3	2.4	75	5	**15**
	19–30 years	30	550	400	16	5	1.3	1.2	900	1.3	2.4	90	5	15
	31–50 years	30	550	400	16	5	1.3	1.2	900	1.3	2.4ʰ	90	5	15
	51–70 years	30	550	400	16	5	1.3	1.2	900	1.7	2.4ʰ	90	10	15
	>70 years	30	550	400	16	5	1.3	1.2	900	1.7	2.4ʰ	90	15	15
Females	9–13 years	20	375	300	12	4	0.9	0.9	600	1.0	1.8	45	5	11
	14–18 years	25	400	400ⁱ	14	5	1.0	1.0	700	1.2	2.4	65	5	15
	19–30 years	30	425	400ⁱ	14	5	1.1	1.1	700	1.3	2.4	75	5	15
	31–50 years	30	425	400ⁱ	14	5	1.1	1.1	700	1.3	2.4	75	5	15
	51–70 years	30	425	400ⁱ	14	5	1.1	1.1	700	1.5	2.4ʰ	75	10	15
	>70 years	30	425	400	14	5	1.1	1.1	700	1.5	2.4ʰ	75	15	15
Pregnancy	≤18 years	30	450	600ʲ	18	6	1.4	1.4	750	1.9	2.6	80	5	15
	19–30 years	30	450	600ʲ	18	6	1.4	1.4	770	1.9	2.6	85	5	15
	31–50 years	30	450	600ʲ	18	6	1.4	1.4	770	1.9	2.6	85	5	15
Lactation	≤18 years	35	550	500	17	7	1.6	1.4	1200	2.0	2.8	115	5	19
	19–30 years	35	550	500	17	7	1.6	1.4	1300	2.0	2.8	120	5	19
	31–50 years	35	550	500	17	7	1.6	1.4	1300	2.0	2.8	120	5	19
Tolerable Upper Intake Levels for Adults (19–70)			3500	1000ᵏ	35ᵏ				3000	100		2000	50	1000ᵏ

NOTE: The table includes values for the type of DRI standard—Adequate Intake (AI) or Recommended Dietary Allowance (RDA)—that has been established for that particular nutrient and life stage; RDAs are shown in **bold type**. The final row of the table shows the Tolerable Upper Intake Levels (ULs) for adults; refer to the full DRI report for information on other ages and life stages. A UL is the maximum level of daily nutrient intake that is likely to pose no risk of adverse effects. There is insufficient data to set ULs for all nutrients, but this does not mean that there is no potential for adverse effects; source of intake should be from food only to prevent high levels of intake of nutrients without established ULs. In healthy individuals, there is no established benefit from nutrient intakes above the RDA or AI.

ᵃAlthough AIs have been set for choline, there are few data to assess whether a dietary supply of choline is needed at all stages of the life cycle, and it may be that the choline requirement can be met by endogenous synthesis at some of these stages.

ᵇAs dietary folate equivalents (DFE): 1 DFE = 1 µg food folate = 0.6 µg folate from fortified food or as a supplement consumed with food = 0.5 µg of a supplement taken on an empty stomach.

ᶜAs niacin equivalents (NE): 1 mg niacin = 60 mg tryptophan.

Table 1   Dietary Reference Intakes (DRIs): Recommended Levels for Individual Intake (Continued)

Life Stage	Group	Vitamin K (μg/day)	Calcium (mg/day)	Chromium (μg/day)	Copper (μg/day)	Fluoride (mg/day)	Iodine (μg/day)	Iron (mg/day)[l]	Magnesium (mg/day)	Manganese (mg/day)	Molybdenum (μg/day)	Phosphorus (mg/day)	Selenium (μg/day)	Zinc (mg/day)[m]
Infants	0–6 months	2.0	210	0.2	200	0.01	110	0.27	30	0.003	2	100	15	2
	7–12 months	2.5	270	5.5	220	0.5	130	11	75	0.6	3	275	20	3
Children	1–3 years	30	500	11	340	0.7	90	7	80	1.2	17	460	20	3
	4–8 years	55	800	15	440	1	90	10	130	1.5	22	500	30	5
Males	9–13 years	60	1300	25	700	2	120	8	240	1.9	34	1250	40	8
	14–18 years	75	1300	35	890	3	150	11	410	2.2	43	1250	55	11
	19–30 years	120	1000	35	900	4	150	8	400	2.3	45	700	55	11
	31–50 years	120	1000	35	900	4	150	8	420	2.3	45	700	55	11
	51–70 years	120	1200	30	900	4	150	8	420	2.3	45	700	55	11
	>70 years	120	1200	30	900	4	150	8	420	2.3	45	700	55	11
Females	9–13 years	60	1300	21	700	2	120	8	240	1.6	34	1250	40	8
	14–18 years	75	1300	24	890	3	150	15	360	1.6	43	1250	55	9
	19–30 years	90	1000	25	900	3	150	18	310	1.8	45	700	55	8
	31–50 years	90	1000	25	900	3	150	18	320	1.8	45	700	55	8
	51–70 years	90	1200	20	900	3	150	8	320	1.8	45	700	55	8
	>70 years	90	1200	20	900	3	150	8	320	1.8	45	700	55	8
Pregnancy	≤18 years	75	1300	29	1000	3	220	27	400	2.0	50	1250	60	13
	19–30 years	90	1000	30	1000	3	220	27	350	2.0	50	700	60	11
	31–50 years	90	1000	30	1000	3	220	27	360	2.0	50	700	60	11
Lactation	≤18 years	75	1300	44	1300	3	290	10	360	2.6	50	1250	70	14
	19–30 years	90	1000	45	1300	3	290	9	310	2.6	50	700	70	12
	31–50 years	90	1000	45	1300	3	290	9	320	2.6	50	700	70	12
Tolerable Upper Intake Levels for Adults (19–70)			2500		10,000	10	1100	45	350[k]	11	2000	4000	400	40

d As retinol activity equivalents (RAEs): 1 RAE = 1 μg retinol, 12 μg β-carotene, or 24 μg α-carotene or β-cryptoxanthin. Preformed vitamin A (retinol) is abundant in animal-derived foods; provitamin A carotenoids are abundant in some dark yellow, orange, red, and deep-green fruits and vegetables. For preformed vitamin A and for provitamin A carotenoids in supplements, 1RE = 1 RAE; for provitamin A carotenoids in foods, divide the REs by 2 to obtain RAEs. The UL applies only to preformed vitamin A.

e Individuals who smoke require an additional 35 mg/day of vitamin C over that needed by nonsmokers; nonsmokers regularly exposed to tobacco smoke should ensure they meet the RDA for vitamin C.

f As cholecalciferol: 1 μg cholecalciferol = 40 IU vitamin D. DRI values are based on the absence of adequate exposure to sunlight.

g As α-tocopherol. Includes naturally occurring RRR-α-tocopherol and the 2R-stereoisomeric forms from supplements; does not include the 2S-stereoisomeric forms from supplements.

h Since 10–30% of older people may malabsorb food-bound B-12, those over age 50 should meet their RDA mainly with supplements or foods fortified with B-12.

i In view of evidence linking folate intake with neural tube defects in the fetus. It is recommended that all women capable of becoming pregnant consume 400 μg from supplements or fortified foods in addition to consuming folate from a varied diet.

j It is assumed that women will continue consuming 400 μg from supplements or fortified food until their pregnancy is confirmed and they enter prenatal care, which ordinarily occurs after the end of the periconceptional period—the critical time for formation of the neural tube.

k The UL applies only to intake from supplements, fortified foods, and/or pharmacological agents and not to intake from foods.

l Because the absorption of iron from plant foods is low compared to that from animal foods, the RDA for strict vegetarians is approximately 1.8 times higher than the values established for omnivores (14 mg/day for adult male vegetarians; 33 mg/day for premenopausal female vegetarians). Oral contraceptives (OCs) reduce menstrual blood losses, so women taking them need less daily iron; the RDA for premenopausal women taking OCs is 10.9 mg/day. For more on iron requirements for other special situations, refer to Dietary Reference Intakes for Vitamin A, Vitamin K, Arsenic, Boron, Chromium, Copper, Iodine, Iron, Manganese, Molybdenum, Nickel, Silicon, Vanadium, and Zinc (visit http://www.nap.edu for the complete report).

m Zinc absorption is lower for those consuming vegetarian diets so the zinc requirement for vegetarians is approximately twofold greater than for those consuming a nonvegetarian diet.

Nutrition Resources

Table 1 Dietary Reference Intakes (DRIs): Recommended Levels for Individual Intake (Continued)

Life Stage Group	Potassium (g/day)	Sodium (g/day)	Chloride (g/day)	Carbohydrate RDA/AI (g/day)	Carbohydrate AMDR[o] (%)	Total Fiber RDA/AI (g/day)	Total Fat AMDR[o] (%)	Linoleic Acid RDA/AI (g/day)	Linoleic Acid AMDR[o] (%)	Alpha-linolenic Acid RDA/AI (g/day)	Alpha-linolenic Acid AMDR[o] (%)	Protein[n] RDA/AI (g/day)	Protein[n] AMDR[o] (%)
Infants													
0–6 months	0.4	0.12	0.18	60	ND[p]	ND	q	4.4	ND[p]	0.5	ND[p]	9.1	ND[p]
7–12 months	0.7	0.37	0.57	95	ND[p]	ND	q	4.6	ND[p]	0.5	ND[p]	13.5	ND[p]
Children													
1–3 years	3.0	1.0	1.5	130	45–65	19	30–40	7	5–10	0.7	0.6–1.2	13	5–20
4–8 years	3.8	1.2	1.9	130	45–65	25	25–35	10	5–10	0.9	0.6–1.2	19	10–30
Males													
9–13 years	4.5	1.5	2.3	130	45–65	31	25–35	12	5–10	1.2	0.6–1.2	34	10–30
14–18 years	4.7	1.5	2.3	130	45–65	38	25–35	16	5–10	1.6	0.6–1.2	52	10–30
19–30 years	4.7	1.5	2.3	130	45–65	38	20–35	17	5–10	1.6	0.6–1.2	56	10–35
31–50 years	4.7	1.5	2.3	130	45–65	38	20–35	17	5–10	1.6	0.6–1.2	56	10–35
51–70 years	4.7	1.3	2.0	130	45–65	30	20–35	14	5–10	1.6	0.6–1.2	56	10–35
>70 years	4.7	1.2	1.8	130	45–65	30	20–35	14	5–10	1.6	0.6–1.2	56	10–35
Females													
9–13 years	4.5	1.5	2.3	130	45–65	26	25–35	10	5–10	1.0	0.6–1.2	34	10–30
14–18 years	4.7	1.5	2.3	130	45–65	26	25–35	11	5–10	1.1	0.6–1.2	46	10–30
19–30 years	4.7	1.5	2.3	130	45–65	25	20–35	12	5–10	1.1	0.6–1.2	46	10–35
31–50 years	4.7	1.5	2.3	130	45–65	25	20–35	12	5–10	1.1	0.6–1.2	46	10–35
51–70 years	4.7	1.3	2.0	130	45–65	21	20–35	11	5–10	1.1	0.6–1.2	46	10–35
>70 years	4.7	1.2	1.8	130	45–65	21	20–35	11	5–10	1.1	0.6–1.2	46	10–35
Pregnancy													
≤18 years	4.7	1.5	2.3	175	45–65	28	20–35	13	5–10	1.4	0.6–1.2	71	10–35
19–30 years	4.7	1.5	2.3	175	45–65	28	20–35	13	5–10	1.4	0.6–1.2	71	10–35
31–50 years	4.7	1.5	2.3	175	45–65	28	20–35	13	5–10	1.4	0.6–1.2	71	10–35
Lactation													
≤18 years	5.1	1.5	2.3	210	45–65	29	20–35	13	5–10	1.3	0.6–1.2	71	10–35
19–30 years	5.1	1.5	2.3	210	45–65	29	20–35	13	5–10	1.3	0.6–1.2	71	10–35
31–50 years	5.1	1.5	2.3	210	45–65	29	20–35	13	5–10	1.3	0.6–1.2	71	10–35
Tolerable Upper Intake Level for Adults (19–70)		2.3	3.6										

[n]Daily protein recommendations are based on body weight for reference body weights: 1.5 g/kg for infants, 1.1 g/kg for 1–3 years, 0.95 g/kg for 4–13 years, 0.85 g/kg for 14–18 years, 0.8 g/kg for adults, and 1.1 g/kg for pregnant (using prepregnancy weight) and lactating women.

[o]Acceptable Macronutrient Distribution Range (AMDR), expressed as a percent of total daily calories, is the range of intake for a particular energy source that is associated with reduced risk of chronic disease while providing intakes of essential nutrients. If an individual consumes in excess of the AMDR, there is a potential for increasing the risk of chronic diseases and/or insufficient intakes of essential nutrients.

[p]Not determinable due to lack of data of adverse effects in this age group and concern with regard to lack of ability to handle excess amounts. Source of intake should be from food only to prevent high levels of intake.

[q]For infants, Adequate Intake of total fat is 31 grams/day (0–6 months) and 30 grams per day (7–12 months) from breast milk and, for infants 7–12 months, complementary foods and beverages.

SOURCES: Food and Nutrition Board, Institute of Medicine, National Academies. 2004. Dietary Reference Intakes: Water, Potassium, Sodium, Chloride, and Sulfate. Washington, D.C.: National Academies Press. Food and Nutrition Board, Institute of Medicine. National Academies. 2002. Dietary Reference Intakes Tables (http://www4.nationalacademies.org/IOM/IOMHome.nsf/Pages/Food+and+Nutrition+Board; retrieved December 2, 2002. The complete Dietary Reference Intake reports are available from the National Academy Press (http://www.nap.edu).

Reprinted with permission from Dietary Reference Intakes: Applications in Dietary Planning, copyright © 2003 by the National Academy of Sciences. Courtesy of the National Academy of Sciences.

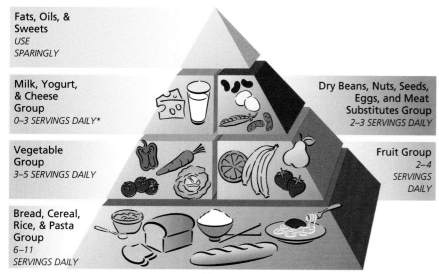

*Vegetarians who choose not to use milk, yogurt, or cheese need to select other food sources rich in calcium.

Figure 1   A Food Pyramid for vegetarian meal planning.   A healthy vegetarian diet includes a variety of foods, including whole grains, vegetables, fruits, legumes, nuts, seeds, and, if desired, dairy products and eggs.   SOURCE: Reprinted from *Journal of the Dietetic Association,* "Vegetarian Diets—Position of ADA," pp. 1317–1321. Copyright ©1997 American Dietetic Association. With permission from the American Dietetic Association.

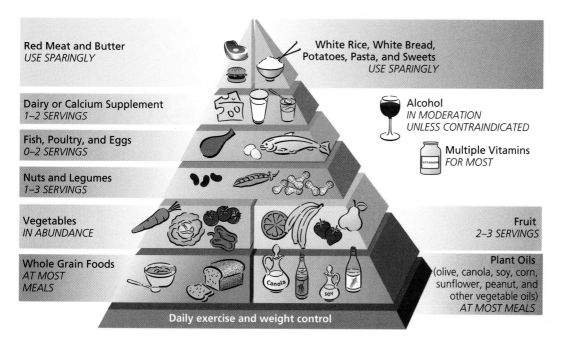

Figure 2   Healthy Eating Pyramid.   The Healthy Eating Pyramid is a alternative food group plan developed by researchers at the Harvard School of Public Health; this pyramid reflects many major research studies that have looked at the relationship between diet and long-term health. The Healthy Eating Pyramid differentiates between the various dietary sources of fat, protein, and carbohydrates, and it emphasizes whole grains, vegetable oils, fruits and vegetables, nuts, and dried peas and beans.   SOURCE: Reprinted by permission of Simon & Schuster Adult Publishing Group from *Eat, Drink, and Be Healthy: The Harvard Medical School Guide to Healthy Eating* by Walter C. Willett, M.D. Copyright © 2001 by the President and Fellows of Harvard College.

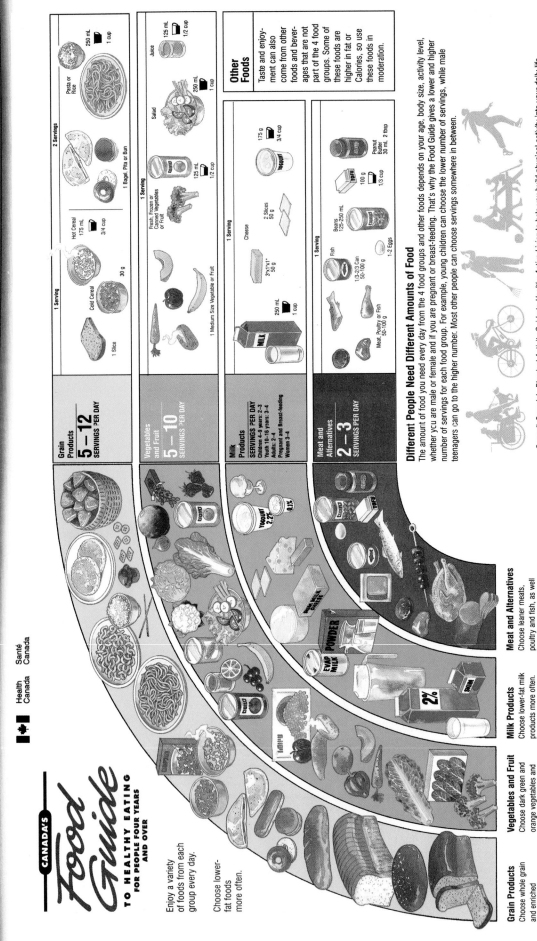

Figure 3 Canada's Food Guide to Healthy Eating. SOURCE: Canada's Food Guide to Healthy Eating for People Four Years and Over, 1997. © Reproduced with the permission of the Minister of Public Works and Government Service Canada, 2004.

Name _____ **Section** _____ **Date** _____

LAB 8.1 *Your Daily Diet Versus the Food Guide Pyramid*

Keep a record of everything you eat for 3 consecutive days. Record all foods and beverages you consume, breaking each food item into its component parts (for example, a turkey sandwich would be listed as 2 slices of bread, 3 oz of turkey, 1 tsp of mayonnaise, and so on). Complete the first two columns of the chart during the course of the day; fill in the remaining information at the end of the day using Figure 8.4 and pp. 235–237 in your text. For fats, oils, and sweets—foods from the tip of the Pyramid—put a star (*) in the Food Group column. (Note: This lab can also be completed using nutritional analysis software or Web sites.)

DAY 1

Food	Your Portion Size	Food Group	Number of Pyramid Servings*

Daily Total

Food Group	Number of Servings
Milk, yogurt, cheese	
Meat, poultry, fish, dry beans, eggs, nuts	
Fruits	
Vegetables	
Breads, cereals, rice, pasta	

*Your portion sizes may be smaller or larger than the serving sizes given in the Food Guide Pyramid; list the actual number of Food Guide Pyramid servings contained in the foods you eat.

DAY 2

Food	Your Portion Size	Food Group	Number of Pyramid Servings*

Daily Total

Food Group	Number of Servings
Milk, yogurt, cheese	
Meat, poultry, fish, dry beans, eggs, nuts	
Fruits	
Vegetables	
Breads, cereals, rice, pasta	

*Your portion sizes may be smaller or larger than the serving sizes given in the Food Guide Pyramid; list the actual number of Food Guide Pyramid servings contained in the foods you eat.

DAY 3

Food	Your Portion Size	Food Group	Number of Pyramid Servings*

Daily Total

Food Group	Number of Servings
Milk, yogurt, cheese	
Meat, poultry, fish, dry beans, eggs, nuts	
Fruits	
Vegetables	
Breads, cereals, rice, pasta	

*Your portion sizes may be smaller or larger than the serving sizes given in the Food Guide Pyramid; list the actual number of Food Guide Pyramid servings contained in the foods you eat.

Next, average your serving totals for the 3 days and enter them in the chart below. Fill in the recommended serving totals that apply to you from Figure 8.4 and Table 8.5.

Food Group	Recommended Number of Daily Servings	Actual (Average) Number of Daily Servings
Milk, yogurt, cheese		
Meat, poultry, fish, dry beans, eggs, nuts		
Fruits		
Vegetables		
Breads, cereals, rice, pasta		

Using Your Results

How did you score? How close is your diet to that recommended by the Food Guide Pyramid? Are you at all surprised by the actual number of servings you're consuming from each food group?

What should you do next? If the results of the assessment indicate that you could boost your level of wellness by improving your diet, set realistic goals for change. Do you need to increase or decrease your consumption of any food groups? List any areas of concern below, along with a goal for change and strategies for achieving the goal you've set. If you see that you are falling short in one food group, such as fruits or vegetables, but have many starred items from the fats, oils, and sweets category, you might try decreasing those items in favor of an apple, a bunch of grapes, or some baby carrots. Think carefully about the reasons behind your food choices. For example, if you eat doughnuts for breakfast every morning because you feel rushed, make a list of ways to save time to allow for a healthier breakfast.

Problem: _____

Goal: _____

Strategies for change: _____

_____

Problem: _____

Goal: _____

Strategies for change: _____

_____

Problem: _____

Goal: _____

Strategies for change: _____

_____

_____

Enter the results of this lab in the Preprogram Assessment column in Appendix D. If you've set goals and identified strategies for change, begin putting your plan into action. After several weeks of your program, complete this lab again and enter the results in the Postprogram Assessment column of Appendix D. How do the results compare?

Name _____ Section _____ Date _____

LAB 8.2 *Dietary Analysis*

You can complete this activity using either a nutrition analysis software program or the food composition data in Appendix B and the charts printed below. Information about the nutrient content of foods is also available online; see the For Further Exploration section for recommended Web sites. (This lab asks you to analyze one day's diet. For a more complete and accurate assessment of your diet, analyze the results from several different days, including a weekday and a weekend day.)

DATE _____   DAY: M Tu W Th F Sa Su

Food	Amount	Calories	Protein (g)	Carbohydrate (g)	Dietary fiber (g)	Fat, total (g)	Saturated fat (g)	Cholesterol (mg)	Sodium (mg)	Vitamin A (mg)	Vitamin C (mg)	Calcium (mg)	Iron (mg)
Recommended totals[a]			10–35%	45–65%	25–38 g	20–35%	<10%	≤300 mg	≤2300 mg	RE	mg	mg	mg
Actual totals[b]		cal	g / %	g / %	g	g / %	g / %	mg	mg	RE	mg	mg	mg

[a]Fill in the appropriate RDA or DRI values for vitamin A, vitamin C, calcium, and iron from Table 1 in the Nutrition Resources section.
[b]Total the values in each column. To calculate the percentage of total calories from protein, carbohydrate, fat, and saturated fat, use the formulas on p. 224. Protein and carbohydrate provide 4 calories per gram; fat provides 9 calories per gram. For example, if you consume a total of 270 grams of carbohydrate and 2000 calories, your percentage of total calories from carbohydrate would be (270 g × 4 cal/g) ÷ 2000 cal = 54%. Do not include data for alcoholic beverages in your calculations. Percentages may not total 100% due to rounding.

Using Your Results

How did you score? How close is your diet to that recommended by the Dietary Guidelines, Dietary Reference Intakes, and other guidelines? Are you surprised by any of the results of this assessment?

What should you do next? Enter the results of this lab in the Preprogram Assessment column in Appendix D. If your daily diet meets all the recommended intakes, congratulations—and keep up the good work. If the results of the assessment pinpoint areas of concern, then work with your food record on the previous page to determine what changes you could make to meet all the guidelines. Make changes, additions, and deletions until it conforms to all or most of the guidelines. Or, if you prefer, start from scratch to create a day's diet that meets the guidelines. Use the chart below to experiment and record your final, healthy sample diet for one day. Then put what you learned from this exercise into practice in your daily life. After several weeks of your program, complete this lab again and enter the results in the Postprogram Assessment column of Appendix D. How do the results compare?

DATE _____   DAY: M Tu W Th F Sa Su

Food	Amount	Calories	Protein (g)	Carbohydrate (g)	Dietary fiber (g)	Fat, total (g)	Saturated fat (g)	Cholesterol (mg)	Sodium (mg)	Vitamin A (RE)	Vitamin C (mg)	Calcium (mg)	Iron (mg)
Recommended totals			10–35%	45–65%	25–38 g	20–38%	<10%	≤300 mg	≤2300 mg	RE	mg	mg	mg
Actual totals		cal	g / %	g / %	g	g / %	g / %	mg	mg	RE	mg	mg	mg

LAB 8.3 *Informed Food Choices*

Part I   Using Food Labels

Choose three food items to evaluate. You might want to select three similar items, such as regular, low-fat, and non-fat salad dressing, or three very different items. Record the information from their food labels in the table below.

Food Items			
Serving size			
Total calories	cal	cal	cal
Total fat—grams	g	g	g
—% Daily Value	%	%	%
Saturated fat—grams	g	g	g
—% Daily Value	%	%	%
Trans fat—grams	g	g	g
Cholesterol—milligrams	mg	mg	mg
—% Daily Value	%	%	%
Sodium—milligrams	mg	mg	mg
—% Daily Value	%	%	%
Carbohydrates (total)—grams	g	g	g
—% Daily Value	%	%	%
Dietary fiber—grams	g	g	g
—% Daily Value	%	%	%
Sugars—grams	g	g	g
Protein—grams	g	g	g
Vitamin A—% Daily Value	%	%	%
Vitamin C—% Daily Value	%	%	%
Calcium—% Daily Value	%	%	%
Iron—% Daily Value	%	%	%

How do the items you chose compare? You can do a quick nutrient check by totaling the Daily Value percentages for nutrients you should limit (total fat, cholesterol, sodium) and the nutrients you should favor (dietary fiber, vitamin A, vitamin C, calcium, iron) for each food. Which food has the largest percent Daily Value sum for nutrients to limit? For nutrients to favor?

Food Items			
Calories	cal	cal	cal
% Daily Value total for nutrients to limit (total fat, cholesterol, sodium)	%	%	%
% Daily Value total for nutrients to favor (fiber, vitamin A, vitamin C, calcium, iron)	%	%	%

Part II   Evaluating Fast Food

Use the information from Appendix C, Nutritional Content of Popular Items from Fast-Food Restaurants, to complete the chart on this page for the last fast-food meal you ate. Add up your totals for the meal. Compare the values for fat, protein, carbohydrate, cholesterol, and sodium content for each food item and for the meal as a whole with the levels suggested by the Dietary Guidelines for Americans. Calculate the percent of total calories derived from fat, saturated fat, protein, and carbohydrate using the formulas given.

If you haven't recently been to one of the restaurants included in the appendix, fill in the chart for any sample meal you might eat. If some of the food items you selected don't appear in Appendix C, ask for a nutrition information brochure when you visit the restaurant, or check out online fast-food information: Arby's (http://www.arbysrestaurant.com), Burger King (http://www.burgerking.com), Domino's Pizza (http://www.dominos.com), Jack in the Box (http://www.jackinthebox.com), KFC (http://www.kfc.com), McDonald's (http://www.mcdonalds.com), Subway (http://www.subway.com), Taco Bell (http://www.tacobell.com), Wendy's (http://www.wendys.com).

FOOD ITEMS

	Dietary Guidelines							Total[b]
Serving size (g)		g	g	g	g	g	g	g
Calories		cal	cal	cal	cal	cal	cal	cal
Total fat—grams		g	g	g	g	g	g	g
—% calories[a]	20–35%	%	%	%	%	%	%	%
Saturated fat—grams		g	g	g	g	g	g	g
—% calories[a]	<10%	%	%	%	%	%	%	%
Protein—grams		g	g	g	g	g	g	g
—% calories[a]	10–35%	%	%	%	%	%	%	%
Carbohydrate—grams		g	g	g	g	g	g	g
—% calories[a]	45–65%	%	%	%	%	%	%	%
Cholesterol[c]	100 mg	mg	mg	mg	mg	mg	mg	mg
Sodium[c]	800 mg	mg	mg	mg	mg	mg	mg	mg

[a]To calculate the percent of total calories from each food energy source (fat, carbohydrate, protein), use the following formula:

$$\frac{(\text{number of grams of energy source}) \times (\text{number of calories per gram of energy source})}{(\text{total calories in serving of food item})}$$

(*Note:* Fat and saturated fat provide 9 calories per gram; protein and carbohydrate provide 4 calories per gram.) For example, the percent of total calories from protein in a 150-calorie dish containing 10 grams of protein is

$$\frac{(10 \text{ grams of protein}) \times (4 \text{ calories per gram})}{(150 \text{ calories})} = \frac{40}{150} = 0.27, \text{ or } 27\% \text{ of total calories from protein}$$

[b]For the Total column, add up the total grams of fat, carbohydrate, and protein contained in your sample meal and calculate the percentages based on the total calories in the meal. (Percentages may not total 100% due to rounding.) For cholesterol and sodium values, add up the total number of milligrams.
[c]Recommended daily limits of cholesterol and sodium are divided by 3 here to give an approximate recommended limit for a single meal.

Injury Prevention and Personal Safety

Unintentional injuries are the fifth leading cause of death among Americans overall and the leading killer of young people. Injuries affect all segments of the population, but they are particularly common among minorities and people with low incomes, primarily due to social, environmental, and economic factors. The economic cost of injuries in the United States is high, with more than $512 billion spent each year for medical care and rehabilitation of injured people, employer losses, vehicle-damage costs, and fire losses.

Injuries are generally classified into four categories, based on where they occur: motor vehicle injuries, home injuries, leisure injuries, and work injuries.

MOTOR VEHICLE INJURIES

Incidents involving motor vehicles are the leading cause of death for people between the ages of 1 and 29, the leading cause of paralysis due to spinal injury, and the leading cause of severe brain injury.

Factors in Motor Vehicle Injuries

Driving Habits   Nearly two-thirds of all motor vehicle injuries are caused by bad driving, especially speeding. As speed increases, momentum and force of impact increase and the time available for the driver to react decreases. Speed limits are posted to establish the safest *maximum* speed limit for a given area under *ideal* conditions. Anything that distracts a driver—sleepiness, bad mood, children or pets in the car, use of a cellular phone—can increase the risk of a crash.

Safety Belts and Air Bags   A person who doesn't wear a safety belt is twice as likely to be injured in a crash as a person who does wear a safety belt. Safety belts not only prevent occupants from being thrown from the car at the time of the crash but also provide protection from the "second collision," which occurs when the occupant of the car hits something inside the car, such as the steering column or windshield. The safety belt also spreads the stopping force of a collision over the body.

Since 1998, all new cars have been equipped with dual air bags—one for the driver and one for the front passenger seat. Although air bags provide some supplemental protection in the event of a collision, most are useful only in head-on collisions. They also deflate immediately after inflating and so do not provide protection in collisions involving multiple impacts. To ensure that air bags work as intended, always follow these basic guidelines: Place infants in rear-facing infant seats in the back seat, transport children age 12 and under in the back seat, always use safety belts or appropriate safety seats, and keep 10 inches between the air bag cover and the breastbone of the driver or passenger. In the rare event that a person cannot comply with these guidelines, he or she can apply to the National Highway Traffic Safety Administration for permission to install an on-off switch that temporarily disables the air bag.

Alcohol and Other Drugs   Alcohol is involved in about half of all fatal crashes. Alcohol-impaired driving, defined by blood alcohol concentration (BAC), is illegal. The legal BAC limit is 0.08% in most states, but driving ability is impaired at much lower BACs. All psychoactive drugs have the potential to impair driving ability.

Preventing Motor Vehicle Injuries

About 75% of all motor vehicle collisions occur within 25 miles of home and at speeds lower than 40 mph. These crashes often occur because the driver believes safety measures are not necessary for short trips. Clearly, the statistics prove otherwise.

To prevent motor vehicle injuries:

- Obey the speed limit. If you have to speed to get to your destination on time, you're not allowing enough time. Try leaving 10–15 minutes earlier.
- Always wear a safety belt. Strap infants and toddlers into government-approved car seats in the back seat. Children under 12 should ride in the back seat.
- Never drive under the influence of alcohol or other drugs. Never ride with a driver who has been drinking or using drugs.
- Keep your car in good working order. Regularly inspect tires, oil and fluid levels, windshield wipers, spare tire, and so on.
- Always allow enough following distance. Follow the "3-second rule": When the vehicle ahead passes a reference point, count out 3 seconds. If you pass the reference point before you finish counting, drop back and allow more following distance.
- Always increase following distance and slow down if weather or road conditions are poor.
- Choose interstate highways rather than rural roads. Highways are much safer because of better visibility, wider lanes, fewer surprises, and other factors.
- Always signal before turning or changing lanes.
- Stop completely at stop signs. Follow all traffic laws.
- Take special care at intersections. Always look left, right, and then left again. Make sure you have plenty of time to complete your maneuver in the intersection.
- Don't pass on two-lane roads unless you're in a designated passing area and have a clear view ahead.

Motorcycles and Mopeds

About one out of every ten traffic fatalities among people age 15–34 involves someone riding a motorcycle. Injuries from motorcycle collisions are generally more severe than those involving automobiles because motorcycles provide little, if any, protection. Moped riders face additional challenges. Mopeds usually have a maximum speed of 30–35 mph and have less power for maneuverability.

To prevent motorcycle and moped injuries:

- Make yourself easier to see by wearing light-colored clothing, driving with your headlights on, and correctly positioning yourself in traffic.
- Develop the necessary skills. Lack of skill, especially when evasive action is needed to avoid a collision, is a major factor in motorcycle and moped injuries. Skidding from improper braking is the most common cause of loss of control.
- Wear a close-fitting helmet, one marked with the symbol DOT (for Department of Transportation).
- Protect your eyes with goggles, a face shield, or a windshield.
- Drive defensively and never assume that other drivers see you.

Pedestrians and Bicycles

Injuries to pedestrians and bicyclists are considered motor vehicle related because they are usually caused by motor vehicles. About one in seven motor vehicle deaths each year involves a pedestrian; more than 90,000 pedestrians are injured each year.

To prevent injuries when walking or jogging:

- Walk or jog in daylight.
- Make yourself easier to see by wearing light-colored, reflective clothing.
- Face traffic when walking or jogging along a roadway, and follow traffic laws.
- Avoid busy roads or roads with poor visibility.
- Cross only at marked crosswalks and intersections.
- Don't listen to a radio, tape, or CD on headphones while walking or jogging.
- Don't hitchhike; it places you in a potentially dangerous situation.

Bicycle injuries result primarily from not knowing or understanding the rules of the road, failing to follow traffic laws, and not having sufficient skill or experience to handle traffic conditions. Bicycles are considered vehicles; bicycle riders must obey all traffic laws that apply to automobile drivers, including stopping at traffic lights and stop signs.

To prevent injuries when riding a bike:

- Wear safety equipment, including a helmet, eye protection, gloves, and proper footwear. Secure the bottom of your pant legs with clips and secure your shoelaces so they don't get tangled in the chain.
- Make yourself easier to see by wearing light-colored, reflective clothing. Equip your bike with reflectors and use lights, especially at night or when riding in wooded or other dark areas.

- Ride with the flow of traffic, not against it, and follow traffic laws. Use bike paths when they are available.
- Ride defensively; never assume that drivers see you. Be especially careful when turning or crossing at corners and intersections. Watch for cars turning right.
- Stop at all traffic lights and stop signs. Know and use hand signals.
- Continue pedaling at all times when moving (don't coast) to help keep the bike stable and to maintain your balance.
- Properly maintain your bike in working condition.

Aggressive Driving

Aggressive driving, known as road rage, has increased more than 50% since 1990. Aggressive drivers increase the risk of crashes for themselves and others. They further increase the risk of injuries if they stop their vehicles and confront each other. Even if you are successful at controlling your own aggressive driving impulses, you may still encounter an aggressive driver.

To avoid being the victim of an aggressive driver:

- *Always keep distance between your car and others.* If you are behind a very slow driver and can't pass, slow down to increase distance in case that driver does something unexpected. If you are being tailgated, do not increase your speed; instead, let the other driver pass you. If you are in the left lane when being tailgated, signal and pull over to let the other driver go by, even if you are traveling at the speed limit. When you are merging, make sure you have plenty of room. If you are being cut off by a merging driver, slow down to make room.
- *Be courteous, even if the other driver is not.* Use your horn rarely, if ever. Avoid making gestures of irritation, even shaking your head. When parking, let the other driver have the space that you both found.
- *Refuse to join in a fight.* Avoid eye contact with an angry driver. If someone makes a rude gesture, ignore it. If you think another car is following you and you have a cellular phone, call the police. Otherwise, drive to a public place and honk your horn to get someone's attention.
- *If you make a mistake while driving, apologize.* Raise or wave your hand or touch or knock your head with the palm of your hand to indicate "What was I thinking?" You can also mouth the words "I'm sorry."

HOME INJURIES

Contrary to popular belief, home is one of the most dangerous places to be. The most common fatal home injuries are caused by falls, poisoning, fires, suffocation and choking, and incidents involving firearms.

Falls

Falls are second only to motor vehicle injuries in terms of causing deaths. They are the fifth leading cause of unintentional death for people under age 25. Most deaths occurring from falls involve falling on stairs or steps or from one level to another. Falls also occur on the same level, from tripping, slipping, or stumbling. Alcohol is a contributing factor in many falls.

To prevent injuries from falls:

- Install handrails and nonslip applications in the shower and bathtub. Place skidproof backing on rugs and carpets.
- Keep floors clear of objects or conditions that could cause slipping or tripping, such as heavy wax coating, electrical cords, and toys.
- Put a light switch by the door of every room so that no one has to walk across a room to turn on a light. Use night-lights in bedrooms, halls, and bathrooms.
- Outside the house, clear dangerous surfaces created by ice, snow, fallen leaves, or rough ground.
- Install handrails on stairs. Keep stairs well lit and clear of objects.
- When climbing a ladder, use both hands. Never stand higher than the third step from the top. When using a stepladder, make sure the spreader brace is in the locked position. With straight ladders, set the base 1 foot out for every 4 feet of height. Don't stand on chairs to reach things.
- If there are small children in the home, place gates at the top and bottom of stairs. Never leave a baby unattended on a bed or table.

Poisoning

More than 2.2 million poisonings occur every year in the United States.

To prevent poisoning:

- Store all medicines out of the reach of children. Use medicines only as directed on the label or by a physician.
- Use cleaners, pesticides, and other dangerous substances only in areas with proper ventilation. Store them out of the reach of children.
- Never operate a vehicle in an enclosed space. Have your furnace inspected yearly. Use caution with any substance that produces potentially toxic fumes, such as kerosene. If appropriate, install carbon monoxide detectors.
- Keep poisonous plants out of the reach of children. These include azalea, oleander, rhododendron, wild mushrooms, daffodil and hyacinth bulbs, mistletoe berries, apple seeds, morning glory seeds, wisteria seeds, and the leaves and stems of potato, rhubarb, and tomato plants.

To be prepared in case of poisoning:

- Keep the number of the nearest Poison Control Center (or emergency room) in an accessible location. A call to the national poison control hotline (800-222-1222) will be routed to a local center.

Emergency first aid for poisonings:

1. Remove the poison from contact with eyes, skin, or mouth, or remove the victim from contact with poisonous fumes or gases.
2. Call the Poison Control Center immediately for instructions. Have the container with you.
3. Do not follow emergency instructions on labels. Some may be out of date and carry incorrect treatment information.
4. If you are instructed to go to an emergency room, take the poisonous substance or its container with you.

Guidelines for specific types of poisons:

- *Swallowed poisons.* If the person is awake and able to swallow, give water only; then call the Poison Control Center or a physician for advice.
- *Poisons on the skin.* Remove any affected clothing. Flood affected parts of the skin with warm water, wash with soap and water, and rinse. Then call for advice.
- *Poisons in the eye.* For children, flood the eye with lukewarm water poured from a pitcher held 3–4 inches above the eye for 15 minutes; alternatively, irrigate the eye under a faucet. For adults, get in the shower and flood the eye with a gentle stream of lukewarm water for 15 minutes. Then call for advice.
- *Inhaled poisons.* Immediately carry or drag the person to fresh air and, if necessary, give mouth-to-mouth resuscitation. If the victim is not breathing easily, call 911 for help. Ventilate the area. Then call for advice.

Fires

Each year about 80% of fire deaths and 65% of fire injuries occur in the home. Careless smoking is the leading cause of fire deaths.

To prevent fires:

- Dispose of all cigarettes in ashtrays. Never smoke in bed.
- Do not overload electrical outlets. Do not place extension cords under rugs or where people walk. Replace worn or frayed extension cords.
- Place a wire screen in front of fireplaces and wood stoves. Remove ashes carefully and store them in airtight metal containers, not paper bags.
- Properly maintain electrical appliances, kerosene heaters, and furnaces. Clean flues and chimneys annually.
- Keep portable heaters at least 3 feet away from curtains, bedding, towels, or anything that might catch fire. Never leave heaters on when you're out of the room or sleeping.

To be prepared for a fire:

- Plan at least two escape routes out of each room. Designate a location outside the home as a meeting place.
- Install a smoke-detection device on every level of your home. Clean the detectors and test batteries once a month and replace the batteries at least once a year.
- Keep a fire extinguisher in your home and know how to use it.

To prevent injuries from fire:

- Get out as quickly as possible and go to the designated meeting place. Don't stop for a keepsake or a pet. Never hide in a closet or under a bed. Once outside, count heads to see if everyone is out. If you think someone is still inside the burning building, tell the firefighters. Never go back inside a burning building.
- If you're trapped in a room, feel the door. If it is hot or if smoke is coming in through the cracks, don't open it; use the alternative escape route. If you can't get out of a room, go to the window and shout or wave for help.
- Smoke inhalation is the largest cause of death and injury in fires. To avoid inhaling smoke, crawl along the floor away

from the heat and smoke. Cover your mouth and nose, ideally with a wet cloth, and take short, shallow breaths.

- If your clothes catch fire, don't run. Drop to the ground, cover your face, and roll back and forth to smother the flames. Remember: stop-drop-roll.

Suffocation and Choking

Suffocation accounts for about 3500 deaths annually in the United States. Young children account for nearly half of these deaths. Children can suffocate if they put small items in their mouths, get tangled in their crib bedding, or get trapped in airtight appliances like old refrigerators. Keep small objects out of reach of children under age 3, and don't give them raw carrots, hot dogs, popcorn, or hard candy. Examine toys carefully for small parts that could come loose; don't give plastic bags or balloons to small children.

Adults can also become choking victims, especially if they fail to chew food properly, eat hurriedly, or try to talk and eat at the same time. Many choking victims can be saved with abdominal thrusts, also called the Heimlich maneuver (Figure A.1, p. A-5). Infants who are choking can be saved with blows to the upper back, followed by chest thrusts if necessary.

Incidents Involving Firearms

Firearms pose a significant threat of unintentional injury, especially to people between ages 15 and 24.

To prevent firearm injuries:

- Never point a loaded gun at something you do not intend to shoot.
- Store unloaded firearms under lock and key in a place separate from ammunition.
- Inspect firearms carefully before handling them.
- Follow the safety procedures advocated in firearm safety courses.

LEISURE INJURIES

Leisure injuries take place in public places (but do not involve motor vehicles) and include recreational, sports, and transportation injuries. Many injuries in this category involve such recreational activities as boating and swimming, playground activities, in-line skating, and sports.

Drowning and Boating Injuries

Although most drownings are reported in lakes, ponds, rivers, and oceans, more than half the drownings of young children take place in residential pools. Among adolescents and adults, alcohol plays a significant role in many boating injuries and drownings.

To prevent drowning and boating injuries:

- Develop adequate swimming skill and make sure children learn to swim.
- Make sure residential pools are fenced and that children are never allowed to swim without supervision.
- Don't swim alone or in unsupervised places.

- Use caution when swimming in unfamiliar surroundings or for an unusual length of time. To avoid being chilled, don't swim in water colder than 70°F.
- Don't swim or boat under the influence of alcohol or other drugs. Don't chew gum or eat while in the water.
- Check the depth of water before diving.
- When on a boat, use a life jacket (personal flotation device).

In-Line Skating and Scooter Injuries

Most in-line skating injuries occur because users are not familiar with the equipment and do not wear appropriate safety gear. Injuries to the wrist and head are the most common. To reduce your risk of being injured while skating, wear a helmet, elbow and knee pads, wrist guards, a long-sleeved shirt, and long pants.

Wearing a helmet and knee and elbow pads is also important for preventing scooter injuries. The rise in popularity of lightweight scooters has seen a corresponding increase in associated injuries. Scooters should not be viewed as toys, and young children should be closely supervised. Be sure that handlebars, steering column, and all nuts and bolts are securely fastened. Ride on smooth, paved surfaces away from motor vehicle traffic. Avoid streets and surfaces with water, sand, gravel, or dirt.

Sports Injuries

Since more people have begun exercising to improve their health, there has been an increase in sports-related injuries.

To prevent sports injuries:

- Develop the skills required for the activity. Recognize and guard against the hazards associated with it.
- Always warm up and cool down.
- Make sure facilities are safe.
- Follow the rules and practice good sportsmanship.
- Use proper safety equipment, including, where appropriate, helmets, eye protection, knee and elbow pads, and wrist guards. Wear correct footwear.
- When it is excessively hot and humid, avoid heat stress by following the guidelines given in the box "Exercising in Hot Weather" in Chapter 3.

WORK INJURIES

Many aspects of workplace safety are monitored by the Occupational Safety and Health Administration (OSHA), a federal agency. The highest rate of work-related injuries occurs among laborers, whose jobs usually involve extensive manual labor and lifting—two areas not addressed by OSHA safety standards. Back injuries are the most common work injury.

To protect your back when lifting:

- Don't try to lift beyond your strength. If you need it, get help.
- Get a firm footing, with your feet shoulder-width apart. Get a firm grip on the object.
- Keep your torso in a relatively upright position and crouch down, bending at the knees and hips. Avoid bending at

American Red Cross **Steps for Choking Emergencies**

Local Emergency Telephone Number

Check
✓ Check the scene for safety
✓ Check the victim for consciousness, breathing and signs of circulation

Call
✓ Dial 9-1-1 or local emergency number
✓ If alone and victim is under 8 years old, give 1 minute of care, then call 9-1-1

Care
✓ Care for conditions you find

INFANTS (birth to 1 year)

If conscious and choking...

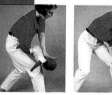

Give 5 back blows | Then give 5 chest thrusts

Repeat back blows and chest thrusts until object comes out or victim becomes unconscious.

If infant becomes unconscious...

Look for and remove any foreign object seen in mouth | Give 1 rescue breath; if air does NOT go in— | Give 5 chest compressions

If air does NOT go in, repeat steps 1, 2 and 3. If air DOES go in, give another breath then check for signs of circulation.

CHILDREN (1 to 8 years old)

If conscious and choking...

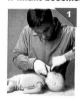

Give abdominal thrusts until object comes out or victim is unconscious

If child becomes unconscious...

Look for and remove any foreign object seen in mouth | Give 1 rescue breath; if air does NOT go in— | Give 5 chest compressions

If air does NOT go in, repeat steps 1, 2 and 3. If air DOES go in, give another breath, then check for signs of circulation.

ADULTS

If conscious and choking...

Give abdominal thrusts until object comes out or victim is unconscious

If adult becomes unconscious...

Look for and remove any foreign object seen in mouth | Give 2 rescue breaths; if air does NOT go in— | Give 15 chest compressions

If air does NOT go in, repeat steps 1, 2 and 3. If air DOES go in, check for signs of circulation.

THE SKILLS TO SAVE A LIFE...

American Red Cross lifesaving training can give you the skills and confidence to safely act in an emergency.

Don't Delay—Get Trained!

First aid, CPR and automated external defibrillation (AED) training can mean the difference between life and death. For more information, contact your local American Red Cross chapter or visit **www.redcross.org**

This poster should not be used as a substitute for training. If you do not have a breathing barrier or disposable gloves available, do not delay care.

 American Red Cross

Together, we can save a life

Figure A.1   Rescue breathing and first aid for choking: procedures recommended by the American Red Cross.

the waist. To lift, stand up or push up with your leg muscles. Lift gradually, keeping your arms straight. Keep the object close to your body.

- Don't twist. If you have to turn with an object, change the position of your feet.
- Put the object down gently, reversing the rules for lifting.

Another type of work-related injury is damage to the musculoskeletal system from repeated strain on the hand, arm, wrist, or other part of the body. Such repetitive-strain injuries are proliferating due to increased use of computers. One type, carpal tunnel syndrome, is characterized by pain and swelling in the tendons of the wrists and sometimes numbness and weakness.

To prevent carpal tunnel syndrome:

- Maintain good posture at the computer. Use a chair that provides back support and place the feet flat on the floor or on a foot rest.
- Position the screen at eye level and the keyboard so the hands and wrists are straight.
- Take breaks periodically to lessen the cumulative effects of stress.

VIOLENCE AND INTENTIONAL INJURIES

With more than 2 million Americans victims of violent injury each year, violence is a major public health concern. It includes assault, sexual assault, homicide, domestic violence, suicide, and child abuse. Compared with rates of violence in other industrialized countries, U.S. rates are abnormally high in two areas: homicide and firearm-related deaths.

Assault

Assault is the use of physical force to inflict injury or death on another person. Most assaults occur during arguments or in connection with another crime, such as robbery. Poverty, urban settings, and the use of alcohol and drugs are associated with higher rates of assault. Homicide is the fifteenth leading cause of death in the United States. Homicide victims are most likely to be male, between ages 19 and 24, and members of minority groups. Most homicides are committed with a firearm; the murderer and the victim usually know each other.

To protect yourself at home:

- Secure your home with good lighting and effective locks, preferably deadbolts. Make sure that all doors and windows are securely locked.
- Get a dog or post "Beware of Dog" signs.
- Don't hide keys in obvious places and don't give anyone the chance to duplicate your keys.
- Install a peephole in your front door. Don't open your door to people you don't know.
- If you or a family member owns a weapon, store it securely. Store guns and ammunition separately.
- If you are a woman living alone, use your initials rather than your full name in the phone directory. Don't use a greeting on your answering machine that implies you live alone or are not home.

- Teach everyone in the household how to obtain emergency assistance.
- Know your neighbors. Work out a system for alerting each other in case of an emergency.
- Establish a neighborhood watch program.

To protect yourself on the street:

- Avoid walking alone, especially at night. Stay where people can see and hear you.
- Walk on the outside of the sidewalk, facing traffic. Walk purposefully. Act alert and confident. If possible, keep at least two arm lengths between yourself and a stranger.
- Know where you are going. Appearing to be lost increases your vulnerability.
- Carry valuables in a fanny pack, pants pocket, or shoulder bag strapped diagonally across the chest.
- Always have your keys ready as you approach your vehicle or home.
- Carry a whistle to blow if you are attacked or harassed. If you feel threatened, run and/or yell. Go into a store or knock on the door of a home. If someone grabs you, yell "Help!" or "Fire!"

To protect yourself in your car:

- Keep your car in good working condition, carry emergency supplies, and keep the gas tank at least half full.
- When driving, keep doors locked and windows rolled up at least three-quarters of the way.
- Park your car in well-lighted areas or parking garages, preferably those with an attendant or a security guard.
- Lock your car when you leave it and check the interior before opening the door when you return.
- Don't pick up strangers. Don't stop for vehicles in distress; drive on and call for help.
- Note the location of emergency call boxes along highways and in public facilities. If you travel alone frequently, consider investing in a cellular phone.
- If your car breaks, down, raise the hood and tie a white cloth to the antenna or door handle. Wait in the car with the doors locked and windows rolled up. If someone approaches to offer help, open a window only a crack and ask the person to call the police or a towing service.
- When you stop at a light or stop sign, leave enough room to maneuver if you need an escape route.
- If you are involved in a minor automobile crash and you think you have been bumped intentionally, don't leave your car. Motion to the other driver to follow you to the nearest police station. If confronted by a person with a weapon, give up your car.

To protect yourself on public transportation:

- While waiting, stand in a populated, well-lighted area.
- Make sure that the bus, subway, or train is bound for your destination before you board it. Sit near the driver or conductor in a single seat or an outside seat.
- If you flag down a taxi, ensure that it's from a legitimate service. When you reach your destination, ask the driver to wait until you are safely inside the building.

To protect yourself on campus:

- Ensure that door and window locks are secure and that halls and stairwells have adequate lighting.
- Don't give dorm or residence keys to anybody.
- Don't leave your door unlocked or allow strangers into your room.
- Avoid solitary late-night trips to the library or laundry room. Take advantage of on-campus escort services.
- Don't exercise outside alone at night. Don't take shortcuts across campus that are unfamiliar or seem unsafe.
- If security guards patrol the campus, know the areas they cover and stay where they can see or hear you.

Sexual Assault—Rape and Date Rape

The use of force and coercion in sexual relationships is one of the most serious problems in human interactions. The most extreme manifestation of sexual coercion—forcing a person to submit to another's sexual desires—is rape. Taking advantage of circumstances that render a person incapable of giving consent (such as when drunk) is also considered sexual assault or rape. Coerced sexual activity in which the victim knows or is dating the rapist is often referred to as date rape.

At least 3.5 million females are raped annually in the United States, and some males—perhaps 10,000 annually—are raped each year by other males. Rape victims suffer both physical and psychological injury. The psychological pain can be substantial and long-lasting.

To protect yourself against rape:

- Following the guidelines listed earlier for protecting yourself against assault.
- Trust your gut feeling. If you feel you are in danger, don't hesitate to run and scream.
- Think out in advance what you would do if you were threatened with rape. However, no one knows what he or she will do when scared to death. Trust that you will make the best decision at the time—whether to scream, run, fight, or give in to avoid being injured or killed.

To protect yourself against date rape:

- Believe in your right to control what you do. Set limits and communicate them clearly, firmly, and early. Be assertive; men often interpret passivity as permission.
- If you are unsure of a new acquaintance, go on a group date or double date. If possible, provide your own transportation.
- Remember that some men think flirtatious behavior or sexy clothing indicates an interest in having sex.
- Remember that alcohol and drugs interfere with judgment, perception, and communication about sex. In a bar or at a party, don't leave your drink unattended, and don't accept opened beverages; watch your drinks being poured.
- Use the statement that has proven most effective in stopping date rape: "This is rape and I'm calling the cops!"

If you are raped:

- Tell what happened to the first friendly person you meet.
- Call the police. Tell them you were raped and give your location.

- Try to remember everything you can about your attacker and write it down.
- Don't wash or douche before the medical exam. Don't change your clothes, but bring a new set with you if you can.
- At the hospital you will have a complete exam. Show the physician any bruises or scratches.
- Tell the police exactly what happened. Be honest and stick to your story.
- If you do not want to report the rape to the police, see a physician as soon as possible. Be sure you are checked for pregnancy and STDs.
- Contact an organization with skilled counselors so you can talk about the experience. Look in the telephone directory under "Rape" or "Rape Crisis Center" for a hotline number.

Guidelines for men:

- Be aware of social pressure. It's OK not to "score."
- Understand that "No" means "No." Stop making advances when your date says to stop. Remember that she has the right to refuse sex.
- Don't assume that flirtatious behavior or sexy clothing means a woman is interested in having sex, that previous permission for sex applies to the current situation, or that your date's relationships with other men constitute sexual permission for you.
- Remember that alcohol and drugs interfere with judgment, perception, and communication about sex.

Stalking and Cyberstalking

Stalking is characterized by harassing behaviors such as following or spying on a person and making verbal, written, or implied threats. It is estimated that 1 million U.S. women and 400,000 men are stalked each year; most stalkers are men. Cyberstalking, the use of electronic communications devices to stalk another person, is becoming more common. Cyberstalkers may send harassing or threatening e-mails or chat room messages to the victim, or they may encourage others to harass the victim by posting inflammatory messages and personal information on bulletin boards or chat rooms.

To protect yourself online:

- Never use your real name as an e-mail user name or chat room nickname. Select an age-and gender-neutral identity.
- Avoid filling out profiles for accounts related to e-mail use or chat room activities with information that could be used to identify you.
- Do not share personal information in public spaces anywhere online or give it to strangers.
- Learn how to filter unwanted e-mail messages.
- If you do experience harassment online, do not respond to the harasser. Log off or surf elsewhere. Save all communications for evidence. If harassment continues, report it to the harasser's Internet service provider, your Internet service provider, and the local police.
- Don't agree to meet someone you've met online face to face unless you feel completely comfortable about it. Schedule a series of phone conversations first. Meet initially in a very public place and bring along a friend to increase your safety.

Coping after Terrorism or Mass Violence

For many Americans, the September 11, 2001, terrorist attacks were the first major national catastrophe they have experienced. Some people suffered the loss of relatives or friends; many others were robbed of their sense of security. Each person reacts differently to this type of traumatic disaster, and it is normal to experience a variety of responses. Reactions may include disbelief and shock, fear, anger and resentment, anxiety about the future, difficulty concentrating or making decisions, mood swings, irritability, sadness and depression, panic, guilt, apathy, feelings of isolation or powerlessness, and many of the behavioral signs such as headaches or insomnia that are associated with excess stress (see Chapter 10). Reactions may occur immediately or may be delayed until weeks or months after the event.

Taking positive steps can help you cope with powerful emotions. Consider the following strategies:

- Share your experiences and emotions with friends and family members. Be a supportive listener. Reassure children and encourage them to talk about what they are feeling.
- Take care of your mind and body. Choose a healthy diet, exercise regularly, get plenty of sleep, and practice relaxation techniques. Don't turn to unhealthy coping techniques such as using alcohol or other drugs.
- Take a break from media reports and images, and try not to develop nightmare scenarios for possible future events.
- Reestablish your routines at home, school, and work.
- Find ways to help others. Donating money, blood, food, clothes, or time can ease difficult emotions and give you a greater sense of control.

Everyone copes with tragedy in a different way and recovers at a different pace. If you feel overwhelmed by your emotions, seek professional help. Additional information about coping with terrorism and violence is available from the Federal Emergency Management Agency (www.fema.gov), the U.S. Department of Justice (www.usdoj.gov), and the National Mental Health Association (www.nmha.org).

PROVIDING EMERGENCY CARE

You can improve someone else's chances of surviving if you are prepared to provide emergency help. A course in first aid offered by the American Red Cross and on many college campuses can teach you to respond appropriately when someone needs help. Emergency rescue techniques can save the lives of people who have stopped breathing, who are choking, or whose hearts have stopped beating. Pulmonary resuscitation (also known as rescue breathing, artificial respiration, or mouth-to-mouth resuscitation) is used when a person is not breathing (see Figure A.1). Cardiopulmonary resuscitation (CPR) is used when a pulse can't be found. Training is required before a person can perform CPR. Courses are offered by the American Red Cross and the American Heart Association.

When you have to provide emergency care:

- Remain calm and act sensibly. The basic pattern for providing emergency care is check-call-care.
- *Check the situation.* Make sure the scene is safe for both you and the injured person. Don't put yourself in danger; if you get hurt too, you will be of little help to the injured person.
- *Check the victim.* Conduct a quick head-to-toe examination. Assess the victim's signs and symptoms, such as level of responsiveness, pulse, and breathing rate. Look for bleeding and any indications of broken bones or paralysis.
- *Call for help.* Call 911 or a local emergency number. Identify yourself and give as much information as you can about the condition of the victim and what happened.
- *Care for the victim.* If the situation requires immediate action (no pulse, shock, etc.), provide first aid if you are trained to do so (see Figure A.1).

SELECTED BIBLIOGRAPHY

AAA Foundation for Traffic Safety. 1997. *Road Rage: How to Avoid Aggressive Driving.* Washington, D.C.: AAA Foundation for Traffic Safety.

American Academy of Pediatrics. 2004. *Q & A: Poison Treatment in the Home* (http://www.aap.org/advocacy/releases/novpoisonqanda.htm; retrieved February 5, 2004.)

American Academy of Pediatrics. 2002. Skateboard and scooter injuries. *Pediatrics* 103(3): 542–543.

Burt, C. W., and M. D. Overpeck. 2001. Emergency visits for sports-related injuries. *Annals of Emergency Medicine* 37(3): 301–308.

Carpal tunnel syndrome. 2002. *Journal of the American Medical Association* 288(10): 1310.

Centers for Disease Control and Prevention. 2001. Surveillance for fatal and nonfatal firearm-related injuries. *CDC Surveillance Summaries* 50(SS2).

Federal Bureau of Investigation. 2003. *Crime in the United States: Uniform Crime Reports, 2002.* Washington, D.C.: U.S. Department of Justice.

Li, G., et al. 2001. Use of alcohol as a risk factor for bicycling injury. *Journal of the American Medical Association* 285(7): 893–896.

National Institutes of Health. 2001. Coping with terrorism. *Word on Health,* December.

National Mental Health Association. 2001. *Coping with Disaster: Tips for College Students* (http://www.nmha.org/reassurance/collegetips.cfm; retrieved April 30, 2002).

National Safety Council. 2003. *Injury Facts.* Itasca, Ill.: National Safety Council.

New York State Department of Motor Vehicles. 2000. *Aggressive Driving* (http://www.nysgtsc.state.ny.us/aggr-ndx.htm; retrieved December 27, 2000).

Philip, P., et al. 2001. Fatigue, alcohol, and serious road crashes in France. *British Medical Journal* 322(7290): 829–830.

Steenland, K., et al. 2003. Deaths due to injuries among employed adults: The effects of socioeconomic class. *Epidemiology* 14(1): 74–79.

U.S. Department of Justice. 1999. *1999 Report on Cyberstalking: A New Challenge for Law Enforcement and Industry* (http://www.usdoj.gov:80/criminal/cybercrime/cyberstalking.htm; retrieved December 17, 2000).

Williamson, A. M., and A. M. Feyer. 2000. Moderate sleep deprivation produces impairments in cognitive and motor performance equivalent to legally proscribed levels of alcohol intoxication. *Occupational and Environmental Medicine* 57(10): 649–655.

Nutritional Content of Common Foods

For this food composition table, foods are listed within the following groups, corresponding to the Food Guide Pyramid: (1) breads, cereals, rice, and pasta; (2) vegetables; (3) fruit; (4) milk, yogurt, and cheese; (5) meat, poultry, fish, dry beans, eggs, and nuts; and (6) fats, oils, sweets, and alcoholic beverages.

Data are provided for a variety of nutrients. For planning and easy reference, complete the following chart with your approximate daily goals or limits; refer to p. 224 and the Nutrition Resources section that follows Chapter 8. Fill in the daily totals that apply to your approximate daily calorie intake, sex, and age.

TOTAL DAILY GOAL OR LIMIT			
Total energy	_____ calories	Cholesterol	_300_ mg
Protein	_____ grams	Sodium	_2300_ mg
Carbohydrate	_____ grams	Vitamin A	_____ RE
Dietary fiber	_25–38_ grams	Vitamin C	_____ mg
Total fat	_____ grams	Calcium	_____ mg
Saturated fat	_____ grams	Iron	_____ mg

This appendix contains information on the same nutrients found on most food labels, so you can make easy comparisons. On food labels, percent Daily Values without corresponding units are usually provided for vitamins and minerals. For reference, the Daily Values are as follows: 5000 IU of vitamin A, 60 mg of vitamin C, 1000 mg of calcium, and 18 mg of iron.

BREADS, CEREALS, RICE, AND PASTA
The Food Guide Pyramid recommends 6–11 servings per day. One serving is equivalent to 1 slice of bread, about 1 cup of ready-to-eat cereal, or ½ cup of cooked cereal, rice, or pasta.

Name	Amount	Weight g	Energy calories	Protein g	Carb. g	Fiber g	Total fat g	Sat. fat g	Chol. mg	Sod. mg	Vit. A RE	Vit. C mg	Calc. mg	Iron mg
Bagel, plain	1 bagel, 4″ dia.	89	245	9.3	47.5	2.0	1.4	0.2	0	475	0	0	66	3.2
Barley, pearled, cooked	½ cup	79	97	1.8	22.2	3.0	0.3	0.1	0	2	0	0	9	1.0
Bulgur, cooked	½ cup	91	76	2.8	16.9	4.1	0.2	0	0	5	0	0	9	0.8
Biscuit	1 biscuit, 2½″ dia.	35	127	2.2	17.0	0.5	5.8	0.9	0	368	0	0	17	1.2
Bread, corn	1 piece	60	188	4.3	28.9	1.4	6.0	1.6	37	467	26	0	44	1.1
Bread, French	1 slice	64	175	5.6	33.2	1.9	1.9	0.4	0	390	0	0	48	1.6
Bread, oatmeal	1 slice	27	73	2.3	13.1	1.1	1.2	0.2	0	162	1	0	18	0.73
Bread, pita, white	1 pita, 6½″ dia.	60	165	5.5	33.4	1.3	0.7	0.1	0	322	0	0	52	1.6
Bread, pita, whole wheat	1 pita, 6½″ dia.	64	170	6.3	35.2	4.7	1.7	0.3	0	340	0	0	10	2.0
Bread, pumpernickel	1 slice	26	65	2.3	12.4	1.7	0.8	0.1	0	174	0	0	18	0.7
Bread, raisin	1 slice	32	88	2.5	16.7	1.4	1.4	0.3	0	125	0	0	21	0.9
Bread, rye	1 slice	32	83	2.7	15.5	1.9	1.1	0.2	0	211	0	0.1	23	0.9
Bread sticks	2 sticks, 7⅝″ x ⅝″	20	82	2.4	13.6	0.6	1.9	0.3	0	131	0	0	4	0.8
Bread stuffing	½ cup	100	178	3.2	21.7	2.9	8.6	1.7	0	543	118	0	32	1.1
Bread, white	1 slice	30	80	2.3	15.2	0.7	1.0	0.2	0	204	0	0	45	1.1

Name	Amount	Weight g	Energy calories	Protein g	Carb. g	Fiber g	Total fat g	Sat. fat g	Chol. mg	Sod. mg	Vit. A RE	Vit. C mg	Calc. mg	Iron mg
Bread, whole grain	1 slice	32	80	3.2	14.8	2.0	1.2	0.3	0	156	0	0.1	29	1.1
Bread, whole wheat	1 slice	28	69	2.7	12.9	1.9	1.2	0.3	0	148	0	0	20	0.9
Buckwheat groats, cooked	½ cup	84	77	2.8	16.8	2.3	0.5	0.1	0	3	0	0	6	0.7
Bun, hamburger/hot dog	1 roll	43	120	4.1	21.3	0.9	1.9	0.5	0	206	0	0	59	1.4
Cake, angelfood	1/12 of 10" cake	50	129	3.1	29.4	0.1	0.2	0	0	255	0	0	42	0.1
Cake, chocolate w/frosting	1/8 of 18 oz cake	64	235	2.6	34.9	1.8	10.5	3.1	27	214	16	0.1	28	1.4
Cake, yellow w/icing	1/8 of 18 oz cake	64	243	2.4	35.5	1.2	11.1	3.0	35	216	21	0	24	1.3
Cereal, All-Bran	⅓ cup	30	75	2.1	24.0	12.9	0.9	0.1	0	203	153	6.0	19	4.5
Cereal, Cheerios	1 cup	30	111	3.3	22.2	2.7	1.8	0.4	0	273	150	6.0	100	8.1
Cereal, corn flakes	1 cup	28	101	1.8	24.3	1.3	0.1	0	0	203	150	6.2	2	8.4
Cereal, Cream of Wheat	½ cup	126	63	1.9	13.8	0.5	0.3	0	0	168	0	0	56.5	4.8
Cereal, Frosted Flakes	¾ cup	31	114	1.0	28.0	1.0	0.2	0.1	0	148	160	6.2	2	4.5
Cereal, granola	½ cup	51	232	5.4	33.8	3.7	6.5	4.2	1	24	1	0.3	61	1.3
Cereal, raisin bran	1 cup	61	195	5.2	46.5	7.3	3.0	0.6	0	362	155	0.4	29	4.6
Cereal, Total	¾ cup	30	97	2.4	23.0	2.4	0.3	0.2	0	192	150	60.0	1000	18.0
Cereal, Wheat Chex	1 cup	30	104	3.0	24.3	3.3	0.6	0.1	0	267	90	3.6	60	8.7
Cereal, Wheaties	1 cup	30	106	3.0	24.3	3.0	0.3	0.2	0	218	150	6.0	0	8.1
Coffee cake w/topping	1 piece	63	263	4.3	29.4	1.3	14.7	3.7	20	221	21	0.2	34	1.2
Cookie, chocolate chip	1 medium cookie	16	78	0.9	9.3	0.4	4.5	1.3	5	58	26	0	6	0.4
Cookie, fig bar	1 cookie	16	56	0.6	11.3	0.7	1.2	0.2	0	56	1	0	10	0.5
Cookie, fortune	1 cookie	8	30	0.3	6.7	0.1	0.2	0.1	0	22	0	0	1	0.1
Cookie, oatmeal	1 large cookie	18	81	1.1	12.4	0.5	3.3	0.8	0	69	0	0.1	7	0.5
Cookie, sandwich	1 cookie	10	47	0.5	7.0	0.3	0.3	0.4	0	60	0	0	3	0.4
Corn meal, dry	¼ cup	35	126	2.9	26.8	2.6	0.6	0.1	0	1	14	0	2	1.4
Corn grits, cooked	½ cup	121	73	1.7	15.7	0.2	0.2	0	0	0	7	0	0	0.8
Couscous, cooked	½ cup	79	88	3.0	18.2	1.1	0.1	0	0	4	0	0	6	0.3
Cracker, crispbread, rye	3 crispbreads	30	110	2.4	24.7	5.0	0.4	0	0	79	0	0	9	0.7
Cracker, graham	3 squares	28	119	2.0	21.3	1.0	1.6	0.4	0	185	0	0	22	1.2
Cracker, matzo	1 matzo	28	111	2.8	23.4	0.8	0.4	0.1	0	1	0	0	4	0.9
Cracker, melba toast	6 pieces	30	117	3.6	23.0	1.9	1.0	0.1	0	249	0	0	28	1.1
Cracker, Ritz	5 crackers	16	79	1.2	10.3	0.3	3.7	0.6	0	124	0	0	24	0.6
Cracker, saltine	10 squares	30	130	2.8	21.5	0.9	3.5	0.9	0	390	0	0	36	1.6
Cracker, whole wheat	6 crackers	24	106	2.1	16.5	2.5	4.1	0.8	0	158	0	0	24	0.7
Croissant, butter	1 medium	57	231	4.7	26.1	1.5	12.0	6.6	38	424	106	0.1	21	1.2
Danish pastry, cheese	1 pastry	71	266	5.7	26.4	0.7	15.5	4.8	11	320	32	0	25	1.1
Doughnut, glazed	1 medium	45	192	2.3	22.9	0.7	10.3	2.7	14	181	1	0	27	0.5
English muffin, plain	½ muffin	29	67	2.2	13.1	0.8	0.5	0.1	0	132	0	0	50	0.7
French toast	1 slice	65	149	5.0	16.3	0	7.0	1.8	75	311	86	0.2	65	1.1
Macaroni, cooked	½ cup	70	99	3.3	19.8	0.9	0.5	0.1	0	1	0	0	5	1.0
Muffin, blueberry	2" by 2¾"	57	162	3.71	23.2	0	6.2	1.2	21	251	22	0.9	108	1.3
Muffin, oat bran	1 small	66	178	4.6	31.9	3.0	4.8	0.7	0	259	0	0	42	2.7
Noodles, chow mein	½ cup	23	119	1.9	12.9	0.9	6.9	1.0	0	99	2	0	5	1.1
Noodles, egg, cooked	½ cup	80	106	3.8	19.9	0.9	1.2	0.2	53	6	5	0	10	1.3
Noodles, Japanese soba	½ cup	57	56	2.9	12.2	0	0.1	0	0	34	0	0	2	0.3
Oat bran, raw	¼ cup	24	58	4.1	15.6	3.6	1.7	0.3	0	1	0	0	14	1.3
Oatmeal, instant	1 packet	28	103	4.3	17.9	3.1	1.7	0.3	0	80	300	0	100	8.1
Pancake	4" pancake	38	74	2.0	13.9	0.5	1.0	0.2	5	239	12	0.1	48	0.6
Pasta, cooked	2 oz.	57	75	2.9	14.2	0	0.6	0.1	19	3	3	0	3	0.7
Popcorn, air-popped	2 cups	16	61	1.9	12.5	2.4	0.7	0.1	0	1	3	0	2	0.4
Popcorn, oil-popped	2 cups	22	110	1.9	12.6	2.2	6.2	1.0	0	194	3	0	2	0.6
Pretzels	10 twists	60	229	5.5	47.5	1.9	2.1	0.5	0	1029	0	0	22	2.6
Quinoa, uncooked	¼ cup	43	159	5.6	29.3	2.5	2.5	0.3	0	9	0	0	26	3.9
Roll, dinner	1 roll, 2" square	28	84	2.3	14.1	0.8	2.0	0.5	0	146	0	0	33	0.8
Rice, brown, cooked	½ cup	98	108	2.5	22.4	1.8	0.9	0.2	0	5	0	0	10	0.4
Rice cake	1 cake	9	35	0.7	7.3	0.4	0.3	0	0	29	0	0	1	0.1
Rice, white, cooked	½ cup	79	103	2.1	22.3	0.3	0.2	0	0	1	0	0	8	0.9
Rice, wild, cooked	½ cup	82	83	3.3	17.5	1.5	0.3	0	0	3	0	0	2	0.5
Spaghetti, cooked	½ cup	70	99	3.3	19.8	1.2	0.5	0.1	0	70	0	0	5	1.0
Taco shell	1 medium	13	62	1.0	8.3	1.0	3.0	0.4	0	49	0	0	21	0.3
Tortilla chips	1 oz.	28	142	2.0	17.8	1.8	7.4	1.4	0	150	6	0	44	0.4

Name	Amount	Weight g	Energy calories	Protein g	Carb. g	Fiber g	Total fat g	Sat. fat g	Chol. mg	Sod. mg	Vit. A RE	Vit. C mg	Calc. mg	Iron mg
Tortilla, corn	1 medium	24	53	1.4	11.2	1.2	0.6	0.1	0	39	0	0	42	0.3
Tortilla, flour	8" tortilla	51	146	4.4	25.3	0	3.1	0.4	0	249	0	0	97	1.0
Wheat germ, toasted	¼ cup	28	108	8.3	14.1	3.7	3.0	0.5	0	1	0	1.7	13	2.6

VEGETABLES

The Food Guide Pyramid recommends 3–5 servings per day. One serving is equivalent to 1 cup of raw leafy vegetables, ½ cup of other raw or cooked vegetables, or ¾ cup of vegetable juice.

Name	Amount	Weight g	Energy calories	Protein g	Carb. g	Fiber g	Total fat g	Sat. fat g	Chol. mg	Sod. mg	Vit. A RE	Vit. C mg	Calc. mg	Iron mg
Alfalfa sprouts	½ cup	17	5	0.7	0.6	0.4	0.1	0	0	1	1	1.4	5	0.2
Artichoke, cooked	1 medium	120	60	4.2	13.4	6.5	0.2	0	0	114	22	12.0	54	1.5
Arugula, raw	1 cup	20	5	0.5	0.7	0.3	0.1	0	0	3	24	3.0	16	0.1
Asparagus, cooked	6 spears	90	22	2.3	3.8	1.4	0.3	0	0	10	49	9.7	18	0.7
Bamboo shoots, canned	½ cup	66	13	1.1	2.1	0.9	0.3	0.1	0	5	1	0.7	5	0.2
*Beans, baked (plain)	½ cup	127	118	6.1	26.0	6.4	0.6	0.1	0	504	22	3.9	64	0.4
*Beans, black, cooked	½ cup	86	114	7.6	20.4	7.5	0.5	0.1	0	1	1	0	23	1.8
*Beans, fava, raw	½ cup	63	55	4.9	11.1	0	0.5	0.1	0	16	11	2.3	23	0.9
Beans, green snap, cooked	½ cup	63	22	1.2	4.9	2.0	0.2	0	0	2	42	6.1	29	0.8
*Beans, kidney, cooked	½ cup	89	112	7.7	20.2	6.5	0.4	0.1	0	2	0	1.1	25	2.6
*Beans, lentils, cooked	½ cup	99	115	8.9	19.9	7.8	0.4	0.1	0	2	1	1.5	19	3.3
*Beans, lima, cooked	½ cup	94	108	7.3	19.6	6.6	0.4	0.1	0	2	0	0	16	2.2
*Beans, navy, cooked	½ cup	91	129	7.9	23.9	5.8	0.5	0.1	0	1	0	0.8	64	2.3
*Beans, pinto, cooked	½ cup	85.5	120	7.8	21.3	7.0	0.7	0.1	0	9	0	0.7	36	1.8
*Beans, refried	½ cup	126	118	6.9	19.6	6.7	1.6	0.6	10	377	0	7.6	44	2.1
Beans, yellow snap, cooked	½ cup	63	22	1.2	4.9	2.1	0.2	0	0	2	5	6.1	29	0.8
Beet greens, cooked	½ cup	72	19	1.9	3.4	2.1	0.1	0	0	174	276	17.9	82	1.4
Beets, cooked	½ cup	85	37	1.4	8.5	1.7	0.2	0	0	65	3	3.1	14	0.7
Broccoli spears, cooked	2 spears	78	22	2.3	3.9	2.3	0.3	0	0	20	108	58.2	36	0.7
Brussels sprouts, cooked	4 sprouts	84	30	2.1	7.3	2.2	0.4	0.1	0	18	60	52.1	30	1.0
Cabbage, cooked	½ cup	75	17	0.8	3.3	1.7	0.3	0	0	6	10	15.1	23	0.1
Cabbage, raw	½ cup	45	11	0.6	2.4	1.0	0.1	0	0	8	6	14.3	21	0.3
Carrot, juice	¾ cup	177	71	1.7	16.4	1.4	0.3	0	0	51	1938	15.0	42	0.8
Carrots, cooked	½ cup	78	27	0.6	6.4	2.3	0.1	0	0	236	659	2.8	23	0.3
Carrots, raw	1 medium	61	21	0.6	5.8	1.8	0.2	0	0	42	367	3.6	20	0.2
Cauliflower, cooked	½ cup	62	14	1.1	2.5	1.7	0.3	0	0	9	1	27.4	10	0.2
Celery, raw	8 sticks	32	4	0.2	1.0	0.5	0	0	0	26	7	1.0	13	0.1
Chard, cooked	½ cup	88	18	1.6	3.6	1.8	0.1	0	0	156	275	15.8	51	2.0
Coleslaw, homemade	½ cup	60	41	0.8	7.4	0.9	1.6	0.2	5	14	49	19.6	27	0.4
Collards, cooked	½ cup	95	25	2.0	4.7	2.7	0.3	0	0	9	297	17.3	113	0.4
Corn, yellow, cooked	½ cup	82	89	2.7	20.6	2.3	1.1	0.2	0	14	18	5.1	2	0.5
Cucumber, raw	½ cup	52	8	0.3	1.9	0.4	0.1	0	0	1	3	1.5	8	0.2
Eggplant, cooked	½ cup	50	17	0.4	4.3	1.2	0.1	0	0	0	1	0.6	3	0.1
Endive, raw	½ cup	25	4	0.3	0.8	0.8	0.1	0	0	6	51	1.6	13	0.2
Hominy, canned	½ cup	83	59	1.2	11.8	2.1	0.7	0.1	0	173	0	0	8	0.5
Kale, cooked	½ cup	65	18	1.2	3.6	1.3	0.3	0	0	15	481	26.7	47	0.6
Kohlrabi, cooked	½ cup	83	24	1.5	5.5	0.9	0.1	0	0	17	2	44.5	21	0.3
Leeks, raw	½ cup	45	27	0.7	6.3	0.8	0.1	0	0	9	37	5.3	26	0.9
Lettuce, green leaf	1 cup	56	8	0.7	1.6	0.7	0.1	0	0	16	207	10.1	20	0.5
Lettuce, iceberg	1 cup	55	8	0.6	1.2	0.6	0.1	0	0	5	9	2.1	11	0.2
Lettuce, romaine	1 cup	56	10	0.7	1.8	1.2	0.2	0	0	4	162	13.4	18	0.5
Mushrooms, raw	½ cup	35	8	1.1	1.1	0.4	0.1	0	0	1	0	0.8	1	0.2
Mushrooms, cooked	½ cup	78	21	1.7	4.0	1.7	0.3	0	0	2	0	3.1	5	1.4
Mustard greens, cooked	½ cup	70	10	1.6	1.5	1.4	0.2	0	0	11	212	17.7	52	0.5
Okra, cooked	½ cup	80	18	1.5	3.6	2.0	0.1	0	0	5	11	13.0	62	0.2
Onion, raw	½ cup	80	34	0.7	8.0	1.1	0.1	0	0	2	0	5.1	18	0.2
Parsley, raw	2 tablespoons	8	3	0.2	0.5	0.3	0.1	0	0	4	32	10.1	10	0.5
Parsnip, raw	½ cup	67	50	0.8	12.0	3.2	0.2	0	0	7	0	11.3	24	0.4
*Peas, blackeye, cooked	½ cup	86	100	6.6	17.9	5.6	0.5	0.1	0	3	1	0.3	21	2.2
*Peas, chickpeas (garbanzos)	½ cup	82	134	7.3	22.5	6.2	2.1	0.2	0	6	2	1.1	40	2.4

Name	Amount	Weight g	Energy calories	Protein g	Carb. g	Fiber g	Total fat g	Sat. fat g	Chol. mg	Sod. mg	Vit. A RE	Vit. C mg	Calc. mg	Iron mg
Peas, edible, podded	10 pea pods	34	14	1.0	2.6	0.9	0.1	0	0	1	5	20.4	15	0.7
Peas, green	½ cup	80	62	4.1	11.4	4.4	0.2	0	0	70	54	7.9	19	1.2
*Peas, split, cooked	½ cup	98	116	8.2	20.6	8.1	0.4	0.1	0	2	1	0.4	14	1.3
Pepper, green chili, canned	½ cup	70	15	0.5	3.2	1.2	0.2	0	0	276	9	23.8	25	0.9
Pepper, sweet green, raw	1 small	74	20	0.7	4.8	1.2	0.1	0	0	1	47	66.1	7	0.3
Pepper, sweet red, raw	1 small	74	20	0.7	4.8	1.5	0.1	0	0	1	422	140.6	7	0.3
Pickle, dill	1 medium	65	12	0.4	2.7	0.8	0.1	0	0	21	833	1.2	6	0.3
Potato, mashed w/milk	½ cup	105	81	2.0	18.4	1.6	0.6	0.3	2	318	4	7.0	23	0.3
Potato salad	½ cup	125	179	3.4	14.0	1.6	10.3	1.8	85	661	41	12.5	24	0.8
Potato, baked w/skin	1 medium	173	161	4.3	36.6	3.8	0.2	0.1	0	17	17	16.6	26	1.9
Potato, boiled	1 potato, 2½" dia.	136	118	2.5	27.4	2.4	0.1	0	0	5	0	17.7	7	0.4
Potato, french fries	10 fries	50	100	1.6	15.6	1.6	3.8	0.6	0	15	0	5.0	4	0.6
Pumpkin, canned	½ cup	123	42	1.3	9.9	3.6	0.3	0.2	0	6	2702	5.1	32	1.7
Radish, raw	13 medium	56	9	0.4	2.1	0.9	0	0	0	23	0	8.7	15	0.2
Rutabaga, mashed	½ cup	120	47	1.5	10.5	2.2	0.3	0	0	24	67	22.6	58	0.6
Sauerkraut, drained	½ cup	121	13	0.6	3.0	1.8	0.1	0	0	469	1	10.5	21	1.0
Soybeans, green, boiled	½ cup	90	127	11.1	9.9	3.8	5.8	0.7	0	13	14	15.3	131	2.3
Spinach, raw	1 cup	30	7	0.9	1.1	0.8	0.1	0	0	24	202	8.4	30	0.8
Spinach, cooked	½ cup	95	27	3.0	5.1	2.9	0.2	0	0	82	739	11.7	139	1.4
Squash, summer, raw	½ small squash	59	12	0.7	2.6	1.1	0.1	0	0	1	12	8.7	12	0.3
Squash, summer, cooked	½ cup	90	18	0.8	3.9	1.3	0.3	0	0	1	26	5.0	24	0.3
Squash, winter	½ cup	100	39	0.9	8.8	2.8	0.6	0.1	0	1	356	9.6	14	0.3
Sweet potato, baked	½ cup	100	90	2.0	20.7	3.3	0.2	0	0	36	961	19.6	38	0.7
Sweet potato, canned w/syrup	½ cup	98	106	1.3	24.9	2.9	0.3	0.1	0	38	351	10.6	17	1.0
Tomato, red, raw	1 medium	123	22	1.1	4.8	1.5	0.3	0.1	0	6	52	15.6	12	0.3
Tomato sauce	½ cup	123	39	1.6	9.0	1.8	0.3	0	0	642	21	8.6	16	1.3
Tomato juice	¾ cup	182	31	1.4	7.7	1.5	1.4	0	0	18	102	33.3	18	0.1
Turnip, cooked, mashed	½ cup	115	24	0.8	5.6	2.3	0.1	0	0	108	0	13.3	25	0.3
Vegetable juice	¾ cup	182	35	1.1	8.3	1.5	0.2	0	0	491	213	50.4	20	0.8
Vegetables, mixed	½ cup	91	54	2.6	11.9	4.0	0.1	0	0	32	389	2.9	23	0.7
Vegetable soup	1 cup	241	72	2.1	12.0	0.5	1.9	0.3	0	822	301	1.4	22	1.1
Water chestnuts	½ cup	70	35	0.6	8.7	1.8	0	0	0	6	0	0.9	3	0.6

*Dry beans and peas (legumes) can be counted as servings of vegetables or as servings from the meat, poultry, fish, dry beans, eggs, and nuts group. They are listed here and marked with an asterisk.

FRUIT

The Food Guide Pyramid recommends 2–4 servings per day. One serving is equivalent to 1 medium apple, banana, orange, or pear; ½ cup of chopped, cooked, or canned fruit; or ¾ cup of fruit juice.

Name	Amount	Weight g	Energy calories	Protein g	Carb. g	Fiber g	Total fat g	Sat. fat g	Chol. mg	Sod. mg	Vit. A RE	Vit. C mg	Calc. mg	Iron mg
Apple, raw, w/skin	1 medium	138	72	0.4	19.1	3.3	0.2	0	0	1	4	6.3	8	0.2
Apple juice	¾ cup	179	84	0.3	20.7	0.2	0.2	0	0	13	0	44.8	11	0.5
Apple sauce, unsweetened	½ cup	122	52	0.2	13.8	1.5	0.1	0	0	2	4	25.9	4	0.1
Apricots	2 medium	70	34	1.0	7.8	1.7	0.3	0	0	1	67	7.0	10	0.4
Apricots, dried	9 halves	32	75	1.2	19.7	2.3	0.1	0	0	3	228	0.8	14	1.5
Avocado	1 medium	173	289	3.4	15.0	11.8	26.6	3.7	0	14	12	15.2	22	1.1
Banana	1 medium	118	105	1.3	27.0	3.1	0.4	0.1	0	1	4	10.3	6	0.3
Blackberries, raw	½ cup	72	31	1.0	6.9	3.8	0.4	0	0	1	8	15.1	21	0.5
Blueberries	½ cup	73	41	0.5	10.2	2.0	0.3	0	0	1	2	7.0	4	0.2
Cantaloupe	¼ melon, 5" dia.	138	48	1.2	11.5	1.1	0.4	0.1	0	12	444	58.2	12	0.3
Carambola (starfruit)	1 small	70	23	0.4	5.5	1.9	0.2	0	0	1	34	14.8	3	0.2
Cherries, sweet, raw	11 cherries	75	47	0.8	12.0	1.6	0.2	0	0	0	2	5.2	10	0.3
Cherries, canned in syrup	½ cup	127	105	0.8	26.9	1.9	0.2	0	0	4	10	4.6	11	0.4
Cranberries, raw	½ cup	48	23	0.2	6.0	2.0	0.1	0	0	1	2	6.4	3	0.1
Cranberry juice cocktail	¾ cup	190	108	0	27.3	0.2	0.2	0	0	4	0	67.1	6	0.3
Cranberry sauce	¼ cup	139	105	0.1	26.9	0.7	0.1	0	0	20	1	1.4	3	0.2
Currants, dried	¼ cup	36	102	1.5	26.7	2.4	0.1	0	0	3	3	1.7	31	1.2
Dates, dried	¼ cup	45	122	0.9	32.7	3.3	0.2	0.1	0	1	2	0	14	0.5
Figs, raw	2 medium	100	74	0.8	19.2	2.9	0.3	0.1	0	1	7	2.0	35	0.4
Fruit cocktail, heavy syrup	½ cup	124	91	0.5	23.4	1.2	0.1	0	0	7	25	2.4	7	0.4